American Medical Association

Physicians dedicated to the health of America

Outpatient Services

cpt® 2005

Specially annotated for use in hospitals, ambulatory surgery centers, and outpatient provider-based facilities owned by hospitals

Grace M. Kotowicz, RN, BS
Editor, Outpatient Services Content

Joyce A. Dalton
Catherine Duffy, BS, RHIT
Martha Espronceda, AAS
Desiree D. Evans, AAS
Rejina L. Glenn
Gloria Green, BA
DeHandro Hayden, BS
Elizabeth Lumakovska, BS, RHIT
Anita Majerowicz, MS, RHIA
Marie L. Mindeman, BA, RHIT
Karen E. O'Hara, BS, CCS-P
Mary R. O'Heron, RHIA, CCS-P
Danielle Pavloski, BS, RHIT, CCS-P
Dan Reyes, BA
Desiree Rozell, MPA
Lianne Stancik, RHIT
Susan Tracy, BA, RHIT
Jennifer Trajkovski, BS, RHIT
Ada Walker, AAS

AMA press

Current Procedural Terminology for
Outpatient Services
Specially annotated
Current Procedural Terminology,
Fourth Edition, CPT® 2005
for use in hospitals, ambulatory surgery centers, and outpatient provider-based facilities owned by hospitals

For information regarding the reprinting or licensing, or parts hereof, of *CPT® 2005 Outpatient Services: Specially Annotated for Use in Hospitals, Ambulatory Surgery Centers, and Outpatient Provider-Based Facilities Owned by Hospitals,* please contact:

CPT Intellectual Property Services
American Medical Association
515 North State Street
Chicago, Illinois 60610
312 464-5022

Additional copies of this book may be ordered by calling 800 621-8335 or from the secure AMA Press Web site at *www.amapress.com.* Refer to product number OP055005.

ISBN: 1-57947-584-1
AC25:05-P-009:3/05

Foreword

Current Procedural Terminology, Fourth Edition (*CPT*®) is a listing of descriptive terms and identifying codes for reporting medical services and procedures performed by physicians. The purpose of the terminology is to provide a uniform language that will accurately describe medical, surgical, and diagnostic services, and will thereby provide an effective means for reliable nationwide communication among physicians, patients, and third parties. *CPT 2005* is the most recent revision of a work that first appeared in 1966.

CPT descriptive terms and identifying codes currently serve a wide variety of important functions in the field of medical nomenclature. The *CPT* book is useful for administrative management purposes such as claims processing and for the development of guidelines for medical care review. The uniform language is also applicable to medical education and outcomes, health services and quality research by providing a useful basis for local, regional, and national utilization comparisons. The *CPT* book is the most widely accepted nomenclature for the reporting of physician procedures and services under government and private health insurance programs. In 2000 the CPT Code Set was designated by the Department of Health and Human Services as the national coding standard for physician and other health care professional services and procedures under the Health Insurance Portability and Accountability Act (HIPAA). This means that for all financial and administrative health care transactions sent electronically, the CPT Code Set will need to be used.

The changes that appear in this revision have been prepared by the CPT Editorial Panel with the assistance of physicians representing all specialties of medicine, and with important contributions from many third party payors and governmental agencies.

The American Medical Association trusts that this revision will continue the usefulness of its predecessors in identifying, describing, and coding medical, surgical, and diagnostic services.

Michael D. Maves, MD, MBA
Executive Vice President, CEO

Acknowledgments

Publication of the annual *CPT* book represents many challenges and opportunities. From reconciling the many differences of opinion about the best way to describe a procedure, to the last details on placement of a semicolon, many individuals and organizations devote their energies and expertise to the preparation of this revision.

The editorial staff wishes to express sincere thanks to the many national medical specialty societies, health insurance organizations and agencies, and to the many individual physicians and other health professionals who have made contributions.

Thanks are due to Robert A. Musacchio, PhD, Sr VP, American Medical Association; Claudia Bonnell, Blue Cross and Blue Shield Association; Nelly Leon-Chisen, Danelle Kelly RN, American Hospital Association; Thomas Musco, Health Insurance Association of America; and Sue Bowman, RHIA, American Health Information Management Association, for their invaluable assistance in enhancing the CPT Code Set.

And finally, our gratitude to AMA Press of the American Medical Association for their assistance in producing the books, diskettes, and CD-ROMs that contain the CPT Code Set: Anthony J. Frankos, Vice President, Business Products; Mike Desposito, Publisher; Elise Schumacher, Senior Acquisition Editor; J. D. Kinney, Director of Marketing; Jean Roberts, Director, Production and Manufacturing; Erin Kalitowski, Marketing Manager; Pat Lee, Developmental Editor; Rosalyn Carlton, Senior Production Coordinator; Boon Ai Tan, Senior Production Coordinator; Ronnie Summers, Senior Print Coordinator; and Todd Feinstein, Application Developer.

AMA CPT Editorial Panel

AMA CPT Advisory Committee

American Roentgen Ray Society
Geraldine B. McGinty, MD
American Society for Aesthetic Plastic Surgery
Paul R. Weiss, MD
American Society for Clinical Pathology
Mark S. Synovec, MD
American Society for Dermatologic Surgery
Pamela K. Phillips, MD
American Society for Gastrointestinal Endoscopy
Klaus Mergener, MD
American Society for Reproductive Medicine
John T. Queenan, Jr, MD
American Society for Surgery of the Hand
Daniel J. Nagle, MD
American Society for Therapeutic Radiology and Oncology
Michael L. Steinberg, MD
American Society of Abdominal Surgeons
Louis F. Alfano, Jr, MD
American Society of Anesthesiologists
H. J. Przybylo, MD
American Society of Cataract and Refractive Surgery
Stephen S. Lane, MD
American Society of Clinical Oncology
Dean Gesme, MD
William C. Penley, MD*
American Society of Colon and Rectal Surgeons
David A. Margolin, MD
American Society of Cytopathology
David C. Hoak, MD
American Society of General Surgeons
Charles Drueck, MD, FACS
American Society of Hematology
Samuel M. Silver, MD, PhD
American Society of Neuroimaging
Mircea A. Morariu, Jr, MD
American Society of Neuroradiology
Robert A. Murray, MD
American Society of Ophthalmic Plastic and Reconstructive Surgery
L. Neal Freeman, MD*
American Society of Plastic Surgeons
Raymond V. Janevicius, MD
American Thoracic Society
Scott Manaker, MD
American Urological Association
Jeffrey A. Dann, MD
Association of University Radiologists
Bob W. Gayler, MD
College of American Pathologists
Stephen N. Bauer, MD
Congress of Neurological Surgeons
R. Patrick Jacob, MD
Contact Lens Association of Ophthalmologists
Charles B. Slonim, MD, FACS
International Spinal Injection Society
Claire Tibiletti, MD*
National Association of Medical Examiners
Paul A. Raslavicus, MD*
North American Spine Society
William Mitchell, MD*
Radiologic Society of North America
Richard E. Fulton, MD
Renal Physicians Association
Richard J. Hamburger, MD
Society for Investigative Dermatology
Stephen P. Stone, MD
Society for Vascular Surgery
Anton N. Sidawy, MD
Society of Radiologists in Ultrasound
Robert L. Bree, MD
Society of American Gastrointestinal Endoscopic Surgeons
Eric G. Weiss, MD
Paresh C. Shah, MD*
Society of Critical Care Medicine
George A. Sample, MD
Society of Interventional Radiology
Gary S. Dorfman, MD
Society of Nuclear Medicine
Kenneth A. McKusick, MD
Society of Radiologists in Ultrasound
Robert L. Bree, MD
Society of Thoracic Surgeons
Keith S. Naunheim, MD
The Endocrine Society
Richard A. Dickey, MD
The Triological Society
James H. Kelly, MD*
*New Advisors June 2004

AMA Health Care Professionals Advisory Committee (HCPAC)

Tracy R. Gordy, MD, Co-Chair
AMA CPT Editorial Panel
Helene Fearon, PT, Co-Chair
AMA CPT Editorial Panel
American Academy of Physician Assistants
Patrick J. Cafferty, MPAS, PA-C
American Association of Naturopathic Physicians
William B. Milliman, N.D.
American Association for Respiratory Care
Susan Rinaldo-Gallo, Med, RRT
American Chiropractic Association
Craig S. Little, DC
American Dietetic Association
Jane V. White, PhD, RD, FADA
American Massage Therapy Association
Whitney W. Lowe
American Nurses Association
Ann M. Thrailkill, RN
American Occupational Therapy Association
Linda Botten, OTR, CHT, ATP
Leslie F. Davison, Ed.D, OTR/L*
American Optometric Association
Mike Todd, OD
Douglas C. Morrow, OD*
X12 Pharmacy Advisory Panel
Daniel E. Buffington, PharmD, MBA
American Physical Therapy Association
Paul Rockar PT
American Podiatric Medical Association
Michael J. King, DPM
American Psychological Association
Antonio Puente, PhD
American Speech-Language Hearing Association
R. Wayne Holland, Ed.D
National Association of Social Workers
Nelda Spyres, ACSW, LCSW
National Society of Genetic Counselors
Debra L. Doyle, MS, CGC

Contents

Introduction

Current Procedural Terminology, Fourth Edition (*CPT*®) is a systematic listing and coding of procedures and services performed by health care professionals. Each procedure or service is identified with an alphanumeric code. The use of CPT codes simplifies the reporting of services. With this coding and recording system, the procedure or service rendered by the physician is accurately identified.

Inclusion of a descriptor and its associated specific identifying code number in the *CPT* book is generally based upon the procedure being consistent with contemporary medical practice and being performed by many physicians in clinical practice in multiple locations. Inclusion in the *CPT* nomenclature does not represent endorsement by the American Medical Association of any particular diagnostic or therapeutic procedure. Inclusion or exclusion of a procedure does not imply any health insurance coverage or reimbursement policy.

The main body of the material is listed in six sections. Within each section are subsections with anatomic, procedural, condition, or descriptor subheadings. The procedures and services with their identifying codes are presented in numeric order with one exception—the entire **Evaluation and Management** section (99201-99499) has been placed at the beginning of the listed procedures, because these items are used by most physicians in reporting a significant portion of their services. The **Medicine** (procedures) section now follows **Pathology and Laboratory**.

Section Numbers and Their Sequences

Evaluation and Management . . . . .99201 to 99499

Anesthesiology . . . . .00100 to 01999, 99100 to 99140

Surgery . . . . .10021 to 69990

Radiology (Including Nuclear Medicine and Diagnostic Ultrasound) .70010 to 79999

Pathology and Laboratory . . . . .80048 to 89399

Medicine (except Anesthesiology) .90281-99199, 99500-99569

The first and last code numbers and the subsection name of the items appear at the top of each page (eg, "11000-11313 Surgery/Integumentary System"). The page number and the section name are printed on the lower, outer margin of each page.

Hospital Use of the CPT Code Set for the Medicare Program

Disclaimer

This specially annotated version of CPT codes has been prepared for use by hospitals, ambulatory surgery centers, and outpatient provider-based facilities owned by hospitals, and ambulatory surgery centers incorporating information provided by the Centers for Medicare and Medicaid Services (CMS). It is designed to provide accurate and authoritative information. The content highlights important changes excerpted from the CMS final rule and in no way suggests or infers that the published content represents the vast amount of Medicare statutory requirements, regulations, Program Memoranda/Transmittal instruction, and policy associated with the use of OPPS. The final rule document can be found in its entirety at the CMS website at www.cms.hhs.gov/regulations/hopps. Although not listed in this publication, CMS also requires the reporting of certain Level II (HCPCS National) codes and modifiers to describe covered services, ensure correct reporting, track utilization, and establish payment policy. For a specific list of new/existing ►2005◄ Level II Healthcare Common Procedure Coding System (HCPCS) codes, see Addendum B of the ►November 15, 2004◄, *Federal Register.* Electronic copy(s) of this *Federal Register* document is also available on the US Government Printing Office website at www. gpoaccess.gov/fr/index.html. For specific CMS OPPS policy, you may also visit either the CMS web site at www.cms.hhs.gov or visit CPT on the AMA web site at www.ama-assn.org/cpt

The identification of an ambulatory payment classification (APC) service and status indicators for each CPT code is based upon the most recent information available as of the date of publication. Every reasonable effort has been made to assure the accuracy of the information provided. However, the ultimate responsibility for correct coding lies with the provider of services pertaining to the use of Hospital Outpatient Prospective Payment System (OPPS) for Medicare reporting purposes. Specific CMS OPPS policy can be found on the Hospital Outpatient Prospective Payment web site at: **www.cms.hhs.gov/providers/hopps/2005fc/**

Summary of Rulemaking for the Outpatient Prospective Payment System

CPT coding for hospital outpatient claims was necessary to implement section 9343(a) of the Omnibus Budget Reconciliation Act of 1986 (OBRA) which required that for cost reporting periods beginning on or after October 1, 1987, Medicare payment for certain ambulatory surgical procedures performed in a hospital on an outpatient basis, be based in part on what the program would have paid for the same surgery if it were performed in an approved Ambulatory Surgical Center (ASC). Because ASC payment rates were paid based on CPT coded procedures, comparable coding for procedures performed by a hospital on an outpatient basis was needed in order to compare hospital reasonable cost and customary charges to the ASC payment rates as required by section 9343(a) of OBRA 1986. Further, Section 4066 of OBRA 1987 required a new payment methodology for hospital outpatient radiology services, which also required the use of CPT codes after September 30, 1988.

The use of CPT codes enables the CMS to accumulate a database for use in development of a full prospective payment system for hospital outpatient surgical procedures and for all hospital outpatient services as required under section 9343(f) of OBRA.

►When the Medicare statute was originally enacted, Medicare payment for hospital outpatient services was based on hospital-specific costs. In an effort to ensure that Medicare and its beneficiaries pay appropriately for services and to encourage more efficient delivery of care, the Congress mandated replacement of the cost-based payment methodology with a prospective payment system (PPS). The Balanced Budget Act of 1997 (BBA) (Pub. L. 105-33), enacted on August 5, 1997, added section 1833(t) to the Social Security Act (the Act) authorizing implementation of a PPS for hospital outpatient services. The Balanced Budget Refinement Act of 1999 (BBRA) (Pub. L. 106-113), enacted on November 29, 1999, made major changes that affected the hospital outpatient PPS (OPPS). The Medicare, Medicaid, and SCHIP Benefits Improvement and Protection Act of 2000 (BIPA) (Pub. L. 106-554), enacted on December 21, 2000, made further changes in the OPPS. ►The Medicare, Medicaid, and SCHIP Benefits Improvement and Protection Act of 2000 (BIPA) (Pub. L. 106-554), enacted on December 21, 2000, made further changes in the OPPS. Section 1833(t) of the Act was also recently amended by the Medicare Prescription Drug, Improvement, and Modernization Act of 2003, Pub. L. 108-173, enacted on December 8, 2003◄.

The CMS announced its new Medicare payment system for hospital outpatient services, with implementation effective for claims with dates of service on or after August 1, 2000. The provisions for provider-based facilities owned by hospitals, including physician office practices, were effective six months from the April 7, 2000, publication date. Section 1833 (t) of the social Security Act (the Act) as added to the Act by §4523 of the Balanced Budget Act of 1997, authorized CMS to implement a Medicare prospective payment system. The Balanced Budget Refinement Act (BBRA) of 1999 adjusted certain provisions of the Hospital OPPS. To provide for the annual update to the amounts and factors for OPPS payment rates effective for services furnished on or after January 1, 2001, CMS published an interim final rule with comment period (65 FR 67798) on November 13, 2000. A complete summary of rulemaking for the OPPS, is outlined in the ►November 15, 2004◄, *Federal Register*. Electronic copy(s) of this Federal Register document is available on the U. S. Government Printing Office web site at **www.gpoaccess.gov/fr/index/html**

►Ambulatory Payment Classification (APC) Groups◄

►Under the OPPS, CMS pays for hospital outpatient services on a rate-per-service basis that varies according to the ambulatory payment classification (APC) group to which the service is assigned. CMS uses Healthcare Common Procedure Coding System (HCPCS) codes (which include certain Current Procedural Terminology (CPT) codes) and descriptors to identify and group the services within each APC.◄ Outpatient services typically are performed at a hospital and include clinical visits, emergency room visits, x-rays, and surgical procedures not performed as part of an inpatient stay. By statute, outpatient services exclude physical and speech therapies and ambulance services. Similarly, the individual physicians are not paid under the outpatient system, but are paid under the physician fee schedule.

According to CMS, the primary objective of the Hospital Outpatient Prospective Payment system is to simplify the payment system, encourage efficient delivery of care, and encourage hospital efficiency in providing outpatient services, while ensuring adequate compensation, and reducing the Medicare beneficiary share of outpatient hospital payment(s).

For Medicare reporting purposes, previous ASC payment was based on eight ambulatory groups without clinical coherence. The new payment system is based on groups of services called "ambulatory payment classifications" (APCs), that divide all outpatient services included in the new payment schedule. The services within each group are clinically similar and require comparable resources. APCs group together services, supplies, drugs, and devices that are used in particular procedures. Each APC has a separate payment rate that is meant to account for all of the items used in the procedure. Each APC is assigned a relative payment weight, based on the median costs of the services within the APC. A hospital receives multiple APC payments for a single visit if multiple services are delivered in that visit. ►Section 1833(t)(9) of the Act requires the Secretary to review certain components of the OPPS not less often than annually and to revise the groups, relative payment weights, and other adjustments to take into account changes in medical practice, changes in technology, and the addition of new services, new cost data, and other relevant information and factors. (A list of CPT codes and their respective APC assignment is included in **Appendix J**)◄.

The APC groups are refined based on public comment, wherein CMS modifies the proposed regulation to allow a smoother transition to the new fee system for providers. A payment rate is established for each APC. Depending on the services provided, hospitals may be paid for more than one APC for an encounter. The APC payment rate established for each group applies to all services within the group. Although national payment rates are established for each group, payments are wage adjusted to reflect geographic differences.

Section 1833(t) (9)(A) of the Social Security Act (the Act) requires that CMS consult with an outside panel of experts, the Panel, to review the clinical integrity of the APC groups and their weights. The Act specifies that the Panel will act in an advisory capacity. This expert panel, which is to be composed of ►15◄ representatives of providers subject to the OPPS (currently employed full-time, in their respective areas of expertise), reviews and advises us about the clinical integrity of the APC groups and their weights. The Panel is not restricted to using ►CMS◄ data and may use data collected or developed by organizations outside the Department in conducting its review.

On November 21, 2000, the Secretary signed the charter establishing an "Advisory Panel on APC Groups." The Panel is technical in nature and is governed by the provisions of the Federal Advisory Committee Act (FACA) as amended (Pub. L. 92-463). On November 1, 2002, the Secretary renewed the charter. The new charter indicates that the Panel continues to be technical in nature, is governed by the provisions of the FACA, may convene "up to three meetings per year," and is chaired by a Federal official. ►The entire APC Panel membership is identified on the CMS website at **www.cms.hhs.gov/faca/apc/apcmem.asp**. Information about each APC Panel meeting is available on the CMS website: **www.cms.hhs.gov/faca/apc/panel**. As a result of requests from the public, the Packaging Subcommittee of the APC Panel was established to review all the CPT codes with a status indicator of "N." Status indicator "N" indicates that payment for packaged codes is bundled into the payment that providers receive for separately payable codes for items or services provided on the same day. The Packaging Subcommittee reviewed every code that was packaged in 2004. CMS encourages submission of clinical scenarios involving currently packaged codes to the Packaging Subcommittee for review at future meetings. Submissions should be sent to the **APCPanel@cms.hhs.gov** with "Packaging Subcommittee" in the subject line.◄

►Payment Status Indicators (Special Symbols)◄

►To assist in ascertaining which ambulatory payment classification has been assigned to a particular procedure or service, the Hospital OPPS includes payment status "indicators." The status indicators CMS assigns to CPT Level I and HCPCS Level II codes and APCs under the OPPS have an important role in payment for services under the OPPS because they indicate if a service represented by a CPT/HCPCS code is payable under the OPPS or another payment system or if a particular OPPS policy applies to the CPT or HCPCS code. The OPPS is based on CPT and HCPCS codes for medical and other health services. These codes are used for a wide variety of payment systems under Medicare, including, but not limited to, the Medicare fee schedule for physician services, the Medicare fee schedule for durable medical equipment and prosthetic devices, and the Medicare clinical laboratory fee schedule. For purposes of making payment under the OPPS, CMS requires a means to discern the claims processing system for CPT/HCPCS codes that are paid under the OPPS and for those codes to which particular OPPS payment policies apply. CMS accomplishes this identification in the OPPS through the establishment of a system of "status indicators" with specific meanings. CMS assigns one and only one status indicator to each APC, to each CPT or HCPCS code. Each CPT or HCPCS code that is assigned to an APC has the same status indicator as the APC to which it is assigned (See **Appendix J**). The software that controls Medicare payment looks to the status indicators attached to the HCPCS codes and APCs for direction in the processing of the claim. Therefore, the assignment of the status indicators has significance for the payment of services.◄

►The specifications for the January 1, 2004, outpatient code editor (OCE) and PRICER, are pivotal in determining how hospital claims for outpatient services are processed and paid. CMS determined that claims would be processed more accurately if two additional payment status indicators were established CMS added status indicator "B" and status indicator "Y" to designate with greater specificity the appropriate disposition of certain codes for which payment is not made under the OPPS. CMS also revised and refined the status indicator definitions and clarified the explanation of what each status indicator means. None of these changes affects how services are paid under the OPPS. Rather, the changes are intended to clarify how the status indicators relate to existing payment policy and rules and to assist hospitals and our contractors in determining the disposition of individual HCPCS/CPT codes when they are billed to Medicare. The status indicator "Y" designate codes for non-implantable Durable Medical Equipment (DME) to assist hospitals in identifying codes that they must bill directly to the Durable Medical Equipment Regional Carrier (DMERC) rather than to the fiscal intermediary. Addendum D1 of the final rule contains the definitions of each status indicator for the 2005 OPPS.◄

►Historically, CMS has used status indicator "E" to identify certain HCPCS codes that are recognized by Medicare but that are not payable under the OPPS when they are submitted on an outpatient hospital Part B bill type (12x, 13x, or 14x). Beginning with implementation of the 2004 final rule, CMS has assigned status indicator

OPPS APC Status Indicator	CPT Symbol	Service/Procedure
A	♠	Paid/Not Paid Under Other Fee Schedule
B	✤	Not Paid Under OPPS. • May be paid by Intermediaries when submitted on a different bill type, e.g., 75x (CORF), but not paid under OPPS. • An alternate code that is recognized by OPPS when submitted on an Outpatient Hospital Part B bill type (12x, 13x, and 14x) may be available.
C	✿	Inpatient Procedure
E	☐	Not Paid Under Outpatient OPPS Codes Not Reportable in Hospital Outpatient Settings
K	■	Non Pass-through Drug/Biological
L	✪	Influenza Vaccine; Pneumococcal Pneumonia Vaccine—Paid Reasonable Cost; Not Subject to Deductible or Coinsurance
N	☆	Incidental Services Packaged into APC Rate Payment Is Packaged into Payment for Other Services
P	◇	Partial Hospitalization
S	❖	Significant Procedure—Not Discounted When Multiple
T	§	Significant Procedure—Multiple Procedure Reduction Applies
V	➧	Visit to Clinic or Emergency Department Paid Under OPPS
X	♣	Ancillary Service
►Other Indicator◄	**CPT Symbol**	**Service/Procedure**
Conditional Bilateral Procedure	♦	Bilateral Procedure Modifier Reportable—Conditional Bilateral – Procedure Considered Bilateral If Modifier –50 Is Appended*
Inherently Bilateral Procedure	✶	Bilateral Procedure Modifier Not Reportable—**Inherently Bilateral**—Procedure in and of Itself Is Bilateral.*
Independent Bilateral Procedure	✛	Bilateral Procedure Modifier Reportable—Procedure Considered Bilateral If Modifier –50 Is Appended
Unilateral Procedure	⌘	Bilateral Procedure Modifier Not Reportable—Use Existing Bilateral Procedure Code

►*For further clarification, see Modifiers Approved for Hospital Outpatient Use and **Appendix A**◄

"B" to HCPCS codes that are not payable under OPPS when submitted on an outpatient hospital Part B bill type (12x, 13x, and 14x), but that may be payable by intermediaries to other provider types when submitted on an appropriate bill type, such as bill type 75x submitted by a CORF. In some cases, another code may be submitted by hospitals on an outpatient hospital Part B bill type (12x, 13x, and 14x) to receive payment for a service or code that is assigned status indicator "B" in Addendum B. For the purposes of this publication, the table on this page shows the payment status indicators and description of the particular services each indicator identifies for each CPT code. The symbols are used only in this specially annotated version of CPT. (**Note:** For payment status indicators for Level II HCPCS codes, visit either the CMS web site at **www.cms.hhs.gov/regulations/hopps/2005f/** or visit the AMA CPT web site at **www.ama-assn.org/cpt**◄

►Effective January 1, 2003, CMS created a new status indicator "L" "Influenza vaccine; pneumococcal pneumonia vaccine" to indicate that these vaccines are paid on a reasonable cost basis but deductible and coinsurance do not apply to the payment. Therefore, the status indicator "K" was replaced by the status indicator "L" for influenza and pneumoccocal pneumonia vaccines (eg, 90657, 90658, 90659, 90732). Also effective January 1, 2005, CMS assigned the "E" status indicator (Not Paid Under Outpatient OPPS—Codes not Reportable in Hospital Outpatient Settings) to the diphtheria, tetanus toxoids, and acellular pertussis vaccine, Hepatitis B, and poliovirus vaccine, inactivated, CPT code 90723. Please bear in mind that these symbols relate to the CMS imposed regulations on reporting for the Medicare hospital outpatient prospective system ambulatory payment classification indicators, and have no meaning in any other third party payment system.◄

►Reporting CPT/HCPCS Codes◄

►How does a coder readily discern which "HCPCS" (Level I or Level II) code to report as the procedure/service may be identified in two or even three coding levels? When both a CPT and a HCPCS Level II code have virtually identical narratives for a procedure or service, the CPT code should be used. If, however, the narratives are not identical (for example, the CPT code narrative is generic, whereas the HCPCS Level II code is specific), the Level II code should be used." [Since CMS has eliminated certain unofficial Level III (local) codes, it is suggested you check with your local fiscal intermediary.]◄

►During the first two quarters of 2004, CMS created 85 HCPCS codes that were not addressed in the November 7, 2003, final rule that updated the 2004 OPPS. CMS has designated the payment status of those codes. Thirty of the new codes were created to enable providers to bill for brand name drugs and to receive payments at a rate that differs from that for generic equivalents, as mandated in new section 1833(t)(14)(A)(i) of the Act as added by Pub. L. 108-173. CMS publishes proposed/interim/final rules reflecting changes to OPPS. Instructional information usually precedes tables outlining proposed/final payment rates, new CPT and HCPCS codes assigned to APC groups, movement of certain CPT and HCPCS codes to different APC groups, current status indicators with definitions for a given calendar year, new technology category codes (HCPCS "C" codes), and new HCPCS Level II codes for a given calendar year. If the payment rate and status indicators are assigned to a CPT code versus a HCPCS Level II code, then the CPT code should be reported. Conversely, if the CPT code status indicator assignment reflects it is a "noncovered" service, but the HCPCS code is listed in a given APC and assigned a status indicator and payment rate, then the HCPCS code is to be reported. There is no single answer, except to urge users that is essential to continue to be diligent to any revised or new OPPS policy. (**Note:** For further instruction, please refer to the January-October 2003 editions of the *CPT Assistant*. See page xxx for information to obtain this referenced publication.)◄

Hospitals/Services Included/Excluded from OPPS

The Hospital Outpatient Payment System applies to covered hospital outpatient services furnished by all hospitals participating in the Medicare program. The OPPS final rule for 2002 clarified that effective January 1, 2002, CMS excludes from the OPPS, hospitals that are located outside the 50 States or the District of Columbia or Puerto Rico; that is, hospitals in Guam, Saipan, American Samoa, and the Virgin Islands. Section 413.65 (b) (2) states: "a provider or a facility or organization must contact CMS and the facility or organization must be determined by CMS to be provider-based before the main provider begins billing for services of the facility or for service (s) of the facility or organization as if they were furnished by a department of the provider-based entity." The regulation also addresses the criteria a facility must meet to be designated "provider-based." In recent years, provider-based facilities have expanded, including an increase in hospitals acquiring physician office practices to use as hospital outpatient departments. The regulation also includes requirements for hospitals to furnish an appropriate level of physician supervision in off-site clinics.

Having clear criteria for provider-based status is important because this designation can result in additional Medicare payments for services furnished at the provider-based facility, and may also increase the coinsurance liability of Medicare for those services. The regulations at Section 413.65 (b) (2) define provider-based status as "the relationship between a main provider and a provider-based entity or a department of a provider, remote location of hospital, or satellite facility, that complies with the provisions in this section." Among these criteria are the requirements that the main provider and the facility must have common licensure (when appropriate), the facility must operate under the ownership and control of the main provider, and the facility must be located in the immediate vicinity of the main provider. (See also *Federal Register*, April 7, 2000.)

Section 404 (a) of BIPA includes a grandfathering provision for facilities treated as provider-based on October 1, 2000; alternative criteria for meeting the geographic location requirement; and criteria for temporary treatment as provider-based. Under section 404 (a) of BIPA, any facilities or organizations that were "treated" as provider-based in relation to any hospital on October 1, 2000, continued to be treated as such until October 1, 2002. Thus, the provider-based facilities and organizations affected under section 404 (a) of BIPA were not required to submit an application for or obtain a provider-based status determination in order to continue receiving reimbursement as provider-based during this period. (**Note:** For further information pertaining to issues related to provider-based status, you may access the CMS web site at **www.cms.hhs.gov**)

The OPPS also applies to limited services provided by Comprehensive Outpatient Rehabilitation Facilities (CORFs), Home Health Agencies (HHAs), or to hospice patients for the treatment of a non-terminal illness. It does not apply to Critical Access Hospitals. The Indian health care system was initially excluded from the OPPS, but effective July 1, 2002, section 432 of the BIPA extended the exception to permit Medicare payments to hospitals and outpatient clinics (provider-based or free-standing), operated by the Indian Health Service (IHS) or by a tribe or tribal organization, for services furnished by physicians and specified non-physician practitioners in or at the direction of an IHS hospital or outpatient clinic. Payments for these services are made to the IHS or tribal hospital or outpatient clinic, not to the physician or other practitioner.

►Partial Hospitalization◄

►Partial hospitalization is an intensive outpatient program of psychiatric services provided to patients in the place of inpatient care. Under OPPS, a partial hospitalization program (PHP)may be provided by a hospital to its outpatients or by a Medicare-certified Community Mental Health Center. (See also *Federal Register*, April 7, 2000, November 1, 2002, November 7, 2003.) Exclusions from outpatient PPS are different and more limited than exclusions from inpatient PPS. Thus, hospitals or distinct parts of hospitals that are excluded from the inpatient PPS are included in the outpatient PPS, to the extent that the hospital or distinct part furnishes outpatient services. The following list of current CPT/HCPCS codes are as follows:◄

Revenue Codes	Description	HCPCS Codes
250* (*Limited to Medicare covered, ie, not usually self-administered drugs)	Pharmacy HCPS code not required	
43X	Occupational Therapy	G0129
904	Activity Therapy	G0176
910	Psychiatric General Services	90801, 90802, 90899
914	Individual Psychotherapy	90816, 90817, 90818, 90819, 90821, 90822, 90823, 90824, 90826, 90827, 90828, 90829
915	Group Therapy	90849, 90853, 90857
916	Family Psychotherapy	90846, 90847, 90849
918	Psychiatric Testing	96100, 96115, 96117
942	Education/Training	G0177

►Blood and Blood Products◄

►From the onset of the OPPS, CMS has developed separate APCs to reimburse for blood, other blood products, and anti-hemophilic factors either in APCs with status indicator "K" or as pass-through drugs and biologicals with status indicator "G" rather than packaging them into payment for the procedures with which they were administered. For 2005, CMS will continue to pay separately for blood and blood products. CMS is also establishing new APCs that would allow each blood product to be in its own separate APC and to implement proposed APC reassignments for such blood and blood products.◄

►Administrative costs for the processing and storage specific to the transfused blood product are included in the APC payment, which is based on hospitals' charges. Payment for the collection, processing, and storage of autologous blood, as described by CPT 86890 and used in transfusion is made through APC 347 (Level III Transfusion Laboratory Procedures). Other than for autologous blood products, the costs for collection, processing, storage, wastage, and other administrative costs for blood products that are not transfused are reported in the appropriate cost centers on hospitals' cost reports.◄

►Reporting New Drugs, Biologicals and Radiopharmaceuticals Before HCPCS/CPT Codes Are Assigned◄

►Section 621(a)(1) of Pub. L. 108-173 amended section 1833(t) of the Act by adding paragraph (15) to provide for payment for new drugs and biologicals until HCPCS Level II codes are assigned under the OPPS. Under this provision, CMS is required to make payment for an outpatient drug or biological that is furnished as part of covered outpatient services for which a HCPCS Level II code has not been assigned. Historically, hospitals have used a code for an unlisted or unclassified drug, biological, or radiopharmaceutical or used an appropriate revenue code to report drugs, biologicals, and radiopharmaceuticals furnished in the outpatient department that do not have an assigned HCPCS code. The codes for not otherwise classified drugs, biologicals, (CMS-1427-P 169) and radiopharmaceuticals are assigned packaged status under the OPPS. That is, separate payment is not made for the code, but charges for the code would be eligible for an outlier payment and, in future updates, the charges for the code are packaged with the separately payable service with which the code is reported for the same date of service. Drugs and biologicals that are newly approved by the FDA and for which a HCPCS code has not yet been assigned by the National HCPCS Alpha-Numeric Workgroup could qualify for pass-through payment under the OPPS.◄

►Exception to CMS Packaging Rule◄

►CMS has applied an exception to its packaging rule to one particular class of drugs, the injectible and oral forms of anti-emetic treatments. CMS recognizes that for beneficiaries to achieve the maximum therapeutic benefit from chemotherapy and other therapies with side effects of nausea and vomiting, anti-emetic use is often an integral part of the treatment regimen. CMS has worked to ensure that its payment rules do not impede a beneficiary's access to the particular antiemetic that is most effective for him or her as determined by the beneficiary and his or her physician. Therefore, CMS will pay separately for all six injectible and oral forms of anti-emetic products for 2005 (CMS-1427-P 149).◄

►CMS decided to apply its equitable adjustment authority to establish several exceptions to the packaging threshold. CMS noted that there were seven drugs and biologicals that it proposed to pay separately for in the proposed rule. Table 24 of the final rule (69 FR 50506) lists the seven drugs and biologicals to which this policy will apply along with the 2004 and 2005 payment status indicators. Table 25 lists the drugs and biologicals that were proposed as packaged drugs and biologicals but will be paid separately in 2005. The table also indicates the methodology that will be used to determine APC payment rates in 2005.◄

►Payment for Brachytherapy Sources◄

►Sections 621(b)(1) and (b)(2) of Pub. L. 108-173 amended the Act by adding section 1833(t)(16)(C) and section 1833(t)(2)(H), respectively, to establish separate payment for devices of brachytherapy consisting of a seed or seeds (or radioactive source) based on a hospital's charges for the service, adjusted to cost. The period of payment under this provision is for brachytherapy sources furnished from January 1, 2004 through December 31, 2006. In the OPPS interim final rule with comment period published on January 6, 2004 (69 FR 827), CMS implemented sections 621(b)(1) and 621(b)(2)(C) of Pub. L. 108-173. CMS stated that it will pay for the brachytherapy sources listed in Table 4 of the interim final rule with comment period (69 FR 828) on a cost basis, as required by the statute.◄

►Accordingly, the status indicator for brachytherapy sources was changed to "H." The definition of status indicator "H" was for pass-through payment only for devices, but the brachytherapy sources affected by new sections 1833(t)(16)(C) and 1833(t)(2)(H) of the Act are not pass-through device categories. Therefore, CMS also changed for 2004 the definition of payment status indicator "H" to include nonpass-through brachytherapy sources paid on a cost basis. According to CMS, this use of status indicator "H" allows CMS to pay for brachytherapy sources in accordance with new section 1833(t)(16)(C) of the Act, effective January 1, 2004, without having to modify its claims processing systems. CMS stated in the January 6, 2004 interim final rule with comment period that it would revisit the use and definition of status indicator "H" for this purpose in the OPPS update for 2005.◄

►As indicated in the January 6, 2004 interim final rule with comment period, CMS began payment for the brachytherapy source in HCPCS code C1717 (Brachytx source, HCR Ir-192) based on the hospital's charge adjusted to cost beginning January 1, 2004. Prior to enactment of Pub. L. 108-173, these sources were paid as packaged services in APC 0313. For 2004, CMS invited the public to submit recommendations for new codes to describe brachytherapy sources in a manner reflecting the number, radioisotope, and radioactivity intensity of the sources (69 FR 828). CMS requested that commenters provide a detailed rationale to support recommended new codes. The public may send such recommendations to the Division of Outpatient Care, Mailstop C4-05-17, Centers for Medicare and Medicaid Services, 7500 Security Blvd., 21244. CMS indicates it will endeavor to add new brachytherapy source codes and descriptors to its systems for payment on a quarterly rather than an annual basis.◄

►Based on concurrence of a recommendation from the APC Panel, CMS established two new brachytherapy source codes for 2005: C2634 Brachytherapy source, high activity Iodine-125, greater than 1.01 mCi (NIST), per source and C2635 Brachytherapy source, high activity Palladium-103, greater than 2.2 mCi (NIST), per source. Since new brachytherapy sources may be added more frequently than annually (when CMS is able to add new codes and payment instructions to its electronic claims processing systems), CMS did not create a new code of miscellaneous brachytherapy sources. (**Note:** Table 40 of the final rule provides a complete listing of the HCPCS codes, long descriptors, APC assignments and status indicators that CMS will use for separately payable brachytherapy sources under the OPPS in 2005).◄

Transitional Pass-Through Payments

Section 1833 (t) (6)(B) (i) of the Act provides for temporary additional payments or "transitional pass-through payments" for certain medical devices, drugs, and biologicals. As originally enacted by the BBRA, this provision required the Secretary to make additional payments to hospitals for "current" orphan drugs, biologic agents, and brachytherapy devices used for the treatment of cancer; and current radiopharmaceutical drugs and biological products. For those drugs, biological agents, and devices referred to as "current" the transitional pass-through payment began on the first date the hospital OPPS was implemented ►(before enactment of BIPA (Pub. L. 106-554), on December 21, 2000))◄. Transitional pass-through payments are also required for certain "new" medical devices, drugs, and biological agents that were not being paid for as a hospital outpatient service as of December 31, 1996. Under the statute, transitional pass-through payments are to be made for at least 2 years but not more than 3 years ► and whose cost is "not insignificant" in relation to the OPPS payment for the procedures or services associated with the new drug, device, or biological.◄ (**Note:** For a list of those devices, drugs, and biological agents with proposed expiration dates, see Table 21 of the ►November 15, 2004,◄ *Federal Register.*)

Since the inception of OPPS, transitional pass-through payments have been reported using the Healthcare Common Procedure Coding System (HCPCS). Initially, the HCPCS C codes were device-specific (eg, dual chamber pacemaker). Section 1833 (t) (6) (B) (8) of the Act, as amended, required CMS to establish by April 1, 2001, HCPCS C codes representing devicecategories to be used for the purposes of determining which medical devices are eligible for transitional pass-through payments. This requirement was met through the issuance on March 22, 2001, of two Program Memoranda, Transmittals A-01-40 and A-01-41, which were published on the CMS website at **www.hcfa.gov/pubforms/transmit/A0140.pdf** and **www.hcfa.gov/pubforms/transmit/A0141.pdf**, respectively. Transitional pass-through categories are for devices only; they do not apply to drugs or biological agents. C codes have been assigned by CMS exclusively for this purpose, and were effective for reporting April 1, 2001. Items eligible for transitional pass-through payments are generally reported using a Level II HCPCS code with an alpha prefix of "C". Pass-through device categories are identified by status indicator "H" and pass-through drugs and biologicals are identified by status indicator "G"). CMS added two additional categories and made clarifications to some of the categories' long descriptors found in transmittal A-01-73. (**Note:** A current list of device category codes in effect as of July 1, 2002, can be found in Transmittal A-02-050, issued on June 17, 2002. This Program Memorandum can be accessed at the CMS web site at **www.cms.hhs.gov.manuals**.)

To qualify for a transitional pass-through payment, a device must meet all the requirements as defined by Medicare. Medicare only makes transitional pass-through payments for a device in conjunction with a procedure for its implantation or insertion. For example, scalpels and coagulators are considered supplies because they are neither implanted (like a pacemaker) nor surgically inserted (like an ablation catheter) in a patient. These and other supplies are "packaged" into the APC payment rates for surgeries, and they do not qualify for separate transitional pass-through payments. (**Note:** The process to apply for transitional pass-through payment for eligible drugs and biological agents or for additional device categories can be found on respective pages of the CMS web site at **www.cms.hhs.gov**. Notification of new drug, biological, or device category application processes are generally posted on the OPPS web site at **www.cms.hhs.gov/hopps**.)

Expiring Pass-Through Status for Drugs and Devices

Drugs, biologicals, and devices, to the extent they are eligible to receive pass-through payments, must receive such payments for at least two, but no more than three years. January of 2003 was the first time that transitional pass-through status of drugs or categories of devices expired. These drugs and devices ►are◄ generally packaged into the APCs for which they are used. In some cases, certain drugs and biological agents are paid in separate APCs.

Device eligibility for pass-through status is based upon the category to which the device belongs, rather than on an individual device. Once the device category's eligibility for pass-through payments expires, all devices in that category expire with it (see Table 21, of the ►November 15 2004,◄ *Federal Register*). All devices in that category will be incorporated into the payment rate for the procedures that use those devices. (**Note:** For drugs and biological agents for which pass-through status expires ►on December 31,◄ 2004, see Table 21 of the ►November 15, 2004,◄ *Federal Register*).

Separate APCs for Drugs Not Eligible for Transitional Pass-Through Payment

Under the OPPS, CMS currently pays for radiopharmaceuticals, drugs, and biologicals including blood and blood products, which do not have pass-through status, in one of three ways: packaged payment, separate payment (individual APCs), and reasonable cost. As explained in the April 7, 2000, final rule (65 FR 18450), CMS generally packages the cost of drugs and radiopharmaceuticals into the APC payment rate for the procedure or treatment with which the products are usually furnished. OPPS rule policy includes the packaging of services into the APC "when they are directly related and integral to performing a procedure or furnishing a service." Therefore, hospitals do not receive separate payment from Medicare for packaged items and supplies, and hospitals may not bill beneficiaries separately for any such packaged items and supplies whose costs are recognized and paid for within the national OPPS payment rate for the associated procedure or service. (**Note:** Transmittal A-01-133, a Program Memorandum issued to Intermediaries on November 20, 2001, explains in greater detail the rules regarding separate payment for packaged services by accessing the CMS web site at **www.cms.hhs.gov**)

Under OPPS, the status indicator "K" is used to denote the APCs for drugs and biological agents (including blood and blood products) and certain brachytherapy seeds that are paid separately from and in addition to the procedure or treatment with which they are associated, but that are not eligible for transitional pass-through payment.

Drugs for which separate payment is allowed are designated by status indicator "K" in Addendum B of the ►2005◄ final rule. Hospitals should continue to bill for packaged drugs, which are assigned status indicator "N," using any of the drug revenue codes that are packaged revenue codes under the OPPS: 250, 251, 252, 254, 255, 257, 258, 259, 631, 632, or 633. Hospitals are not required to use HCPCS codes when billing for packaged drugs, unless revenue code 636 is used. Although CMS ►does◄ not require hospitals to report HCPCS codes for packaged drugs, it is essential that hospitals continue to bill charges for packaged drugs by including the charge for packaged drugs in the charge for the procedure or service with which the drug is used, or as a separate drug charge (whether or not it is separately payable). Reporting charges for packaged drugs is critical because packaged drug costs are used for calculating outlier payments and are also identified when we calculate hospital costs for the procedures and services with which the drugs are used in the course of the annual OPPS updates.

New Technology

In the April 7, 2000, final rule (68 FR 18477), CMS created a set of new technology APCs to pay for certain new technology services under OPPS.

►CMS proposed to limit eligibility for placement in new technology APCs only to comprehensive services or procedures. New technology APCs are reported using certain CPT Category I and Category III codes or HCPCS Level II codes, and represent technology services not addressed by the transitional pass-through provisions of the BBRA 1999 and BIPA 2000. Therefore, to assist in the use of this publication, only certain CPT Category III codes are recognized for payment under OPPS have been assigned a payment status indicator. For example, CPT Category III code 0003T has a status indicator of "N" identified using symbol (☆), while Category III code 0009T has a status indicator of "T" identified using symbol (§). CMS does not recognize under the OPPS new CPT Category III codes released on a mid-year basis. Even though the CPT Editorial Panel may assign new Category III codes mid-year, CMS only assigns new CPT codes on an annual basis, effective with its January 1 updates to the OPPS.◄

►In the November 30, 2001 final rule, CMS made final its proposal to change the period of time during which a service may be p aid under a new technology APC (66 FR 59903), initially established in the April 7, 2000, final rule. That is, beginning in 2002, CMS retained a service within a new technology APC group until it had acquired adequate data that allow CMS to assign the service to a clinically appropriate APC. This policy allows CMS to move a service from a new technology APC in less than 2 years if sufficient data are available, and it also allows CMS to retain a service in a new technology APC for more than 3 years if sufficient data upon which to base a decision for reassignment have not been collected. (**Note:** For a complete listing of the APCs, see **Appendix J**, or Addendum C of the November 2004, final rule, or period updates on the CMS website **www.cms.hhs.gov/manuals**.)◄

Evaluation and Management (E/M Services Approved for Hospital Outpatient Use)

With the implementation of OPPS on August 1, 2001, for emergency and clinic visits, the OPPS requires correct reporting of services using certain CPT and HCPCS Level II codes as a prerequisite to payment. The OPPS distinguishes three levels of service for payment purposes which are referred to as "low-level," "midlevel," and "high-level" emergency or clinic visits. Again, for 2003 OPPS reporting purposes, low-level clinic and emergency visits include CPT codes for level one and two services (for example, CPT codes 92012,99201, 99202, 99211, 99212, 99241, 99242, 99271, 99272, 99281, 99282, 99431, and HCPCS codes G0101, G0245, G0246, and G0264); mid-level visits include level three services (for example, CPT codes 92002, 99203, 99213, 99243, 99273 and 99283), and high-level visits include level four and five services (for example, CPT codes 92004, 92014,99204, 99205, 99214, 99215, 99244, 99245, 99274, 99275, 99284, 99285, and HCPCS code G0175). There is a single APC for critical care services (99291), as hospitals are required to use CPT code 99291 to report outpatient encounters in which critical care services are furnished. The hospital is required to use CPT code 99291 in place of, but not in addition to, a code for a medical visit or for an emergency department service.

To address the need for facilities to comply with the requirements of the Health Insurance Portability and Accountability Act (HIPAA) and audit and compliance program issues, CMS has proposed development of new Level II HCPCS codes for facility visits in the emergency department and clinic setting to ensure accurate payment. CMS proposes to implement new evaluation and management codes only when it is also ready to implement guidelines for their use, after allowing ample opportunity for public comment, systems change, and provider education. CMS will continue to work with hospitals to develop documentation guidelines for the use of the new facility emergency and clinic visit Level II HCPCS codes. CMS plans to make any proposed guidelines available to the public for comment on the OPPS web site as soon as they are complete. ►CMS anticipates providing at least 6 to 12 months notice prior to implementation of the new evaluation and management codes and guidelines. CMS will continue working to develop and test the new codes even though it has not yet made plans for their implementation.◄ CMS will notify the public through listserve when these proposed guidelines become available. To subscribe to this listserve, please go to the following web site: **www.cms.hhs.gov/medlearn/listserv.asp** and follow the directions to the OPPS listserve.

►Initial Preventive Physical Examinations◄

►Section 611 of Pub. 108-173 provides for coverage under Medicare Part B of an initial preventive physical examination for new beneficiaries, effective for services furnished on or after January 1, 2005. CMS proposes to amend §419.21 of the OPPS regulations to add a new paragraph (e) to specify payment for an initial preventive physical examination as a Medicare Part B covered service under the OPPS if the examination is furnished within the first 6 months of the beneficiary's first Medicare Part B coverage. CMS noted that the initial preventive physical examination is also addressed in detail in its proposed rule to update the 2005 Medicare Physician's Fee Schedule. However, because CMS believes the same elements of the initial physical examination furnished in a physician's office would also apply when the examination is performed in a hospital outpatient clinic, CMS proposed to revise the applicable regulations to reflect this requirement. (**Note:** Definitions to interpret the term "initial preventive physical examination" for purposes of this new benefit include all of the services furnished by a doctor of medicine or osteopathy or a qualified nonphysician practitioner. Section 611(d)(2) of Pub. L 108-173 amended section 1861(s)(2)(K)(i) and (ii) of the Act specify the services identified as physicians' services and referred in the definition of initial preventive physical examination to include services furnished by a physician assistant, a nurse practitioner, or a clinical nurse specialist. CMS refers to these professionals as "qualified nonphysician practitioners" (CMS-1427-P 74). For a complete listing of the education, counseling, and referral services with respect to the screening and other preventive services authorized under Medicare Part B including the definition of the term "initial preventive physical examination", refer to the November 15, 2004, final rule, at the CMS website, **www.cms.hhs.gov**).◄

►CMS indicated there is no current CPT code that contains the specific elements included in the initial preventive physical examination. Therefore, CMS has established four new HCPCS codes, to be used to bill for the new service under both the Medicare physician fee schedule and the OPPS. As required by the statute, this code includes an electrocardiogram, but does not include the other preventive services that are currently separately covered and paid under the Medicare Part B screening benefits. When these other preventive services are performed, they should be identified using the existing appropriate codes. Section 611 of Pub. L. 108-173 does require a screening EKG to be performed as part of the initial preventive physical examination visit. In view of the different circumstances that may occur when performing the full initial preventive physical examination, CMS established four new G codes for the initial preventative physical examination for CY 2005.◄

- G0344: Initial preventive physical examination; face-to-face visit, services listed to new beneficiary during the first 6 months of Medicare Part B enrollment. (This code is assigned a status indicator "V" for the OPPS.)
- G0366: Electrocardiogram, routine EKG with at least 12 leads; performed as a component of the initial preventive physical examination with interpretation and report. (This code is assigned a status indicator "B" for the OPPS.)
- G0367: Electrocardiogram, tracing only, without interpretation and report, performed as a component of the initial preventive physical examination. (This code is assigned status indicator "S" for the OPPS.)
- G0368: Electrocardiogram, interpretation and report only, performed as a component of the initial preventive physical examination. (This code is assigned status indicator "A" for the OPPS.)

►In the hospital, performance of the complete initial preventive physical examination service would be coded using both the G0344 and G0367 codes. As required by the statute, the new codes describe the visit and the EKG, but not other preventive services currently separately covered and paid under the Medicare Part B screening benefits. When these other preventive services are performed, they should be billed using the existing appropriate HCPCS and CPT codes.◄

►According to CMS, the initial preventive physical examination will not be subject to each hospital's internal set of evaluation and management guidelines that hospitals were instructed to develop at the implementation of the OPPS in the August 7, 2000, final rule (65 FR 18451) because CMS defined one explicit service, without levels. CMS will release appropriate manual and transmittal instructions and information from the CMS educational components for the medical community, including a MedLearn Matters article and fact sheets such as the "2005 Payment Changes for Physicians and Other Providers: News From Medicare for 2005." Information on the new benefit will also be made available to the public through its website, **www.medicare.gov**, the partner website to **www.cms.hhs.gov**◄

Observation Services

Under the OPPS, hospitals are required to bill for observation services in one of two ways: as packaged services, or as a separately payable APC when certain conditions are met for patients having diagnoses of chest pain, asthma, or congestive heart failure, for whom observation services are furnished. Hospitals are required to report observation charges under revenue code 762 "Observation Room." CPT coding is not required, but if reported, the "packaged" CPT observation services are reported using codes 99218, 99219, 99220, 99234, 99235, or 99236. In the units field, hospitals should enter the number of hours the outpatient is in observation status. Hospitals should report laboratory, radiology, or other diagnostic services under revenue codes 30X, 31X, 32X, etc., as appropriate. (**Note:** For further CMS instructions, see January 3, 2003, Program Memorandum (Transmittal A-02-129) at the CMS website **www.cms.hhs.gov/manuals.**)

Criteria for Separate Reporting of Observation Services

►Frequently, beneficiaries are placed in "observation status" in order to receive treatment or to be monitored before making a decision concerning their next placement (that is, admit to the hospital or discharge). This status assignment occurs most frequently after surgery or a visit to the emergency department. With the initiation of the OPPS, observation services were no longer paid separately; that is, they were not assigned to a separate APC. Instead, costs for observation services were packaged into payments for the services with which the observation care was associated.◄

►For 2002 OPPS, CMS implemented separate payment for observation services (APC 0339) under the OPPS for three medical conditions: chest pain, congestive heart failure, and asthma. CMS agreed that specifying which diagnostic tests must be performed as a prerequisite for payment of APC 0339 may be imposing an unreasonable reporting burden on hospitals and may, in some cases, result in unnecessary tests being performed. Effective January 1, 2005, the following tests would no longer be required to receive payment for APC 0339 (Observation): For congestive heart failure, a chest x-ray (71010, 71020, 71030), and electrocardiogram (93005) and pulse oximetry (94760, 94761, 94762) 94762). For chest pain, two sets of cardiac enzyme tests; either two CPK (82550, 82552, 82553) or two troponins (84484, 84512) and two sequential electrocardiograms (93005). Beginning April 1, 2005, hospitals must report a qualifying ICD-9 CM diagnosis code in Form Locator (FL) 76, Patient Reason for Visit, and/or FL 67, principal diagnosis, in order for the hospital to receive separate payment for APC 0339. If a qualifying ICD-9 diagnosis code(s) is reported in the secondary diagnosis field but is not reported in either the Patient Reason for Visit field (FL 76) or the principal diagnosis field (FL 67), separate payment for APC 0339 will not be allowed. (For a complete listing of eligible diagnoses codes to be used for reporting observation services for 2005, see Table 38 in the final rule preamble.)◄

►In an effort to allay apparent confusion regarding reporting observation stays that exceed 48 hours, CMS has changed the descriptor for HCPCS code G0244 to read as follows: G0244, Observation care provided by a facility to a patient with CHF, chest pain or asthma, minimum 8 hours. CMS indicates hospitals should report one unit of G0244 for each hour of observation care provided to patients for congestive heart failure, chest pain, or asthma, with a minimum 8 units billed to be eligible for separate observation payment. Currently, hospitals report the time in observation beginning with the admission of the beneficiary to observation and ending with the physician's order to discharge the patient from observation. To clarify use of G0244, CMS reiterates in provider education materials developed for the 2005 OPPS update that observation time begins at the clock time documented in the patient's medical record, which coincides with the time the patient is placed in a bed for the purpose of initiating observation care in accordance with a physician's order.◄

►CMS has outlined the following requirements to receive separate payment for HCPCS code G0244 in APC 0339 for medically necessary observation services involving specific goals and a plan of care that are distinct from the goals and plan of care for an emergency department, physician office, or clinic visit:

- The beneficiary must have one of three medical conditions: congestive heart failure, chest pain, or asthma. (The hospital bill must report as the admitting or principal diagnosis an appropriate ICD-9-CM code to reflect the condition. The eligible ICD-9-CM diagnosis codes for 2005 are shown in Table 38 of the final rule preamble.)
- The hospital must provide and report on the bill an emergency department visit (APC 0610, 0611, or 0612), clinic visit (APC 0600, 0601, or 0602), or critical care (APC 0620) on the same day or the day before the separately payable observation care (G0244) is provided.◄

If the observation services furnished by a hospital do not meet the requirements for separate APC payment, the hospital must bill observation services using revenue code 762 only or using revenue code 762 with one of the CPT/HCPCS codes for packaged observation services (CPT observation services 99218, 99219, 99220, 99234, 99235, or 99236). Because the status indicator on HCPCS G0244 is an "S," any claim with an E/M visit on the same day as the observation will be subject to OPPS OCE edit 21 (medical visit on same day as type T or S procedure without modifier -25). Therefore, the E/M code for the visit must be reported with modifier -25 in order for the observation to be paid. Since critical care may be furnished in a clinic or an emergency department and may appropriately precede admission to observation for chest pain, asthma, or congestive heart failure, the critical care CPT code 99291 must also be listed on the same claim in order to receive separate payment for observation services.

Direct Admission to Observation

For observation services *without* an associated hospital clinic visit or emergency department visit furnished on or after January 1, 2003, CMS modified the criteria and the codes used under OPPS. Specifically, CMS has created two new HCPCS Level II codes. According to CMS, these additional codes would allow data collection on the extent to which patients are directly admitted to hospital observation services *without* an associated hospital clinic visit or emergency department. As outlined above, the current requirement that the hospital bill an emergency department visit (APC 0600, 0601, or 0602) or a clinic visit (APC 0610, 0611, or 0612) or a critical care service (APC 0620) in order to receive separate payment for observation services for patients not admitted directly from a physician's office would remain in effect.

According to CMS, a "direct admission" occurs when a physician in the community refers a patient to the hospital for observation, bypassing the clinic or emergency department (ED). Hospitals must use modifier -25 with G0263 in order to receive payment for G0244. Hospitals should bill G0263 and G0264 with revenue code 762. Certain diagnoses are required to qualify for separate observation payment.

►For direct admissions to observation, in lieu of an emergency department visit, clinic visit, or critical care, G0263 (Admission with congestive heart failure, chest pain, asthma) must be billed on the same day as G0244, as outlined by CMS:

- HCPCS code G0244 must be billed for a minimum of 8 hours.
- No procedures with a 'T' status indicator, except the code for infusion therapy of other than a chemotherapy drug (CPT code 90780) can be reported on the same day or day before observation care is provided.
- Observation time must be documented in the medical record and begins with the beneficiary's admission to an observation bed and ends when he or she is discharged from the hospital.
- The beneficiary must be in the care of a physician during the period of observation, as documented in the medical record by admission, discharge, and other appropriate progress notes that are timed, written, and signed by the physician.
- The medical record must include documentation that the physician explicitly assessed patient risk to determine that the beneficiary would benefit from observation care.◄

As of January 1, 2003, if a hospital directly admits to observation from a physician's office a patient with a diagnosis of congestive heart failure, asthma, or chest pain, hospitals may report HCPCS Level II code G0263—"Direct admission of patient with diagnosis of congestive heart failure, chest pain, or asthma for observation" with HCPCS Level II code G0244. Payment for G0263 will be packaged into the payment for APC 339. The determination of whether use of G0263 is appropriate will be made after reviewing all diagnoses submitted on the claim (e.g., admission, principal, and secondary diagnoses). Code G0263 must be billed with G0244. Although code G0263 is treated as a packaged service and will not generate a payment under OPPS, the code will be recognized as taking the place of a visit or critical care code in meeting the observation criteria for patients directly admitted to observation.

Intravenous Infusion During Observation Stay

►CMS recognizes the costs of space, utilities, and staff attendance are duplicated when the beneficiary is receiving another service at the same time as infusion therapy, in particular when the patient is in observation. According to CMS, it is appropriate to apply a multiple procedure reduction to infusion therapy particularly when the patient is in observation status. CMS indicates it is necessary to understand how the Outpatient Code Editor (OCE) multiple procedure discounting logic functions. Line-items with a service indicator of "T" are subject to multiple procedure discounting unless CPT modifiers 76, 77, 78, and/or 79 are present on the claim. The "T" line-item with the highest payment amount will not be discounted but all other "T" line items will be discounted as multiple procedures. All line-items that do not have a service indicator of "T" will be ignored in determining the discount. Therefore, if the only other services reported with infusion therapy are an emergency department or other visit code, or diagnostic tests and services assigned status indicator "S," the infusion therapy code would not be subject to the multiple procedure discounting.◄

►Drug Administration in the Outpatient Department◄

►Since implementation of the OPPS, Medicare OPPS payment for administration of cancer chemotherapy drugs and infusion of other drugs has been made using HCPCS Level II codes Q0081, Q0083, Q0084, and Q0085 (CMS-1427-P 182). In the 2004 proposed rule, CMS proposed to change coding and payment for these services to enable it to pay more accurately for the wide range of services and the drugs that CMS packages into these "per visit" codes. (See August 12, 2003, proposed rule (68 FR 47998) for background discussion on these codes.)◄

►For 2005, CMS is implementing the existing CPT codes for drug administration rather than the new G-codes that will be used for the Medicare Physician Fee Schedule payments. CMS does not intend to use the new HCPCS G-codes for the OPPS drug administration services until such time as the new CPT codes for those services are issued in 2006. CMS will require use of the CPT codes for drug administration, but will crosswalk the CPT codes into APCs that reflect how the services would have been paid under the Q codes. Although hospitals would bill the CPT codes and include the charges for each CPT code on the claim, payment would be made on a "per visit" basis. It is critical for hospitals to bill the charges for the packaged CPT codes for drug administration for 2005 (that is, the CPT codes with status indicator N), even though there would be no separate payment for them in 2005. For 2007 OPPS, the 2005 claims data would be used as the basis for setting median costs for each CPT code, based on the reported charges reduced to cost, and would determine what APC configuration ensures most appropriate payment for the CPT drug administration codes. If hospitals do not bill charges in 2005 for the packaged drug administration CPT codes such as CPT codes 96412, 96423, 96545, or 90781, they would jeopardize CMS' ability to make accurate payments for services billed and paid under these codes for OPPS 2007 when the 2005 data is used to set the payment weights (CMS-1427-P 186).◄

►CMS recognizes multiple "visits" for chemotherapy are possible and multiple visits per day for antibiotic infusion are common. CMS indicates the reporting and payment for these multiple visits and services will not be an issue once payment for drug administration under the OPPS is made based on CPT code-specific data. However, until such time, for OPPS reporting, hospitals are to append the CPT modifier 59 (distinct procedure) when reporting services furnished during multiple visits that follow the initial visit. For CPT codes 90780 and 90781, in the event there are multiple visits for infusion on the same day, the hospital should report CPT code 90780 with modifier 59 and CPT code 90781, if appropriate, with modifier 59 for each separate visit for infusion. With modifier 59 appended to CPT codes 90780 and 90781, the Outpatient Code Editor (OCE) will allow up to 4 units of APC 0120 (Infusion of nonchemotherapy drugs) to be paid. Similarly, for the chemotherapy administration codes, where there is no modifier 59 reported, the OCE will collapse all codes that map to a particular APC into one unit of that APC and will pay one unit of each applicable APC. The system will assume that all services were furnished in one single encounter. Where the chemotherapy services are provided in multiple encounters, the hospital will need to show modifier 59 on the service furnished in the second encounter. The OCE will map those services into an additional unit of each applicable APC and will pay for each visit. The OCE will not, for a single date of service, pay more than 4 units of APC 120, nor more than 2 units of APCs 116 and 117 (chemotherapy by route other than infusion and infusion of chemotherapy drugs).◄

►CMS affirms that hospitals may report CPT codes 90780 (intravenous infusion for therapy/diagnosis administered by physician or under direct supervision of physician; up to one hour) and 90781 (each additional hour up to (8) hours), notwithstanding that the administration is not done by a physician or under the direct supervision of a physician. Although such services are typically administered in hospitals by nurses without direct physician supervision, CMS does not view the language of these CPT codes' definitions as being an obstacle to or inconsistent with the use of the codes by hospitals for Medicare reporting. CMS views its general requirements regarding physician supervision (with respect to payment for services that are incident to a physician's service in the outpatient hospital setting) as meeting the physician supervision aspect of the codes and thus, do not believe that use of the codes in the hospital outpatient setting would be prevented by the inclusion of the language in the code definition.◄

►Payment for Vaccines◄

►Outpatient hospital departments administer large amounts of the vaccines for influenza (flu) and pneumococcal pneumonia (PPV), typically by participating in immunization programs. In recent years, the availability and cost of some vaccines (particularly the flu vaccine) have fluctuated considerably. As discussed in the November 1, 2002, final rule (67 FR 66718), CMS was advised by providers that OPPS payment was insufficient to cover the costs of the flu vaccine and that access of Medicare beneficiaries to flu vaccines might be limited. Hospitals, home health agencies (HHAs), and hospices, which were paid for these vaccines under the OPPS in 2002, have been receiving payment at reasonable cost for these vaccines since 2003. For 2005, CMS will continue paying for influenza and pneumococcal pneumonia vaccines under the reasonable cost methodology.◄

►CMS noted that for 2005 a new CPT code for an influenza vaccine was created. The new CPT code 90656 (Influenza virus vaccine, split virus, preservative free, for use in individuals 3 years and above, for intramuscular use) will be paid at reasonable cost in 2005. CMS assigned status indicator "L" (Not Paid under OPPS. Paid at reasonable cost) to this new CPT code.◄

►Unlisted Codes◄

►Certain CPT codes have descriptors that do not define the exact service furnished. They are commonly called "unlisted" codes. The code descriptors often contain phrases such as: "unlisted procedure," "not otherwise classified," or "not otherwise specified" (CMS-1427-P 65). The unlisted codes typically fall within a clinical or procedural category, but they lack the specificity needed to describe the resources used in the service. For example, CPT code 17999 is defined as, "Unlisted procedure, skin, mucous membrane and subcutaneous tissue." The unlisted codes provide a way for providers to report services for which there is no CPT code that specifically describes the service furnished. However, the lack of specificity in describing the service prevents CMS from assigning the code to an APC based on clinical homogeneity and median cost. In most cases, the unlisted codes are assigned to the lowest level, clinically appropriate APC under the Medicare OPPS. This creates an incentive for providers to select the appropriate, specific CPT code to describe the service where one is available. According to CMS, if there is no CPT code that accurately describes the service, placing the unlisted code in the lowest level APC provides an incentive for interested parties to secure a code through the AMA's CPT process that will describe the service. Once a code that accurately describes the service is created, CMS can collect data on the service and place it in the correct APC based on the clinical nature of the service and its median cost.◄

►Services Excluded from OPPS◄

►Certain procedures/services/equipment are reportable to Medicare, but are excluded from OPPS payment because they are paid under other fee schedules. While most hospital outpatient services are payable under the OPPS, section 1833(t)(1)(B)(iv) of the Act excluded payment for ambulance, physical and occupational therapy, and speech-language pathology services, for which payment is made under a fee schedule. The Secretary exercised the broad authority granted under the statute to exclude from the OPPS those services that are already paid under fee schedules or other payment systems. Such excluded services include, for example, the professional services of physicians and nonphysician practitioners paid under the Medicare physician fee schedule; laboratory services paid under the clinical diagnostic laboratory fee schedule; services for beneficiaries with end-stage renal disease (ESRD) that are paid under the ESRD composite rate; and services and procedures that require an inpatient stay that are paid under the hospital inpatient prospective payment system (IPPS) (CMS-1427-P 20). CMS set forth the services that are excluded from payment under the OPPS in §419.22 of the regulations.

►Effective January 1, 2003, CMS allowed payment under OPPS for dialysis treatments for ESRD patients in the outpatient department of a non-ESRD hospital in specific situations and limited to unscheduled dialysis for ESRD patients in exceptional circumstances. (Outpatient dialysis for acute patients are not included in this payment mechanism.) CMS limits payment to medical situations in which the ESRD patient cannot obtain her or his regularly scheduled dialysis treatment at a certified ESRD facility: 1) dialysis performed following or in connection with a vascular access procedure; 2) dialysis performed following treatment for an unrelated medical emergency. (eg, if a patient goes to the emergency room for chest pains and misses a regularly scheduled dialysis treatment that cannot be rescheduled, CMS allows the hospital to provide and bill Medicare for the dialysis treatment; or 3) emergency dialysis for ESRD patients would otherwise have to be admitted as inpatients in order for the hospital to receive payment.) For Medicare reporting purposes, non-ESRD certified hospital outpatient facilities CMS is required to use Level II HCPCS G code G0257—"Unscheduled or emergency treatment for dialysis for ESRD patient in the outpatient department of a hospital that does not have a certified ESRD facility" as opposed to any CPT dialysis code to report this circumstance. CMS indicates that code G0257 has a status indicator "S" and is assigned to APC 0170. CMS instructs hospitals not to use G0257 to bill for the provision of dialysis treatment to patients with acute renal failure.◄

►Inpatient Procedures/Services◄

►In the April 7, 2000, final rule, CMS identified procedures that are typically provided only in an inpatient setting and, therefore, would not be paid by Medicare under the OPPS (65 FR 18455). These procedures comprise what is referred to as the "inpatient list," representing services that require inpatient care because of the nature of the procedure, the need for at least 24 hours of postoperative recovery time or monitoring before the patient can be safely discharged, or the underlying physican condition of the patient. CMS updates the inpatient list as often as quarterly through program memoranda to reflect current advances in medical practice. (**Note:** To assist in the use of this publication, see the "Special Symbols" table on page [folio] to identify those CPT codes having an inpatient procedure status indicator "C" using the symbol (✿)).◄

►In preparing the 2003 OPPS, CMS compared procedures with status indicator "C" (status indicator "C" is assigned to inpatient procedures that are not payable under the OPPS to the list of procedures that are currently on the Ambulatory Surgical Center (ASC) list of approved procedures and other published and recommended procedures. A review of 2001 physician claims data revealed that physicians were performing some of the "C" status indicator procedures on Medicare beneficiaries on an outpatient basis. CMS concluded that it was appropriate to remove certain procedures currently on the OPPS inpatient list that are being performed on an outpatient basis and/or that CMS determined could be safely and appropriately performed on a Medicare beneficiary in an ASC under the applicable ASC rules set forth in 42 CFR 416.22. CMS determined that payment policies for surgical procedures provided in an outpatient hospital setting and in the ASC setting should be consistent to the extent possible within the limitations imposed by statutory or regulatory requirements.◄

►CMS reiterated in the November 7, 2003, final rule "the inpatient list is rooted in section 1833(t)(1)(B)(i) of the Act, which gives the Secretary broad authority to determine the services to be covered and paid for under the OPPS. The authority in this section of the Act does not extend to services that are covered and paid for under the Medicare physician fee schedule, which is a separate benefit and payment system. Section 1833(t)(1)(B)(i) of the Act gives the Secretary broad authority to determine the services to be covered and paid for under the OPPS." In the April 7, 2000, final rule, CMS identified procedures that are typically provided only in an inpatient setting and, therefore, would not be paid by Medicare under the OPPS (65 FR 18455). These procedures comprise what is referred to as the "inpatient list." The inpatient list specifies those services that are only paid when provided in an inpatient setting. These are services that require inpatient care because of the nature of the procedure, the need for at least 24 hours of postoperative recovery time or monitoring before the patient can be safely discharged, or the underlying physical condition of the patient. As discussed in the April 7, 2000, and the November 30, 2001, final rule, CMS uses the following criteria when reviewing procedures to determine whether or not they should be moved from the inpatient list and assigned to an APC group for payment under the OPPS:◄

- Most outpatient departments are equipped to provide the services to the Medicare population.
- The simplest procedure described by the code may be performed in most outpatient departments.
- The procedure is related to codes moved off the inpatient list.

►For the 2003 OPPS update, CMS added the following criteria for use in reviewing procedures to determine whether they should be removed from the inpatient list and assigned to an APC group for payment under the OPPS:◄

- The procedure is being performed in numerous hospitals on an outpatient basis; or
- The procedure can be appropriately and safely performed in an ASC and is on the list of approved ASC procedures or proposed by us for addition to the ASC list.

►CMS recognizes that as hospitals and physicians continue to gain experience and become more knowledgeable about how Medicare pays for services under the OPPS, problems associated with the existence of the inpatient list will continue to diminish. Therefore, CMS invites recommendations from hospitals and/or physicians regarding procedures currently on the inpatient list that are being safely and appropriately performed on an outpatient basis. Requests for review of a code or group of codes on the inpatient list should be sent to the Director, Division of Outpatient Care, Centers for Medicare & Medicaid Services, Mailstop C4-05-17, 7500 Security Boulevard, Baltimore, MD 21244-1850. Such requests should include supporting information and data to demonstrate that the code meets the five criteria for payment under the OPPS that are listed above, and that are also discussed in the November 1, 2002, final rule (67 FR 66739). In addition, CMS asks that evidence be submitted, including operative reports of actual cases and peer-reviewed medical literature, to demonstrate that the procedure is being performed on an outpatient basis in a safe and appropriate manner in a variety of different types of hospitals.◄

►For 2005, CMS did not accept the APC Panel's recommendation to completely eliminate the inpatient list. CMS has removed 22 procedures from the 2004 list. Those codes being removed from the inpatient list and their APC assignments effective January 1, 2005, can be found in Table 39 of the final rule preamble. A complete listing of those CPT codes assigned with the status indicator "C" can be found Addendum E of the November 15, 2004, *Federal Register*.◄

►CMS continues to instruct the use of HCPCS Level II modifier –CA "Procedure payable only in the inpatient setting when performed emergently on an outpatient who dies prior to admission". This modifier is intended to identify the circumstances when a surgical procedure on the inpatient list is performed on an emergency basis or when a patient whose status is "outpatient" dies. The –CA modifier is not to be used to bill for a procedure with the status indicator "C" that is performed on an elective basis or scheduled to be performed on a patient whose status is that of an outpatient (**Note:** For further CMS instructions, see January 3, 2003, Program Memorandum (Transmittal A-02-129) or access the CMS website at **www.cms.hhs.gov/manuals**)◄

Modifiers Approved for Hospital Outpatient Use

A modifier provides the means by which the reporting physicians and hospitals can indicate that a service or procedure that has been performed has been altered by some specific circumstances but has not changed the definition of the code. The judicious application of modifiers obviates the necessity for separate procedure listings that may describe the modifying circumstance. Modifiers may be used to indicate to the recipient of a report that:

- A service or procedure has both a professional and technical component.
- A service or procedure was performed by more than one physician and/or in more than one location.
- A service or procedure has been increased or reduced.
- Only part of a service was performed.
- An adjunctive service was performed.
- A bilateral procedure was performed.
- A service or procedure was provided more than once.
- Unusual events occurred.
- The National Uniform Billing committee approved certain

Level I CPT and Level II HCPCS modifiers applicable to outpatient hospital reporting. CMS required Medicare fiscal intermediaries to accept certain CPT modifiers beginning April 1, 1998, with providers required to use them for Medicare reporting purposes by July 1, 1998. However, these implementation dates were delayed until August 1, 2000.

CPT Level I Modifiers

(See Appendix A for Definition)

25 Significant, Separately Identifiable Evaluation and Management Service by the Same Physician on the Same Day of the Procedure or Other Service

27 Multiple Outpatient Hospital Encounters on the Same Date

50 Bilateral Procedure

52 Reduced Services

58 Staged or Related Procedure or Service by the Same Physician During the Postoperative Period

59 Distinct Procedural Service
73 Discontinued Out-Patient Procedure Prior to Anesthesia Administration
74 Discontinued Out-Patient Procedure After Anesthesia Administration
76 Repeat Procedure by Same Physician
77 Repeat Procedure by Another Physician
78 Return to the Operating Room for a Related Procedure During the Postoperative Period
79 Unrelated Procedure or Service by the Same Physician During the Postoperative Period
91 Repeat Laboratory Procedure

Level II (HCPCS/National) Modifiers

Effective January 1, 2003, CMS has added a new Level II modifier -CA Procedure payable only in the inpatient setting when performed emergently on an outpatient who expires prior to admission, to the list of reportable modifiers under the OPPS.

LT Left side (used to identify procedures performed on the left side of the body)
RT Right side (used to identify procedures performed on the right side of the body)
CA Procedure payable only in the inpatient setting when performed emergently on an outpatient who expires prior to admission
E1 Upper left, eyelid
E2 Lower left, eyelid
E3 Upper right, eyelid
E4 Lower right, eyelid
FA Left hand, thumb
F1 Left hand, second digit
F2 Left hand, third digit
F3 Left hand, fourth digit
F4 Left hand, fifth digit
F5 Right hand, thumb
F6 Right hand, second digit
F7 Right hand, third digit
F8 Right hand, fourth digit
F9 Right hand, fifth digit
GA Waiver of liability statement on file
GG Performance and payment of a screening mammogram and diagnostic mammogram on the same patient, same day
GH Diagnostic mammogram converted from screening mammogram on same day
LC Left circumflex coronary artery (Hospitals use with codes 92980-92984, 92995, 92996)
LD Left anterior descending coronary artery (Hospitals use with codes 92980-92984, 92995, 92996)
RC Right coronary artery (Hospitals use with codes 92980-92984, 92995, 92996)
QM Ambulance service provided under arrangement by a provider of services
QN Ambulance service furnished directly by a provider of services
TA Left foot, great toe
T1 Left foot, second digit
T2 Left foot, third digit
T3 Left foot, fourth digit
T4 Left foot, fifth digit
T5 Right foot, great toe
T6 Right foot, second digit
T7 Right foot, third digit
T8 Right foot, fourth digit
T9 Right foot, fifth digit

Instruction relevant to certain outpatient hospital modifier usage is outlined below. A complete listing of modifiers is found in **Appendix A.** *CPT Assistant and CPT Changes: An Insider's View* references are cited following the CPT modifiers.

OPPS Computation of Discounting Fraction for Modifier Usage

According to the August 21, 2002, Program Memorandum for the October Outpatient Code Editor (CE) Specifications (TR A-02-082) CMS outlines the eight different discount formulas that can be applied to a line. Line items with a service indicator of "T" are subject to multiple procedure discounting unless modifiers 76, 77, 78, and/or 79 are present. The "T" line item with the highest payment amount will not be multiple procedure discounted, and all other "T" line items will be multiple procedure discounted. All line items that do not have a service indicator of "T" will be ignored in determining the discount. A modifier of 73 indicates that a procedure was terminated prior to anesthesia. A terminated procedure will also be discounted although not necessarily at the same level as the discount for multiple type "T" procedures. Terminated bilateral procedures or terminated procedures with units greater than one for type "T" procedures should not occur and have the discounting factor set so as to result in the equivalent of a single procedure.

Bilateral procedures are identified from the "bilateral" field in the physician fee schedule. For non-type "T" procedures there is no terminated procedure or multiple bilateral discounting performed. (For further information, see Modifier 50 instruction below.)

Multiple Outpatient Hospital E/M Encounters on the Same Date (Modifier 27)

CMS indicated that October 1, 2001, was the implementation date for use of the CPT Multiple Outpatient Hospital E/M Encounters on the Same Date Modifier 27. The modifier 27 is intended to facilitate hospital outpatient reporting to delineate a circumstance wherein a patient receives multiple evaluation and management services performed by the same or differing physician(s) in multiple outpatient hospital settings. Modifier 27 should be used to report separate and distinct E/M encounters performed on the same patient and provided by the same or different physician(s) in more than one (different, multiple) outpatient hospital setting(s) (eg, hospital emergency department, clinic) on the same date.

For Medicare reporting purposes, the following are general guidelines for reporting modifiers 25 and 27 under the hospital OPPS, effective October 1, 2001:

—Modifier 25 should be appended only to E/M codes 92002-92014, 99201-99499, and with HCPCS code G0175;

—To append the modifier 25 appropriately to an E/M code, the service provided must meet the definition of "significant, separately identifiable E/M service," as defined by *Current Procedural Terminology*®;

—Although CMS stated in Transmittal A-00-40 that Medicare requires that modifier 25 "always be appended to the Emergency Department E/M codes when provided . . .", the Outpatient Code Editor (OCE) only requires the use of modifier 25 on an E/M code when it is reported with a procedure code that has a status indicator of "S" or "T". Nevertheless, such an edit does not preclude the reporting of modifier 25 on E/M codes that are reported with procedure codes asigned to other than "S" or "T" status indicators, if the procedure meets the definition of "significant, separately reportable E/M service."

The August 21, 2002, Program Memorandum for the October Outpatient Code Editor (CE) Specifications (TR A-02-082) updates the "Rules for Medical and Procedure Visits on the Same Day and for Multiple Medical Visits on the Same Day." According to CMS, "Under some circumstances, medical visits on the same date as a procedure will result in additional payments. A modifier of 25 with an Evaluation and Management (E/M) (service indicator V) code is used to indicate that a medical visit was unrelated to any procedure that was performed with a type of T or S [status indicator]. E/M codes on the same day and same claim as a procedure of type T or S will have the medical APC assigned to all lines with E/M codes. However, if any E/M code that occurs on a claim with a type T or S procedure does not have a modifier of 25, then edit 21 will apply and there will be a line item rejection. If there are multiple E/M codes on the same day on the same claim, the rules associated with multiple visits are shown in the following table."

"Condition code G0 specifies that multiple medical visits occurred on the same day with the same revenue center, and these visits were distinct and constituted independent visits (eg, two visits to the ER, one for a broken arm and one for chest pain)."

—Modifier 27 should be appended only to E/M service codes 92002-92014, 99201-99499, and with Level II HCPCS code G0175;

—Hospitals may append modifier 27 to the **second and subsequent** E/M code when more than one E/M service is provided to indicate that the E/M service is a "separate and distinct E/M encounter" from the service previously provided that same day in the same or different hospital outpatient setting;

—When reporting modifier 27, report the condition code G0 when multiple medical visits occur on the same day in the same revenue centers; use of the modifiers 25 and 27 must be substantiated in the patient's medical record.

E & M	Revenue Center	Condition Code	Action	Edit
2 or more	Revenue center is different for each E&M code, and all E&M codes have units equal to 1	Not G0	Assign medical APC to each line item with E&M code	–
2 or more	Two or more E&M codes have the same revenue center OR One or more E&M codes with units greater than 1 had same revenue center	Not G0	Assign medical APC to each line item with E&M code and RTP	Edit 42
2 or more	Two or more E&M codes have the same revenue center OR One or more E&M codes with units greater than 1 had same revenue center	G0	Assign medical APC to each line item with E&M code	–

Bilateral Surgery (Modifier 50)

Based on the 2003 National Physician Fee Schedule Relative Value File the bilateral surgery modifier 50 has several reporting usages due to differing payment policy. Although the modifier 50 language refers to an *operative session*, these words are used in a broad context since diagnostic as well as therapeutic procedures may require the use of the bilateral modifier.

According to an August 21, 2002, CMS Program Memorandum for the October Outpatient Code Editor (OCE) (Transmittal A-02-082), Bilateral procedures have the following values in the "bilateral" field:

1. Conditional bilateral (ie, procedure is considered bilateral if the modifier 50 is present);
2. Inherent bilateral (ie, procedure in and of itself is bilateral);
3. Independent bilateral (ie, procedure is considered a bilateral if the modifier 50 is present, but full payment should be made for each procedure (eg, certain radiological procedures)).

For the discounting process, CMS will utilize an APC payment amount file. The discounting factor for bilateral procedures is the same as the discounting factor for multiple type "T" procedures. Inherent bilateral procedures will be treated as a non-bilateral procedure since the bilaterality of the procedure is encompassed in the code. For bilateral procedures the type "T" procedure discounting rules will take precedence over the discounting specified in the physician fee schedule. All line items for which the line item denial or reject indicator is 1 and the line item action flag is zero, or the line item action flag is 2, 3, or 4 will be ignored in determining the discount.

For the purpose of this publication, certain CPT codes are identified using symbols to indicate one of three CMS payment policies:

The (♦) symbol is used to identify those CPT codes having a "conditional bilateral" designation, indicating it is appropriate to append the modifier 50 such as to certain surgical procedures (eg, 15822—Revision of upper eyelid; 25505—Treat fracture of radius).

The (✶) symbol is used to identify those CPT codes having an "inherent bilateral" designation, indicating it is **not** appropriate to append the modifier 50. For these codes, the procedure/service is being performed as a bilateral procedure since the technique may inherently involve physiology or anatomy on both the left and right side of the body. You will also note that the CPT/HCPCS descriptors for these procedures/services may either: a) specifically state the procedure/service may be performed either unilaterally or bilaterally (eg, 58900—Biopsy of ovary(s)); b) specify the procedure is "bilateral" (eg, 78458—Vein thrombosis images, bilateral); or, reflect multiple anatomy (eg, 73520—X-ray exam of hips).

The symbol (✢) is used to identify CPT codes having an "independent bilateral" designation (eg, certain radiological procedures). For these codes, it is appropriate to append the modifier 50 to each procedure performed, as the anatomic structures exist bilaterally and the identical procedure is performed independent of the other, on both sides of the body (eg, 73100—X-ray exam of wrist; 92135—Ophthalmic diagnostic imaging).

The symbol (⌘) is used to identify CPT codes that describe "unilateral" procedures for which a correlating "bilateral"procedure code exists. For these codes, it is **not** appropriate to append the modifier 50 to each procedure performed, as the bilateral procedure is accurately described by a specific CPT code (eg, 70328—Radiologic examination, temporomandibular joint, open and closed mouth; unilateral and 70330 – bilateral).

Multiple Procedures (Modifier 51)

For OPPS reporting, the CPT Multiple Procedure Modifier 51 is not used. Instead, OPPS uses the status indicator "T" to indicate surgical services for which payment is allowed. Services with this payment indicator are the only services to which the OPPS multiple procedure payment reduction applies. (**Note:** Since the CPT codes currently serve a wide variety of important functions in the field of medical nomenclature, users will note that the "modifier 51 exempt" symbol (⊘) and references to the use of the Multiple Procedure Modifier 51 found in *Current Procedural Termininology (CPT®)* are not applicable for OPPS reporting.)

►CMS indicates it is necessary to understand how the Outpatient Code Editor (OCE) multiple procedure discounting logic functions. Line-items with a service indicator of "T" are subject to multiple procedure discounting unless CPT modifiers 76, 77, 78, and/or 79 are present on the claim. The "T" line-item with the highest payment amount will not be discounted but all other "T" line items will be discounted as multiple procedures. All line-items that do not have a service indicator of "T" will be ignored in determining the discount. Therefore, if the only other services reported with infusion therapy are an emergency department or other visit code, or diagnostic tests and services assigned status indicator "S," the infusion therapy code would not be subject to the multiple procedure discounting.◄

Reduced Services (Modifier 52)

Due to the varying nature of procedures described by the CPT codes, the modifier 52 has several reporting usages. The modifier 52 may be used to represent:

- a service or procedure that is partially reduced or eliminated at the provider's discretion;
- when a service is not performed for the entire time specified in the code descriptor;
- that an inherently bilateral procedure cannot be performed as such.

Staged or Related Procedure or Service by the Same Physician During the Postoperative Period (Modifier 58)

A common question asked about Modifier 58 is why and how is the modifier 58 used for hospital outpatient reporting. It is recognized that the reference to the "post-operative period" in the language of modifier 58 does not have strict relevance in hospital outpatient reporting. However, the individual circumstance depicted by modifier 58 continues to have reimbursement or tracking relevance to the fiscal intermediary (FI). The intent and use of modifier 58 precludes its use to report the treatment of a problem that requires a return to the operating room. For that circumstance, use the modifier 78. Modifier 58 is not used to report a related or unrelated procedure performed on the same date as the original procedure. To report that circumstance, use modifier 59. (**Note:** Please check with your fiscal intermediary regarding local policy associated with the use of the modifier 58 for staged procedures on the same date.)

Distinct Procedural Service (Modifier 59)/ Repeat Clinical Diagnostic Laboratory Test (Modifier 91)

These two modifiers are discussed together to allay confusion in differentiating usage. By identifying procedures/services that are not normally reported together, but are appropriate under the circumstances, the distinct procedural service modifier 59 is used to clearly designate instances when distinct and separate multiple services are provided to a patient on a single date of service. Although the modifier 59 has several reporting usages, it is only to be used if no more descriptive modifier is available, and its use best explains the circumstances. As the description of this modifier indicates, some examples of common uses of the 59 modifier include separate sessions or patient encounters, different procedures or surgeries, surgery directed to different sites or organ systems, surgery directed to separate incision/excision or separate lesions, or treatment to separate injuries.

The modifier 59 is also intended to assist in reporting those procedures/services that may be considered a component of another procedure, but have been carried out independently or considered unrelated or distinct from other procedures/services provided at that time. In this instance, the procedure/service may be reported by itself, or in addition to other procedures/services, by appending the modifier 59 to the specific procedure code reported.

Both modifier 59 and modifier 91 are used to report repeat clinical diagnostic laboratory tests performed on the same patient on the same day. As indicated in the descriptor language for use of modifier 91, it is used to identify repeat performance of the same laboratory test on the same day to obtain subsequent (multiple) test results. For example, if a second culture was performed of the same wound site on the same day, then modifier 91 would be appended. Modifier 91 is not intended to be used when tests are rerun to confirm initial results due to testing problems with the specimen(s) or equipment, or for any other reason when a normal, one-time reportable result is all that is required. In addition, modifier 91 is not intended for use when there are CPT codes available to describe the series of results (eg, glucose tolerance tests, evocative/suppression testing, etc).

According to CMS, the modifier 59 is appropriate for reporting multiple claims submissions by a clinical laboratory for the same CPT code for the same patient on the same day. For example to report procedures that are distinct or independent, such as performing the same procedure (which uses the same procedure code) for testing of a different specimen (eg, aerobic culture of two independent wound site specimens). To clarify, according to the NCCI guidelines, it would not be appropriate to append the modifier 59 "If after a test is ordered and performed, additional related procedures are necessary to provide or confirm the result, these would be considered part of the ordered test. As another example, if a patient has an abnormal test result and repeat performance of the test is done to verify the result, the test is reported as one unit of service rather than two." NCCI also directs, "Multiple tests to identify the same analyte marker, or infectious agent should not be reported separately. For example, it would not be appropriate to report both direct probe and amplified probe technique tests for the same infectious agent."

Modifier 91 is appropriate when in the course of treatment of the patient it is necessary to repeat the same laboratory test on the same day to obtain subsequent test results. For example, repeated blood testing for the same patient, using the same CPT code, performed at different intervals during the same day (eg, initial and three subsequent blood potassium levels). The CPT microbiology guidelines in the Pathology and Laboratory section state: "Presumptive identification of microorganisms is defined as identification by colony morphology, growth on selective media, Gram stains, or up to three tests (eg, catalase, oxidase, indole, urease). Definitive identification of microorganisms is defined as an identification to the genus or species level that requires additional tests (eg, biochemical panels, slide cultures). If additional studies involve molecular probes, chromatography, or immunologic techniques, these should be separately codedin addition to definitive identification codes (87140-87158). For multiple specimens/sites use modifier 59. For repeat laboratory tests performed on the same day, use modifier 91."

Discontinued Outpatient Hospital/ Ambulatory Surgery Center (ASC) Procedure Prior to the Administration of Anesthesia (Modifier 73)

Effective January 1, 1999, CPT modifier 73 was established to clarify and differentiate specific CMS policy. Modifier 73 was specifically established to assist hospital outpatient reporting associated with the use of resources in the event a surgical or diagnostic procedure is cancelled due to extenuating circumstances, or those that threaten the well-being of the patient. In this instance, the cancellation occurs:

- after the patient's surgical preparation (including sedation when provided);
- after the patient was brought to the room where the procedure was to be performed; and
- before the administration of anesthesia (local, regional block(s) or general).

Discontinued Out-Patient Hospital/ Ambulatory Surgery (ASC) Procedure After Administration of Anesthesia (Modifier 74)

Also effective January 1, 1999, CPT modifier 74 was established specifically to assist hospital outpatient reporting associated with the use of resources in the event a surgical or diagnostic procedure is terminated due to extenuating circumstances or those that threaten the well-being of the patient after the procedure is started (incision made, intubation started, scope inserted, etc). (**Note:** Modifiers 73 and 74 are not used to indicate discontinued radiology procedures.)

Modifiers for "Repeat" Procedures (Modifier 76 and Modifier 77)

The "repeat" procedures modifiers, 76 and 77, are also discussed together looking first at some specific CMS policy issues. The original intent and use of modifiers 76 and 77 is not altered for hospital outpatient reporting:

- Modifier 76 is used to indicate that a procedure or service was repeated in a separate operative session on the same day by the same physician.
- Modifier 77 is used to indicate that a procedure or service was repeated in a separate operative session on the same day by another physician.

Similar to modifier 58, the reference to the "postoperative period" in the language of the "repeat" procedure modifiers does not have strict relevance in hospital outpatient reporting. But the individual circumstances depicted by modifiers 76, 77, 78, and 79 continue to have reimbursement or tracking relevance to the fiscal intermediary (FI), which enables the FI or other payers/carriers to appropriately pay for the procedure per se and other associated postoperative services performed within or subsequent to its assigned global period (eg, 0 days, 10 days, 90 days).

In addition, the modifier usage allows to electronically differentiate the instance where duplicate billing or duplicate services may have been reported.

As outlined in the October 5, 2000, Program Memorandum, CMS implemented the two repeat procedure modifiers for hospital use. CMS directs that should there be a question regarding whom the ordering physician was and whether or not the same physician ordered the second procedure, code choice is based on whether or not the physician performing the procedure is the same. The procedure must be the same procedure. It is listed once and then listed again with the appropriate modifier.

Return to the Operating Room for a Related Procedure During the Postoperative Period (Modifier 78)

Modifier 78 is appended to procedures that are performed during the postoperative period that require a patient to return to the operating room and are directly associated with the performance of the initial operation. To illustrate, if a patient's operative site bleeds after an initial surgery and requires a return to the operating room to stop the bleeding, the same procedure is not repeated. As with the modifiers 76 and 77, for OPPS purposes, the postoperative period is the same day.

Unrelated Procedure or Service by the Same Physician During the Postoperative Period (Modifier 79)

The use of this modifier is described in its title. However, the issues surrounding its use, occur when providers and carriers disagree as to whether the procedure is actually "unrelated" to the original procedure. To illustrate usage, portions of the preceding two examples are used. As with the modifiers 76 and 77, for OPPS purposes, the ostoperative period is the same day.

Instructions for Use of the CPT Code Set

Select the name of the procedure or service that most accurately identifies the service performed. In surgery, it may be an operation; in medicine, a diagnostic or therapeutic procedure; in radiology, a radiograph. Other additional procedures performed or pertinent special services are also listed. When necessary, any modifying or extenuating circumstances are added. Any service or procedure should be adequately documented in the medical record. It is important to recognize that the listing of a service or procedure and its code number in a specific section of this book does not restrict its use to a specific specialty group. Any procedure or service in any section of this book may be used to designate the services rendered by any qualified physician or other qualified health care professional.

Format of the Terminology

The CPT nomenclature has been developed as standalone descriptions of medical procedures. However, some of the procedures in the CPT code set are not printed in their entirety, but refer back to a common portion of the procedure listed in a preceding entry. This is evident when an entry is followed by one or more indentations. This is done in an effort to conserve space.

Example

25100 Arthrotomy, wrist joint; for biopsy

25105 for synovectomy

Note that the common part of code 25100 (that part before the semicolon) should be considered part of code 25105. Therefore the full procedure represented by code 25105 should read:

25105 Arthrotomy, wrist joint; for synovectomy

Requests to Update the CPT Code Set

The effectiveness of the CPT nomenclature is dependent upon constant updating to reflect changes in medical practice. This can only be accomplished through the interest and timely suggestions of practicing physicians, medical specialty societies, state medical associations, and other organizations and agencies. Accordingly, the American Medical Association welcomes correspondence, inquiries, and suggestions concerning old and new procedures, as well as other matters such as codes and indices.

For suggestions concerning the introduction of new procedures, or the coding, deleting, or revising of procedures contained in *CPT 2005*, correspondence requesting an application for coding change should be directed to:

CPT Editorial Research & Development
American Medical Association
515 North State Street
Chicago, Illinois 60610

All proposed additions to, or modifications of, *CPT 2005* will be by decision of the CPT Editorial Panel after consultation with appropriate medical specialty societies.

Guidelines

Specific "Guidelines" are presented at the beginning of each of the six sections. These Guidelines define items that are necessary to appropriately interpret and report the procedures and services contained in that section. For example, in the **Medicine** section, specific instructions are provided for handling unlisted services or procedures, special reports, and supplies and materials provided. Guidelines also provide explanations regarding terms that apply only to a particular section. For instance, **Surgery Guidelines** provide an explanation of the use of the star, while in **Radiology**, the unique term, "radiological supervision and interpretation" is defined.

Add-on Codes

Some of the listed procedures are commonly carried out in addition to the primary procedure performed. These additional or supplemental procedures are designated as "add-on" codes with a "✚" symbol, and are listed in **Appendix D** of the *CPT* book. Add-on codes in *CPT 2005* can be readily identified by specific descriptor nomenclature which includes phrases such as "each additional" or "(List separately in addition to primary procedure)". For OPPS reporting purposes, all add-on codes found in the *CPT* book are exempt from the use of the CPT Multiple Procedure Modifier 51. Therefore, certain add-on codes have a "T" status indicator (ie, they are subject to the OPPS multiple procedure reduction rules), while other add-on codes have an "S" status indicator (ie, they are not subject to the OPPS multiple procedure reduction rules).

The CPT "add-on" code concept in *CPT 2005* applies only to add-on procedures/services performed: a) by the same physician or qualified health care professional (for reporting physician services); or b) at the same setting (for OPPS reporting). Add-on codes describe additional intra-service work associated with the primary procedure (eg, additional digit(s), lesion(s), neurorrhaphy(s), vertebral segment(s), tendon(s), joint(s)). Add-on codes are always performed in addition to the primary service/procedure, and must never be reported as a stand-alone code, since CMS uses only single procedure claims to determine APC payments.

For OPPS reporting, CMS also uses the phrase "add-on codes" when discussing those procedures that should never be reported without the code for the associated procedure. In this instance, the code(s) may not necessarily be designated as CPT add-on procedures (ie, having standard CPT add-on code language and the "✚" symbol). A CMS "add-on" procedure example would be the reporting of a code for a biopsy when the radiological guidance is necessary only when that specific biopsy procedure is performed. To further illustrate, when performing tissue ablation, the appropriate code from the 47370-47382 series must be reported in addition to code 76490 for the ultrasound guidance used to perform the tissue ablation.

According to the final rule published November 1, 2002, for calendar year 2003, CMS will continue to pay for add-on codes separately, setting relative weights with the use of single procedure claims. CMS will continue to explore ways to most appropriately pay for these services.

Unlisted Procedure or Service

It is recognized that there may be services or procedures performed by physicians that are not found in the CPT code set. Therefore, a number of specific code numbers have been designated for reporting unlisted procedures. When an unlisted procedure number is used, the service or procedure should be described. Each of these unlisted procedural code numbers (with the appropriate accompanying topical entry) relates to a specific section of the book and is presented in the Guidelines of that section.

Special Report

A service that is rarely provided, unusual, variable, or new may require a special report in determining medical appropriateness of the service. Pertinent information should include an adequate definition or description of the nature, extent, and need for the procedure; and the time, effort, and equipment necessary to provide the service. Additional items which may be included are: Complexity of symptoms, final diagnosis, pertinent physical findings, diagnostic and therapeutic procedures, concurrent problems, and follow-up care.

Code Changes

A summary listing of additions, deletions, and revisions applicable to *CPT 2005* is found in **Appendix B**. New procedure numbers added to the CPT code set are identified throughout the text with the symbol "●" placed before the code number. In instances where a code revision has resulted in a substantially altered procedure descriptor, the symbol "▲" is placed before the code number. The symbols "▶ ◀" are used to indicate new and revised text other than the procedure descriptors. CPT add-on codes are annotated by a "✚" symbol and are listed in **Appendix D**.

Alphabetical Reference Index

A new expanded alphabetical index is found in the back of the book. It includes listings by procedure and anatomic site. Procedures and services commonly known by their eponyms or other designations are also included.

CPT in Electronic Formats

CPT 2005 procedure codes and descriptions are also available in CD-ROM formats. For more information call 800 621-8335. These files can also be purchased for immeditae download at:
www.ama-assn.org/CPT/online

Visit CPT on the AMA Website
www.ama-assn.org/cpt

CPT Assistant Newsletter and *CPT 2005 Changes: An Insider's View* References

When using your *CPT 2005 Outpatient Services* book you will notice the symbol "➲" below many codes throughout the body of the book. This symbol has been included to indicate that the American Medical Association (AMA) has published reference material on that particular code.

The "➲" symbol refers to two AMA publications—the *CPT Assistant* monthly newsletter and *CPT Changes: An Insider's View,* an annual book with all of the coding changes for the current year.

How to Read the References

Example

34808 Endovascular placement of iliac artery occlusion device (List separately in addition to code for primary procedure)
➲ *CPT Assistant* Dec 00:1; *CPT Changes: An Insider's View* 2001

This reference indicates that in the *CPT Assistant* newsletter, December 2000 issue, page 1, and in *CPT Changes: An Insider's View* 2001 edition, there is material that may assist you in understanding the application of the code.

How to Obtain the Referenced Publications

CPT Assistant annual subscriptions can be purchased by calling the AMA's Customer Service Department at 800 623-8335. Individual back issues are available online at **www.ama-assn.org/go/cpt/online**.

Current and past editions of *CPT Changes: An Insider's View* can be purchased by calling the AMA's Customer Service Department at 800 621-8335, or online at **www.amapress.com**.

Evaluation and Management (E/M) Services Guidelines

In addition to the information presented in the **Introduction,** several other items unique to this section are defined or identified here.

Classification of Evaluation and Management (E/M) Services

The E/M section is divided into broad categories such as office visits, hospital visits, and consultations. Most of the categories are further divided into two or more subcategories of E/M services. For example, there are two subcategories of office visits (new patient and established patient) and there are two subcategories of hospital visits (initial and subsequent). The subcategories of E/M services are further classified into levels of E/M services that are identified by specific codes. This classification is important because the nature of physician work varies by type of service, place of service, and the patient's status.

The basic format of the levels of E/M services is the same for most categories. First, a unique code number is listed. Second, the place and/or type of service is specified, eg, office consultation. Third, the content of the service is defined, eg, comprehensive history and comprehensive examination. (See "Levels of E/M Services," page 2, for details on the content of E/M services.) Fourth, the nature of the presenting problem(s) usually associated with a given level is described. Fifth, the time typically required to provide the service is specified. (A detailed discussion of time is provided on page 3.)

Definitions of Commonly Used Terms

Certain key words and phrases are used throughout the E/M section. The following definitions are intended to reduce the potential for differing interpretations and to increase the consistency of reporting by physicians in differing specialties.

New and Established Patient

Solely for the purposes of distinguishing between new and established patients, **professional services** are those face-to-face services rendered by a physician and reported by a specific CPT code(s). A new patient is one who has not received any professional services from the physician or another physician of the same specialty who belongs to the same group practice, within the past three years.

An established patient is one who has received professional services from the physician or another physician of the same specialty who belongs to the same group practice, within the past three years.

In the instance where a physician is on call for or covering for another physician, the patient's encounter will be classified as it would have been by the physician who is not available.

No distinction is made between new and established patients in the emergency department. E/M services in the emergency department category may be reported for any new or established patient who presents for treatment in the emergency department.

Chief Complaint

A concise statement describing the symptom, problem, condition, diagnosis or other factor that is the reason for the encounter, usually stated in the patient's words.

Concurrent Care

Concurrent care is the provision of similar services, eg, hospital visits, to the same patient by more than one physician on the same day. When concurrent care is provided, no special reporting is required. Modifier 75 has been deleted.

Counseling

Counseling is a discussion with a patient and/or family concerning one or more of the following areas:

- diagnostic results, impressions, and/or recommended diagnostic studies;
- prognosis;
- risks and benefits of management (treatment) options;
- instructions for management (treatment) and/or follow-up;

- importance of compliance with chosen management (treatment) options;
- risk factor reduction; and
- patient and family education.

(For psychotherapy, see 90804-90857)

Family History

A review of medical events in the patient's family that includes significant information about:

- the health status or cause of death of parents, siblings, and children;
- specific diseases related to problems identified in the Chief Complaint or History of the Present Illness, and/or System Review;
- diseases of family members which may be hereditary or place the patient at risk.

History of Present Illness

A chronological description of the development of the patient's present illness from the first sign and/or symptom to the present. This includes a description of location, quality, severity, timing, context, modifying factors and associated signs and symptoms significantly related to the presenting problem(s).

Levels of E/M Services

Within each category or subcategory of E/M service, there are three to five levels of E/M services available for reporting purposes. Levels of E/M services are **not** interchangeable among the different categories or subcategories of service. For example, the first level of E/M services in the subcategory of office visit, new patient, does not have the same definition as the first level of E/M services in the subcategory of office visit, established patient.

The levels of E/M services include examinations, evaluations, treatments, conferences with or concerning patients, preventive pediatric and adult health supervision, and similar medical services, such as the determination of the need and/or location for appropriate care. Medical screening includes the history, examination, and medical decision-making required to determine the need and/or location for appropriate care and treatment of the patient (eg, office and other outpatient setting, emergency department, nursing facility, etc.). The levels of E/M services encompass the wide variations in skill, effort, time, responsibility and medical knowledge required for the prevention or diagnosis and treatment of illness or injury and the promotion of optimal health. Each level of E/M services may be used by all physicians.

The descriptors for the levels of E/M services recognize seven components, six of which are used in defining the levels of E/M services. These components are:

- history;
- examination;
- medical decision making;
- counseling;
- coordination of care;
- nature of presenting problem; and
- time.

The first three of these components (history, examination, and medical decision making) are considered the **key** components in selecting a level of E/M services. (See "Determine the Extent of History Obtained," page 5.)

The next three components (counseling, coordination of care, and the nature of the presenting problem) are considered **contributory** factors in the majority of encounters. Although the first two of these contributory factors are important E/M services, it is not required that these services be provided at every patient encounter.

Coordination of care with other providers or agencies without a patient encounter on that day is reported using the case management codes.

The final component, time, is discussed in detail (see page 3).

Any specifically identifiable procedure (ie, identified with a specific CPT code) performed on or subsequent to the date of initial or subsequent "E/M Services" should be reported separately.

The actual performance and/or interpretation of diagnostic tests/studies ordered during a patient encounter are not included in the levels of E/M services. Physician performance of diagnostic tests/studies for which specific CPT codes are available may be reported separately, in addition to the appropriate E/M code. The physician's interpretation of the results of diagnostic tests/studies (ie, professional component) with preparation of a separate distinctly identifiable signed written report may also be reported separately, using the appropriate CPT code with modifier 26 appended.

The physician may need to indicate that on the day a procedure or service identified by a CPT code was performed, the patient's condition required a significant separately identifiable E/M service above and beyond other services provided or beyond the usual preservice and postservice care associated with the procedure that was performed. The E/M service may be caused or prompted by the symptoms or condition for which the procedure and/or service was provided. This circumstance may be reported by adding modifier 25 to the appropriate level of E/M service. As such, different diagnoses are not required for reporting of the procedure and the E/M services on the same date.

Nature of Presenting Problem

A presenting problem is a disease, condition, illness, injury, symptom, sign, finding, complaint, or other reason for encounter, with or without a diagnosis being established at the time of the encounter. The E/M codes recognize five types of presenting problems that are defined as follows:

Minimal: A problem that may not require the presence of the physician, but service is provided under the physician's supervision.

Self-limited or minor: A problem that runs a definite and prescribed course, is transient in nature, and is not likely to permanently alter health status OR has a good prognosis with management/compliance.

Low severity: A problem where the risk of morbidity without treatment is low; there is little to no risk of mortality without treatment; full recovery without functional impairment is expected.

Moderate severity: A problem where the risk of morbidity without treatment is moderate; there is moderate risk of mortality without treatment; uncertain prognosis OR increased probability of prolonged functional impairment.

High severity: A problem where the risk of morbidity without treatment is high to extreme; there is a moderate to high risk of mortality without treatment OR high probability of severe, prolonged functional impairment.

Past History

A review of the patient's past experiences with illnesses, injuries, and treatments that includes significant information about:

- prior major illnesses and injuries;
- prior operations;
- prior hospitalizations;
- current medications;
- allergies (eg, drug, food);
- age appropriate immunization status;
- age appropriate feeding/dietary status.

Social History

An age appropriate review of past and current activities that includes significant information about:

- marital status and/or living arrangements;
- current employment;
- occupational history;
- use of drugs, alcohol, and tobacco;
- level of education;
- sexual history;
- other relevant social factors.

System Review (Review of Systems)

An inventory of body systems obtained through a series of questions seeking to identify signs and/or symptoms which the patient may be experiencing or has experienced. For the purposes of *CPT* the following elements of a system review have been identified:

- Constitutional symptoms (fever, weight loss, etc.)
- Eyes
- Ears, Nose, Mouth, Throat
- Cardiovascular
- Respiratory
- Gastrointestinal
- Genitourinary
- Musculoskeletal
- Integumentary (skin and/or breast)
- Neurological
- Psychiatric
- Endocrine
- Hematologic/Lymphatic
- Allergic/Immunologic

The review of systems helps define the problem, clarify the differential diagnosis, identify needed testing, or serves as baseline data on other systems that might be affected by any possible management options.

Time

The inclusion of time in the definitions of levels of E/M services has been implicit in prior editions of *CPT.* The inclusion of time as an explicit factor beginning in *CPT 1992* is done to assist physicians in selecting the most appropriate level of E/M services. It should be recognized that the specific times expressed in the visit code descriptors are averages, and therefore represent a range of times which may be higher or lower depending on actual clinical circumstances.

Time is **not** a descriptive component for the emergency department levels of E/M services because emergency department services are typically provided on a variable intensity basis, often involving multiple encounters with several patients over an extended period of time. Therefore, it is often difficult for physicians to provide accurate estimates of the time spent face-to-face with the patient.

Studies to establish levels of E/M services employed surveys of practicing physicians to obtain data on the amount of time and work associated with typical E/M services. Since "work" is not easily quantifiable, the codes must rely on other objective, verifiable measures that correlate with physicians' estimates of their "work". It has been demonstrated that physicians' estimations of **intraservice** time (as explained on the next page), both within and across specialties, is a variable that is predictive of the "work" of E/M services. This same research has shown there is a strong relationship between intra-service time and total time for E/M services. Intra-service time, rather than total time, was chosen for inclusion with the codes because of its relative ease of measurement and because of its direct correlation with measurements of the total amount of time and work associated with typical E/M services.

Intra-service times are defined as **face-to-face** time for office and other outpatient visits and as **unit/floor** time for hospital and other inpatient visits. This distinction is necessary because most of the work of typical office visits takes place during the face-to-face time with the patient, while most of the work of typical hospital visits takes place during the time spent on the patient's floor or unit.

Face-to-face time (office and other outpatient visits and office consultations): For coding purposes, face-to-face time for these services is defined as only that time that the physician spends face-to-face with the patient and/or family. This includes the time in which the physician performs such tasks as obtaining a history, performing an examination, and counseling the patient.

Physicians also spend time doing work before or after the face-to-face time with the patient, performing such tasks as reviewing records and tests, arranging for further services, and communicating further with other professionals and the patient through written reports and telephone contact.

This **non-face-to-face** time for office services—also called pre- and post-encounter time—is not included in the time component described in the E/M codes. However, the pre- and post-face-to-face work associated with an encounter was included in calculating the total work of typical services in physician surveys.

Thus, the face-to-face time associated with the services described by any E/M code is a valid proxy for the total work done before, during, and after the visit.

Unit/floor time (hospital observation services, inpatient hospital care, initial and follow-up hospital consultations, nursing facility): For reporting purposes, intra-service time for these services is defined as unit/floor time, which includes the time that the physician is present on the patient's hospital unit and at the bedside rendering services for that patient. This includes the time in which the physician establishes and/or reviews the patient's chart, examines the patient, writes notes and communicates with other professionals and the patient's family.

In the hospital, pre- and post-time includes time spent off the patient's floor performing such tasks as reviewing pathology and radiology findings in another part of the hospital.

This pre- and post-visit time is not included in the time component described in these codes. However, the pre- and post-work performed during the time spent off the floor or unit was included in calculating the total work of typical services in physician surveys.

Thus, the unit/floor time associated with the services described by any code is a valid proxy for the total work done before, during, and after the visit.

Unlisted Service

An E/M service may be provided that is not listed in this section of *CPT*. When reporting such a service, the appropriate "Unlisted" code may be used to indicate the service, identifying it by "Special Report", as discussed in the following paragraph. The "Unlisted Services" and accompanying codes for the E/M section are as follows:

99429 **Unlisted preventive** medicine service

99499 **Unlisted evaluation and management** service

Special Report

An unlisted service or one that is unusual, variable, or new may require a special report demonstrating the medical appropriateness of the service. Pertinent information should include an adequate definition or description of the nature, extent, and need for the procedure; and the time, effort, and equipment necessary to provide the service. Additional items which may be included are complexity of symptoms, final diagnosis, pertinent physical findings, diagnostic and therapeutic procedures, concurrent problems, and follow-up care.

Clinical Examples

Clinical examples of the codes for E/M services are provided to assist physicians in understanding the meaning of the descriptors and selecting the correct code. The clinical examples are listed in Appendix C. Each example was developed by physicians in the specialties shown.

The same problem, when seen by physicians in different specialties, may involve different amounts of work. Therefore, the appropriate level of encounter should be reported using the descriptors rather than the examples.

The examples have been tested for validity and approved by the CPT Editorial Panel. Physicians were given the examples and asked to assign a code or assess the amount of time and work involved. Only examples that were rated consistently have been included in Appendix C.

Table 1
Categories and Subcategories of Service

Category/Subcategory	Code Numbers
Office or Other Outpatient Services	
New Patient	99201-99205
Established Patient	99211-99215
Hospital Observation Discharge Services	99217
Hospital Observation Services	99218-99220
Hospital Observation or Inpatient Care Services (Including Admission and Discharge Services)	99234-99236
Hospital Inpatient Services	
Initial Hospital Care	99221-99223
Subsequent Hospital Care	99231-99233
Hospital Discharge Services	99238-99239
Consultations	
Office Consultations	99241-99245
Initial Inpatient Consultations	99251-99255
Follow-up Inpatient Consultations	99261-99263
Confirmatory Consultations	99271-99275
Emergency Department Services	99281-99288
Pediatric Patient Transport	99289-99290
Critical Care Services	
Adult (over 24 months of age)	99291-99292
Pediatric	99293-99294
Neonatal	99295-99296
Intensive Care (Low Birth Weight)	99298-99299
Nursing Facility Services	
Comprehensive Nursing Facility Assessments	99301-99303
Subsequent Nursing Facility Care	99311-99313
Nursing Facility Discharge Services	99315-99316
Domiciliary, Rest Home or Custodial Care Services	
New Patient	99321-99323
Established Patient	99331-99333
Home Services	
New Patient	99341-99345
Established Patient	99347-99350
Prolonged Services	
With Direct Patient Contact	99354-99357
Without Direct Patient Contact	99358-99359
Standby Services	99360
Case Management Services	
Team Conferences	99361-99362
Telephone Calls	99371-99373
Care Plan Oversight Services	99374-99380
Preventive Medicine Services	
New Patient	99381-99387
Established Patient	99391-99397
Individual Counseling	99401-99404
Group Counseling	99411-99412
Other	99420-99429
Newborn Care	99431-99440
Special E/M Services	99450-99456
Other E/M Services	99499

Instructions for Selecting a Level of E/M Service

Identify the Category and Subcategory of Service

The categories and subcategories of codes available for reporting E/M services are shown in Table 1 above.

Review the Reporting Instructions for the Selected Category or Subcategory

Most of the categories and many of the subcategories of service have special guidelines or instructions unique to that category or subcategory. Where these are indicated, eg, "Inpatient Hospital Care," special instructions will be presented preceding the levels of E/M services.

Review the Level of E/M Service Descriptors and Examples in the Selected Category or Subcategory

The descriptors for the levels of E/M services recognize seven components, six of which are used in defining the levels of E/M services. These components are:

- history;
- examination;
- medical decision making;
- counseling;
- coordination of care;
- nature of presenting problem; and
- time.

The first three of these components (ie, history, examination, and medical decision making) should be considered the **key** components in selecting the level of E/M services. An exception to this rule is in the case of visits which consist predominantly of counseling or coordination of care (See numbered paragraph 3, page 7.)

The nature of the presenting problem and time are provided in some levels to assist the physician in determining the appropriate level of E/M service.

Determine the Extent of History Obtained

The extent of the history is dependent upon clinical judgment and on the nature of the presenting problems(s). The levels of E/M services recognize four types of history that are defined as follows:

Problem focused: chief complaint; brief history of present illness or problem.

Expanded problem focused: chief complaint; brief history of present illness; problem pertinent system review.

Detailed: chief complaint; extended history of present illness; problem pertinent system review extended to include a review of a limited number of additional systems; **pertinent** past, family, and/or social history **directly related to the patient's problems.**

Comprehensive: chief complaint; extended history of present illness; review of systems which is directly related to the problem(s) identified in the history of the present illness plus a review of all additional body systems; **complete** past, family, and social history.

The comprehensive history obtained as part of the preventive medicine evaluation and management service is not problem-oriented and does not involve a chief complaint or present illness. It does, however, include a comprehensive system review and comprehensive or interval past, family, and social history as well as a comprehensive assessment/history of pertinent risk factors.

Determine the Extent of Examination Performed

The extent of the examination performed is dependent on clinical judgment and on the nature of the presenting problem(s). The levels of E/M services recognize four types of examination that are defined as follows:

Problem focused: a limited examination of the affected body area or organ system.

Expanded problem focused: a limited examination of the affected body area or organ system and other symptomatic or related organ system(s).

Detailed: an extended examination of the affected body area(s) and other symptomatic or related organ system(s).

Comprehensive: a general multi-system examination or a complete examination of a single organ system. **Note:** The comprehensive examination performed as part of the preventive medicine evaluation and management service is multisystem, but its extent is based on age and risk factors identified.

For the purposes of these CPT definitions, the following body areas are recognized:

- Head, including the face
- Neck
- Chest, including breasts and axilla
- Abdomen
- Genitalia, groin, buttocks
- Back
- Each extremity

For the purposes of these CPT definitions, the following organ systems are recognized:

- Eyes
- Ears, Nose, Mouth, and Throat
- Cardiovascular
- Respiratory
- Gastrointestinal
- Genitourinary
- Musculoskeletal
- Skin
- Neurologic
- Psychiatric
- Hematologic/Lymphatic/Immunologic

Determine the Complexity of Medical Decision Making

Medical decision making refers to the complexity of establishing a diagnosis and/or selecting a management option as measured by:

- the number of possible diagnoses and/or the number of management options that must be considered;
- the amount and/or complexity of medical records, diagnostic tests, and/or other information that must be obtained, reviewed, and analyzed; and
- the risk of significant complications, morbidity, and/or mortality, as well as comorbidities, associated with the patient's presenting problems(s), the diagnostic procedure(s) and/or the possible management options.

Four types of medical decision making are recognized: straightforward; low complexity; moderate complexity; and high complexity. To qualify for a given type of decision making, two of the three elements in Table 2 on the following page must be met or exceeded.

Comorbidities/underlying diseases, in and of themselves, are not considered in selecting a level of E/M services *unless* their presence significantly increases the complexity of the medical decision making.

Select the Appropriate Level of E/M Services Based on the Following

1. For the following categories/subcategories, **all of the key components,** ie, history, examination, and medical decision making, must meet or exceed the stated requirements to qualify for a particular level of E/M service: office, new patient; hospital observation services; initial hospital care; office consultations; initial inpatient consultations; confirmatory consultations; emergency department services; comprehensive nursing facility assessments; domiciliary care, new patient; and home, new patient.

Table 2
Complexity of Medical Decision Making

Number of Diagnoses or Management Options	Amount and/or Complexity of Data to be Reviewed	Risk of Complications and/or Morbidity or Mortality	Type of Decision Making
minimal	minimal or none	minimal	**straightforward**
limited	limited	low	**low complexity**
multiple	moderate	moderate	**moderate complexity**
extensive	extensive	high	**high complexity**

2. For the following categories/subcategories, **two of the three key components** (ie, history, examination, and medical decision making) must meet or exceed the stated requirements to qualify for a particular level of E/M services: office, established patient; subsequent hospital care; follow-up inpatient consultations; subsequent nursing facility care; domiciliary care, established patient; and home, established patient.

3. When counseling and/or coordination of care dominates (more than 50%) the physician/patient and/or family encounter (face-to-face time in the office or other outpatient setting or floor/unit time in the hospital or nursing facility), then **time** may be considered the key or controlling factor to qualify for a particular level of E/M services. This includes time spent with parties who have assumed responsibility for the care of the patient or decision making whether or not they are family members (eg, foster parents, person acting in locum parentis, legal guardian). The extent of counseling and/or coordination of care must be documented in the medical record.

Notes

Evaluation and Management

Office or Other Outpatient Services

The following codes are used to report evaluation and management services provided in the physician's office or in an outpatient or other ambulatory facility. A patient is considered an outpatient until inpatient admission to a health care facility occurs.

To report services provided to a patient who is admitted to a hospital or nursing facility in the course of an encounter in the office or other ambulatory facility, see the notes for initial hospital inpatient care (page 12) or comprehensive nursing facility assessments (page 23).

For services provided by physicians in the emergency department, see 99281-99285.

For observation care, see 99217-99220.

For observation or inpatient care services (including admission and discharge services), see 99234-99236.

New Patient

➧ **99201** **Office or other outpatient visit** for the evaluation and management of a new patient, which requires these three key components:

- **a problem focused history;**
- **a problem focused examination; and**
- **straightforward medical decision making.**

Counseling and/or coordination of care with other providers or agencies are provided consistent with the nature of the problem(s) and the patient's and/or family's needs.

Usually, the presenting problems are self limited or minor. Physicians typically spend 10 minutes face-to-face with the patient and/or family.

➲ *CPT Assistant* Jan 01:3, 5, Apr 02:5, Jul 02:4, Jan 03:10, 12, May 03:13

➧ **99202** **Office or other outpatient visit** for the evaluation and management of a new patient, which requires these three key components:

- **an expanded problem focused history;**
- **an expanded problem focused examination; and**
- **straightforward medical decision making.**

Counseling and/or coordination of care with other providers or agencies are provided consistent with the nature of the problem(s) and the patient's and/or family's needs.

Usually, the presenting problem(s) are of low to moderate severity. Physicians typically spend 20 minutes face-to-face with the patient and/or family.

➲ *CPT Assistant* Jan 01:5, Apr 02:5, Jul 02:4, Jan 03:10, 12, May 03:13

➧ **99203** **Office or other outpatient visit** for the evaluation and management of a new patient, which requires these three key components:

- **a detailed history;**
- **a detailed examination; and**
- **medical decision making of low complexity.**

Counseling and/or coordination of care with other providers or agencies are provided consistent with the nature of the problem(s) and the patient's and/or family's needs.

Usually, the presenting problem(s) are of moderate severity. Physicians typically spend 30 minutes face-to-face with the patient and/or family.

➲ *CPT Assistant* Jan 01:5, Apr 02:5, Jul 02:4, Jan 03:10, 12, May 03:13

➧ **99204** **Office or other outpatient visit** for the evaluation and management of a new patient, which requires these three key components:

- **a comprehensive history;**
- **a comprehensive examination; and**
- **medical decision making of moderate complexity.**

Counseling and/or coordination of care with other providers or agencies are provided consistent with the nature of the problem(s) and the patient's and/or family's needs.

Usually, the presenting problem(s) are of moderate to high severity. Physicians typically spend 45 minutes face-to-face with the patient and/or family.

➲ *CPT Assistant* Jan 01:5, Apr 02:5, Jul 02:4, Jan 03:10, 12, May 03:13

➧ **99205** **Office or other outpatient visit** for the evaluation and management of a new patient, which requires these three key components:

- **a comprehensive history;**
- **a comprehensive examination; and**
- **medical decision making of high complexity.**

Counseling and/or coordination of care with other providers or agencies are provided consistent with the nature of the problem(s) and the patient's and/or family's needs.

Usually, the presenting problem(s) are of moderate to high severity. Physicians typically spend 60 minutes face-to-face with the patient and/or family.

➲ *CPT Assistant* Jan 01:5, Jul 02:4, Jan 03:10, 12, May 03:13

Established Patient

➤ **99211** **Office or other outpatient visit** for the evaluation and management of an established patient, that may not require the presence of a physician. Usually, the presenting problem(s) are minimal. Typically, 5 minutes are spent performing or supervising these services.

➲ *CPT Assistant* Jan 03:10, 12, Apr 03:15, May 03:13, Mar 04:9, Apr 04:14

➤ **99212** **Office or other outpatient visit** for the evaluation and management of an established patient, which requires at least two of these three key components:

- **a problem focused history;**
- **a problem focused examination;**
- **straightforward medical decision making.**

Counseling and/or coordination of care with other providers or agencies are provided consistent with the nature of the problem(s) and the patient's and/or family's needs.

Usually, the presenting problem(s) are self limited or minor. Physicians typically spend 10 minutes face-to-face with the patient and/or family.

➲ *CPT Assistant* Jan 03:10, 12, Apr 03:15, May 03:13, Mar 04:9, Apr 04:14

➤ **99213** **Office or other outpatient visit** for the evaluation and management of an established patient, which requires at least two of these three key components:

- **an expanded problem focused history;**
- **an expanded problem focused examination;**
- **medical decision making of low complexity.**

Counseling and coordination of care with other providers or agencies are provided consistent with the nature of the problem(s) and the patient's and/or family's needs.

Usually, the presenting problem(s) are of low to moderate severity. Physicians typically spend 15 minutes face-to-face with the patient and/or family.

➲ *CPT Assistant* Jan 03:10, 12, May 03:13, Mar 04:9, Apr 04:14

➤ **99214** **Office or other outpatient visit** for the evaluation and management of an established patient, which requires at least two of these three key components:

- **a detailed history;**
- **a detailed examination;**
- **medical decision making of moderate complexity.**

Counseling and/or coordination of care with other providers or agencies are provided consistent with the nature of the problem(s) and the patient's and/or family's needs.

Usually, the presenting problem(s) are of moderate to high severity. Physicians typically spend 25 minutes face-to-face with the patient and/or family.

➲ *CPT Assistant* Jan 03:10, 12, May 03:13, Mar 04:9, Apr 04:14

➤ **99215** **Office or other outpatient visit** for the evaluation and management of an established patient, which requires at least two of these three key components:

- **a comprehensive history;**
- **a comprehensive examination;**
- **medical decision making of high complexity.**

Counseling and/or coordination of care with other providers or agencies are provided consistent with the nature of the problem(s) and the patient's and/or family's needs.

Usually, the presenting problem(s) are of moderate to high severity. Physicians typically spend 40 minutes face-to-face with the patient and/or family.

➲ *CPT Assistant* Jan 03:10, 12, May 03:13, Mar 04:9, Apr 04:14

Hospital Observation Services

The following codes are used to report evaluation and management services provided to patients designated/admitted as "observation status" in a hospital. It is not necessary that the patient be located in an observation area designated by the hospital.

If such an area does exist in a hospital (as a separate unit in the hospital, in the emergency department, etc.), these codes are to be utilized if the patient is placed in such an area.

For definitions of key components and commonly used terms, please see **Evaluation and Management Services Guidelines.**

Typical times have not yet been established for this category of services.

Observation Care Discharge Services

Observation care discharge of a patient from "observation status" includes final examination of the patient, discussion of the hospital stay, instructions for continuing care, and preparation of discharge records. For observation or inpatient hospital care including the admission and discharge of the patient on the same date, see codes 99234-99236 as appropriate.

☆ **99217** **Observation care discharge** day management (This code is to be utilized by the physician to report all services provided to a patient on discharge from "observation status" if the discharge is on other than the initial date of "observation status." To report services to a patient designated as "observation status" or "inpatient status" and discharged on the same date, use the codes for Observation or Inpatient Care Services [including Admission and Discharge Services, 99234-99236 as appropriate.])

➔ *CPT Assistant* May 03:13

Initial Observation Care

New or Established Patient

The following codes are used to report the encounter(s) by the supervising physician with the patient when designated as "observation status." This refers to the initiation of observation status, supervision of the care plan for observation and performance of periodic reassessments. For observation encounters by other physicians, see Office or Other Outpatient Consultation codes (99241-99245).

To report services provided to a patient who is admitted to the hospital after receiving hospital observation care services on the same date, see the notes for initial hospital inpatient care (page 12). For a patient admitted to the hospital on a date subsequent to the date of observation status, the hospital admission would be reported with the appropriate Initial Hospital Care code (99221-99223). For a patient admitted and discharged from observation or inpatient status on the same date, the services should be reported with codes 99234-99236 as appropriate. Do not report observation discharge (99217) in conjunction with a hospital admission.

When "observation status" is initiated in the course of an encounter in another site of service (eg, hospital emergency department, physician's office, nursing facility) all evaluation and management services provided by the supervising physician in conjunction with initiating "observation status" are considered part of the initial observation care when performed on the same date. The observation care level of service reported by the supervising physician should include the services related to initiating "observation status" provided in the other sites of service as well as in the observation setting.

Evaluation and management services on the same date provided in sites that are related to initiating "observation status" should NOT be reported separately.

These codes may not be utilized for post-operative recovery if the procedure is considered part of the surgical "package." These codes apply to all evaluation and management services that are provided on the same date of initiating "observation status."

☆ **99218** **Initial observation care,** per day, for the evaluation and management of a patient which requires these three key components:

- **a detailed or comprehensive history;**
- **a detailed or comprehensive examination; and**
- **medical decision making that is straightforward or of low complexity.**

Counseling and/or coordination of care with other providers or agencies are provided consistent with the nature of the problem(s) and the patient's and/or family's needs.

Usually, the problem(s) requiring admission to "observation status" are of low severity.

➔ *CPT Assistant* Jan 03:10, 12, 13, May 03:13

☆ **99219** **Initial observation care,** per day, for the evaluation and management of a patient, which requires these three key components:

- **a comprehensive history;**
- **a comprehensive examination; and**
- **medical decision making of moderate complexity.**

Counseling and/or coordination of care with other providers or agencies are provided consistent with the nature of the problem(s) and the patient's and/or family's needs.

Usually, the problem(s) requiring admission to "observation status" are of moderate severity.

➔ *CPT Assistant* Jan 03:10, 13, May 03:13

☆ **99220** **Initial observation care,** per day, for the evaluation and management of a patient, which requires these three key components:

- **a comprehensive history;**
- **a comprehensive examination; and**
- **medical decision making of high complexity.**

Counseling and/or coordination of care with other providers or agencies are provided consistent with the nature of the problem(s) and the patient's and/or family's needs.

Usually, the problem(s) requiring admission to "observation status" are of high severity.

➔ *CPT Assistant* Jan 03:10, 13, May 03:13

Hospital Inpatient Services

The following codes are used to report evaluation and management services provided to hospital inpatients. Hospital inpatient services include those services provided to patients in a "partial hospital" setting. These codes are to be used to report these partial hospitalization services. See also psychiatry notes in the full text of *CPT.*

For definitions of key components and commonly used terms, please see **Evaluation and Management Services Guidelines.** For Hospital Observation Services, see 99218-99220. For a patient admitted and discharged from observation or inpatient status on the same date, the services should be reported with codes 99234-99236 as appropriate.

Initial Hospital Care

New or Established Patient

The following codes are used to report the first hospital inpatient encounter with the patient by the admitting physician.

For initial inpatient encounters by physicians other than the admitting physician, see initial inpatient consultation codes (99251-99255) or subsequent hospital care codes (99231-99233) as appropriate.

When the patient is admitted to the hospital as an inpatient in the course of an encounter in another site of service (eg, hospital emergency department, observation status in a hospital, physician's office, nursing facility) all evaluation and management services provided by that physician in conjunction with that admission are considered part of the initial hospital care when performed on the same date as the admission. The inpatient care level of service reported by the admitting physician should include the services related to the admission he/she provided in the other sites of service as well as in the inpatient setting.

Evaluation and management services on the same date provided in sites that are related to the admission "observation status" should NOT be reported separately. For a patient admitted and discharged from observation or inpatient status on the same date, the services should be reported with codes 99234-99236 as appropriate.

☐ **99221** **Initial hospital care,** per day, for the evaluation and management of a patient which requires these three key components:

- **a detailed or comprehensive history;**
- **a detailed or comprehensive examination; and**
- **medical decision making that is straightforward or of low complexity.**

Counseling and/or coordination of care with other providers or agencies are provided consistent with the nature of the problem(s) and the patient's and/or family's needs.

Usually, the problem(s) requiring admission are of low severity. Physicians typically spend 30 minutes at the bedside and on the patient's hospital floor or unit.

➲ *CPT Assistant* May 00:2, Jan 01:5, Mar 04:9, Apr 04:14

☐ **99222** **Initial hospital care,** per day, for the evaluation and management of a patient, which requires these three key components:

- **a comprehensive history;**
- **a comprehensive examination; and**
- **medical decision making of moderate complexity.**

Counseling and/or coordination of care with other providers or agencies are provided consistent with the nature of the problem(s) and the patient's and/or family's needs.

Usually, the problem(s) requiring admission are of moderate severity. Physicians typically spend 50 minutes at the bedside and on the patient's hospital floor or unit.

➲ *CPT Assistant* May 00:2, Jan 01:5, Mar 04:9, Apr 04:14

☐ **99223** **Initial hospital care,** per day, for the evaluation and management of a patient, which requires these three key components:

- **a comprehensive history;**
- **a comprehensive examination; and**
- **medical decision making of high complexity.**

Counseling and/or coordination of care with other providers or agencies are provided consistent with the nature of the problem(s) and the patient's and/or family's needs.

Usually, the problem(s) requiring admission are of high severity. Physicians typically spend 70 minutes at the bedside and on the patient's hospital floor or unit.

➲ *CPT Assistant* May 00:2, Jan 01:5, Mar 04:9, Apr 04:14

Subsequent Hospital Care

All levels of subsequent hospital care include reviewing the medical record and reviewing the results of diagnostic studies and changes in the patient's status, (ie, changes in history, physical condition and response to management) since the last assessment by the physician.

☐ **99231** **Subsequent hospital care,** per day, for the evaluation and management of a patient, which requires at least two of these three key components:

- **a problem focused interval history;**
- **a problem focused examination;**
- **medical decision making that is straightforward or of low complexity.**

Counseling and/or coordination of care with other providers or agencies are provided consistent with the nature of the problem(s) and the patient's and/or family's needs.

Usually, the patient is stable, recovering or improving. Physicians typically spend 15 minutes at the bedside and on the patient's hospital floor or unit.

☐ **99232** **Subsequent hospital care,** per day, for the evaluation and management of a patient, which requires at least two of these three key components:

- **an expanded problem focused interval history;**
- **an expanded problem focused examination;**
- **medical decision making of moderate complexity.**

Counseling and/or coordination of care with other providers or agencies are provided consistent with the nature of the problem(s) and the patient's and/or family's needs.

Usually, the patient is responding inadequately to therapy or has developed a minor complication. Physicians typically spend 25 minutes at the bedside and on the patient's hospital floor or unit.

☐ **99233** **Subsequent hospital care,** per day, for the evaluation and management of a patient, which requires at least two of these three key components:

- **a detailed interval history;**
- **a detailed examination;**
- **medical decision making of high complexity.**

Counseling and/or coordination of care with other providers or agencies are provided consistent with the nature of the problem(s) and the patient's and/or family's needs.

Usually, the patient is unstable or has developed a significant complication or a significant new problem. Physicians typically spend 35 minutes at the bedside and on the patient's hospital floor or unit.

Observation or Inpatient Care Services (Including Admission and Discharge Services)

The following codes are used to report observation or inpatient hospital care services provided to patients admitted and discharged on the same date of service. When a patient is admitted to the hospital from observation status on the same date, the physician should report only the initial hospital care code. The initial hospital care code reported by the admitting physician should include the services related to the observation status services he/she provided on the same date of inpatient admission.

When "observation status" is initiated in the course of an encounter in another site of service (eg, hospital emergency department, physician's office, nursing facility) all evaluation and management services provided by the supervising physician in conjunction with initiating "observation status" are considered part of the initial observation care when performed on the same date. The observation care level of service should include the services related to initiating "observation status" provided in the other sites of service as well as in the observation setting when provided by the same physician.

For patients admitted to observation or inpatient care and discharged on a different date, see codes 99218-99220 and 99217, or 99221-99223 and 99238, 99239.

☆ **99234** **Observation or inpatient hospital care,** for the evaluation and management of a patient including admission and discharge on the same date which requires these three key components:

- **a detailed or comprehensive history;**
- **a detailed or comprehensive examination; and**
- **medical decision making that is straightforward or of low complexity.**

Counseling and/or coordination of care with other providers or agencies are provided consistent with the nature of the problem(s) and the patient's and/or family's needs.

Usually the presenting problem(s) requiring admission are of low severity.

➲ *CPT Assistant* Jan 03:10, 13, May 03:13, Mar 04:9, Apr 04:14

☆ **99235** **Observation or inpatient hospital care,** for the evaluation and management of a patient including admission and discharge on the same date which requires these three key components:

- **a comprehensive history;**
- **a comprehensive examination; and**
- **medical decision making of moderate complexity.**

Counseling and/or coordination of care with other providers or agencies are provided consistent with the nature of the problem(s) and the patient's and/or family's needs.

Usually the presenting problem(s) requiring admission are of moderate severity.

➲ *CPT Assistant* Jan 03:10, 13, May 03:13, Mar 04:9, Apr 04:14

☆ **99236** **Observation or inpatient hospital care,** for the evaluation and management of a patient including admission and discharge on the same date which requires these three key components:

- **a comprehensive history;**
- **a comprehensive examination; and**
- **medical decision making of high complexity.**

Counseling and/or coordination of care with other providers or agencies are provided consistent with the nature of the problem(s) and the patient's and/or family's needs.

Usually the presenting problem(s) requiring admission are of high severity.

➲ *CPT Assistant* Jan 03:10, 13, May 03:13, Mar 04:9, Apr 04:14

Hospital Discharge Services

The hospital discharge day management codes are to be used to report the total duration of time spent by a physician for final hospital discharge of a patient. The codes include, as appropriate, final examination of the patient, discussion of the hospital stay, even if the time spent by the physician on that date is not continuous, instructions for continuing care to all relevant caregivers, and preparation of discharge records, prescriptions and referral forms. For a patient admitted and discharged from observation or inpatient status on the same date, the services should be reported with codes 99234-99236 as appropriate.

☐ **99238** **Hospital discharge day management;** 30 minutes or less

☐ **99239** more than 30 minutes

(These codes are to be utilized by the physician to report all services provided to a patient on the date of discharge, if other than the initial date of inpatient status. To report services to a patient who is admitted as an inpatient, and discharged on the same date, see codes 99234-99236 for observation or inpatient hospital care including the admission and discharge of the patient on the same date. To report concurrent care services provided by a physician(s) other than the attending physician, use subsequent hospital care codes (99231-99233) on the day of discharge.)

(For Observation Care Discharge, use 99217)

(For observation or inpatient hospital care including the admission and discharge of the patient on the same date, see 99234-99236)

(For Nursing Facility Care Discharge, see 99315, 99316)

(For discharge services provided to newborns admitted and discharged on the same date, use 99435)

Consultations

A consultation is a type of service provided by a physician whose opinion or advice regarding evaluation and/or management of a specific problem is requested by another physician or other appropriate source.

A physician consultant may initiate diagnostic and/or therapeutic services at the same or subsequent visit.

The written or verbal request for a consult may be made by a physician or other appropriate source and documented in the patient's medical record. The consultant's opinion and any services that were ordered or performed must also be documented in the patient's medical record and communicated by written report to the requesting physician or other appropriate source.

A "consultation" initiated by a patient and/or family, and not requested by a physician, is not reported using the initial consultation codes but may be reported using the codes for confirmatory consultation or office visits, as appropriate.

If a confirmatory consultation is required, eg, by a third party payor, modifier 32 should also be reported.

Any specifically identifiable procedure (ie, identified with a specific CPT code) performed on or subsequent to the date of the initial consultation should be reported separately.

If subsequent to the completion of a consultation, the consultant assumes responsibility for management of a portion or all of the patient's condition(s), the follow-up consultation codes should not be used. In the hospital setting, the consulting physician should use the appropriate inpatient hospital consultation code for the initial encounter and then subsequent hospital care codes (not follow-up consultation codes). In the office setting, the appropriate established patient code should be used.

There are four subcategories of consultations: office, initial inpatient, follow-up inpatient, and confirmatory. See each subcategory for specific reporting instructions.

For definitions of key comp onents and commonly used terms, please see **Evaluation and Management Services Guidelines.**

Office or Other Outpatient Consultations

New or Established Patient

The following codes are used to report consultations provided in the physician's office or in an outpatient or other ambulatory facility, including hospital observation services, home services, domiciliary, rest home, custodial care, or emergency department (see consultation definition, above). Follow-up visits in the consultant's office or other outpatient facility that are initiated by the physician consultant are reported using office visit codes for established patients (99211-99215). If an additional request for an opinion or advice regarding the same or a new problem is received from the attending physician and documented in the medical record, the office consultation codes may be used again.

➧ **99241** **Office consultation** for a new or established patient, which requires these three key components:

- **a problem focused history;**
- **problem focused examination; and**
- **straightforward medical decision making.**

Counseling and/or coordination of care with other providers or agencies are provided consistent with the nature of the problem(s) and the patient's and/or family's needs.

Usually, the presenting problem(s) are self limited or minor. Physicians typically spend 15 minutes face-to-face with the patient and/or family.

➲ *CPT Assistant* Jul 02:3, May 03:13, Mar 04:9, Apr 04:14

99242 **Office consultation** for a new or established patient, which requires these three key components:

- **an expanded problem focused history;**
- **an expanded problem focused examination; and**
- **straightforward medical decision making.**

Counseling and/or coordination of care with other providers or agencies are provided consistent with the nature of the problem(s) and the patient's and/or family's needs.

Usually, the presenting problem(s) are of low severity. Physicians typically spend 30 minutes face-to-face with the patient and/or family.

➲ *CPT Assistant* May 03:13, Mar 04:9, Apr 04:14

99243 **Office consultation** for a new or established patient, which requires these three key components:

- **a detailed history;**
- **a detailed examination; and**
- **medical decision making of low complexity.**

Counseling and/or coordination of care with other providers or agencies are provided consistent with the nature of the problem(s) and the patient's and/or family's needs.

Usually, the presenting problem(s) are of moderate severity. Physicians typically spend 40 minutes face-to-face with the patient and/or family.

➲ *CPT Assistant* May 03:13, Mar 04:9, Apr 04:14

99244 **Office consultation** for a new or established patient, which requires these three key components:

- **a comprehensive history;**
- **a comprehensive examination; and**
- **medical decision making of moderate complexity.**

Counseling and/or coordination of care with other providers or agencies are provided consistent with the nature of the problem(s) and the patient's and/or family's needs.

Usually, the presenting problem(s) are of moderate to high severity. Physicians typically spend 60 minutes face-to-face with the patient and/or family.

➲ *CPT Assistant* May 03:13, Mar 04:9, Apr 04:14

99245 **Office consultation** for a new or established patient, which requires these three key components:

- **a comprehensive history;**
- **a comprehensive examination; and**
- **medical decision making of high complexity.**

Counseling and/or coordination of care with other providers or agencies are provided consistent with the nature of the problem(s) and the patient's and/or family's needs.

Usually, the presenting problem(s) are of moderate to high severity. Physicians typically spend 80 minutes face-to-face with the patient and/or family.

➲ *CPT Assistant* May 03:13, Mar 04:9, Apr 04:14

Initial Inpatient Consultations

New or Established Patient

The following codes are used to report physician consultations provided to hospital inpatients, residents of nursing facilities, or patients in a partial hospital setting. Only one initial consultation should be reported by a consultant per admission.

✿ **99251** **Initial inpatient consultation** for a new or established patient, which requires these three key components:

- **a problem focused history;**
- **a problem focused examination; and**
- **straightforward medical decision making.**

Counseling and/or coordination of care with other providers or agencies are provided consistent with the nature of the problem(s) and the patient's and/or family's needs.

Usually, the presenting problem(s) are self limited or minor. Physicians typically spend 20 minutes at the bedside and on the patient's hospital floor or unit.

✿ **99252** **Initial inpatient consultation** for a new or established patient, which requires these three key components:

- **an expanded problem focused history;**
- **an expanded problem focused examination; and**
- **straightforward medical decision making.**

Counseling and/or coordination of care with other providers or agencies are provided consistent with the nature of the problem(s) and the patient's and/or family's needs.

Usually, the presenting problem(s) are of low severity. Physicians typically spend 40 minutes at the bedside and on the patient's hospital floor or unit.

✿ 99253 **Initial inpatient consultation** for a new or established patient, which requires these three key components:

- **a detailed history;**
- **a detailed examination; and**
- **medical decision making of low complexity.**

Counseling and/or coordination of care with other providers or agencies are provided consistent with the nature of the problem(s) and the patient's and/or family's needs.

Usually, the presenting problem(s) are of moderate severity. Physicians typically spend 55 minutes at the bedside and on the patient's hospital floor or unit.

✿ 99254 **Initial inpatient consultation** for a new or established patient, which requires three key components:

- **a comprehensive history;**
- **a comprehensive examination; and**
- **medical decision making of moderate complexity.**

Counseling and/or coordination of care with other providers or agencies are provided consistent with the nature of the problem(s) and the patient's and/or family's needs.

Usually, the presenting problem(s) are of moderate to high severity. Physicians typically spend 80 minutes at the bedside and on the patient's hospital floor or unit.

✿ 99255 **Initial inpatient consultation** for a new or established patient, which requires these three key components:

- **a comprehensive history;**
- **a comprehensive examination; and**
- **medical decision making of high complexity.**

Counseling and/or coordination of care with other providers or agencies are provided consistent with the nature of the problem(s) and the patient's and/or family's needs.

Usually, the presenting problem(s) are of moderate to high severity. Physicians typically spend 110 minutes at the bedside and on the patient's hospital floor or unit.

Follow-Up Inpatient Consultations

Established Patient

Follow-up consultations are visits to complete the initial consultation OR subsequent consultative visits requested by the attending physician.

A follow-up consultation includes monitoring progress, recommending management modifications or advising on a new plan of care in response to changes in the patient's status.

If the physician consultant has initiated treatment at the initial consultation, and participates thereafter in the patient's management, the codes for subsequent hospital care should be used (99231-99233).

The following codes are used to report follow-up consultations provided to hospital inpatients or nursing facility residents only. For consultative services provided in other settings, the codes for office or other outpatient consultations should be reported (99241-99245).

✿ 99261 **Follow-up inpatient consultation** for an established patient, which requires at least two of these three key components:

- **a problem focused interval history;**
- **a problem focused examination;**
- **medical decision making that is straightforward or of low complexity.**

Counseling and/or coordination of care with other providers or agencies are provided consistent with nature of the problem(s) and the patient's and/or family's needs.

Usually, the patient is stable, recovering or improving. Physicians typically spend 10 minutes at the bedside and on the patient's hospital floor or unit.

✿ 99262 **Follow-up inpatient consultation** for an established patient which requires at least two of these three key components:

- **an expanded problem focused interval history;**
- **an expanded problem focused examination;**
- **medical decision making of moderate complexity.**

Counseling and/or coordination of care with other providers or agencies are provided consistent with the nature of the problem(s) and the patient's and/or family's needs.

Usually, the patient is responding inadequately to therapy or has developed a minor complication. Physicians typically spend 20 minutes at the bedside and on the patient's hospital floor or unit.

✿ 99263 **Follow-up inpatient consultation** for an established patient which requires at least two of these three key components:

- **a detailed interval history;**
- **a detailed examination;**
- **medical decision making of high complexity.**

Counseling and/or coordination of care with other providers or agencies are provided consistent with the nature of the problem(s) and the patient's and/or family's needs.

Usually, the patient is unstable or has developed a significant complication or a significant new problem. Physicians typically spend 30 minutes at the bedside and on the patient's hospital floor or unit.

Confirmatory Consultations

New or Established Patient

The following codes are used to report the evaluation and management services provided to patients when the consulting physician is aware of the confirmatory nature of the opinion sought (eg, when a second/third opinion is requested or required on the necessity or appropriateness of a previously recommended medical treatment or surgical procedure).

Confirmatory consultations may be provided in any setting.

A physician consultant providing a confirmatory consultation is expected to provide an opinion and/or advice only. Any services subsequent to the opinion are coded at the appropriate level of office visit, established patient, or subsequent hospital care. If a confirmatory consultation is required, eg, by a third party payor, modifier 32 should also be reported. (See also Consultation notes, page 14.) Typical times have not yet been established for this subcategory of services.

➧ **99271** **Confirmatory consultation** for a new or established patient, which requires these three key components:

- **a problem focused history;**
- **a problem focused examination; and**
- **straightforward medical decision making.**

Counseling and/or coordination of care with other providers or agencies are provided consistent with the nature of the problem(s) and the patient's and/or family's needs.

Usually, the presenting problem(s) are self limited or minor.

➲ *CPT Assistant* May 03:13, Mar 04:9, Apr 04:14

➧ **99272** **Confirmatory consultation** for a new or established patient, which requires these three key components:

- **an expanded problem focused history;**
- **an expanded problem focused examination; and**
- **straightforward medical decision making.**

Counseling and/or coordination of care with other providers or agencies are provided consistent with the nature of the problem(s) and the patient's and/or family's needs.

Usually, the presenting problem(s) are of low severity.

➧ **99273** **Confirmatory consultation** for a new or established patient, which requires these three key components:

- **a detailed history;**
- **a detailed examination; and**
- **medical decision making of low complexity.**

Counseling and/or coordination of care with other providers or agencies are provided consistent with the nature of the problem(s) and the patient's and/or family's needs.

Usually, the presenting problem(s) are of moderate severity.

➧ **99274** **Confirmatory consultation** for a new or established patient, which requires these three key components:

- **a comprehensive history;**
- **a comprehensive examination; and**
- **medical decision making of moderate complexity.**

Counseling and/or coordination of care with other providers or agencies are provided consistent with the nature of the problem(s) and the patient's and/or family's needs.

Usually, the presenting problem(s) are of moderate to high severity.

➧ **99275** **Confirmatory consultation** for a new or established patient, which requires these three key components:

- **a comprehensive history;**
- **a comprehensive examination; and**
- **medical decision making of high complexity.**

Counseling and/or coordination of care with other providers or agencies are provided consistent with the nature of the problem(s) and the patient's and/or family's needs.

Usually, the presenting problem(s) are of moderate to high severity.

Emergency Department Services

New or Established Patient

The following codes are used to report evaluation and management services provided in the emergency department. No distinction is made between new and established patients in the emergency department.

An emergency department is defined as an organized hospital-based facility for the provision of unscheduled episodic services to patients who present for immediate medical attention. The facility must be available 24 hours a day.

For critical care services provided in the emergency department, see Critical Care notes and 99291, 99292.

For evaluation and management services provided to a patient in an observation area of a hospital, see 99217-99220.

For observation or inpatient care services (including admission and discharge services), see 99234-99236.

99281 **Emergency department visit** for the evaluation and management of a patient, which requires these three key components:

- **a problem focused history;**
- **a problem focused examination; and**
- **straightforward medical decision making.**

Counseling and/or coordination of care with other providers or agencies are provided consistent with the nature of the problem(s) and the patient's and/or family's needs.

Usually, the presenting problem(s) are self limited or minor.

CPT Assistant Apr 02:5, Jul 02:3, Jan 03:10, 12, Mar 03:17, 19, May 03:13, Mar 04:9, Apr 04:14

99282 **Emergency department visit** for the evaluation and management of a patient, which requires these three key components:

- **an expanded problem focused history;**
- **an expanded problem focused examination; and**
- **medical decision making of low complexity.**

Counseling and/or coordination of care with other providers or agencies are provided consistent with the nature of the problem(s) and the patient's and/or family's needs.

Usually, the presenting problem(s) are of low to moderate severity.

CPT Assistant Apr 02:5, Jul 02:3, Jan 03:10, 12, Mar 03:17, 19, May 03:13, Mar 04:9, Apr 04:14

99283 **Emergency department visit** for the evaluation and management of a patient, which requires these three key components:

- **an expanded problem focused history;**
- **an expanded problem focused examination; and**
- **medical decision making of moderate complexity.**

Counseling and/or coordination of care with other providers or agencies are provided consistent with the nature of the problem(s) and the patient's and/or family's needs.

Usually, the presenting problem(s) are of moderate severity.

CPT Assistant Apr 02:5, Jul 02:3, Jan 03: 12, Mar 03:17, 19, May 03:13, Mar 04:9, Apr 04:14

99284 **Emergency department visit** for the evaluation and management of a patient, which requires these three key components:

- **a detailed history;**
- **a detailed examination; and**
- **medical decision making of moderate complexity.**

Counseling and/or coordination of care with other providers or agencies are provided consistent with the nature of the problem(s) and the patient's and/or family's needs.

Usually, the presenting problem(s) are of high severity, and require urgent evaluation by the physician but do not pose an immediate significant threat to life or physiologic function.

CPT Assistant Apr 02:5, Jul 02:3, Jan 03:10, 12, Mar 03:17, 19, May 03:13, Mar 04:9, Apr 04:14

99285 **Emergency department visit** for the evaluation and management of a patient, which requires these three key components within the constraints imposed by the urgency of the patient's clinical condition and/or mental status:

- **a comprehensive history;**
- **a comprehensive examination; and**
- **medical decision making of high complexity.**

Counseling and/or coordination of care with other providers or agencies are provided consistent with the nature of the problem(s) and the patient's and/or family's needs.

Usually, the presenting problem(s) are of high severity and pose an immediate significant threat to life or physiologic function.

CPT Assistant Apr 02:5, Jul 02:3, Jan 03:10, 12, Mar 03:17, 19, May 03:13, Mar 04:9, Apr 04:14

Other Emergency Services

In physician directed emergency care, advanced life support, the physician is located in a hospital emergency or critical care department, and is in two-way voice communication with ambulance or rescue personnel outside the hospital. The physician directs the performance of necessary medical procedures, including but not limited to: telemetry of cardiac rhythm; cardiac and/or pulmonary resuscitation; endotracheal or esophageal obturator airway intubation; administration of intravenous fluids and/or administration of intramuscular, intratracheal or subcutaneous drugs; and/or electrical conversion of arrhythmia.

99288 **Physician direction of** emergency medical systems (EMS) emergency care, advanced life support

Pediatric Critical Care Patient Transport

The following codes 99289 and 99290 are used to report the physical attendance and direct face-to-face care by a physician during the interfacility transport of a critically ill or critically injured pediatric patient. For the purpose of reporting codes 99289 and 99290, face-to-face care begins when the physician assumes primary responsibility of the pediatric patient at the referring hospital/facility, and ends when the receiving hospital/facility accepts responsibility for the pediatric patient's care. Only the time the physician spends in direct face-to-face contact with the patient during the transport should be reported. Pediatric patient transport services involving less than 30 minutes of face-to-face physician care should not be reported using codes 99289, 99290. Procedure(s) or service(s) performed by other members of the transporting team may not be reported by the supervising physician.

The following services are included when performed during the pediatric patient transport by the physician providing critical care and may not be reported separately: routine monitoring evaluations (eg, heart rate, respiratory rate, blood pressure, and pulse oximetry), the interpretation of cardiac output measurements (93561, 93562), chest x-rays (71010, 71015, 71020), pulse oximetry (94760, 94761, 94762), blood gases and information data stored in computers (eg, ECGs, blood pressures, hematologic data) (99090), gastric intubation (43752, 91105), temporary transcutaneous pacing (92953), ventilatory management (94656, 94660, 94662) and vascular access procedures (36000, 36400, 36405, 36406, 36410, 36415, 36540, 36600). Any services performed which are not listed above should be reported separately.

Critical care is the direct delivery by a physician(s) of medical care for a critically ill or critically injured patient. A critical illness or injury acutely impairs one or more vital organ systems such that there is a high probability of imminent or life threatening deterioration in the patient's condition. Critical care involves high complexity decision making to assess, manipulate, and support vital system function(s) to treat single or multiple vital organ system failure and/or to prevent further life threatening deterioration of the patient's condition. Examples of vital organ system failure include, but are not limited to: central nervous system failure, circulatory failure, shock, renal, hepatic, metabolic, and/or respiratory failure.

Providing medical care to a critically ill, injured, or post-operative patient qualifies as a critical care service only if both the illness or injury and the treatment being provided meet the above requirements.

The direction of emergency care to transporting staff by a physician located in a hospital or other facility by two-way communication is not considered direct face-to-face care and should not be reported with codes 99289, 99290. Physician directed emergency care through outside voice communication to transporting staff personnel is reported with code 99288.

The emergency department services codes (99281-99285), initial hospital care codes (99221-99223), hourly critical care codes (99291, 99292), or initial date neonatal intensive care code (99295) are only reported after the patient has been admitted to the emergency department, the inpatient floor or the critical care unit of the receiving facility.

Code 99289 is used to report the first 30-74 minutes of direct face-to-face time with the transport pediatric patient and should be reported only once on a given date. Code 99290 is used to report each additional 30 minutes provided on a given date. Face-to-face services less than 30 minutes should not be reported with these codes.

☆ **99289** Critical care services delivered by a physician, face-to-face, during an interfacility transport of critically ill or critically injured pediatric patient, 24 months of age or less; first 30-74 minutes of hands on care during transport

☆+ **99290** each additional 30 minutes (List separately in addition to code for primary service)

(Use 99290 in conjunction with 99289)

(Critical care of less than 30 minutes total duration should be reported with the appropriate E/M code)

Critical Care Services

Critical care is the direct delivery by a physician(s) of medical care for a critically ill or critically injured patient. A critical illness or injury acutely impairs one or more vital organ systems such that there is a high probability of imminent or life threatening deterioration in the patient's condition. Critical care involves high complexity decision making to assess, manipulate, and support vital system function(s) to treat single or multiple vital organ system failure and/or to prevent further life threatening deterioration of the patient's condition. Examples of vital organ system failure include, but are not limited to: central nervous system failure, circulatory failure, shock, renal, hepatic, metabolic, and/or respiratory failure. Although critical care typically requires interpretation of multiple physiologic parameters and/or application of advanced technology(s), critical care may be provided in life threatening situations when these elements are not present. Critical care may be provided on multiple days, even if no changes are made in the treatment rendered to the patient, provided that the patient's condition continues to require the level of physician attention described above.

Providing medical care to a critically ill, injured, or post-operative patient qualifies as a critical care service only if both the illness or injury and the treatment being provided meet the above requirements. Critical care is usually, but not always, given in a critical care area, such as the coronary care unit, intensive care unit, pediatric intensive care unit, respiratory care unit, or the emergency care facility.

Inpatient critical care services provided to infants ►29◄ days through 24 months of age are reported with pediatric critical care codes 99293 and 99294. The pediatric critical care codes are reported as long as the infant/young child qualifies for critical care services during the hospital stay through 24 months of age. Inpatient critical care services provided to neonates (►28◄ days of age or less) are reported with the neonatal critical care codes 99295 and 99296. The neonatal critical care codes are reported as long as the neonate qualifies for critical care services during the hospital stay through the ►28◄th postnatal day. The reporting of the pediatric and neonatal critical care services is not based on time or the type of unit (eg, pediatric or neonatal critical care unit) and it is not dependent upon the type of provider delivering the care. To report critical care services provided in the outpatient setting (eg, emergency department or office), for neonates and pediatric patients up through 24 months of age, see the hourly Critical Care codes 99291, 99292. If the same physician provides critical care services for a neonatal or pediatric patient in both the outpatient and inpatient settings on the same day, report only the appropriate Neonatal or Pediatric Critical Care code (99293-99296) for all critical care services provided on that day. For additional instructions on reporting these services, see the Neonatal and Pediatric Critical Care section and codes 99293-99296.

Services for a patient who is not critically ill but happens to be in a critical care unit are reported using other appropriate E/M codes.

Critical care and other E/M services may be provided to the same patient on the same date by the same physician.

The following services are included in reporting critical care when performed during the critical period by the physician(s) providing critical care: the interpretation of cardiac output measurements (93561, 93562), chest x-rays (71010, 71015, 71020), pulse oximetry (94760, 94761, 94762), blood gases, and information data stored in computers (eg, ECGs, blood pressures, hematologic data (99090)); gastric intubation (43752, 91105); temporary transcutaneous pacing (92953); ventilatory management (94656, 94657, 94660, 94662); and vascular access procedures (36000, 36410, 36415, 36540, 36600). Any services performed which are not listed above should be reported separately.

Codes 99291, 99292 should be reported for the physician's attendance during the transport of critically ill or critically injured patients over 24 months of age to or from a facility or hospital. For physician transport services of critically ill or critically injured pediatric patients 24 months of age or less see 99289, 99290.

The critical care codes 99291 and 99292 are used to report the total duration of time spent by a physician providing critical care services to a critically ill or critically injured patient, even if the time spent by the physician on that date is not continuous. For any given period of time spent providing critical care services, the physician must devote his or her full attention to the patient and, therefore, cannot provide services to any other patient during the same period of time.

Time spent with the individual patient should be recorded in the patient's record. The time that can be reported as critical care is the time spent engaged in work directly related to the individual patient's care whether that time was spent at the immediate bedside or elsewhere on the floor or unit. For example, time spent on the unit or at the nursing station on the floor reviewing test results or imaging studies, discussing the critically ill patient's care with other medical staff or documenting critical care services in the medical record would be reported as critical care, even though it does not occur at the bedside. Also, when the patient is unable or clinically incompetent to participate in discussions, time spent on the floor or unit with family members or surrogate decision makers obtaining a medical history, reviewing the patient's condition or prognosis, or discussing treatment or limitation(s) of treatment may be reported as critical care, provided that the conversation bears directly on the management of the patient.

Time spent in activities that occur outside of the unit or off the floor (eg, telephone calls, whether taken at home, in the office, or elsewhere in the hospital) may not be reported as critical care since the physician is not immediately available to the patient. Time spent in activities that do not directly contribute to the treatment of the patient may not be reported as critical care, even if they are performed in the critical care unit (eg, participation in administrative meetings or telephone calls to discuss other patients). Time spent performing separately reportable procedures or services should not be included in the time reported as critical care time.

Code 99291 is used to report the first 30-74 minutes of critical care on a given date. It should be used only once per date even if the time spent by the physician is not continuous on that date. Critical care of less than 30 minutes total duration on a given date should be reported with the appropriate E/M code.

Code 99292 is used to report additional block(s) of time, of up to 30 minutes each beyond the first 74 minutes. (See table below.)

The following examples illustrate the correct reporting of critical care services:

Total Duration of Critical Care	Codes
less than 30 minutes (less than 1/2 hour)	appropriate E/M codes
30-74 minutes (1/2 hr. - 1 hr. 14 min.)	99291 X 1
75-104 minutes (1 hr. 15 min. - 1 hr. 44 min.)	99291 X 1 AND 99292 X 1
105-134 minutes (1 hr. 45 min. - 2 hr. 14 min.)	99291 X 1 AND 99292 X 2
135 - 164 minutes (2 hr. 15 min. - 2 hr. 44 min.)	99291 X 1 AND 99292 X 3
165 - 194 minutes (2 hr. 45 min. - 3 hr. 14 min.)	99291 X 1 AND 99292 X 4
194 minutes or longer (3 hr. 14 min. - etc.)	99291 and 99292 as appropriate (see illustrated reporting examples above)

❖ **99291** **Critical care, evaluation and management** of the critically ill or critically injured patient; first 30-74 minutes

➲ *CPT Assistant* Jan 01:5, Jan 03:10, 11, 12, Feb 03:15, Oct 03:1, Mar 04:9

☆+ **99292** each additional 30 minutes (List separately in addition to code for primary service)

(Use 99292 in conjunction with 99291)

Inpatient Neonatal and Pediatric Critical Care Services

The following codes (99293-99296) are used to report services provided by a physician directing the inpatient care of a critically ill neonate/infant. The same definitions for critical care services apply for the adult, child, and neonate.

The initial day neonatal critical care code (99295) can be used in addition to codes 99360, 99436 or 99440 as appropriate, when the physician is present for the delivery (99360 or 99436) and newborn resuscitation (99440) is required. Other procedures performed as a necessary part of the resuscitation (eg, endotracheal intubation (31500)) are also reported separately when performed as part of the pre-admission delivery room care. In order to report these procedures separately, they must be performed as a necessary component of the resuscitation and not simply as a convenience before admission to the neonatal intensive care unit.

Codes 99295, 99296 are used to report services provided by a physician directing the inpatient care of a critically ill neonate through the first ►28◄ days of life. They represent care starting with the date of admission (99295) and subsequent day(s) (99296) and may be reported only once per day, per patient. Once the neonate is no longer considered to be critically ill, the Intensive Low Birth Weight Services codes for those with present body weight of less than 2500 grams (99298, 99299) or the codes for Subsequent Hospital Care (99231-99233) for those with present body weight over 2500 grams should be utilized.

Codes 99293, 99294 are used to report services provided by a physician directing the inpatient care of a critically ill infant or young child from ►29◄ days of postnatal age through 24 months of age. They represent care starting with the date of admission (99293) and subsequent day(s) (99294) and may be reported by a single physician only once per day, per patient in a given setting. The critically ill or critically injured child older than 24 months of age would be reported with hourly critical care service codes (99291, 99292). Once an infant is no longer considered to be critically ill but continues to require intensive care, the Intensive Low Birth Weight Services codes (99298, 99299) should be used to report services for infants with present body weight of less than 2500 grams. When the present body weight of those infants exceeds 2500 grams, the Subsequent Hospital Care (99231-99233) codes should be utilized. To report critical care services provided in the outpatient setting (eg, emergency department or office), for neonates and pediatric patients up through 24 months of age, see the hourly Critical Care codes 99291, 99292. If the same physician provides critical care services for a neonatal or pediatric patient in both the outpatient and inpatient settings on the same day, report only the appropriate Neonatal or Pediatric Critical Care code (99293-99296) for all critical care services provided on that day.

Care rendered under 99293-99296 includes management, monitoring, and treatment of the patient including respiratory, pharmacologic control of the circulatory system, enteral and parenteral nutrition, metabolic and hematologic maintenance, parent/family counseling, case management services, and personal direct supervision of the health care team in the performance of cognitive and procedural activities.

The pediatric and neonatal critical care codes include those procedures listed above for the hourly critical care codes (99291, 99292). In addition, the following procedures are also included in the bundled (global) pediatric and neonatal critical care service codes (99293-99296): umbilical venous (36510) and umbilical arterial (36660) catheters, central (36555) or peripheral vessel catheterization (36000), other arterial catheters (36140, 36620), oral or nasogastric tube placement (43752), endotracheal intubation (31500), lumbar puncture (62270), suprapubic bladder aspiration (51000), bladder catheterization (►51701, 51702◄), initiation and management of mechanical ventilation (94656, 94657) or continuous positive airway pressure (CPAP) (94660), surfactant administration, intravascular fluid administration (90780, 90781), transfusion of blood components (36430, 36440), vascular punctures (36420, 36600), invasive or non-invasive electronic monitoring of vital signs, bedside pulmonary function testing (94375), and/or monitoring or interpretation of blood gases or oxygen saturation (94760-94762). Any services performed which are not listed above should be reported separately.

For additional instructions, see descriptions listed for 99293-99296

Inpatient Pediatric Critical Care

✿▲ 99293 **Initial inpatient pediatric critical care,** per day, for the evaluation and management of a critically ill infant or young child, 29 days through 24 months of age

✿▲ 99294 **Subsequent inpatient pediatric critical care,** per day, for the evaluation and management of a critically ill infant or young child, 29 days through 24 months of age

Inpatient Neonatal Critical Care

✿▲ 99295 **Initial inpatient neonatal critical care,** per day, for the evaluation and management of a critically ill neonate, 28 days of age or less

This code is reserved for the date of admission for neonates who are critically ill. Critically ill neonates require cardiac and/or respiratory support (including ventilator or nasal CPAP when indicated), continuous or frequent vital sign monitoring, laboratory and blood gas interpretations, follow-up physician reevaluations, and constant observation by the health care team under direct physician supervision. Immediate preoperative evaluation and stabilization of neonates with life threatening surgical or cardiac conditions are included under this code. Neonates with life threatening surgical or cardiac conditions are included under this code.

Care for neonates who require an intensive care setting but who are not critically ill is reported using the initial hospital care codes (99221-99223).

✿▲ 99296 **Subsequent inpatient neonatal critical care,** per day, for the evaluation and management of a critically ill neonate, 28 days of age or less

A critically ill neonate will require cardiac and/or respiratory support (including ventilator or nasal CPAP when indicated), continuous or frequent vital sign monitoring, laboratory and blood gas interpretations, follow-up physician re-evaluations throughout a 24-hour period, and constant observation by the health care team under direct physician supervision.

(Subsequent care for neonates who require an intensive setting but who are not critically ill is reported using either the intensive low birth weight services codes (99298, 99299) or the subsequent hospital care codes (99231-99233))

(99297 has been deleted. To report, use 99296)

Intensive (Non-Critical) Low Birth Weight Services

Codes 99298, 99299 are used to report services subsequent to the day of admission provided by a physician directing the continuing intensive care of the low birth weight (LBW) or very low birth weight (VLBW) infant who no longer meets the definition of critically ill. They represent subsequent day(s) of care and may be reported only once per day, per patient. Low birth weight services are reported for those neonates less than 2500 grams who do not meet the definition of critical care but continue to require intensive observation and frequent services and interventions only available in an intensive care setting. The level and frequency of services required for the LBW and the VLBW infant exceed those available in less intensive hospital areas or medical floors. Codes 99298, 99299 are global 24-hour codes with the same services bundled as outlined under codes 99293-99296.

For additional instructions, see descriptions listed for 99298, 99299.

✿ 99298 **Subsequent intensive care,** per day, for the evaluation and management of the recovering very low birth weight infant (present body weight less than 1500 grams)

Infants with present body weight less than 1500 grams who are no longer critically ill continue to require intensive cardiac and respiratory monitoring, continuous and/or frequent vital sign monitoring, heat maintenance, enteral and/or parenteral nutritional adjustments, laboratory and oxygen monitoring and constant observation by the health care team under direct physician supervision.

✿ 99299 **Subsequent intensive care,** per day, for the evaluation and management of the recovering low birth weight infant (present body weight of 1500-2500 grams)

Infants with present body weight of 1500-2500 grams who are no longer critically ill continue to require intensive cardiac and respiratory monitoring, continuous and/or frequent vital sign monitoring, heat maintenance, enteral and/or parenteral nutritional adjustments, laboratory and oxygen monitoring, and constant observation by the health care team under direct physician supervision.

Nursing Facility Services

The following codes are used to report evaluation and management services to patients in Nursing Facilities (formerly called Skilled Nursing Facilities (SNFs), Intermediate Care Facilities (ICFs) or Long Term Care Facilities (LTCFs)).

These codes should also be used to report evaluation and management services provided to a patient in a psychiatric residential treatment center (a facility or a distinct part of a facility for psychiatric care, which provides a 24-hour therapeutically planned and professionally staffed group living and learning environment). If procedures such as medical psychotherapy are provided in addition to evaluation and management services, these should be reported in addition to the evaluation and management services provided.

Nursing facilities that provide convalescent, rehabilitative, or long term care are required to conduct comprehensive, accurate, standardized, and reproducible assessments of each resident's functional capacity using a Resident Assessment Instrument (RAI). All RAIs include the Minimum Data Set (MDS), Resident Assessment Protocols (RAPs) and utilization guidelines. The MDS is the primary screening and assessment tool; the RAPs trigger the identification of potential problems and provide guidelines for follow-up assessments.

Physicians have a central role in assuring that all residents receive thorough assessments and that medical plans of care are instituted or revised to enhance or maintain the residents' physical and psychosocial functioning.

Two subcategories of nursing facility services are recognized: Comprehensive Nursing Facility Assessments and Subsequent Nursing Facility Care. Both subcategories apply to new or established patients. Comprehensive Assessments may be performed at one or more sites in the assessment process: the hospital, observation unit, office, nursing facility, domiciliary/non-nursing facility or patient's home.

For definitions of key components and commonly used terms, please see Evaluation and Management Services Guidelines.

Comprehensive Nursing Facility Assessments

New or Established Patient

When the patient is admitted to the nursing facility in the course of an encounter in another site of service (eg, hospital emergency department, physician's office), all evaluation and management services provided by that physician in conjunction with that admission are considered part of the initial nursing facility care when performed on the same date as the admission or readmission. The nursing facility care level of service reported by the admitting physician should include the services related to the admission he/she provided in the other sites of service as well as in the nursing facility setting.

Hospital discharge or observation discharge services performed on the same date of nursing facility admission or readmission may be reported separately. For a patient discharged from inpatient status on the same date of nursing facility admission or readmission, the hospital discharge services should be reported with codes 99238, 99239 as appropriate. For a patient discharged from observation status on the same date of nursing facility admission or readmission, the observation care discharge services should be reported with code 99217. For a patient admitted and discharged from observation or inpatient status on the same date, see codes 99234-99236.

(For nursing facility care discharge, see 99315, 99316)

More than one comprehensive assessment may be necessary during an inpatient confinement.

✣ **99301** **Evaluation and management** of a new or established patient involving an annual nursing facility assessment which requires these three key components:

- **a detailed interval history;**
- **a comprehensive examination; and**
- **medical decision making that is straightforward or of low complexity.**

Counseling and/or coordination of care with other providers or agencies are provided consistent with the nature of the problem(s) and the patient's and/or family's needs.

Usually, the patient is stable, recovering or improving. The review and affirmation of the medical plan of care is required. Physicians typically spend 30 minutes at the bedside and on the patient's facility floor or unit.

✣ **99302** **Evaluation and management** of a new or established patient involving a nursing facility assessment which requires these three key components:

- **a detailed interval history;**
- **a comprehensive examination; and**
- **medical decision making of moderate to high complexity.**

Counseling and/or coordination of care with other providers or agencies are provided consistent with the nature of the problem(s) and the patient's and/or family's needs.

Usually, the patient has developed a significant complication or a significant new problem and has had a major permanent change in status.

The creation of a new medical plan of care is required. Physicians typically spend 40 minutes at the bedside and on the patient's facility floor or unit.

✣ **99303** **Evaluation and management** of a new or established patient involving a nursing facility assessment at the time of initial admission or readmission to the facility, which requires these three key components:

- **a comprehensive history;**
- **a comprehensive examination; and**
- **medical decision making of moderate to high complexity.**

Counseling and/or coordination of care with other providers or agencies are provided consistent with the nature of the problem(s) and the patient's and/or family's needs.

The creation of a medical plan of care is required. Physicians typically spend 50 minutes at the bedside and on the patient's facility floor or unit.

Subsequent Nursing Facility Care

New or Established Patient

The following codes are used to report the services provided to residents of nursing facilities who do not require a comprehensive assessment, and/or who have not had a major, permanent change of status.

All levels include reviewing the medical record, noting changes in the resident's status since the last visit, and reviewing and signing orders.

✣ **99311** **Subsequent nursing facility care,** per day, for the evaluation and management of a new or established patient, which requires at least two of these three key components:

- **a problem focused interval history;**
- **a problem focused examination;**
- **medical decision making that is straightforward or of low complexity.**

Counseling and/or coordination of care with other providers or agencies are provided consistent with the nature of the problem(s) and the patient's and/or family's needs.

Usually, the patient is stable, recovering or improving. Physicians typically spend 15 minutes at the bedside and on the patient's facility floor or unit.

✣ **99312** **Subsequent nursing facility care,** per day, for the evaluation and management of a new or established patient, which requires at least two of these three key components:

- **an expanded problem focused interval history;**
- **an expanded problem focused examination;**
- **medical decision making of moderate complexity.**

Counseling and/or coordination of care with other providers or agencies are provided consistent with the nature of the problem(s) and the patient's and/or family's needs.

Usually, the patient is responding inadequately to therapy or has developed a minor complication. Physicians typically spend 25 minutes at the bedside and on the patient's facility floor or unit.

✣ **99313** **Subsequent nursing facility care,** per day, for the evaluation and management of a new or established patient, which requires at least two of these three key components:

- **a detailed interval history;**
- **a detailed examination;**
- **medical decision making of moderate to high complexity.**

Counseling and/or coordination of care with other providers or agencies are provided consistent with the nature of the problem(s) and the patient's and/or family's needs.

Usually, the patient has developed a significant complication or a significant new problem. Physicians typically spend 35 minutes at the bedside and on the patient's facility floor or unit.

Nursing Facility Discharge Services

The nursing facility discharge day management codes are to be used to report the total duration of time spent by a physician for the final nursing facility discharge of a patient. The codes include, as appropriate, final examination of the patient, discussion of the nursing facility stay, even if the time spent by the physician on that date is not continuous. Instructions are given for continuing care to all relevant caregivers, and preparation of discharge records, prescriptions and referral forms.

✣ **99315** Nursing facility discharge day management; 30 minutes or less

✣ **99316** more than 30 minutes

Domiciliary, Rest Home (eg, Boarding Home), or Custodial Care Services

The following codes are used to report evaluation and management services in a facility which provides room, board and other personal assistance services, generally on a long-term basis. The facility's services do not include a medical component.

For definitions of key components and commonly used terms, please see **Evaluation and Management Services Guidelines.**

Typical times have not yet been established for this category of services.

New Patient

✣ 99321 **Domiciliary or rest home visit** for the evaluation and management of a new patient which requires these three key components:

- **a problem focused history;**
- **a problem focused examination; and**
- **medical decision making that is straightforward or of low complexity.**

Counseling and/or coordination of care with other providers or agencies are provided consistent with the nature of the problem(s) and the patient's and/or family's needs.

Usually, the presenting problem(s) are of low severity.

✣ 99322 **Domiciliary or rest home visit** for the evaluation and management of a new patient, which requires these three key components:

- **an expanded problem focused history;**
- **an expanded problem focused examination; and**
- **medical decision making of moderate complexity.**

Counseling and/or coordination of care with other providers or agencies are provided consistent with the nature of the problem(s) and the patient's and/or family's needs.

Usually, the presenting problem(s) are of moderate severity.

✣ 99323 **Domiciliary or rest home visit** for the evaluation and management of a new patient, which requires these three key components:

- **a detailed history;**
- **a detailed examination; and**
- **medical decision making of high complexity.**

Counseling and/or coordination of care with other providers or agencies are provided consistent with the nature of the problem(s) and the patient's and/or family's needs.

Usually, the presenting problem(s) are of high complexity.

Established Patient

✣ 99331 **Domiciliary or rest home visit** for the evaluation and management of an established patient, which requires at least two of these three key components:

- **a problem focused interval history;**
- **a problem focused examination;**
- **medical decision making that is straightforward or of low complexity.**

Counseling and/or coordination of care with other providers or agencies are provided consistent with the nature of the problem(s) and the patient's and/or family's needs.

Usually, the patient is stable, recovering or improving.

✣ 99332 **Domiciliary or rest home visit** for the evaluation and management of an established patient, which requires at least two of these three key components:

- **an expanded problem focused interval history;**
- **an expanded problem focused examination;**
- **medical decision making of moderate complexity.**

Counseling and/or coordination of care with other providers or agencies are provided consistent with the nature of the problem(s) and the patient's and/or family's needs.

Usually, the patient is responding inadequately to therapy or has developed a minor complication.

✣ 99333 **Domiciliary or rest home visit** for the evaluation and management of an established patient, which requires at least two of these three key components:

- **a detailed interval history;**
- **a detailed examination;**
- **medical decision making of high complexity.**

Counseling and/or coordination of care with other providers or agencies are provided consistent with the nature of the problem(s) and the patient's and/or family's needs.

Usually, the patient is unstable or has developed a significant complication or a significant new problem.

Home Services

The following codes are used to report evaluation and management services provided in a private residence.

For definitions of key components and commonly used terms, please see **Evaluation and Management Services Guidelines.**

New Patient

✣ **99341** **Home visit** for the evaluation and management of a new patient, which requires these three key components:

- **a problem focused history;**
- **a problem focused examination; and**
- **straightforward medical decision making.**

Counseling and/or coordination of care with other providers or agencies are provided consistent with the nature of the problem(s) and the patient's and/or family's needs.

Usually, the presenting problem(s) are of low severity. Physicians typically spend 20 minutes face-to-face with the patient and/or family.

✣ **99342** **Home visit** for the evaluation and management of a new patient, which requires these three key components:

- **an expanded problem focused history;**
- **an expanded problem focused examination; and**
- **medical decision making of low complexity.**

Counseling and/or coordination of care with other providers or agencies are provided consistent with the nature of the problem(s) and the patient's and/or family's needs.

Usually, the presenting problem(s) are of moderate severity. Physicians typically spend 30 minutes face-to-face with the patient and/or family.

✣ **99343** **Home visit** for the evaluation and management of a new patient, which requires these three key components:

- **a detailed history;**
- **a detailed examination; and**
- **medical decision making of moderate complexity.**

Counseling and/or coordination of care with other providers or agencies are provided consistent with the nature of the problem(s) and the patient's and/or family's needs.

Usually, the presenting problem(s) are of moderate to high severity. Physicians typically spend 45 minutes face-to-face with the patient and/or family.

✣ **99344** **Home visit** for the evaluation and management of a new patient, which requires these three components:

- **a comprehensive history;**
- **a comprehensive examination; and**
- **medical decision making of moderate complexity.**

Counseling and/or coordination of care with other providers or agencies are provided consistent with the nature of the problem(s) and the patient's and/or family's needs.

Usually, the presenting problem(s) are of high severity. Physicians typically spend 60 minutes face-to-face with the patient and/or family.

✣ **99345** **Home visit** for the evaluation and management of a new patient, which requires these three key components:

- **a comprehensive history;**
- **a comprehensive examination; and**
- **medical decision making of high complexity.**

Counseling and/or coordination of care with other providers or agencies are provided consistent with the nature of the problem(s) and the patient's and/or family's needs.

Usually, the patient is unstable or has developed a significant new problem requiring immediate physician attention. Physicians typically spend 75 minutes face-to-face with the patient and/or family.

Established Patient

✣ **99347** **Home visit** for the evaluation and management of an established patient, which requires at least two of these three key components:

- **a problem focused interval history;**
- **a problem focused examination;**
- **straightforward medical decision making.**

Counseling and/or coordination of care with other providers or agencies are provided consistent with the nature of the problem(s) and the patient's and/or family's needs.

Usually, the presenting problem(s) are self limited or minor. Physicians typically spend 15 minutes face-to-face with the patient and/or family.

✣ **99348** **Home visit** for the evaluation and management of an established patient, which requires at least two of these three key components:

- **an expanded problem focused interval history;**
- **an expanded problem focused examination;**
- **medical decision making of low complexity.**

Counseling and/or coordination of care with other providers or agencies are provided consistent with the nature of the problem(s) and the patient's and/or family's needs.

Usually, the presenting problem(s) are of low to moderate severity. Physicians typically spend 25 minutes face-to-face with the patient and/or family.

✣ **99349** **Home visit** for the evaluation and management of an established patient, which requires at least two of these three key components:

- **a detailed interval history;**
- **a detailed examination;**
- **medical decision making of moderate complexity.**

Counseling and/or coordination of care with other providers or agencies are provided consistent with the nature of the problem(s) and the patient's and/or family's needs.

Usually, the presenting problem(s) are moderate to high severity. Physicians typically spend 40 minutes face-to-face with the patient and/or family.

✣ **99350** **Home visit** for the evaluation and management of an established patient, which requires at least two of these three key components:

- **a comprehensive interval history;**
- **a comprehensive examination;**
- **medical decision making of moderate to high complexity.**

Counseling and/or coordination of care with other providers or agencies are provided consistent with the nature of the problem(s) and the patient's and/or family's needs.

Usually, the presenting problem(s) are of moderate to high severity. The patient may be unstable or may have developed a significant new problem requiring immediate physician attention. Physicians typically spend 60 minutes face-to-face with the patient and/or family.

Prolonged Services

Prolonged Physician Service With Direct (Face-To-Face) Patient Contact

Codes 99354-99357 are used when a physician provides prolonged service involving direct (face-to-face) patient contact that is beyond the usual service in either the inpatient or outpatient setting. This service is reported in addition to other physician services, including evaluation and management services at any level. Appropriate codes should be selected for supplies provided or procedures performed in the care of the patient during this period.

Codes 99354-99357 are used to report the total duration of face-to-face time spent by a physician on a given date providing prolonged service, even if the time spent by the physician on that date is not continuous.

Code 99354 or 99356 is used to report the first hour of prolonged service on a given date, depending on the place of service.

Either code also may be used to report a total duration of prolonged service of 30-60 minutes on a given date. Either code should be used only once per date, even if the time spent by the physician is not continuous on that date. Prolonged service of less than 30 minutes total duration on a given date is not separately reported because the work involved is included in the total work of the evaluation and management codes.

Code 99355 or 99357 is used to report each additional 30 minutes beyond the first hour, depending on the place of service. Either code may also be used to report the final 15-30 minutes of prolonged service on a given date. Prolonged service of less than 15 minutes beyond the first hour or less than 15 minutes beyond the final 30 minutes is not reported separately.

The following examples illustrate the correct reporting of prolonged physician service with direct patient contact in the office setting:

Total Duration of Prolonged Services	Code(s)
less than 30 minutes (less than 1/2 hour)	Not reported separately
30-74 minutes (1/2 hr. - 1 hr. 14 min.)	99354 X 1
75-104 minutes (1 hr. 15 min. - 1 hr. 44 min.)	99354 X 1 AND 99355 X 1
105-134 minutes (1 hr. 45 min. - 2 hr. 14 min.)	99354 X 1 AND 99355 X 2
135-164 minutes (2 hr. 15 min. - 2 hr. 44 min.)	99354 X 1 AND 99355 X 3
165-194 minutes (2 hr. 45 min. - 3 hr. 14 min.)	99354 X 1 AND 99355 X 4

☆+ 99354 Prolonged physician service in the office or other outpatient setting requiring direct (face-to-face) patient contact beyond the usual service (eg, prolonged care and treatment of an acute asthmatic patient in an outpatient setting); first hour (List separately in addition to code for office or other outpatient Evaluation and Management service)

(Use 99354 in conjunction with 99201-99215, 99241-99245, 99301-99350)

☆+ 99355 each additional 30 minutes (List separately in addition to code for prolonged physician service)

(Use 99355 in conjunction with 99354)

✿+ 99356 Prolonged physician service in the inpatient setting, requiring direct (face-to-face) patient contact beyond the usual service (eg, maternal fetal monitoring for high risk delivery or other physiological monitoring, prolonged care of an acutely ill inpatient); first hour (List separately in addition to code for inpatient Evaluation and Management service)

(Use 99356 in conjunction with 99221-99233, 99251-99255, 99261-99263)

✿+ 99357 each additional 30 minutes (List separately in addition to code for prolonged physician service)

(Use 99357 in conjunction with 99356)

Prolonged Physician Service Without Direct (Face-To-Face) Patient Contact

Codes 99358 and 99359 are used when a physician provides prolonged service not involving direct (face-to-face) care that is beyond the usual service in either the inpatient or outpatient setting.

This service is to be reported in addition to other physician service, including evaluation and management services at any level.

Codes 99358 and 99359 are used to report the total duration of non-face-to-face time spent by a physician on a given date providing prolonged service, even if the time spent by the physician on that date is not continuous. Code 99358 is used to report the first hour of prolonged service on a given date regardless of the place of service.

It may also be used to report a total duration of prolonged service of 30-60 minutes on a given date. It should be used only once per date even if the time spent by the physician is not continuous on that date.

Prolonged service of less than 30 minutes total duration on a given date is not separately reported.

Code 99359 is used to report each additional 30 minutes beyond the first hour regardless of the place of service. It may also be used to report the final 15-30 minutes of prolonged service on a given date.

Prolonged service of less than 15 minutes beyond the first hour or less than 15 minutes beyond the final 30 minutes is not reported separately.

☆+ 99358 **Prolonged evaluation and management service** before and/or after direct (face-to-face) patient care (eg, review of extensive records and tests, communication with other professionals and/or the patient/family); first hour (List separately in addition to code(s) for other physician service(s) and/or inpatient or outpatient Evaluation and Management service)

☆+ 99359 each additional 30 minutes (List separately in addition to code for prolonged physician service)

(Use 99359 in conjunction with 99358)

(To report telephone calls, see 99371-99373)

Physician Standby Services

Code 99360 is used to report physician standby service that is requested by another physician and that involves prolonged physician attendance without direct (face-to-face) patient contact. The physician may not be providing care or services to other patients during this period. This code is not used to report time spent proctoring another physician. It is also not used if the period of standby ends with the performance of a procedure subject to a "surgical" package by the physician who was on standby.

Code 99360 is used to report the total duration of time spent by a physician on a given date on standby. Standby service of less than 30 minutes total duration on a given date is not reported separately.

Second and subsequent periods of standby beyond the first 30 minutes may be reported only if a full 30 minutes of standby was provided for each unit of service reported.

✤ 99360 **Physician standby service,** requiring prolonged physician attendance, each 30 minutes (eg, operative standby, standby for frozen section, for cesarean/high risk delivery, for monitoring EEG)

(For hospital mandated on call services, see 99026, 99027)

(99360 may be reported in addition to 99431, 99440 as appropriate)

(Do not report 99360 in conjunction with 99436)

Case Management Services

Physician case management is a process in which a physician is responsible for direct care of a patient, and for coordinating and controlling access to or initiating and/or supervising other health care services needed by the patient.

Team Conferences

□ **99361** **Medical conference** by a physician with interdisciplinary team of health professionals or representatives of community agencies to coordinate activities of patient care (patient not present); approximately 30 minutes

➔ *CPT Assistant* Feb 03:9, May 03:13, Mar 04:9, Apr 04:14

□ **99362** approximately 60 minutes

➔ *CPT Assistant* Feb 03:9, May 03:13, Mar 04:9, Apr 04:14

Telephone Calls

✣ **99371** **Telephone call** by a physician to patient or for consultation or medical management or for coordinating medical management with other health care professionals (eg, nurses, therapists, social workers, nutritionists, physicians, pharmacists); simple or brief (eg, to report on tests and/or laboratory results, to clarify or alter previous instructions, to integrate new information from other health professionals into the medical treatment plan, or to adjust therapy)

✣ **99372** intermediate (eg, to provide advice to an established patient on a new problem, to initiate therapy that can be handled by telephone, to discuss test results in detail, to coordinate medical management of a new problem in an established patient, to discuss and evaluate new information and details, or to initiate new plan of care)

✣ **99373** complex or lengthy (eg, lengthy counseling session with anxious or distraught patient, detailed or prolonged discussion with family members regarding seriously ill patient, lengthy communication necessary to coordinate complex services of several different health professionals working on different aspects of the total patient care plan)

Care Plan Oversight Services

Care Plan Oversight Services are reported separately from codes for office/outpatient, hospital, home, nursing facility or domiciliary services. The complexity and approximate physician time of the care plan oversight services provided within a 30-day period determine code selection. Only one physician may report services for a given period of time, to reflect that physician's sole or predominant supervisory role with a particular patient. These codes should not be reported for supervision of patients in nursing facilities or under the care of home health agencies unless they require recurrent supervision of therapy.

The work involved in providing very low intensity or infrequent supervision services is included in the pre- and post-encounter work for home, office/outpatient and nursing facility or domiciliary visit codes.

✣ **99374** **Physician supervision** of a patient under care of home health agency (patient not present) in home, domiciliary or equivalent environment (eg, Alzheimer's facility) requiring complex and multidisciplinary care modalities involving regular physician development and/or revision of care plans, review of subsequent reports of patient status, review of related laboratory and other studies, communication (including telephone calls) for purposes of assessment or care decisions with health care professional(s), family member(s), surrogate decision maker(s) (eg, legal guardian) and/or key caregiver(s) involved in patient's care, integration of new information into the medical treatment plan and/or adjustment of medical therapy, within a calendar month; 15-29 minutes

□ **99375** 30 minutes or more

✣ **99377** **Physician supervision** of a hospice patient (patient not present) requiring complex and multidisciplinary care modalities involving regular physician development and/or revision of care plans, review of subsequent reports of patient status, review of related laboratory and other studies, communication (including telephone calls) for purposes of assessment or care decisions with health care professional(s), family member(s), surrogate decision maker(s) (eg, legal guardian) and/or key caregiver(s) involved in patient's care, integration of new information into the medical treatment plan and/or adjustment of medical therapy, within a calendar month; 15-29 minutes

□ **99378** 30 minutes or more

✣ **99379** **Physician supervision** of a nursing facility patient (patient not present) requiring complex and multidisciplinary care modalities involving regular physician development and/or revision of care plans, review of subsequent reports of patient status, review of related laboratory and other studies, communication (including telephone calls) for purposes of assessment or care decisions with health care professional(s), family member(s), surrogate decision maker(s) (eg, legal guardian) and/or key caregiver(s) involved in patient's care, integration of new information into the medical treatment plan and/or adjustment of medical therapy, within a calendar month; 15-29 minutes

✣ **99380** 30 minutes or more

Preventive Medicine Services

The following codes are used to report the preventive medicine evaluation and management of infants, children, adolescents and adults.

The extent and focus of the services will largely depend on the age of the patient.

If an abnormality/ies is encountered or a preexisting problem is addressed in the process of performing this preventive medicine evaluation and management service, and if the problem/abnormality is significant enough to require additional work to perform the key components of a problem-oriented E/M service, then the appropriate Office/Outpatient code 99201-99215 should also be reported. Modifier 25 should be added to the Office/Outpatient code to indicate that a significant, separately identifiable Evaluation and Management service was provided by the same physician on the same day as the preventive medicine service. The appropriate preventive medicine service is additionally reported.

An insignificant or trivial problem/abnormality that is encountered in the process of performing the preventive medicine evaluation and management service and which does not require additional work and the performance of the key components of a problem-oriented E/M service should not be reported.

The "comprehensive" nature of the Preventive Medicine Services codes 99381-99397 reflects an age and gender appropriate history/exam and is NOT synonymous with the "comprehensive" examination required in Evaluation and Management codes 99201-99350.

Codes 99381-99397 include counseling/anticipatory guidance/risk factor reduction interventions which are provided at the time of the initial or periodic comprehensive preventive medicine examination. (Refer to codes 99401-99412 for reporting those counseling/anticipatory guidance/risk factor reduction interventions that are provided at an encounter separate from the preventive medicine examination.)

Immunizations and ancillary studies involving laboratory, radiology, other procedures, or screening tests identified with a specific CPT code are reported separately. For immunizations, see ►90465◄-90474 and 90476-90749.

New Patient

☐ **99381** **Initial comprehensive preventive medicine** evaluation and management of an individual including an age and gender appropriate history, examination, counseling/anticipatory guidance/risk factor reduction interventions, and the ordering of appropriate immunization(s), laboratory/diagnostic procedures, new patient; infant (age under 1 year)

☐ **99382** early childhood (age 1 through 4 years)

☐ **99383** late childhood (age 5 through 11 years)

☐ **99384** adolescent (age 12 through 17 years)

☐ **99385** 18-39 years

☐ **99386** 40-64 years

☐ **99387** 65 years and over

Established Patient

☐ **99391** **Periodic comprehensive preventive medicine** reevaluation and management of an individual including an age and gender appropriate history, examination, counseling/anticipatory guidance/risk factor reduction interventions, and the ordering of appropriate immunization(s), laboratory/diagnostic procedures, established patient; infant (age under 1 year)

☐ **99392** early childhood (age 1 through 4 years)

☐ **99393** late childhood (age 5 through 11 years)

☐ **99394** adolescent (age 12 through 17 years)

☐ **99395** 18-39 years

☐ **99396** 40-64 years

☐ **99397** 65 years and over

Counseling and/or Risk Factor Reduction Intervention

New or Established Patient

These codes are used to report services provided to individuals at a separate encounter for the purpose of promoting health and preventing illness or injury.

Preventive medicine counseling and risk factor reduction interventions provided as a separate encounter will vary with age and should address such issues as family problems, diet and exercise, substance abuse, sexual practices, injury prevention, dental health, and diagnostic and laboratory test results available at the time of the encounter.

These codes are not to be used to report counseling and risk factor reduction interventions provided to patients with symptoms or established illness. For counseling individual patients with symptoms or established illness, use the appropriate office, hospital or consultation or other evaluation and management codes. For counseling groups of patients with symptoms or established illness, use 99078.

Preventive Medicine, Individual Counseling

☐ **99401** **Preventive medicine counseling** and/or risk factor reduction intervention(s) provided to an individual (separate procedure); approximately 15 minutes

☐ **99402** approximately 30 minutes

☐ **99403** approximately 45 minutes

☐ **99404** approximately 60 minutes

Preventive Medicine, Group Counseling

☐ **99411** **Preventive medicine counseling** and/or risk factor reduction intervention(s) provided to individuals in a group setting (separate procedure); approximately 30 minutes

☐ **99412** approximately 60 minutes

Other Preventive Medicine Services

☐ **99420** **Administration and interpretation** of health risk assessment instrument (eg, health hazard appraisal)

☐ **99429** **Unlisted preventive** medicine service

Newborn Care

The following codes are used to report the services provided to newborns in several different settings.

For newborn hospital discharge services provided on a date subsequent to the admission date of the newborn, use 99238.

For discharge services provided to newborns admitted and discharged on the same date, use 99435.

➧ **99431** **History and examination** of the normal newborn infant, initiation of diagnostic and treatment programs and preparation of hospital records. (This code should also be used for birthing room deliveries.)

☆ **99432** **Normal newborn care** in other than hospital or birthing room setting, including physical examination of baby and conference(s) with parent(s)

✿ **99433** **Subsequent hospital care,** for the evaluation and management of a normal newborn, per day

☐ **99435** **History and examination** of the normal newborn infant, including the preparation of medical records. (This code should only be used for newborns assessed and discharged from the hospital or birthing room on the same date.)

☆ **99436** **Attendance** at delivery (when requested by delivering physician) and initial stabilization of newborn

(99436 may be reported in addition to 99431)

(Do not report 99436 in conjunction with 99440)

❖ **99440** **Newborn resuscitation**: provision of positive pressure ventilation and/or chest compressions in the presence of acute inadequate ventilation and/or cardiac output

Special Evaluation and Management Services

The following codes are used to report evaluations performed to establish baseline information prior to life or disability insurance certificates being issued. This service is performed in the office or other setting, and applies to both new and established patients. When using these codes, no active management of the problem(s) is undertaken during the encounter.

If other evaluation and management services and/or procedures are performed on the same date, the appropriate E/M or procedure code(s) should be reported in addition to these codes.

Basic Life and/or Disability Evaluation Services

☐ **99450** **Basic life** and/or disability examination that includes:

- **measurement of height, weight and blood pressure;**
- **completion of a medical history following a life insurance pro forma;**

- **collection of blood sample and/or urinalysis complying with "chain of custody" protocols; and**
- **completion of necessary documentation/certificates.**

Work Related or Medical Disability Evaluation Services

⚘ **99455** **Work related** or medical disability examination by the treating physician that includes:

- **completion of a medical history commensurate with the patient's condition;**
- **performance of an examination commensurate with the patient's condition;**
- **formulation of a diagnosis, assessment of capabilities and stability, and calculation of impairment;**
- **development of future medical treatment plan; and**
- **completion of necessary documentation/certificates and report.**

⚘ **99456** **Work related** or medical disability examination by other than the treating physician that includes:

- **completion of a medical history commensurate with the patient's condition;**
- **performance of an examination commensurate with the patient's condition;**
- **formulation of a diagnosis, assessment of capabilities and stability, and calculation of impairment;**
- **development of future medical treatment plan; and**
- **completion of necessary documentation/certificates and report.**

(Do not report 99455, 99456 in conjunction with 99080 for the completion of Workman's Compensation forms)

Other Evaluation and Management Services

⚘ **99499** **Unlisted evaluation and management** service

Anesthesia Guidelines

Services involving administration of anesthesia are reported by the use of the anesthesia five digit procedure code (00100-01999) plus modifier codes (defined under "Anesthesia Modifiers" later in these Guidelines).

The reporting of anesthesia services is appropriate by or under the responsible supervision of a physician. These services may include but are not limited to general, regional, supplementation of local anesthesia, or other supportive services in order to afford the patient the anesthesia care deemed optimal by the anesthesiologist during any procedure. These services include the usual preoperative and postoperative visits, the anesthesia care during the procedure, the administration of fluids and/or blood and the usual monitoring services (eg, ECG, temperature, blood pressure, oximetry, capnography, and mass spectrometry). Unusual forms of monitoring (eg, intra-arterial, central venous, and Swan-Ganz) are not included.

Items used by all physicians in reporting their services are presented in the **Introduction.** Some of the commonalities are repeated here for the convenience of those physicians referring to this section on **Anesthesia.** Other definitions and items unique to anesthesia are also listed.

To report sedation with or without analgesia (conscious sedation) provided by a physician also performing the service for which conscious sedation is being provided, see codes 99141, 99142. ►When any physician, other than the physician performing the procedure, provides anesthesia services as specified in *CPT* guidelines (conscious sedation or otherwise), the Anesthesia codes should be reported.◄

To report regional or general anesthesia provided by a physician also performing the services for which the anesthesia is being provided, see modifier 47 in Appendix A.

Time Reporting

Time for anesthesia procedures may be reported as is customary in the local area. Anesthesia time begins when the anesthesiologist begins to prepare the patient for the induction of anesthesia in the operating room or in an equivalent area and ends when the anesthesiologist is no longer in personal attendance, that is, when the patient may be safely placed under postoperative supervision.

Physician's Services

Physician's services rendered in the office, home, or hospital, consultation, and other medical services are listed in the section entitled **Evaluation and Management Services** (99200 series) found in the front of the book, beginning on page 1. "Special Services and Reporting" (99000 series) are presented in the **Medicine** section.

Materials Supplied by Physician

Supplies and materials provided by the physician (eg, sterile trays, drugs) over and above those usually included with the office visit or other services rendered may be listed separately. List drugs, tray supplies, and materials provided. Identify as 99070.

Separate or Multiple Procedures

When multiple surgical procedures are performed during a single anesthetic administration, the anesthesia code representing the most complex procedure is reported. The time reported is the combined total for all procedures.

Special Report

A service that is rarely provided, unusual, variable, or new may require a special report in determining medical appropriateness of the service. Pertinent information should include an adequate definition or description of the nature, extent, and need for the procedure; and the time, effort, and equipment necessary to provide the service. Additional items which may be included are:

- complexity of symptoms;
- final diagnosis;
- pertinent physical findings;
- diagnostic and therapeutic procedures;
- concurrent problems;
- follow-up care.

Anesthesia Modifiers

All anesthesia services are reported by use of the anesthesia five digit procedure code (00100-01999) plus the addition of a physical status modifier. The use of other optional modifiers may be appropriate.

Physical Status Modifiers

Physical Status modifiers are represented by the initial letter 'P' followed by a single digit from 1 to 6 defined below.

P1-A normal healthy patient.

P2-A patient with mild systemic disease.

P3-A patient with severe systemic disease.

P4-A patient with severe systemic disease that is a constant threat to life.

P5-A moribund patient who is not expected to survive without the operation.

P6-A declared brain-dead patient whose organs are being removed for donor purposes.

The above six levels are consistent with the American Society of Anesthesiologists (ASA) ranking of patient physical status. Physical status is included in *CPT* to distinguish among various levels of complexity of the anesthesia service provided.

Example: 00100-P1

Qualifying Circumstances

More than one may be selected.

Many anesthesia services are provided under particularly difficult circumstances, depending on factors such as extraordinary condition of patient, notable operative conditions, and/or unusual risk factors. This section includes a list of important qualifying circumstances that significantly impact on the character of the anesthesia service provided. These procedures would not be reported alone but would be reported as additional procedure numbers qualifying an anesthesia procedure or service.

✣+ 99100 Anesthesia for patient of extreme age, under 1 year and over 70 (List separately in addition to code for primary anesthesia procedure)

(For procedure performed on infants less than 1 year of age at time of surgery, see 00326, 00834, 00836)

✣+ 99116 Anesthesia complicated by utilization of total body hypothermia (List separately in addition to code for primary anesthesia procedure)

✣+ 99135 Anesthesia complicated by utilization of controlled hypotension (List separately in addition to code for primary anesthesia procedure)

✣+ 99140 Anesthesia complicated by emergency conditions (specify) (List separately in addition to code for primary anesthesia procedure)

(An emergency is defined as existing when delay in treatment of the patient would lead to a significant increase in the threat to life or body part.)

Anesthesia

Head

☆ 00100 Anesthesia for procedures on salivary glands, including biopsy

☆ 00102 Anesthesia for procedures involving plastic repair of cleft lip
➔ *CPT Changes: An Insider's View* 2000

☆ 00103 Anesthesia for reconstructive procedures of eyelid (eg, blepharoplasty, ptosis surgery)

☆ 00104 Anesthesia for electroconvulsive therapy

☆ 00120 Anesthesia for procedures on external, middle, and inner ear including biopsy; not otherwise specified

☆ 00124 otoscopy

☆ 00126 tympanotomy

☆ 00140 Anesthesia for procedures on eye; not otherwise specified

☆ 00142 lens surgery

☆ 00144 corneal transplant

☆ 00145 vitreoretinal surgery
➔ *CPT Changes: An Insider's View* 2001

☆ 00147 iridectomy

☆ 00148 ophthalmoscopy

☆ 00160 Anesthesia for procedures on nose and accessory sinuses; not otherwise specified

☆ 00162 radical surgery

☆ 00164 biopsy, soft tissue

☆ 00170 Anesthesia for intraoral procedures, including biopsy; not otherwise specified

☆ 00172 repair of cleft palate

☆ 00174 excision of retropharyngeal tumor

✿ 00176 radical surgery

☆ 00190 Anesthesia for procedures on facial bones or skull; not otherwise specified

✿ 00192 radical surgery (including prognathism)

☆ 00210 Anesthesia for intracranial procedures; not otherwise specified

☆ 00212 subdural taps

✿ 00214 burr holes, including ventriculography
➔ *CPT Changes: An Insider's View* 2000

✿ 00215 cranioplasty or elevation of depressed skull fracture, extradural (simple or compound)

☆ 00216 vascular procedures

☆ 00218 procedures in sitting position

☆ 00220 cerebrospinal fluid shunting procedures

☆ 00222 electrocoagulation of intracranial nerve

Neck

☆ 00300 Anesthesia for all procedures on the integumentary system, muscles and nerves of head, neck, and posterior trunk, not otherwise specified

☆ 00320 Anesthesia for all procedures on esophagus, thyroid, larynx, trachea and lymphatic system of neck; not otherwise specified, age 1 year or older

☆ 00322 needle biopsy of thyroid

(For procedures on cervical spine and cord, see 00600, 00604, 00670)

☆ 00326 Anesthesia for all procedures on the larynx and trachea in children less than 1 year of age

(Do not report 00326 in conjunction with 99100)

☆ 00350 Anesthesia for procedures on major vessels of neck; not otherwise specified

☆ 00352 simple ligation

(For arteriography, use 01916)

Thorax (Chest Wall and Shoulder Girdle)

☆ 00400 Anesthesia for procedures on the integumentary system on the extremities, anterior trunk and perineum; not otherwise specified

☆ 00402 reconstructive procedures on breast (eg, reduction or augmentation mammoplasty, muscle flaps)

✿ 00404 radical or modified radical procedures on breast

✿ 00406 radical or modified radical procedures on breast with internal mammary node dissection

☆ 00410 electrical conversion of arrhythmias

☆ 00450 Anesthesia for procedures on clavicle and scapula; not otherwise specified

✿ 00452 radical surgery

☆ 00454 biopsy of clavicle

☆ 00470 Anesthesia for partial rib resection; not otherwise specified

☆ 00472 thoracoplasty (any type)

✿ 00474 radical procedures (eg, pectus excavatum)

Intrathoracic

☆ 00500 Anesthesia for all procedures on esophagus

☆ 00520 Anesthesia for closed chest procedures; (including bronchoscopy) not otherwise specified
➲ *CPT Changes: An Insider's View* 2000

☆ 00522 needle biopsy of pleura

✿ 00524 pneumocentesis

☆ 00528 mediastinoscopy and diagnostic thoracoscopy not utilizing one lung ventilation

(For tracheobronchial reconstruction, use 00539)

☆ 00529 mediastinoscopy and diagnostic thoracoscopy utilizing one lung ventilation
➲ *CPT Changes: An Insider's View* 2004

☆ 00530 Anesthesia for permanent transvenous pacemaker insertion
➲ *CPT Changes: An Insider's View* 2001

☆ 00532 Anesthesia for access to central venous circulation

☆ 00534 Anesthesia for transvenous insertion or replacement of pacing cardioverter-defibrillator

(For transthoracic approach, use 00560)

☆ 00537 Anesthesia for cardiac electrophysiologic procedures including radiofrequency ablation
➲ *CPT Changes: An Insider's View* 2001

☆ 00539 Anesthesia for tracheobronchial reconstruction

✿ 00540 Anesthesia for thoracotomy procedures involving lungs, pleura, diaphragm, and mediastinum (including surgical thoracoscopy); not otherwise specified

☆ 00541 utilizing one lung ventilation

✿ 00542 decortication

(00544 has been deleted. To report, use 00542)

✿ 00546 pulmonary resection with thoracoplasty

☆ 00548 intrathoracic procedures on the trachea and bronchi

☆ 00550 Anesthesia for sternal debridement

✿ 00560 Anesthesia for procedures on heart, pericardial sac, and great vessels of chest; without pump oxygenator

✿● 00561 with pump oxygenator, under one year of age

►(Do not report 00561 in conjunction with 99100, 99116, and 99135)◄

✿ 00562 with pump oxygenator

☆ 00563 with pump oxygenator with hypothermic circulatory arrest

☆ 00566 Anesthesia for direct coronary artery bypass grafting without pump oxygenator

✿ 00580 Anesthesia for heart transplant or heart/lung transplant

Spine and Spinal Cord

☆ 00600 Anesthesia for procedures on cervical spine and cord; not otherwise specified

(For myelography and diskography, see radiological procedures 01905)

✿ 00604 procedures with patient in the sitting position

☆ 00620 Anesthesia for procedures on thoracic spine and cord; not otherwise specified

✿ 00622 thoracolumbar sympathectomy

☆ 00630 Anesthesia for procedures in lumbar region; not otherwise specified

✿ 00632 lumbar sympathectomy

✿ 00634 chemonucleolysis

☆ 00635 diagnostic or therapeutic lumbar puncture
➲ *CPT Changes: An Insider's View* 2001

☆ 00640 Anesthesia for manipulation of the spine or for closed procedures on the cervical, thoracic or lumbar spine
➲ *CPT Changes: An Insider's View* 2003

✿ 00670 Anesthesia for extensive spine and spinal cord procedures (eg, spinal instrumentation or vascular procedures)

Upper Abdomen

☆ **00700** Anesthesia for procedures on upper anterior abdominal wall; not otherwise specified

☆ **00702** percutaneous liver biopsy

☆ **00730** Anesthesia for procedures on upper posterior abdominal wall

☆ **00740** Anesthesia for upper gastrointestinal endoscopic procedures, endoscope introduced proximal to duodenum
➲ *CPT Changes: An Insider's View* 2000

☆ **00750** Anesthesia for hernia repairs in upper abdomen; not otherwise specified

☆ **00752** lumbar and ventral (incisional) hernias and/or wound dehiscence

☆ **00754** omphalocele

☆ **00756** transabdominal repair of diaphragmatic hernia

☆ **00770** Anesthesia for all procedures on major abdominal blood vessels

☆ **00790** Anesthesia for intraperitoneal procedures in upper abdomen including laparoscopy; not otherwise specified

✿ **00792** partial hepatectomy or management of liver hemorrhage (excluding liver biopsy)

✿ **00794** pancreatectomy, partial or total (eg, Whipple procedure)

✿ **00796** liver transplant (recipient)

(For harvesting of liver, use 01990)

☆ **00797** gastric restrictive procedure for morbid obesity

Lower Abdomen

☆ **00800** Anesthesia for procedures on lower anterior abdominal wall; not otherwise specified

✿ **00802** panniculectomy

☆ **00810** Anesthesia for lower intestinal endoscopic procedures, endoscope introduced distal to duodenum
➲ *CPT Changes: An Insider's View* 2000

☆ **00820** Anesthesia for procedures on lower posterior abdominal wall

☆ **00830** Anesthesia for hernia repairs in lower abdomen; not otherwise specified

☆ **00832** ventral and incisional hernias

(For hernia repairs in the infant 1 year of age or younger, see 00834, 00836)

☆ **00834** Anesthesia for hernia repairs in the lower abdomen not otherwise specified, under 1 year of age
➲ *CPT Changes: An Insider's View* 2003

(Do not report 00834 in conjunction with 99100)

☆ **00836** Anesthesia for hernia repairs in the lower abdomen not otherwise specified, infants less than 37 weeks gestational age at birth and less than 50 weeks gestational age at time of surgery
➲ *CPT Changes: An Insider's View* 2003

(Do not report 00836 in conjunction with 99100)

☆ **00840** Anesthesia for intraperitoneal procedures in lower abdomen including laparoscopy; not otherwise specified

☆ **00842** amniocentesis

✿ **00844** abdominoperineal resection

✿ **00846** radical hysterectomy

✿ **00848** pelvic exenteration

☆ **00851** tubal ligation/transection
➲ *CPT Changes: An Insider's View* 2002

☆ **00860** Anesthesia for extraperitoneal procedures in lower abdomen, including urinary tract; not otherwise specified

☆ **00862** renal procedures, including upper 1/3 of ureter, or donor nephrectomy

✿ **00864** total cystectomy

✿ **00865** radical prostatectomy (suprapubic, retropubic)

✿ **00866** adrenalectomy

✿ **00868** renal transplant (recipient)

(For donor nephrectomy, use 00862)

(For harvesting kidney from brain-dead patient, use 01990)

(00869 has been deleted. To report, use 00921)

☆ **00870** cystolithotomy

☆ **00872** Anesthesia for lithotripsy, extracorporeal shock wave; with water bath

☆ **00873** without water bath

☆ **00880** Anesthesia for procedures on major lower abdominal vessels; not otherwise specified

✿ **00882** inferior vena cava ligation

Perineum

(For perineal procedures on integumentary system, muscles and nerves, see 00300, 00400)

☆ **00902** Anesthesia for; anorectal procedure
➔ *CPT Changes: An Insider's View* 2001

✿ **00904** radical perineal procedure

☆ **00906** vulvectomy

✿ **00908** perineal prostatectomy

☆ **00910** Anesthesia for transurethral procedures (including urethrocystoscopy); not otherwise specified

☆ **00912** transurethral resection of bladder tumor(s)

☆ **00914** transurethral resection of prostate

☆ **00916** post-transurethral resection bleeding

☆ **00918** with fragmentation, manipulation and/or removal of ureteral calculus
➔ *CPT Changes: An Insider's View* 2000

☆ **00920** Anesthesia for procedures on male genitalia (including open urethral procedures); not otherwise specified

☆ **00921** vasectomy, unilateral or bilateral
➔ *CPT Changes: An Insider's View* 2003

☆ **00922** seminal vesicles

☆ **00924** undescended testis, unilateral or bilateral

☆ **00926** radical orchiectomy, inguinal

☆ **00928** radical orchiectomy, abdominal

☆ **00930** orchiopexy, unilateral or bilateral

✿ **00932** complete amputation of penis

✿ **00934** radical amputation of penis with bilateral inguinal lymphadenectomy

✿ **00936** radical amputation of penis with bilateral inguinal and iliac lymphadenectomy

☆ **00938** insertion of penile prosthesis (perineal approach)

☆ **00940** Anesthesia for vaginal procedures (including biopsy of labia, vagina, cervix or endometrium); not otherwise specified

☆ **00942** colpotomy, vaginectomy, colporrhaphy, and open urethral procedures
➔ *CPT Changes: An Insider's View* 2001, 2002

✿ **00944** vaginal hysterectomy

☆ **00948** cervical cerclage

☆ **00950** culdoscopy

☆ **00952** hysteroscopy and/or hysterosalpingography
➔ *CPT Changes: An Insider's View* 2000

Pelvis (Except Hip)

☆ **01112** Anesthesia for bone marrow aspiration and/or biopsy, anterior or posterior iliac crest
➔ *CPT Changes: An Insider's View* 2001

☆ **01120** Anesthesia for procedures on bony pelvis

☆ **01130** Anesthesia for body cast application or revision

✿ **01140** Anesthesia for interpelviabdominal (hindquarter) amputation

✿ **01150** Anesthesia for radical procedures for tumor of pelvis, except hindquarter amputation

☆ **01160** Anesthesia for closed procedures involving symphysis pubis or sacroiliac joint

☆ **01170** Anesthesia for open procedures involving symphysis pubis or sacroiliac joint

☆ **01173** Anesthesia for open repair of fracture disruption of pelvis or column fracture involving acetabulum
➔ *CPT Changes: An Insider's View* 2004

☆ **01180** Anesthesia for obturator neurectomy; extrapelvic

✿ **01190** intrapelvic

Upper Leg (Except Knee)

☆ **01200** Anesthesia for all closed procedures involving hip joint

☆ **01202** Anesthesia for arthroscopic procedures of hip joint

☆ **01210** Anesthesia for open procedures involving hip joint; not otherwise specified

✿ **01212** hip disarticulation

✿ **01214** total hip arthroplasty

☆ **01215** revision of total hip arthroplasty

☆ **01220** Anesthesia for all closed procedures involving upper 2/3 of femur

☆ **01230** Anesthesia for open procedures involving upper 2/3 of femur; not otherwise specified

✿ **01232** amputation

✿ **01234** radical resection

☆ **01250** Anesthesia for all procedures on nerves, muscles, tendons, fascia, and bursae of upper leg

☆ **01260** Anesthesia for all procedures involving veins of upper leg, including exploration

☆ 01270 Anesthesia for procedures involving arteries of upper leg, including bypass graft; not otherwise specified

✿ 01272 femoral artery ligation

✿ 01274 femoral artery embolectomy

Knee and Popliteal Area

Surgical endoscopy/arthroscopy always includes a diagnostic endoscopy/arthroscopy.

☆ 01320 Anesthesia for all procedures on nerves, muscles, tendons, fascia, and bursae of knee and/or popliteal area

☆ 01340 Anesthesia for all closed procedures on lower 1/3 of femur

☆ 01360 Anesthesia for all open procedures on lower 1/3 of femur

☆ 01380 Anesthesia for all closed procedures on knee joint

☆ 01382 Anesthesia for diagnostic arthroscopic procedures of knee joint

☆ 01390 Anesthesia for all closed procedures on upper ends of tibia, fibula, and/or patella

☆ 01392 Anesthesia for all open procedures on upper ends of tibia, fibula, and/or patella

☆ 01400 Anesthesia for open or surgical arthroscopic procedures on knee joint; not otherwise specified

✿ 01402 total knee arthroplasty

✿ 01404 disarticulation at knee

☆ 01420 Anesthesia for all cast applications, removal, or repair involving knee joint

☆ 01430 Anesthesia for procedures on veins of knee and popliteal area; not otherwise specified

☆ 01432 arteriovenous fistula

☆ 01440 Anesthesia for procedures on arteries of knee and popliteal area; not otherwise specified

✿ 01442 popliteal thromboendarterectomy, with or without patch graft

✿ 01444 popliteal excision and graft or repair for occlusion or aneurysm

Lower Leg (Below Knee, Includes Ankle and Foot)

Surgical endoscopy/arthroscopy always includes a diagnostic endoscopy/arthroscopy.

☆ 01462 Anesthesia for all closed procedures on lower leg, ankle, and foot

☆ 01464 Anesthesia for arthroscopic procedures of ankle and/or foot

☆ 01470 Anesthesia for procedures on nerves, muscles, tendons, and fascia of lower leg, ankle, and foot; not otherwise specified

☆ 01472 repair of ruptured Achilles tendon, with or without graft

☆ 01474 gastrocnemius recession (eg, Strayer procedure)

☆ 01480 Anesthesia for open procedures on bones of lower leg, ankle, and foot; not otherwise specified

☆ 01482 radical resection (including below knee amputation)

☆ 01484 osteotomy or osteoplasty of tibia and/or fibula

✿ 01486 total ankle replacement

☆ 01490 Anesthesia for lower leg cast application, removal, or repair

☆ 01500 Anesthesia for procedures on arteries of lower leg, including bypass graft; not otherwise specified

✿ 01502 embolectomy, direct or with catheter

☆ 01520 Anesthesia for procedures on veins of lower leg; not otherwise specified

☆ 01522 venous thrombectomy, direct or with catheter

Shoulder and Axilla

Surgical endoscopy/arthroscopy always includes a diagnostic endoscopy/arthroscopy.

Includes humeral head and neck, sternoclavicular joint, acromioclavicular joint, and shoulder joint.

☆ 01610 Anesthesia for all procedures on nerves, muscles, tendons, fascia, and bursae of shoulder and axilla

☆ 01620 Anesthesia for all closed procedures on humeral head and neck, sternoclavicular joint, acromioclavicular joint, and shoulder joint

☆ 01622 Anesthesia for diagnostic arthroscopic procedures of shoulder joint
➲ *CPT Changes: An Insider's View* 2003

☆ 01630 Anesthesia for open or surgical arthroscopic procedures on humeral head and neck, sternoclavicular joint, acromioclavicular joint, and shoulder joint; not otherwise specified
➲ *CPT Changes: An Insider's View* 2003

✿ 01632 radical resection

✿ 01634 shoulder disarticulation

✿ 01636 interthoracoscapular (forequarter) amputation

✿ 01638 total shoulder replacement

☆ 01650 Anesthesia for procedures on arteries of shoulder and axilla; not otherwise specified

✿ 01652 axillary-brachial aneurysm

✿ 01654 bypass graft

✿ 01656 axillary-femoral bypass graft

☆ 01670 Anesthesia for all procedures on veins of shoulder and axilla

☆ 01680 Anesthesia for shoulder cast application, removal or repair; not otherwise specified

☆ 01682 shoulder spica

Upper Arm and Elbow

Surgical endoscopy/arthroscopy always includes a diagnostic endoscopy/arthroscopy.

☆ 01710 Anesthesia for procedures on nerves, muscles, tendons, fascia, and bursae of upper arm and elbow; not otherwise specified

☆ 01712 tenotomy, elbow to shoulder, open

☆ 01714 tenoplasty, elbow to shoulder

☆ 01716 tenodesis, rupture of long tendon of biceps

☆ 01730 Anesthesia for all closed procedures on humerus and elbow

☆ 01732 Anesthesia for diagnostic arthroscopic procedures of elbow joint
➲ *CPT Changes: An Insider's View* 2003

☆ 01740 Anesthesia for open or surgical arthroscopic procedures of the elbow; not otherwise specified
➲ *CPT Changes: An Insider's View* 2003

☆ 01742 osteotomy of humerus

☆ 01744 repair of nonunion or malunion of humerus

✿ 01756 radical procedures

☆ 01758 excision of cyst or tumor of humerus

☆ 01760 total elbow replacement

☆ 01770 Anesthesia for procedures on arteries of upper arm and elbow; not otherwise specified

☆ 01772 embolectomy

☆ 01780 Anesthesia for procedures on veins of upper arm and elbow; not otherwise specified

☆ 01782 phleborrhaphy

Forearm, Wrist, and Hand

☆ 01810 Anesthesia for all procedures on nerves, muscles, tendons, fascia, and bursae of forearm, wrist, and hand

☆ 01820 Anesthesia for all closed procedures on radius, ulna, wrist, or hand bones

☆ 01829 Anesthesia for diagnostic arthroscopic procedures on the wrist
➲ *CPT Changes: An Insider's View* 2003

☆ 01830 Anesthesia for open or surgical arthroscopic/endoscopic procedures on distal radius, distal ulna, wrist, or hand joints; not otherwise specified
➲ *CPT Changes: An Insider's View* 2003

☆ 01832 total wrist replacement

☆ 01840 Anesthesia for procedures on arteries of forearm, wrist, and hand; not otherwise specified

☆ 01842 embolectomy

☆ 01844 Anesthesia for vascular shunt, or shunt revision, any type (eg, dialysis)

☆ 01850 Anesthesia for procedures on veins of forearm, wrist, and hand; not otherwise specified

☆ 01852 phleborrhaphy

☆ 01860 Anesthesia for forearm, wrist, or hand cast application, removal, or repair

Radiological Procedures

☆ 01905 Anesthesia for myelography, diskography, vertebroplasty
➲ *CPT Changes: An Insider's View* 2002

☆ 01916 Anesthesia for diagnostic arteriography/venography
➲ *CPT Changes: An Insider's View* 2002

(Do not report 01916 in conjunction with therapeutic codes 01924-01926, 01930-01933)

☆ **01920** Anesthesia for cardiac catheterization including coronary angiography and ventriculography (not to include Swan-Ganz catheter)

☆ **01922** Anesthesia for non-invasive imaging or radiation therapy

☆ **01924** Anesthesia for therapeutic interventional radiologic procedures involving the arterial system; not otherwise specified
➔ *CPT Changes: An Insider's View* 2002

☆ **01925** carotid or coronary

☆ **01926** intracranial, intracardiac, or aortic

☆ **01930** Anesthesia for therapeutic interventional radiologic procedures involving the venous/lymphatic system (not to include access to the central circulation); not otherwise specified
➔ *CPT Changes: An Insider's View* 2002

☆ **01931** intrahepatic or portal circulation (eg, transcutaneous porto-caval shunt (TIPS))

☆ **01932** intrathoracic or jugular

☆ **01933** intracranial

Burn Excisions or Debridement

☆ **01951** Anesthesia for second and third degree burn excision or debridement with or without skin grafting, any site, for total body surface area (TBSA) treated during anesthesia and surgery; less than four percent total body surface area

☆ **01952** between four and nine percent of total body surface area

☆+ **01953** each additional nine percent total body surface area or part thereof (List separately in addition to code for primary procedure)

(Use 01953 in conjunction with 01952)

Obstetric

☆ **01958** Anesthesia for external cephalic version procedure
➔ *CPT Changes: An Insider's View* 2004

☆ **01960** Anesthesia for vaginal delivery only

☆ **01961** Anesthesia for cesarean delivery only

☆ **01962** Anesthesia for urgent hysterectomy following delivery

☆ **01963** Anesthesia for cesarean hysterectomy without any labor analgesia/anesthesia care

☆ **01964** Anesthesia for abortion procedures

☆ **01967** Neuraxial labor analgesia/anesthesia for planned vaginal delivery (this includes any repeat subarachnoid needle placement and drug injection and/or any necessary replacement of an epidural catheter during labor)

☆+ **01968** Anesthesia for cesarean delivery following neuraxial labor analgesia/anesthesia (List separately in addition to code for primary procedure performed)

(Use 01968 in conjunction with 01967)

☆+ **01969** Anesthesia for cesarean hysterectomy following neuraxial labor analgesia/anesthesia (List separately in addition to code for primary procedure performed)

(Use 01969 in conjunction with 01967)

Other Procedures

✿ **01990** Physiological support for harvesting of organ(s) from brain-dead patient

☆ **01991** Anesthesia for diagnostic or therapeutic nerve blocks and injections (when block or injection is performed by a different provider); other than the prone position
➔ *CPT Changes: An Insider's View* 2003

☆ **01992** prone position
➔ *CPT Changes: An Insider's View* 2003

(Do not report 01991or 01992 in conjunction with 99141)

☆ **01995** Regional intravenous administration of local anesthetic agent or other medication (upper or lower extremity)
➔ *CPT Changes: An Insider's View* 2002

(For intra-arterial or intravenous therapy for pain management, see 90783, 90784)

☆ **01996** Daily hospital management of epidural or subarachnoid continuous drug administration
➔ *CPT Changes: An Insider's View* 2003

(Report code 01996 for daily hospital management of continuous epidural or subarachnoid drug administration performed after insertion of an epidural or subarachnoid catheter)

☆ **01999** Unlisted anesthesia procedure(s)

Notes

Surgery Guidelines

Items used by all physicians in reporting their services are presented in the **Introduction.** Some of the commonalities are repeated here for the convenience of those physicians referring to this section on **Surgery.** Other definitions and items unique to Surgery are also listed.

Physicians' Services

Physicians' services rendered in the office, home, or hospital, consultations, and other medical services are listed in the section entitled **Evaluation and Management Services** (►99201-99499◄) found in the front of the book, beginning on page 9. "Special Services and Reports" (99000 series) is presented in the **Medicine** section.

CPT Surgical Package Definition

The services provided by the physician to any patient by their very nature are variable. The CPT codes that represent a readily identifiable surgical procedure thereby include, on a procedure-by-procedure basis, a variety of services. In defining the specific services "included" in a given CPT surgical code, the following services are always included in addition to the operation per se:

- local infiltration, metacarpal/metatarsal/digital block or topical anesthesia;
- subsequent to the decision for surgery, one related E/M encounter on the date immediately prior to or on the date of procedure (including history and physical);
- immediate postoperative care, including dictating operative notes, talking with the family and other physicians;
- writing orders;
- evaluating the patient in the postanesthesia recovery area;
- typical postoperative follow-up care.

Follow-Up Care for Diagnostic Procedures

Follow-up care for diagnostic procedures (eg, endoscopy, arthroscopy, injection procedures for radiography) includes only that care related to recovery from the diagnostic procedure itself. Care of the condition for which the diagnostic procedure was performed or of other concomitant conditions is not included and may be listed separately.

Follow-Up Care for Therapeutic Surgical Procedures

Follow-up care for therapeutic surgical procedures includes only that care which is usually a part of the surgical service. Complications, exacerbations, recurrence, or the presence of other diseases or injuries requiring additional services should be separately reported.

Materials Supplied by Physician

Supplies and materials provided by the physician (eg, sterile trays/drugs), over and above those usually included with the procedure(s) rendered are reported separately. List drugs, trays, supplies, and materials provided. Identify as 99070 or specific supply code.

Reporting More Than One Procedure/Service

When a physician performs more than one procedure/service on the same date, same session or during a post-operative period (subject to the "surgical package" concept), several CPT modifiers may apply. (See Appendix A for definition.)

27 Multiple Outpatient Hospital E/M Encounters on the Same Date

For hospital outpatient reporting purposes, utilization of hospital resources related to separate and distinct E/M encounters performed in multiple outpatient hospital settings on the same date may be reported by adding modifier 27 to each appropriate level outpatient and/or emergency department E/M code(s). This modifier provides a means of reporting circumstances involving evaluation and management services provided by physician(s) in more than one (multiple) outpatient hospital setting(s) (eg, hospital emergency department, clinic). **Note:** This modifier is not to be used for physician reporting of multiple E/M services performed by the same physician on the same date. For physician reporting of all outpatient evaluation and management services provided by the same physician on the same date and performed in multiple outpatient setting(s) (eg, hospital emergency department, clinic), see **Evaluation and Management, Emergency Department,** or **Preventive Medicine Services** codes.

51 Multiple Procedures

When multiple procedures/services (other than evaluation and management) are performed at the same session, report the most significant procedure first, with all other procedures listed with modifier 51 appended. For a list of procedures exempt from the use of modifier 51, see Appendices D and E.

58 Staged or Related Procedure or Service by the Same Physician During the Postoperative Period

When a procedure(s) is prospectively planned as a staged procedure, or when the secondary and subsequent procedure(s) is more extensive, or to indicate therapy following a diagnostic surgical procedure, use modifier 58 with the staged procedure(s).

59 Distinct Procedural Service

For procedure(s)/service(s) not ordinarily performed or encountered on the same day by the same physician, but appropriate under certain circumstances (eg, different site or organ system, separate excision or lesion), use modifier 59.

76 Repeat Procedure by Same Physician

When a procedure or service is repeated by the same physician subsequent to the original service, use modifier 76.

77 Repeat Procedure by Another Physician

When a procedure is repeated by another physician subsequent to the original service, use modifier 77.

78 Return to the Operating Room for a Related Procedure During the Postoperative Period

When a procedure, related to the initial procedure, requires a return to the operating room during the postoperative period of that initial procedure, use modifier 78.

79 Unrelated Procedure or Service by the Same Physician During the Postoperative Period

When a procedure, unrelated to the initial procedure, is performed by the same physician during the postoperative period of the initial procedure, use modifier 79.

91 Repeat Clinical Diagnostic Laboratory Test

In the course of treatment of the patient, it may be necessary to repeat the same laboratory test on the same day to obtain subsequent (multiple) test results. Under these circumstances, the laboratory test performed can be identified by its usual procedure number and the addition of modifier 91. **Note:** This modifier may not be used when tests are rerun to confirm initial results; due to testing problems with specimens or equipment; or for any other reason when a normal, one-time, reportable result is all that is required. This modifier may not be used when other code(s) describe a series of test results (eg, glucose tolerance tests, evocative/suppression testing). This modifier may only be used for laboratory test(s) performed more than once on the same day on the same patient.

Separate Procedure

Some of the procedures or services listed in *CPT* that are commonly carried out as an integral component of a total service or procedure have been identified by the inclusion of the term "separate procedure." The codes designated as "separate procedure" should not be reported in addition to the code for the total procedure or service of which it is considered an integral component.

However, when a procedure or service that is designated as a "separate procedure" is carried out independently or considered to be unrelated or distinct from other procedures/services provided at that time, it may be reported by itself, or in addition to other procedures/services by appending modifier 59 to the specific "separate procedure" code to indicate that the procedure is not considered to be a component of another procedure, but is a distinct, independent procedure. This may represent a different session or patient encounter, different procedure or surgery, different site or organ system, separate incision/excision, separate lesion, or separate injury (or area of injury in extensive injuries).

Subsection Information

Several of the subheadings or subsections have special needs or instructions unique to that section. Where these are indicated (eg, "Maternity Care and Delivery"), special **"Notes"** will be presented preceding those procedural terminology listings, referring to that subsection specifically. If there is an "Unlisted Procedure" code number (see below) for the individual subsection, it will also be shown. Those subsections within the **Surgery** section that have **"Notes"** are as follows:

Biopsy 11100-11101

Removal of Skin Tags 11200-11201

Shaving of Lesions 11300-11313

Excision—Benign Lesions 11400-11471

Excision—Malignant Lesions 11600-11646

Repair (Closure) 12001-13160

Adjacent Tissue Transfer or Rearrangement 14000-14350

Free Skin Grafts 15000-15401

Flaps (Skin and/or Deep Tissue) 15570-15999

Burns, Local Treatment 16000-16036

Destruction 17000-17286

Mohs Micrographic Surgery 17304-17310

►**Breast—Excision** .... 19100-19272◄

Musculoskeletal 20000-29999

Wound Exploration—Trauma 20100-20103

Grafts (or Implants) 20900-20999

Introduction or Removal 21076-21116

Spine: (Vertebral Column) 22100-22855

Spine: Excision 22100-22116

Spine: Osteotomy 22210-22226

Spine: Fracture/Dislocation 22305-22328

Spine: Arthrodesis 22548-22812

►**Spine: Exploration** .... 22830◄

Spinal Instrumentation 22840-22855

Casting and Strapping 29000-29750

Musculoskeletal: Endoscopy/Arthroscopy 29800-29999

Respiratory: Endoscopy 31231-31294, 31505-31579, 31615-31656, 32601-32665

Cardiovascular System 33010-37799

Pacing Cardioverter-Pacemaker or Defibrillator 33200-33249

Venous—CABG 33510-33516

Arteries and Veins 34001-35907

Endovascular Repair of Abdominal Aortic Aneurysm 34800-34826

Endovascular Repair of Illiac Aneurysm 34900

Transluminal Angioplasty 35450-35476

Transluminal Atherectomy 35480-35495

Bypass Graft 35500-35572

Composite Grafts 35681-35683

Adjuvant Techniques 35685-35686

Vascular Injection Procedures: Intravenous 36000-36015

Central Venous Access Procedures ... 36555-36597

Transcatheter Procedures: Intravenous 37195-37216

Intravascular Ultrasound 37250-37251

Bone Marrow or Stem Cell Services/Procedures 38204-38242

Hemic and Lymphatic Systems: Laparoscopy 38570-38589

Digestive: Endoscopy/Laparoscopy 43200-43272, 43280-43289, 43651-43659, 44200-44239, 44360-44397, 44970-44979, 45300-45387, 46600-46615, 47370-47379, 47550-47556, 47560-47562, 49320-49329, 49650-49659

►**Pancreas Transplantation** .... 48550-48556◄

Herniotomy 49491-49611

►**Renal Transplantation** .... 50300-50380◄

Urodynamics 51725-51798

Endoscopy/Laparoscopy

- **Male Genital** 54690-54699, 55550-55559, 55866
- **Urinary** 50541-50545, 50945-50980, 51990-52648
- **Female Genital** 58545-58579, 58660-58679
- **Endocrine** 60650-60659

Maternity Care and Delivery 59000-59899

Nervous System: Surgery of Skull Base 61580-61619

Neurostimulators (Intracranial) 61850-61888, 62160-62319

Neurostimulators (Spinal) 63650-63688

Neurostimulators (Peripheral Nerve) . 64553-64595

Secondary Implants(s) 65125-65175

Removal Cataract 66830-66999

Prophylaxis 67141-67145

Unlisted Service or Procedure

A service or procedure may be provided that is not listed in this edition of *CPT*. When reporting such a service, the appropriate "Unlisted Procedure" code may be used to indicate the service, identifying it by "Special Report" as discussed in the section below. The "Unlisted Procedures" and accompanying codes for **Surgery** are as follows:

15999	Unlisted procedure, excision pressure ulcer
17999	Unlisted procedure, skin, mucous membrane and subcutaneous tissue
19499	Unlisted procedure, breast
20999	Unlisted procedure, musculoskeletal system, general
21089	Unlisted maxillofacial prosthetic procedure
21299	Unlisted craniofacial and maxillofacial procedure
21499	Unlisted musculoskeletal procedure, head
21899	Unlisted procedure, neck or thorax
22899	Unlisted procedure, spine
22999	Unlisted procedure, abdomen, musculoskeletal system
23929	Unlisted procedure, shoulder
24999	Unlisted procedure, humerus or elbow
25999	Unlisted procedure, forearm or wrist
26989	Unlisted procedure, hands or fingers
27299	Unlisted procedure, pelvis or hip joint
27599	Unlisted procedure, femur or knee
27899	Unlisted procedure, leg or ankle
28899	Unlisted procedure, foot or toes
29799	Unlisted procedure, casting or strapping
29999	Unlisted procedure, arthroscopy
30999	Unlisted procedure, nose
31299	Unlisted procedure, accessory sinuses
31599	Unlisted procedure, larynx
31899	Unlisted procedure, trachea, bronchi
32999	Unlisted procedure, lungs and pleura
33999	Unlisted procedure, cardiac surgery
36299	Unlisted procedure, vascular injection
37501	Unlisted vascular endoscopy procedure
37799	Unlisted procedure, vascular surgery
38129	Unlisted laparoscopy procedure, spleen
38589	Unlisted laparoscopy procedure, lymphatic system
38999	Unlisted procedure, hemic or lymphatic system
39499	Unlisted procedure, mediastinum
39599	Unlisted procedure, diaphragm
40799	Unlisted procedure, lips
40899	Unlisted procedure, vestibule of mouth
41599	Unlisted procedure, tongue, floor of mouth
41899	Unlisted procedure, dentoalveolar structures
42299	Unlisted procedure, palate, uvula
42699	Unlisted procedure, salivary glands or ducts
42999	Unlisted procedure, pharynx, adenoids, or tonsils
43289	Unlisted laparoscopy procedure, esophagus
43499	Unlisted procedure, esophagus
43659	Unlisted laparoscopy procedure, stomach
43999	Unlisted procedure, stomach
44238	Unlisted laparoscopy procedure, intestine (except rectum)
44239	Unlisted laparoscopy procedure, rectum
44799	Unlisted procedure, intestine
44899	Unlisted procedure, Meckel's diverticulum and the mesentery
44979	Unlisted laparoscopy procedure, appendix
45999	Unlisted procedure, rectum
46999	Unlisted procedure, anus
47379	Unlisted laparoscopic procedure, liver
47399	Unlisted procedure, liver
47579	Unlisted laparoscopy procedure, biliary tract
47999	Unlisted procedure, biliary tract
48999	Unlisted procedure, pancreas
49329	Unlisted laparoscopy procedure, abdomen, peritoneum and omentum
49659	Unlisted laparoscopy procedure, hernioplasty, herniorrhaphy, herniotomy
49999	Unlisted procedure, abdomen, peritoneum and omentum
50549	Unlisted laparoscopy procedure, renal
50949	Unlisted laparoscopy procedure, ureter
53899	Unlisted procedure, urinary system
54699	Unlisted laparoscopy procedure, testis
55559	Unlisted laparoscopy procedure, spermatic cord
55899	Unlisted procedure, male genital system
58578	Unlisted laparoscopy procedure, uterus
58579	Unlisted hysteroscopy procedure, uterus
58679	Unlisted laparoscopy procedure, oviduct, ovary
58999	Unlisted procedure, female genital system (nonobstetrical)
59897	Unlisted fetal invasive procedure, including ultrasound guidance
59898	Unlisted laparoscopy procedure, maternity care and delivery
59899	Unlisted procedure, maternity care and delivery
60659	Unlisted laparoscopy procedure, endocrine system
60699	Unlisted procedure, endocrine system
64999	Unlisted procedure, nervous system
66999	Unlisted procedure, anterior segment of eye
67299	Unlisted procedure, posterior segment
67399	Unlisted procedure, ocular muscle
67599	Unlisted procedure, orbit
67999	Unlisted procedure, eyelids
68399	Unlisted procedure, conjunctiva
68899	Unlisted procedure, lacrimal system

69399	Unlisted procedure, external ear
69799	Unlisted procedure, middle ear
69949	Unlisted procedure, inner ear
69979	Unlisted procedure, temporal bone, middle fossa approach

Special Report

A service that is rarely provided, unusual, variable, or new may require a special report in determining medical appropriateness of the service. Pertinent information should include an adequate definition or description of the nature, extent, and need for the procedure, and the time, effort, and equipment necessary to provide the service. Additional items which may be included are:

- complexity of symptoms;
- final diagnosis;
- pertinent physical findings (such as size, locations, and number of lesion(s), if appropriate);
- diagnostic and therapeutic procedures (including major and supplementary surgical procedures, if appropriate);
- concurrent problems;
- follow-up care.

Surgical Destruction

Surgical destruction is a part of a surgical procedure and different methods of destruction are not ordinarily listed separately unless the technique substantially alters the standard management of a problem or condition. Exceptions under special circumstances are provided for by separate code numbers.

Notes

Surgery

General

§ **10021** Fine needle aspiration; without imaging guidance
➔ *CPT Changes: An Insider's View* 2002

§ **10022** with imaging guidance
➔ *CPT Changes: An Insider's View* 2002

(For radiological supervision and interpretation, see 76003, 76360, 76393, 76942)

(For percutaneous needle biopsy other than fine needle aspiration, see 20206 for muscle, 32400 for pleura, 32405 for lung or mediastinum, 42400 for salivary gland, 47000, 47001 for liver, 48102 for pancreas, 49180 for abdominal or retroperitoneal mass, 60100 for thyroid, 62269 for spinal cord)

(For evaluation of fine needle aspirate, see 88172, 88173)

Integumentary System

Skin, Subcutaneous and Accessory Structures

Incision and Drainage

(For excision, see 11400, et seq)

§ **10040** Acne surgery (eg, marsupialization, opening or removal of multiple milia, comedones, cysts, pustules)

§ **10060** Incision and drainage of abscess (eg, carbuncle, suppurative hidradenitis, cutaneous or subcutaneous abscess, cyst, furuncle, or paronychia); simple or single

§ **10061** complicated or multiple

§ **10080** Incision and drainage of pilonidal cyst; simple

§ **10081** complicated

(For excision of pilonidal cyst, see 11770-11772)

§ **10120** Incision and removal of foreign body, subcutaneous tissues; simple

§ **10121** complicated

(To report wound exploration due to penetrating trauma without laparotomy or thoracotomy, see 20100-20103, as appropriate)

(To report debridement associated with open fracture(s) and/or dislocation(s), use 11010-11012, as appropriate)

§ **10140** Incision and drainage of hematoma, seroma or fluid collection
➔ *CPT Changes: An Insider's View* 2002

(If imaging guidance is performed, see 76360, 76393, 76942)

§ **10160** Puncture aspiration of abscess, hematoma, bulla, or cyst
➔ *CPT Changes: An Insider's View* 2002

(If imaging guidance is performed, see 76360, 76393, 76942)

§ **10180** Incision and drainage, complex, postoperative wound infection

(For secondary closure of surgical wound, see 12020, 12021, 13160)

Excision—Debridement

(For dermabrasions, see 15780-15783)

(For nail debridement, see 11720-11721)

(For burn(s), see 16000-16035)

§ **11000** Debridement of extensive eczematous or infected skin; up to 10% of body surface

►(For abdominal wall or genitalia debridement for necrotizing soft tissue infection, see 11004-11006)◄

§+ **11001** each additional 10% of the body surface (List separately in addition to code for primary procedure)
➔ *CPT Assistant* Feb 03:7

(Use 11001 in conjunction with 11000)

✿● **11004** Debridement of skin, subcutaneous tissue, muscle and fascia for necrotizing soft tissue infection; external genitalia and perineum
➔ *CPT Changes: An Insider's View* 2005

✿● **11005** abdominal wall, with or without fascial closure
➔ *CPT Changes: An Insider's View* 2005

✿● **11006** external genitalia, perineum and abdominal wall, with or without fascial closure
➔ *CPT Changes: An Insider's View* 2005

✿+● **11008** Removal of prosthetic material or mesh, abdominal wall for necrotizing soft tissue infection (List separately in addition to code for primary procedure)
➔ *CPT Changes: An Insider's View* 2005

►(Use 11008 in conjunction with 11004-11006)◄

►(Do not report 11008 in conjunction with 11000-11001, 11010-11044)◄

►(Report skin grafts or flaps separately when performed for closure at the same session as 11004-11008)◄

►(If orchiectomy is performed, use 54520)◄

►(If testicular transplantation is performed, use 54680)◄

✶§ **11010** Debridement including removal of foreign material associated with open fracture(s) and/or dislocation(s); skin and subcutaneous tissues
➔ *CPT Assistant* Oct 03:10

✶§ **11011** skin, subcutaneous tissue, muscle fascia, and muscle

✶§ **11012** skin, subcutaneous tissue, muscle fascia, muscle, and bone
➔ *CPT Assistant* Oct 03:10

§ **11040** Debridement; skin, partial thickness

§ **11041** skin, full thickness

§ **11042** skin, and subcutaneous tissue

§ **11043** skin, subcutaneous tissue, and muscle

§ **11044** skin, subcutaneous tissue, muscle, and bone

(Do not report 11040-11044 in conjunction with ►97597-◄97602)

Paring or Cutting

(To report destruction, see 17000-17004)

§ **11055** Paring or cutting of benign hyperkeratotic lesion (eg, corn or callus); single lesion

§ **11056** two to four lesions
➔ *CPT Assistant* May 03:10

§ **11057** more than four lesions

Biopsy

During certain surgical procedures in the integumentary system, such as excision, destruction, or shave removals, the removed tissue is often submitted for pathologic examination. The obtaining of tissue for pathology during the course of these procedures is a routine component of such procedures. This obtaining of tissue is not considered a separate biopsy procedure and is not separately reported. The use of a biopsy procedure code (eg, 11100, 11101) indicates that the procedure to obtain tissue for pathologic examination was performed independently, or was unrelated or distinct from other procedures/services provided at that time. Such biopsies are not considered components of other procedures when performed on different lesions or different sites on the same date, and are to be reported separately.

(For biopsy of conjunctiva, use 68100; eyelid, use 67810)

§ **11100** Biopsy of skin, subcutaneous tissue and/or mucous membrane (including simple closure), unless otherwise listed; single lesion
➔ *CPT Changes: An Insider's View* 2004

§+ **11101** each separate/additional lesion (List separately in addition to code for primary procedure)

(Use 11101 in conjunction with 11100)

Removal of Skin Tags

Removal by scissoring or any sharp method, ligature strangulation, electrosurgical destruction or combination of treatment modalities including chemical or electrocauterization of wound, with or without local anesthesia.

§ **11200** Removal of skin tags, multiple fibrocutaneous tags, any area; up to and including 15 lesions

§+ **11201** each additional ten lesions (List separately in addition to code for primary procedure)

(Use 11201 in conjunction with 11200)

Shaving of Epidermal or Dermal Lesions

Shaving is the sharp removal by transverse incision or horizontal slicing to remove epidermal and dermal lesions without a full-thickness dermal excision. This includes local anesthesia, chemical or electrocauterization of the wound. The wound does not require suture closure.

§ **11300** Shaving of epidermal or dermal lesion, single lesion, trunk, arms or legs; lesion diameter 0.5 cm or less

§ **11301** lesion diameter 0.6 to 1.0 cm

§ **11302** lesion diameter 1.1 to 2.0 cm

§ **11303** lesion diameter over 2.0 cm

§ **11305** Shaving of epidermal or dermal lesion, single lesion, scalp, neck, hands, feet, genitalia; lesion diameter 0.5 cm or less

§ **11306** lesion diameter 0.6 to 1.0 cm

§ **11307** lesion diameter 1.1 to 2.0 cm

§ **11308** lesion diameter over 2.0 cm

§ **11310** Shaving of epidermal or dermal lesion, single lesion, face, ears, eyelids, nose, lips, mucous membrane; lesion diameter 0.5 cm or less

§ **11311** lesion diameter 0.6 to 1.0 cm

§ **11312** lesion diameter 1.1 to 2.0 cm

§ **11313** lesion diameter over 2.0 cm

Excision—Benign Lesions

Excision (including simple closure) of benign lesions of skin (eg, neoplasm, cicatricial, fibrous, inflammatory, congenital, cystic lesions), includes local anesthesia. See appropriate size and area below. For shave removal, see 11300 et seq., and for electrosurgical and other methods see 17000 et seq.

Excision is defined as full-thickness (through the dermis) removal of a lesion, including margins, and includes simple (non-layered) closure when performed. Report separately each benign lesion excised. Code selection is determined by measuring the greatest clinical diameter of the apparent lesion plus that margin required for complete excision (lesion diameter plus the most narrow margins required equals the excised diameter). The margins refer to the most narrow margin required to adequately excise the lesion, based on the physician's judgment. The measurement of lesion plus margin is made prior to excision. The excised diameter is the same whether the surgical defect is repaired in a linear fashion, or reconstructed (eg, with a skin graft).

The closure of defects created by incision, excision, or trauma may require intermediate or complex closure. Repair by intermediate or complex closure should be reported separately. For excision of benign lesions requiring more than simple closure, ie, requiring intermediate or complex closure, report 11400-11446 in addition to appropriate intermediate (12031-12057) or complex closure (13100-13153) codes. For reconstructive closure, see 14000-14300, 15000-15261, 15570-15770. See page 54 for definition of intermediate or complex closure.

§ **11400** Excision, benign lesion including margins, except skin tag (unless listed elsewhere), trunk, arms or legs; excised diameter 0.5 cm or less
➲ *CPT Changes: An Insider's View* 2003

§ **11401** excised diameter 0.6 to 1.0 cm
➲ *CPT Changes: An Insider's View* 2003

§ **11402** excised diameter 1.1 to 2.0 cm
➲ *CPT Changes: An Insider's View* 2003

§ **11403** excised diameter 2.1 to 3.0 cm
➲ *CPT Changes: An Insider's View* 2003

§ **11404** excised diameter 3.1 to 4.0 cm
➲ *CPT Changes: An Insider's View* 2003

§ **11406** excised diameter over 4.0 cm
➲ *CPT Changes: An Insider's View* 2003

(For unusual or complicated excision, add modifier 22)

§ **11420** Excision, benign lesion including margins, except skin tag (unless listed elsewhere), scalp, neck, hands, feet, genitalia; excised diameter 0.5 cm or less
➲ *CPT Changes: An Insider's View* 2003

§ **11421** excised diameter 0.6 to 1.0 cm
➲ *CPT Changes: An Insider's View* 2003

§ **11422** excised diameter 1.1 to 2.0 cm
➲ *CPT Changes: An Insider's View* 2003

§ **11423** excised diameter 2.1 to 3.0 cm
➲ *CPT Changes: An Insider's View* 2003

§ **11424** excised diameter 3.1 to 4.0 cm
➲ *CPT Changes: An Insider's View* 2003

§ **11426** excised diameter over 4.0 cm
➲ *CPT Changes: An Insider's View* 2003

(For unusual or complicated excision, add modifier 22)

§ **11440** Excision, other benign lesion including margins (unless listed elsewhere), face, ears, eyelids, nose, lips, mucous membrane; excised diameter 0.5 cm or less
➲ *CPT Changes: An Insider's View* 2003

§ **11441** excised diameter 0.6 to 1.0 cm
➲ *CPT Changes: An Insider's View* 2003

§ **11442** excised diameter 1.1 to 2.0 cm
➲ *CPT Changes: An Insider's View* 2003

§ **11443** excised diameter 2.1 to 3.0 cm
➲ *CPT Changes: An Insider's View* 2003

§ **11444** excised diameter 3.1 to 4.0 cm
➲ *CPT Changes: An Insider's View* 2003

§ **11446** excised diameter over 4.0 cm
➲ *CPT Changes: An Insider's View* 2003

(For unusual or complicated excision, add modifier 22)

(For eyelids involving more than skin, see also 67800 et seq)

§ **11450** Excision of skin and subcutaneous tissue for hidradenitis, axillary; with simple or intermediate repair

§ **11451** with complex repair

§ **11462** Excision of skin and subcutaneous tissue for hidradenitis, inguinal; with simple or intermediate repair

§ **11463** with complex repair

§ **11470** Excision of skin and subcutaneous tissue for hidradenitis, perianal, perineal, or umbilical; with simple or intermediate repair

§ **11471** with complex repair

(When skin graft or flap is used for closure, use appropriate procedure code in addition)

(For bilateral procedure, add modifier 50)

Excision—Malignant Lesions

Excision (including simple closure) of malignant lesions of skin (eg, basal cell carcinoma, squamous cell carcinoma, melanoma) includes local anesthesia. (See appropriate size and body area below.) For destruction of malignant lesions of skin, see destruction codes 17260-17286.

Excision is defined as full-thickness (through the dermis) removal of a lesion including margins, and includes simple (non-layered) closure when performed. Report separately each malignant lesion excised. Code selection is determined by measuring the greatest clinical diameter of the apparent lesion plus that margin required for complete excision (lesion diameter plus the most narrow margins required equals the excised diameter). The margins refer to the most narrow margin required to adequately excise the lesion, based on the physician's judgment. The measurement of lesion plus margin is made prior to excision. The excised diameter is the same whether the surgical defect is repaired in a linear fashion, or reconstructed (eg, with a skin graft).

The closure of defects created by incision, excision, or trauma may require intermediate or complex closure. Repair by intermediate or complex closure should be reported separately. For excision of malignant lesions requiring more than simple closure, ie, requiring intermediate or complex closure, report 11600-11646 in addition to appropriate intermediate (12031-12057) or complex closure (13100-13153) codes. For reconstructive closure, see 14000-14300, 15000-15261, 15570-15770. See page 54 for definition of intermediate or complex closure.

When frozen section pathology shows the margins of excision were not adequate, an additional excision may be necessary for complete tumor removal. Use only one code to report the additional excision and re-excision(s) based on the final widest excised diameter required for complete tumor removal at the same operative session. To report a re-excision procedure performed to widen margins at a subsequent operative session, see codes 11600-11646, as appropriate. Append modifier 58 if the re-excision procedure is performed during the postoperative period of the primary excision procedure.

§ **11600** Excision, malignant lesion including margins, trunk, arms, or legs; excised diameter 0.5 cm or less
➲ *CPT Assistant* May 03:10; *CPT Changes: An Insider's View* 2003

§ **11601** excised diameter 0.6 to 1.0 cm
➲ *CPT Changes: An Insider's View* 2003

§ **11602** excised diameter 1.1 to 2.0 cm
➲ *CPT Changes: An Insider's View* 2003

§ **11603** excised diameter 2.1 to 3.0 cm
➲ *CPT Changes: An Insider's View* 2003

§ **11604** excised diameter 3.1 to 4.0 cm
➲ *CPT Changes: An Insider's View* 2003

§ **11606** excised diameter over 4.0 cm
➲ *CPT Changes: An Insider's View* 2003

§ **11620** Excision, malignant lesion including margins, scalp, neck, hands, feet, genitalia; excised diameter 0.5 cm or less
➲ *CPT Changes: An Insider's View* 2003

§ **11621** excised diameter 0.6 to 1.0 cm
➲ *CPT Changes: An Insider's View* 2003

§ **11622** excised diameter 1.1 to 2.0 cm
➲ *CPT Changes: An Insider's View* 2003

§ **11623** excised diameter 2.1 to 3.0 cm
➲ *CPT Changes: An Insider's View* 2003

§ **11624** excised diameter 3.1 to 4.0 cm
➲ *CPT Changes: An Insider's View* 2003

§ **11626** excised diameter over 4.0 cm
➲ *CPT Changes: An Insider's View* 2003

§ **11640** Excision, malignant lesion including margins, face, ears, eyelids, nose, lips; excised diameter 0.5 cm or less
➲ *CPT Assistant* May 03:10; *CPT Changes: An Insider's View* 2003

§ **11641** excised diameter 0.6 to 1.0 cm
➲ *CPT Changes: An Insider's View* 2003

§ **11642** excised diameter 1.1 to 2.0 cm
➲ *CPT Changes: An Insider's View* 2003

§ **11643** excised diameter 2.1 to 3.0 cm
➲ *CPT Changes: An Insider's View* 2003

§ **11644** excised diameter 3.1 to 4.0 cm
➲ *CPT Changes: An Insider's View* 2003

§ **11646** excised diameter over 4.0 cm
➲ *CPT Changes: An Insider's View* 2003

(For eyelids involving more than skin, see also 67800 et seq)

Nails

(For drainage of paronychia or onychia, see 10060, 10061)

§ **11719** Trimming of nondystrophic nails, any number

§ **11720** Debridement of nail(s) by any method(s); one to five

§ **11721** six or more

§ **11730** Avulsion of nail plate, partial or complete, simple; single

§+ **11732** each additional nail plate (List separately in addition to code for primary procedure)

(Use 11732 in conjunction with 11730)

§ **11740** Evacuation of subungual hematoma

§ **11750** Excision of nail and nail matrix, partial or complete, (eg, ingrown or deformed nail) for permanent removal;

§ **11752** with amputation of tuft of distal phalanx

(For skin graft, if used, use 15050)

§ **11755** Biopsy of nail unit (eg, plate, bed, matrix, hyponychium, proximal and lateral nail folds) (separate procedure)
➲ *CPT Changes: An Insider's View* 2002

§ **11760** Repair of nail bed

§ **11762** Reconstruction of nail bed with graft

§ **11765** Wedge excision of skin of nail fold (eg, for ingrown toenail)

Pilonidal Cyst

§ **11770** Excision of pilonidal cyst or sinus; simple

§ **11771** extensive

§ **11772** complicated

(For incision of pilonidal cyst, see 10080, 10081)

Introduction

§ **11900** Injection, intralesional; up to and including seven lesions

§ **11901** more than seven lesions

(11900, 11901 are not to be used for preoperative local anesthetic injection)

(For veins, see 36470, 36471)

(For intralesional chemotherapy administration, see 96405, 96406)

§ 11920 Tattooing, intradermal introduction of insoluble opaque pigments to correct color defects of skin, including micropigmentation; 6.0 sq cm or less

§ 11921 6.1 to 20.0 sq cm

§+ 11922 each additional 20.0 sq cm (List separately in addition to code for primary procedure)

(Use 11922 in conjunction with 11921)

§ 11950 Subcutaneous injection of filling material (eg, collagen); 1 cc or less

§ 11951 1.1 to 5.0 cc

§ 11952 5.1 to 10.0 cc

§ 11954 over 10.0 cc

§ 11960 Insertion of tissue expander(s) for other than breast, including subsequent expansion

(For breast reconstruction with tissue expander(s), use 19357)

§ 11970 Replacement of tissue expander with permanent prosthesis

§ 11971 Removal of tissue expander(s) without insertion of prosthesis

□ 11975 Insertion, implantable contraceptive capsules

§ 11976 Removal, implantable contraceptive capsules

□ 11977 Removal with reinsertion, implantable contraceptive capsules

♣ 11980 Subcutaneous hormone pellet implantation (implantation of estradiol and/or testosterone pellets beneath the skin)
➲ *CPT Changes: An Insider's View* 2000

♣ 11981 Insertion, non-biodegradable drug delivery implant
➲ *CPT Changes: An Insider's View* 2000

♣ 11982 Removal, non-biodegradable drug delivery implant
➲ *CPT Changes: An Insider's View* 2000

♣ 11983 Removal with reinsertion, non-biodegradable drug delivery implant
➲ *CPT Changes: An Insider's View* 2000

Repair (Closure)

Use the codes in this section to designate wound closure utilizing sutures, staples, or tissue adhesives (eg, 2-cyanoacrylate), either singly or in combination with each other, or in combination with adhesive strips. Wound closure utilizing adhesive strips as the sole repair material should be coded using the appropriate E/M code.

Definitions

The repair of wounds may be classified as Simple, Intermediate, or Complex.

Simple repair is used when the wound is superficial; eg, involving primarily epidermis or dermis, or subcutaneous tissues without significant involvement of deeper structures, and requires simple one layer closure. This includes local anesthesia and chemical or electrocauterization of wounds not closed.

Intermediate repair includes the repair of wounds that, in addition to the above, require layered closure of one or more of the deeper layers of subcutaneous tissue and superficial (non-muscle) fascia, in addition to the skin (epidermal and dermal) closure. Single-layer closure of heavily contaminated wounds that have required extensive cleaning or removal of particulate matter also constitutes intermediate repair.

Complex repair includes the repair of wounds requiring more than layered closure, viz., scar revision, debridement, (eg, traumatic lacerations or avulsions), extensive undermining, stents or retention sutures. Necessary preparation includes creation of a defect for repairs (eg, excision of a scar requiring a complex repair) or the debridement of complicated lacerations or avulsions. Complex repair does not include excision of benign (11400-11446) or malignant (11600-11646) lesions.

Instructions for listing services at time of wound repair:

1. The repaired wound(s) should be measured and recorded in centimeters, whether curved, angular, or stellate.

2. When multiple wounds are repaired, add together the lengths of those in the same classification (see above) and from all anatomic sites that are grouped together into the same code descriptor. For example, add together the lengths of intermediate repairs to the trunk and extremities. Do not add lengths of repairs from different groupings of anatomic sites (eg, face and extremities). Also, do not add together lengths of different classifications (eg, intermediate and complex repairs).

When more than one classification of wounds is repaired, list the more complicated as the primary procedure and the less complicated as the secondary procedure, using modifier 51.

3. Decontamination and/or debridement: Debridement is considered a separate procedure only when gross contamination requires prolonged cleansing, when appreciable amounts of devitalized or contaminated tissue are removed, or when debridement is carried out separately without immediate primary closure. (For extensive debridement of soft tissue and/or bone, see 11040-11044.)

(For extensive debridement of soft tissue and/or bone, not associated with open fracture(s) and/or dislocation(s) resulting from penetrating and/or blunt trauma, see 11040-11044.)

(For extensive debridement of subcutaneous tissue, muscle fascia, muscle, and/or bone associated with open fracture(s) and/or dislocation(s), see 11010-11012.)

4. Involvement of nerves, blood vessels and tendons: Report under appropriate system (Nervous, Cardiovascular, Musculoskeletal) for repair of these structures. The repair of these associated wounds is included in the primary procedure unless it qualifies as a complex wound, in which case modifier 51 applies.

Simple ligation of vessels in an open wound is considered as part of any wound closure.

Simple "exploration" of nerves, blood vessels or tendons exposed in an open wound is also considered part of the essential treatment of the wound and is not a separate procedure unless appreciable dissection is required. If the wound requires enlargement, extension of dissection (to determine penetration), debridement, removal of foreign body(s), ligation or coagulation of minor subcutaneous and/or muscular blood vessel(s) of the subcutaneous tissue, muscle fascia, and/or muscle, not requiring thoracotomy or laparotomy, use codes 20100-20103, as appropriate.

Repair—Simple

Sum of lengths of repairs for each group of anatomic sites.

§ **12001** Simple repair of superficial wounds of scalp, neck, axillae, external genitalia, trunk and/or extremities (including hands and feet); 2.5 cm or less

§ **12002** 2.6 cm to 7.5 cm

§ **12004** 7.6 cm to 12.5 cm

§ **12005** 12.6 cm to 20.0 cm

§ **12006** 20.1 cm to 30.0 cm

§ **12007** over 30.0 cm

§ **12011** Simple repair of superficial wounds of face, ears, eyelids, nose, lips and/or mucous membranes; 2.5 cm or less

§ **12013** 2.6 cm to 5.0 cm

§ **12014** 5.1 cm to 7.5 cm

§ **12015** 7.6 cm to 12.5 cm

§ **12016** 12.6 cm to 20.0 cm

§ **12017** 20.1 cm to 30.0 cm

§ **12018** over 30.0 cm

§ **12020** Treatment of superficial wound dehiscence; simple closure

§ **12021** with packing

(For extensive or complicated secondary wound closure, use 13160)

Repair—Intermediate

Sum of lengths of repairs for each group of anatomic sites.

§ **12031** Layer closure of wounds of scalp, axillae, trunk and/or extremities (excluding hands and feet); 2.5 cm or less

§ **12032** 2.6 cm to 7.5 cm

§ **12034** 7.6 cm to 12.5 cm

§ **12035** 12.6 cm to 20.0 cm

§ **12036** 20.1 cm to 30.0 cm

§ **12037** over 30.0 cm

§ **12041** Layer closure of wounds of neck, hands, feet and/or external genitalia; 2.5 cm or less

§ **12042** 2.6 cm to 7.5 cm

§ **12044** 7.6 cm to 12.5 cm

§ **12045** 12.6 cm to 20.0 cm

§ **12046** 20.1 cm to 30.0 cm

§ **12047** over 30.0 cm

§ **12051** Layer closure of wounds of face, ears, eyelids, nose, lips and/or mucous membranes; 2.5 cm or less

§ **12052** 2.6 cm to 5.0 cm

§ **12053** 5.1 cm to 7.5 cm

§ **12054** 7.6 cm to 12.5 cm

§ **12055** 12.6 cm to 20.0 cm

§ **12056** 20.1 cm to 30.0 cm

§ **12057** over 30.0 cm

Repair—Complex

Reconstructive procedures, complicated wound closure.

Sum of lengths of repairs for each group of anatomic sites.

(For full thickness repair of lip or eyelid, see respective anatomical subsections)

§ **13100** Repair, complex, trunk; 1.1 cm to 2.5 cm

➲ *CPT Assistant* May 03:10-11

(For 1.0 cm or less, see simple or intermediate repairs)

§ **13101** 2.6 cm to 7.5 cm

➲ *CPT Assistant* May 03:10-11

§+ **13102** each additional 5 cm or less (List separately in addition to code for primary procedure)

➲ *CPT Assistant* May 03:10-11; *CPT Changes: An Insider's View* 2000

(Use 13102 in conjunction with 13101)

§ **13120** Repair, complex, scalp, arms, and/or legs; 1.1 cm to 2.5 cm

➲ *CPT Assistant* May 03:10-11

(For 1.0 cm or less, see simple or intermediate repairs)

§ **13121** 2.6 cm to 7.5 cm

➲ *CPT Assistant* May 03:10-11

§+ **13122** each additional 5 cm or less (List separately in addition to code for primary procedure)

➲ *CPT Assistant* May 03:10-11; *CPT Changes: An Insider's View* 2000

(Use 13122 in conjunction with 13121)

§ **13131** Repair, complex, forehead, cheeks, chin, mouth, neck, axillae, genitalia, hands and/or feet; 1.1 cm to 2.5 cm

➲ *CPT Assistant* May 03:10-11

(For 1.0 cm or less, see simple or intermediate repairs)

§ **13132** 2.6 cm to 7.5 cm

➲ *CPT Assistant* May 03:10-11

§+ **13133** each additional 5 cm or less (List separately in addition to code for primary procedure)

➲ *CPT Assistant* May 03:10-11; *CPT Changes: An Insider's View* 2000

(Use 13133 in conjunction with 13132)

§ **13150** Repair, complex, eyelids, nose, ears and/or lips; 1.0 cm or less

➲ *CPT Assistant* May 03:10-11

(See also 40650-40654, 67961-67975)

§ **13151** 1.1 cm to 2.5 cm

➲ *CPT Assistant* May 03:10-11

§ **13152** 2.6 cm to 7.5 cm

➲ *CPT Assistant* May 03:10-11

§+ **13153** each additional 5 cm or less (List separately in addition to code for primary procedure)

➲ *CPT Assistant* May 03:10-11; *CPT Changes: An Insider's View* 2000

(Use 13153 in conjunction with 13152)

§ **13160** Secondary closure of surgical wound or dehiscence, extensive or complicated

(For packing or simple secondary wound closure, see 12020, 12021)

Adjacent Tissue Transfer or Rearrangement

For full thickness repair of lip or eyelid, see respective anatomical subsections.

Excision (including lesion) and/or repair by adjacent tissue transfer or rearrangement (eg, Z-plasty, W-plasty, V-Y plasty, rotation flap, advancement flap, double pedicle flap). When applied in repairing lacerations, the procedures listed must be developed by the surgeon to accomplish the repair. They do not apply when direct closure or rearrangement of traumatic wounds incidentally result in these configurations.

Skin graft necessary to close secondary defect is considered an additional procedure. For purposes of code selection, the term "defect" includes the primary and secondary defects. The primary defect resulting from the excision and the secondary defect resulting from flap design to perform the reconstruction are measured together to determine the code.

§ **14000** Adjacent tissue transfer or rearrangement, trunk; defect 10 sq cm or less

§ **14001** defect 10.1 sq cm to 30.0 sq cm

§ **14020** Adjacent tissue transfer or rearrangement, scalp, arms and/or legs; defect 10 sq cm or less

§ **14021** defect 10.1 sq cm to 30.0 sq cm

§ **14040** Adjacent tissue transfer or rearrangement, forehead, cheeks, chin, mouth, neck, axillae, genitalia, hands and/or feet; defect 10 sq cm or less

§ **14041** defect 10.1 sq cm to 30.0 sq cm

§ **14060** Adjacent tissue transfer or rearrangement, eyelids, nose, ears and/or lips; defect 10 sq cm or less

§ **14061** defect 10.1 sq cm to 30.0 sq cm

(For eyelid, full thickness, see 67961 et seq)

§ **14300** Adjacent tissue transfer or rearrangement, more than 30 sq cm, unusual or complicated, any area

§ **14350** Filleted finger or toe flap, including preparation of recipient site

Free Skin Grafts

Identify by size and location of the defect (recipient area) and the type of graft; includes simple debridement of granulations or recent avulsion.

When a primary procedure such as orbitectomy, radical mastectomy, or deep tumor removal requires skin graft for definitive closure, see appropriate anatomical subsection for primary procedure and this section for skin graft.

Use 15000 for initial wound preparation.

Use 15100-15261 for autogenous skin grafts. For autogenous tissue-cultured skin grafts, use 15100-15121. These codes include harvesting of keratinocytes and their subsequent application. Procedures are coded by recipient site. Use codes 15342 and 15343 for application of skin substitute/neodermis. Use modifier 58 for staged application procedure(s).

Repair of donor site requiring skin graft or local flaps is to be added as an additional procedure.

Codes 15000, 15001, 15350, 15351, 15400, 15401 describe burn and wound preparation and management procedures. The following definition should be applied to codes 15000, 15001, 15100, 15101, 15120, 15121 when determining the involvement of body size. The measurement of 100 sq cm is applicable to adults and children age 10 and over, percentages apply to infants and children under the age of 10.

(For microvascular flaps, see 15756-15758)

§ **15000** Surgical preparation or creation of recipient site by excision of open wounds, burn eschar, or scar (including subcutaneous tissues); first 100 sq cm or one percent of body area of infants and children

➲ *CPT Changes: An Insider's View* 2001

(For appropriate skin grafts, see 15050-15261; list the free graft separately by its procedure number when the graft, immediate or delayed, is applied)

§+ **15001** each additional 100 sq cm or each additional one percent of body area of infants and children (List separately in addition to code for primary procedure)

(Use 15001 in conjunction with 15000)

(For excision of benign lesions, see 11400-11471)

(For excision of malignant lesions, see 11600-11646)

(For excision with alloplastic dressing, use 15000 only)

(For excision with immediate skin grafting use 15050-15261 in addition to 15000)

(For excision with immediate allograft placement use 15350 in addition to 15000)

(For excision with immediate xenograft placement use 15400 in addition to 15000)

§ **15050** Pinch graft, single or multiple, to cover small ulcer, tip of digit, or other minimal open area (except on face), up to defect size 2 cm diameter

§ **15100** Split graft, trunk, arms, legs; first 100 sq cm or less, or one percent of body area of infants and children (except 15050)
➔ *CPT Changes: An Insider's View* 2002

§+ **15101** each additional 100 sq cm, or each additional one percent of body area of infants and children, or part thereof (List separately in addition to code for primary procedure)
➔ *CPT Changes: An Insider's View* 2002

(Use 15101 in conjunction with 15100)

§ **15120** Split graft, face, scalp, eyelids, mouth, neck, ears, orbits, genitalia, hands, feet and/or multiple digits; first 100 sq cm or less, or one percent of body area of infants and children (except 15050)
➔ *CPT Changes: An Insider's View* 2002

§+ **15121** each additional 100 sq cm, or each additional one percent of body area of infants and children, or part thereof (List separately in addition to code for primary procedure)
➔ *CPT Changes: An Insider's View* 2002

(Use 15121 in conjunction with 15120)

(For eyelids, see also 67961 et seq)

§ **15200** Full thickness graft, free, including direct closure of donor site, trunk; 20 sq cm or less
➔ *CPT Changes: An Insider's View* 2002

§+ **15201** each additional 20 sq cm (List separately in addition to code for primary procedure)
➔ *CPT Changes: An Insider's View* 2002

(Use 15201 in conjunction with 15200)

§ **15220** Full thickness graft, free, including direct closure of donor site, scalp, arms, and/or legs; 20 sq cm or less
➔ *CPT Changes: An Insider's View* 2002

§+ **15221** each additional 20 sq cm (List separately in addition to code for primary procedure)
➔ *CPT Changes: An Insider's View* 2002

(Use 15221 in conjunction with 15220)

§ **15240** Full thickness graft, free, including direct closure of donor site, forehead, cheeks, chin, mouth, neck, axillae, genitalia, hands, and/or feet; 20 sq cm or less
➔ *CPT Changes: An Insider's View* 2002

(For finger tip graft, use 15050)

(For repair of syndactyly, fingers, see 26560-26562)

§+ **15241** each additional 20 sq cm (List separately in addition to code for primary procedure)
➔ *CPT Changes: An Insider's View* 2002

(Use 15241 in conjunction with 15240)

§ **15260** Full thickness graft, free, including direct closure of donor site, nose, ears, eyelids, and/or lips; 20 sq cm or less

§+ **15261** each additional 20 sq cm (List separately in addition to code for primary procedure)
➔ *CPT Changes: An Insider's View* 2002

(Use 15261 in conjunction with 15260)

(For eyelids, see also 67961 et seq)

(Repair of donor site requiring skin graft or local flaps, to be added as additional separate procedure)

§ **15342** Application of bilaminate skin substitute/neodermis; 25 sq cm

§+ **15343** each additional 25 sq cm (List separately in addition to code for primary procedure)

(Use 15343 in conjunction with 15342)

§ **15350** Application of allograft, skin; 100 sq cm or less

(For staged tissue graft implantation, use modifier 58)

§+ **15351** each additional 100 sq cm (List separately in addition to code for primary procedure)

(Use 15351 in conjunction with 15350)

§ **15400** Application of xenograft, skin; 100 sq cm or less

§+ **15401** each additional 100 sq cm (List separately in addition to code for primary procedure)

(Use 15401 in conjunction with 15400)

Flaps (Skin and/or Deep Tissues)

Regions listed refer to recipient area (not donor site) when flap is being attached in transfer or to final site.

Regions listed refer to donor site when tube is formed for later or when "delay" of flap is prior to transfer.

Procedures 15570-15738 do not include extensive immobilization (eg, large plaster casts and other immobilizing devices are considered additional separate procedures).

Repair of donor site requiring skin graft or local flaps is considered an additional separate procedure.

(For microvascular flaps, see 15756-15758)

§ **15570** Formation of direct or tubed pedicle, with or without transfer; trunk

§ **15572** scalp, arms, or legs

§ **15574** forehead, cheeks, chin, mouth, neck, axillae, genitalia, hands or feet

§ **15576** eyelids, nose, ears, lips, or intraoral

§ **15600** Delay of flap or sectioning of flap (division and inset); at trunk

§ **15610** at scalp, arms, or legs

§ **15620** at forehead, cheeks, chin, neck, axillae, genitalia, hands, or feet

§ **15630** at eyelids, nose, ears, or lips

§ **15650** Transfer, intermediate, of any pedicle flap (eg, abdomen to wrist, Walking tube), any location

(For eyelids, nose, ears, or lips, see also anatomical area)

(For revision, defatting or rearranging of transferred pedicle flap or skin graft, see 13100-14300)

(Procedures 15732-15738 are described by donor site of the muscle, myocutaneous, or fasciocutaneous flap)

§ **15732** Muscle, myocutaneous, or fasciocutaneous flap; head and neck (eg, temporalis, masseter muscle, sternocleidomastoid, levator scapulae)
➔ *CPT Changes: An Insider's View* 2002

§ **15734** trunk

§ **15736** upper extremity

§ **15738** lower extremity

Other Flaps and Grafts

Repair of donor site requiring skin graft or local flaps should be reported as an additional procedure.

§ **15740** Flap; island pedicle

§ **15750** neurovascular pedicle

✿ **15756** Free muscle or myocutaneous flap with microvascular anastomosis
➔ *CPT Changes: An Insider's View* 2003

(Do not report code 69990 in addition to code 15756)

✿ **15757** Free skin flap with microvascular anastomosis

(Do not report code 69990 in addition to code 15757)

✿ **15758** Free fascial flap with microvascular anastomosis

(Do not report code 69990 in addition to code 15758)

§ **15760** Graft; composite (eg, full thickness of external ear or nasal ala), including primary closure, donor area

§ **15770** derma-fat-fascia

§ **15775** Punch graft for hair transplant; 1 to 15 punch grafts

§ **15776** more than 15 punch grafts

(For strip transplant, use 15220)

Other Procedures

§ **15780** Dermabrasion; total face (eg, for acne scarring, fine wrinkling, rhytids, general keratosis)

§ **15781** segmental, face

§ **15782** regional, other than face

§ **15783** superficial, any site, (eg, tattoo removal)

§ **15786** Abrasion; single lesion (eg, keratosis, scar)

§✚ **15787** each additional four lesions or less (List separately in addition to code for primary procedure)

(Use 15787 in conjunction with 15786)

§ **15788** Chemical peel, facial; epidermal

§ **15789** dermal

§ **15792** Chemical peel, nonfacial; epidermal

§ **15793** dermal

§ **15810** Salabrasion; 20 sq cm or less

§ **15811** over 20 sq cm

§ **15819** Cervicoplasty

♦§ **15820** Blepharoplasty, lower eyelid;

♦§ **15821** with extensive herniated fat pad

♦§ **15822** Blepharoplasty, upper eyelid;
➔ *CPT Assistant* May 03:15

♦§ **15823** with excessive skin weighting down lid

(For bilateral blepharoplasty, add modifier 50)

♦§ **15824** Rhytidectomy; forehead

(For repair of brow ptosis, use 67900)

♦§ **15825** neck with platysmal tightening (platysmal flap, P-flap)

♦§ **15826** glabellar frown lines

♦§ **15828** cheek, chin, and neck

♦§ **15829** superficial musculoaponeurotic system (SMAS) flap

(For bilateral rhytidectomy, add modifier 50)

§ **15831** Excision, excessive skin and subcutaneous tissue (including lipectomy); abdomen (abdominoplasty)

§ **15832** thigh

§ **15833** leg

§ **15834** hip

§ **15835** buttock

§ **15836** arm

§ **15837** forearm or hand

§ **15838** submental fat pad

§ **15839** other area

(For bilateral procedure, add modifier 50)

§ **15840** Graft for facial nerve paralysis; free fascia graft (including obtaining fascia)

(For bilateral procedure, add modifier 50)

§ **15841** free muscle graft (including obtaining graft)

§ **15842** free muscle flap by microsurgical technique
➔ *CPT Changes: An Insider's View* 2001

(Do not report code 69990 in addition to code 15842)

§ **15845** regional muscle transfer

(For intravenous fluorescein examination of blood flow in graft or flap, use 15860)

(For nerve transfers, decompression, or repair, see 64831-64876, 64905, 64907, 69720, 69725, 69740, 69745, 69955)

§ **15850** Removal of sutures under anesthesia (other than local), same surgeon

§ **15851** Removal of sutures under anesthesia (other than local), other surgeon

♣ **15852** Dressing change (for other than burns) under anesthesia (other than local)

♣ **15860** Intravenous injection of agent (eg, fluorescein) to test vascular flow in flap or graft
➔ *CPT Changes: An Insider's View* 2002

§ **15876** Suction assisted lipectomy; head and neck

§ **15877** trunk

§ **15878** upper extremity

§ **15879** lower extremity

Pressure Ulcers (Decubitus Ulcers)

§ **15920** Excision, coccygeal pressure ulcer, with coccygectomy; with primary suture

§ **15922** with flap closure

§ **15931** Excision, sacral pressure ulcer, with primary suture;

§ **15933** with ostectomy

§ **15934** Excision, sacral pressure ulcer, with skin flap closure;

§ **15935** with ostectomy

§ **15936** Excision, sacral pressure ulcer, in preparation for muscle or myocutaneous flap or skin graft closure;

§ **15937** with ostectomy

(For repair of defect using muscle or myocutaneous flap, use code(s) 15734 and/or 15738 in addition to 15936, 15937. For repair of defect using split skin graft, use codes 15100 and/or 15101 in addition to 15936, 15937)

§ **15940** Excision, ischial pressure ulcer, with primary suture;

§ **15941** with ostectomy (ischiectomy)

§ **15944** Excision, ischial pressure ulcer, with skin flap closure;

§ **15945** with ostectomy

§ **15946** Excision, ischial pressure ulcer, with ostectomy, in preparation for muscle or myocutaneous flap or skin graft closure

(For repair of defect using muscle or myocutaneous flap, use code(s) 15734 and/or 15738 in addition to 15946. For repair of defect using split skin graft, use codes 15100 and/or 15101 in addition to 15946)

§ **15950** Excision, trochanteric pressure ulcer, with primary suture;

§ **15951** with ostectomy

§ **15952** Excision, trochanteric pressure ulcer, with skin flap closure;

§ **15953** with ostectomy

§ **15956** Excision, trochanteric pressure ulcer, in preparation for muscle or myocutaneous flap or skin graft closure;

§ **15958** with ostectomy

(For repair of defect using muscle or myocutaneous flap, use code(s) 15734 and/or 15738 in addition to 15956, 15958. For repair of defect using split skin graft, use codes 15100 and/or 15101 in addition to 15956, 15958)

§ **15999** Unlisted procedure, excision pressure ulcer

(For free skin graft to close ulcer or donor site, see 15000 et seq)

Burns, Local Treatment

Procedures 16000-16036 refer to local treatment of burned surface only.

List percentage of body surface involved and depth of burn.

For necessary related medical services (eg, hospital visits, detention) in management of burned patients, see appropriate services in **Evaluation and Management** and **Medicine** sections.

(For skin graft, see 15100-15650)

§ **16000** Initial treatment, first degree burn, when no more than local treatment is required

§ **16010** Dressings and/or debridement, initial or subsequent; under anesthesia, small

§ **16015** under anesthesia, medium or large, or with major debridement

§ **16020** without anesthesia, office or hospital, small

§ **16025** without anesthesia, medium (eg, whole face or whole extremity)

§ **16030** without anesthesia, large (eg, more than one extremity)

✿ **16035** Escharotomy; initial incision

✿+ **16036** each additional incision (List separately in addition to code for primary procedure)

(Use 16036 in conjunction with 16035)

(For debridement, curettement of burn wound, see 16010-16030)

Destruction

Destruction means the ablation of benign, premalignant or malignant tissues by any method, with or without curettement, including local anesthesia, and not usually requiring closure.

Any method includes electrosurgery, cryosurgery, laser and chemical treatment. Lesions include condylomata, papillomata, molluscum contagiosum, herpetic lesions, warts (ie, common, plantar, flat), milia, or other benign, premalignant (eg, actinic keratoses), or malignant lesions.

(For destruction of lesion(s) in specific anatomic sites, see 40820, 46900-46917, 46924, 54050-54057, 54065, 56501, 56515, 57061, 57065, 67850, 68135)

(For paring or cutting of benign hyperkeratotic lesions (eg, corns or calluses), see 11055-11057)

(For sharp removal or electrosurgical destruction of skin tags and fibrocutaneous tags, see 11200, 11201)

(For cryotherapy of acne, use 17340)

(For initiation or follow-up care of topical chemotherapy (eg, 5-FU or similar agents), see appropriate office visits)

(For shaving of epidermal or dermal lesions, see 11300-11313)

Destruction, Benign or Premalignant Lesions

§ **17000** Destruction (eg, laser surgery, electrosurgery, cryosurgery, chemosurgery, surgical curettement), all benign or premalignant lesions (eg, actinic keratoses) other than skin tags or cutaneous vascular proliferative lesions; first lesion
➲ *CPT Changes: An Insider's View* 2002

§+ **17003** second through 14 lesions, each (List separately in addition to code for first lesion)

(Use 17003 in conjunction with 17000)

§⊘ **17004** Destruction (eg, laser surgery, electrosurgery, cryosurgery, chemosurgery, surgical curettement), all benign or premalignant lesions (eg, actinic keratoses) other than skin tags or cutaneous vascular proliferative lesions, 15 or more lesions
➲ *CPT Changes: An Insider's View* 2002

(Do not report 17004 in conjunction with 17000-17003)

§ **17106** Destruction of cutaneous vascular proliferative lesions (eg, laser technique); less than 10 sq cm

§ **17107** 10.0 to 50.0 sq cm

§ **17108** over 50.0 sq cm

§ **17110** Destruction (eg, laser surgery, electrosurgery, cryosurgery, chemosurgery, surgical curettement), of flat warts, molluscum contagiosum, or milia; up to 14 lesions
➲ *CPT Changes: An Insider's View* 2002

§ **17111** 15 or more lesions

(For destruction of common or plantar warts, see 17000, 17003, 17004)

§ **17250** Chemical cauterization of granulation tissue (proud flesh, sinus or fistula)

(17250 is not to be used with removal or excision codes for the same lesion)

Destruction, Malignant Lesions, Any Method

§ **17260** Destruction, malignant lesion (eg, laser surgery, electrosurgery, cryosurgery, chemosurgery, surgical curettement), trunk, arms or legs; lesion diameter 0.5 cm or less
➲ *CPT Changes: An Insider's View* 2002

§ **17261** lesion diameter 0.6 to 1.0 cm

§ **17262** lesion diameter 1.1 to 2.0 cm

§ **17263** lesion diameter 2.1 to 3.0 cm

§ **17264** lesion diameter 3.1 to 4.0 cm

§ **17266** lesion diameter over 4.0 cm

§ **17270** Destruction, malignant lesion (eg, laser surgery, electrosurgery, cryosurgery, chemosurgery, surgical curettement), scalp, neck, hands, feet, genitalia; lesion diameter 0.5 cm or less
➲ *CPT Changes: An Insider's View* 2002

§ **17271** lesion diameter 0.6 to 1.0 cm

§ **17272** lesion diameter 1.1 to 2.0 cm

§ **17273** lesion diameter 2.1 to 3.0 cm

§ **17274** lesion diameter 3.1 to 4.0 cm

§ **17276** lesion diameter over 4.0 cm

§ **17280** Destruction, malignant lesion (eg, laser surgery, electrosurgery, cryosurgery, chemosurgery, surgical curettement), face, ears, eyelids, nose, lips, mucous membrane; lesion diameter 0.5 cm or less
➲ *CPT Changes: An Insider's View* 2002

§ **17281** lesion diameter 0.6 to 1.0 cm

§ **17282** lesion diameter 1.1 to 2.0 cm

§ **17283** lesion diameter 2.1 to 3.0 cm

§ **17284** lesion diameter 3.1 to 4.0 cm

§ **17286** lesion diameter over 4.0 cm

Mohs Micrographic Surgery

Mohs micrographic surgery, for the removal of complex or ill-defined skin cancer, requires a single physician to act in two integrated, but separate and distinct capacities: surgeon and pathologist. If either of these responsibilities are delegated to another physician who reports his services separately, these codes are not appropriate. If repair is performed, use separate repair, flap, or graft codes. If a biopsy of a suspected skin cancer is performed on the same day as Mohs surgery because there was no prior pathology confirmation of a diagnosis, then report diagnostic skin biopsy (11100, 11101) and frozen section pathology (88331) with modifier 59 to distinguish from the subsequent definitive surgical procedure of Mohs surgery.

§⊘ **17304** Chemosurgery (Mohs micrographic technique), including removal of all gross tumor, surgical excision of tissue specimens, mapping, color coding of specimens, microscopic examination of specimens by the surgeon, and complete histopathologic preparation including the first routine stain (eg, hematoxylin and eosin, toluidine blue); first stage, fresh tissue technique, up to 5 specimens

➔ *CPT Changes: An Insider's View* 2003

(If additional special pathology procedures, stains or immunostains are required, use 88311-88314, 88342)

§⊘ **17305** second stage, fixed or fresh tissue, up to 5 specimens

§⊘ **17306** third stage, fixed or fresh tissue, up to 5 specimens

§⊘ **17307** additional stage(s), up to 5 specimens, each stage

§+ **17310** each additional specimen, after the first 5 specimens, fixed or fresh tissue, any stage (List separately in addition to code for primary procedure)

➔ *CPT Changes: An Insider's View* 2003

(Use 17310 in conjunction with 17304-17307)

Other Procedures

§ **17340** Cryotherapy (CO_2 slush, liquid N_2) for acne

§ **17360** Chemical exfoliation for acne (eg, acne paste, acid)

§ **17380** Electrolysis epilation, each 1/2 hour

(For actinotherapy, use 96900)

§ **17999** Unlisted procedure, skin, mucous membrane and subcutaneous tissue

Breast

Incision

§ **19000** Puncture aspiration of cyst of breast;

➔ *CPT Assistant* Feb 03:12, 13

§+ **19001** each additional cyst (List separately in addition to code for primary procedure)

➔ *CPT Assistant* Feb 03:12, 13

(Use 19001 in conjunction with 19000)

(If imaging guidance is performed, see 76095, 76096, 76393, 76942)

♦§ **19020** Mastotomy with exploration or drainage of abscess, deep

➔ *CPT Assistant* Feb 03:12, 13

♦☆ **19030** Injection procedure only for mammary ductogram or galactogram

➔ *CPT Assistant* Feb 03:12, 13

(For radiological supervision and interpretation, see 76086, 76088)

(For catheter lavage of mammary ducts for collection of cytology specimens, use Category III codes 0046T, 0047T)

Excision

(To report bilateral procedures, report modifier 50 with the procedure code)

►Excisional breast surgery includes certain biopsy procedures, the removal of cysts or other benign or malignant tumors or lesions, and the surgical treatment of breast and chest wall malignancies. Biopsy procedures may be percutaneous or open, and they involve the removal of differing amounts of tissue for diagnosis.◄

►Breast biopsies are reported using codes 19100-19103. The open excision of breast lesions (eg, lesions of the breast ducts, cysts, benign or malignant tumors), without specific attention to adequate surgical margins, with or without the preoperative placement of radiological markers, is reported using codes 19110-19126. Partial mastectomy procedures (eg, lumpectomy, tylectomy, quadrantectomy, or segmentectomy) describe open excisions of breast tissue with specific attention to adequate surgical margins.◄

►Partial mastectomy procedures are reported using codes 19160 or 19162 as appropriate. Documentation for partial mastectomy procedures includes attention to the removal of adequate surgical margins surrounding the breast mass or lesion.◄

►Total mastectomy procedures include simple mastectomy, complete mastectomy, subcutaneous mastectomy, modified radical mastectomy, radical mastectomy, and more extended procedures (eg, Urban type operation). Total mastectomy procedures are reported using codes 19180, 19182, 19200, 19220, or 19240 as appropriate.◄

►Excisions or resections of chest wall tumors including ribs, with or without reconstruction, with or without mediastinal lymphadenectomy, are reported using codes 19260, 19271, or 19272. Codes 19260-19272 are not restricted to breast tumors and are used to report resections of chest wall tumors originating from any chest wall component. (For excision of lung or pleura, see 32310 et seq.)◄

♦§ 19100 Biopsy of breast; percutaneous, needle core, not using imaging guidance (separate procedure)
➔ *CPT Assistant* Feb 03:12, 13; *CPT Changes: An Insider's View* 2001

(For fine needle aspiration, use 10021)

(For image guided breast biopsy, see 19102, 19103, 10022)

♦§ 19101 open, incisional
➔ *CPT Assistant* Feb 03:12, 13

♦§ 19102 percutaneous, needle core, using imaging guidance
➔ *CPT Assistant* Feb 03:12, 13; *CPT Changes: An Insider's View* 2001

(For placement of percutaneous localization clip, use 19295)

♦§ 19103 percutaneous, automated vacuum assisted or rotating biopsy device, using imaging guidance
➔ *CPT Assistant* Feb 03:12, 13, Apr 03:7; *CPT Changes: An Insider's View* 2001

(For imaging guidance performed in conjunction with 19102, 19103, see 76095, 76096, 76360, 76393, 76942)

(For placement of percutaneous localization clip, use 19295)

♦§ 19110 Nipple exploration, with or without excision of a solitary lactiferous duct or a papilloma lactiferous duct
➔ *CPT Assistant* Feb 03:12, 13

♦§ 19112 Excision of lactiferous duct fistula
➔ *CPT Assistant* Feb 03:12, 13

§ 19120 Excision of cyst, fibroadenoma, or other benign or malignant tumor, aberrant breast tissue, duct lesion, nipple or areolar lesion (except 19140), open, male or female, one or more lesions
➔ *CPT Assistant* Feb 03:12, 13; *CPT Changes: An Insider's View* 2001

§ 19125 Excision of breast lesion identified by preoperative placement of radiological marker, open; single lesion
➔ *CPT Assistant* Feb 03:12, 13; *CPT Changes: An Insider's View* 2001

§+ 19126 each additional lesion separately identified by a preoperative radiological marker (List separately in addition to code for primary procedure)
➔ *CPT Assistant* Feb 03:12, 13; *CPT Changes: An Insider's View* 2001

(Use 19126 in conjunction with 19125)

♦§ 19140 Mastectomy for gynecomastia
➔ *CPT Assistant* Feb 03:12, 13

♦§▲ 19160 Mastectomy, partial (eg, lumpectomy, tylectomy, quadrantectomy, segmentectomy);
➔ *CPT Assistant* Feb 03:12, 13; *CPT Changes: An Insider's View* 2005

♦§ 19162 with axillary lymphadenectomy
➔ *CPT Assistant* Feb 03:12, 13

►(For placement of radiotherapy afterloading balloon/brachytherapy catheters, see 19296-19298)◄

♦§ 19180 Mastectomy, simple, complete
➔ *CPT Assistant* Feb 03:12, 13

(For immediate or delayed insertion of implant, use 19340 or 19342)

(For gynecomastia, use 19140)

♦§ 19182 Mastectomy, subcutaneous
➔ *CPT Assistant* Feb 03:12, 13

(For immediate or delayed insertion of implant, use 19340 or 19342)

♦✿ 19200 Mastectomy, radical, including pectoral muscles, axillary lymph nodes
➔ *CPT Assistant* Feb 03:13

(For immediate or delayed insertion of implant, use 19340 or 19342)

♦✿ 19220 Mastectomy, radical, including pectoral muscles, axillary and internal mammary lymph nodes (Urban type operation)
➔ *CPT Assistant* Feb 03:13

(For immediate or delayed insertion of implant, use 19340 or 19342)

♦§ 19240 Mastectomy, modified radical, including axillary lymph nodes, with or without pectoralis minor muscle, but excluding pectoralis major muscle

(For immediate or delayed insertion of implant, use 19340 or 19342)

§ 19260 Excision of chest wall tumor including ribs

✿ 19271 Excision of chest wall tumor involving ribs, with plastic reconstruction; without mediastinal lymphadenectomy

✿ 19272 with mediastinal lymphadenectomy

Introduction

☆ 19290 Preoperative placement of needle localization wire, breast;

☆+ 19291 each additional lesion (List separately in addition to code for primary procedure)

(Use 19291 in conjunction with 19290)

(For radiological supervision and interpretation, see 76095, 76096, 76942)

❖+ 19295 Image guided placement, metallic localization clip, percutaneous, during breast biopsy (List separately in addition to code for primary procedure)
➔ *CPT Changes: An Insider's View* 2001

(Use 19295 in conjunction with 19102, 19103)

Surgery: Integumentary System

♦❖● **19296** Placement of radiotherapy afterloading balloon catheter into the breast for interstitial radioelement application following partial mastectomy, includes imaging guidance; on date separate from partial mastectomy
➲ *CPT Changes: An Insider's View* 2005

♦❖ +● **19297** concurrent with partial mastectomy (List separately in addition to code for primary procedure)
➲ *CPT Changes: An Insider's View* 2005

►(Use 19297 in conjunction with 19160 or 19162)◄

♦❖ ⊙● **19298** Placement of radiotherapy afterloading brachytherapy catheters (multiple tube and button type) into the breast for interstitial radioelement application following (at the time of or subsequent to) partial mastectomy, includes imaging guidance
➲ *CPT Changes: An Insider's View* 2005

Repair and/or Reconstruction

(To report bilateral procedures, report modifier 50 with the procedure code)

♦§ **19316** Mastopexy
➲ *CPT Assistant* Jan 03:7

♦§ **19318** Reduction mammaplasty
➲ *CPT Assistant* Jan 03:7

♦§ **19324** Mammaplasty, augmentation; without prosthetic implant
➲ *CPT Assistant* Jan 03:7

♦§ **19325** with prosthetic implant
➲ *CPT Assistant* Jan 03:7

(For flap or graft, use also appropriate number)

♦§ **19328** Removal of intact mammary implant
➲ *CPT Assistant* Jan 03:7

♦§ **19330** Removal of mammary implant material
➲ *CPT Assistant* Jan 03:7

♦§ **19340** Immediate insertion of breast prosthesis following mastopexy, mastectomy or in reconstruction
➲ *CPT Assistant* Jan 03:7

♦§ **19342** Delayed insertion of breast prosthesis following mastopexy, mastectomy or in reconstruction
➲ *CPT Assistant* Jan 03:7

(For supply of implant, use 99070)

(For preparation of custom breast implant, use 19396)

♦§ **19350** Nipple/areola reconstruction
➲ *CPT Assistant* Jan 03:7

♦§ **19355** Correction of inverted nipples
➲ *CPT Assistant* Jan 03:7

♦§ **19357** Breast reconstruction, immediate or delayed, with tissue expander, including subsequent expansion
➲ *CPT Assistant* Jan 03:7

♦✿ **19361** Breast reconstruction with latissimus dorsi flap, with or without prosthetic implant

♦✿ **19364** Breast reconstruction with free flap

(Do not report code 69990 in addition to code 19364)

(19364 includes harvesting of the flap, microvascular transfer, closure of the donor site, and inset shaping the flap into a breast)

♦§ **19366** Breast reconstruction with other technique
➲ *CPT Assistant* Jan 03:7

(For operating microscope, use 69990)

(For insertion of prosthesis, use also 19340 or 19342)

♦✿ **19367** Breast reconstruction with transverse rectus abdominis myocutaneous flap (TRAM), single pedicle, including closure of donor site;

♦✿ **19368** with microvascular anastomosis (supercharging)

(Do not report code 69990 in addition to code 19368)

♦✿ **19369** Breast reconstruction with transverse rectus abdominis myocutaneous flap (TRAM), double pedicle, including closure of donor site

♦§ **19370** Open periprosthetic capsulotomy, breast
➲ *CPT Assistant* Jan 03:7

♦§ **19371** Periprosthetic capsulectomy, breast
➲ *CPT Assistant* Jan 03:7

♦§ **19380** Revision of reconstructed breast
➲ *CPT Assistant* Jan 03:7

♦§ **19396** Preparation of moulage for custom breast implant
➲ *CPT Assistant* Jan 03:7

Other Procedures

(For microwave thermotherapy of the breast, use Category III code 0061T)

♦§ **19499** Unlisted procedure, breast

Musculoskeletal System

Cast and strapping procedures appear at the end of this section.

The services listed below include the application and removal of the first cast or traction device only. Subsequent replacement of cast and/or traction device may require an additional listing.

Definitions

The terms "closed treatment," "open treatment," and "percutaneous skeletal fixation" have been carefully chosen to accurately reflect current orthopaedic procedural treatments.

Closed treatment specifically means that the fracture site is not surgically opened (exposed to the external environment and directly visualized). This terminology is used to describe procedures that treat fractures by three methods: 1) without manipulation 2) with manipulation 3) with or without traction.

Open treatment is used when the fractured bone is either (1) surgically opened (exposed to the external environment) and the fracture (bone ends) visualized and internal fixation may be used or (2) the fractured bone is opened remote from the fracture site in order to insert an intramedullary nail across the fracture site (the fracture site is not opened and visualized).

Percutaneous skeletal fixation describes fracture treatment which is neither open nor closed. In this procedure, the fracture fragments are not visualized, but fixation (eg, pins) is placed across the fracture site, usually under x-ray imaging.

The type of fracture (eg, open, compound, closed) does not have any coding correlation with the type of treatment (eg, closed, open, or percutaneous) provided.

The codes for treatment of fractures and joint injuries (dislocations) are categorized by the type of manipulation (reduction) and stabilization (fixation or immobilization). These codes can apply to either open (compound) or closed fractures or joint injuries.

Skeletal traction is the application of a force (distracting or traction force) to a limb segment through a wire, pin, screw, or clamp that is attached (eg, penetrates) to bone.

Skin traction is the application of a force (longitudinal) to a limb using felt or strapping applied directly to skin only.

External fixation is the usage of skeletal pins plus an attaching mechanism/device used for temporary or definitive treatment of acute or chronic bony deformity.

Codes for obtaining autogenous bone grafts, cartilage, tendon, fascia lata grafts or other tissues through separate incisions are to be used only when the graft is not already listed as part of the basic procedure.

Re-reduction of a fracture and/or dislocation performed by the primary physician may be identified by the addition of the modifier 76 to the usual procedure number to indicate "Repeat Procedure by Same Physician." (See guidelines.)

Codes for external fixation are to be used only when external fixation is not already listed as part of the basic procedure.

All codes for suction irrigation have been deleted. To report, list only the primary surgical procedure performed (eg, sequestrectomy, deep incision).

Manipulation is used throughout the musculoskeletal fracture and dislocation subsections to specifically mean the attempted reduction or restoration of a fracture or joint dislocation to its normal anatomic alignment by the application of manually applied forces.

(For computer assisted musculoskeletal surgical navigational orthopedic procedures, report 0054T-0056T)

General

Incision

§ **20000** Incision of soft tissue abscess (eg, secondary to osteomyelitis); superficial

§ **20005** deep or complicated

Wound Exploration—Trauma (eg, Penetrating Gunshot, Stab Wound)

20100-20103 relate to wound(s) resulting from penetrating trauma. These codes describe surgical exploration and enlargement of the wound, extension of dissection (to determine penetration), debridement, removal of foreign body(s), ligation or coagulation of minor subcutaneous and/or muscular blood vessel(s), of the subcutaneous tissue, muscle fascia, and/or muscle, not requiring thoracotomy or laparotomy. If a repair is done to major structure(s) or major blood vessel(s) requiring thoracotomy or laparotomy, then those specific code(s) would supersede the use of codes 20100-20103. To report Simple, Intermediate, or Complex repair of wound(s) that do not require enlargement of the wound, extension of dissection, etc., as stated above, use specific Repair code(s) in the Integumentary System section.

♦§ **20100** Exploration of penetrating wound (separate procedure); neck

§ **20101** chest

§ **20102** abdomen/flank/back

§ **20103** extremity

Excision

♦§ **20150** Excision of epiphyseal bar, with or without autogenous soft tissue graft obtained through same fascial incision

(For aspiration of bone marrow, use 38220)

§ **20200** Biopsy, muscle; superficial

§ **20205** deep

§ **20206** Biopsy, muscle, percutaneous needle

(If imaging guidance is performed, see 76360, 76393, 76942)

(For fine needle aspiration, use 10021 or 10022)

(For evaulation of fine needle aspirate, see 88172-88173)

(For excision of muscle tumor, deep, see specific anatomic section)

§ **20220** Biopsy, bone, trocar, or needle; superficial (eg, ilium, sternum, spinous process, ribs)

§ **20225** deep (eg, vertebral body, femur)
➲ *CPT Changes: An Insider's View* 2002

(For bone marrow biopsy, use 38221)

(For radiologic supervision and interpretation, see 76003, 76360, 76393)

§ **20240** Biopsy, bone, open; superficial (eg, ilium, sternum, spinous process, ribs, trochanter of femur)
➲ *CPT Changes: An Insider's View* 2004

§ **20245** deep (eg, humerus, ischium, femur)

§ **20250** Biopsy, vertebral body, open; thoracic

§ **20251** lumbar or cervical

(For sequestrectomy, osteomyelitis or drainage of bone abscess, see anatomical area)

Introduction or Removal

(For injection procedure for arthrography, see anatomical area)

§ **20500** Injection of sinus tract; therapeutic (separate procedure)

☆ **20501** diagnostic (sinogram)

(For radiological supervision and interpretation, use 76080)

§ **20520** Removal of foreign body in muscle or tendon sheath; simple

§ **20525** deep or complicated

♦§ **20526** Injection, therapeutic (eg, local anesthetic, corticosteroid), carpal tunnel
➲ *CPT Changes: An Insider's View* 2002

§ **20550** Injection(s); single tendon sheath, or ligament, aponeurosis (eg, plantar "fascia")
➲ *CPT Changes: An Insider's View* 2002, 2003, 2004

§ **20551** single tendon origin/insertion
➲ *CPT Changes: An Insider's View* 2002, 2004

§ **20552** Injection(s); single or multiple trigger point(s), one or two muscle(s)
➲ *CPT Changes: An Insider's View* 2002, 2003, 2004

§ **20553** single or multiple trigger point(s), three or more muscle(s)
➲ *CPT Changes: An Insider's View* 2002

(If imaging guidance is performed, see 76003, 76393, 76942)

♦§ **20600** Arthrocentesis, aspiration and/or injection; small joint or bursa (eg, fingers, toes)
➲ *CPT Changes: An Insider's View* 2003

♦§ **20605** intermediate joint or bursa (eg, temporomandibular, acromioclavicular, wrist, elbow or ankle, olecranon bursa)
➲ *CPT Changes: An Insider's View* 2003

♦§ **20610** major joint or bursa (eg, shoulder, hip, knee joint, subacromial bursa)

(If imaging guidance is performed, see 76003, 76360, 76393, 76942)

§ **20612** Aspiration and/or injection of ganglion cyst(s) any location
➲ *CPT Changes: An Insider's View* 2003

(To report multiple ganglion cyst aspirations/injections, use 20612 and append modifier 59)

§ **20615** Aspiration and injection for treatment of bone cyst

§ **20650** Insertion of wire or pin with application of skeletal traction, including removal (separate procedure)

✿⊘ **20660** Application of cranial tongs, caliper, or stereotactic frame, including removal (separate procedure)

✿ **20661** Application of halo, including removal; cranial

✿ **20662** pelvic

✿ **20663** femoral

✿ **20664** Application of halo, including removal, cranial, 6 or more pins placed, for thin skull osteology (eg, pediatric patients, hydrocephalus, osteogenesis imperfecta), requiring general anesthesia

♣ **20665** Removal of tongs or halo applied by another physician

§ **20670** Removal of implant; superficial, (eg, buried wire, pin or rod) (separate procedure)

§ **20680** deep (eg, buried wire, pin, screw, metal band, nail, rod or plate)

§⊘ **20690** Application of a uniplane (pins or wires in one plane), unilateral, external fixation system

§⊘ **20692** Application of a multiplane (pins or wires in more than one plane), unilateral, external fixation system (eg, Ilizarov, Monticelli type)

§ **20693** Adjustment or revision of external fixation system requiring anesthesia (eg, new pin(s) or wire(s) and/or new ring(s) or bar(s))

§ **20694** Removal, under anesthesia, of external fixation system

Replantation

♦✿ **20802** Replantation, arm (includes surgical neck of humerus through elbow joint), complete amputation

(To report replantation of incomplete arm amputation, see specific code(s) for repair of bone(s), ligament(s), tendon(s), nerve(s), or blood vessel(s) with modifier 52)

♦✿ **20805** Replantation, forearm (includes radius and ulna to radial carpal joint), complete amputation

(To report replantation of incomplete forearm amputation, see specific code(s) for repair of bone(s), ligament(s), tendon(s), nerve(s), or blood vessel(s) with modifier 52)

♦✿ **20808** Replantation, hand (includes hand through metacarpophalangeal joints), complete amputation

(To report replantation of incomplete hand amputation, see specific code(s) for repair of bone(s), ligament(s), tendon(s), nerve(s), or blood vessel(s) with modifier 52)

✿ **20816** Replantation, digit, excluding thumb (includes metacarpophalangeal joint to insertion of flexor sublimis tendon), complete amputation

(To report replantation of incomplete digit amputation, excluding thumb, see specific code(s) for repair of bone(s), ligament(s), tendon(s), nerve(s), or blood vessel(s) with modifier 52)

✿ **20822** Replantation, digit, excluding thumb (includes distal tip to sublimis tendon insertion), complete amputation

(To report replantation of incomplete digit amputation, excluding thumb, see specific code(s) for repair of bone(s), ligament(s), tendon(s), nerve(s), or blood vessel(s) with modifier 52)

♦✿ **20824** Replantation, thumb (includes carpometacarpal joint to MP joint), complete amputation

(To report replantation of incomplete thumb amputation, see specific code(s) for repair of bone(s), ligament(s), tendon(s), nerve(s), or blood vessel(s) with modifier 52)

♦✿ **20827** Replantation, thumb (includes distal tip to MP joint), complete amputation

(To report replantation of incomplete thumb amputation, see specific code(s) for repair of bone(s), ligament(s), tendon(s), nerve(s), or blood vessel(s) with modifier 52)

(To report replantation of complete leg amputation, see specific code(s) for repair of bone(s), ligament(s), tendon(s), nerve(s), or blood vessel(s) with modifier 52)

(To report replantation of incomplete leg amputation, see specific code(s) for repair of bone(s), ligament(s), tendon(s), nerve(s), or blood vessel(s) with modifier 52)

♦✿ **20838** Replantation, foot, complete amputation

(To report replantation of incomplete foot amputation, see specific code(s) for repair of bone(s), ligament(s), tendon(s), nerve(s), or blood vessel(s) with modifier 52)

Grafts (or Implants)

Codes for obtaining autogenous bone, cartilage, tendon, fascia lata grafts, or other tissues through separate skin/fascial incisions should be reported separately unless the code descriptor references the harvesting of the graft or implant (eg, includes obtaining graft).

Do not append modifier 62 to bone graft codes 20900-20938.

(For spinal surgery bone graft(s) see codes 20930-20938)

§⊘ **20900** Bone graft, any donor area; minor or small (eg, dowel or button)

§⊘ **20902** major or large

§⊘ **20910** Cartilage graft; costochondral

§⊘ **20912** nasal septum

(For ear cartilage, use 21235)

§⊘ **20920** Fascia lata graft; by stripper

§⊘ **20922** by incision and area exposure, complex or sheet

§⊘ **20924** Tendon graft, from a distance (eg, palmaris, toe extensor, plantaris)

§⊘ **20926** Tissue grafts, other (eg, paratenon, fat, dermis)

(Codes 20930-20938 are reported in addition to codes for the definitive procedure(s) without modifier 51)

✶✿⊘ **20930** Allograft for spine surgery only; morselized

✶✿⊘ **20931** structural

✶✿⊘ **20936** Autograft for spine surgery only (includes harvesting the graft); local (eg, ribs, spinous process, or laminar fragments) obtained from same incision

♦✿⊘ **20937** morselized (through separate skin or fascial incision)

♦✿⊘ **20938** structural, bicortical or tricortical (through separate skin or fascial incision)

(For needle aspiration of bone marrow for the purpose of bone grafting, use 38220)

Other Procedures

§ **20950** Monitoring of interstitial fluid pressure (includes insertion of device, eg, wick catheter technique, needle manometer technique) in detection of muscle compartment syndrome

✿ **20955** Bone graft with microvascular anastomosis; fibula

✿ **20956** iliac crest

✿ **20957** metatarsal

✿ **20962** other than fibula, iliac crest, or metatarsal

(Do not report code 69990 in addition to codes 20955-20962)

✿ **20969** Free osteocutaneous flap with microvascular anastomosis; other than iliac crest, metatarsal, or great toe

✿ **20970** iliac crest

✿ **20972** metatarsal

✿ **20973** great toe with web space

(Do not report code 69990 in addition to codes 20969-20973)

(For great toe, wrap-around procedure, use 26551)

♠⊘ **20974** Electrical stimulation to aid bone healing; noninvasive (nonoperative)

♣⊘ **20975** invasive (operative)

♠ **20979** Low intensity ultrasound stimulation to aid bone healing, noninvasive (nonoperative)
➲ *CPT Changes: An Insider's View* 2000

♦§⊙ **20982** Ablation, bone tumor(s) (eg, osteoid osteoma, metastasis) radiofrequency, percutaneous, including computed tomographic guidance
➲ *CPT Changes: An Insider's View* 2004

§ **20999** Unlisted procedure, musculoskeletal system, general

Head

Skull, facial bones and temporomandibular joint.

Incision

(For drainage of superficial abscess and hematoma, use 20000)

(For removal of embedded foreign body from dentoalveolar structure, see 41805, 41806)

♦§ **21010** Arthrotomy, temporomandibular joint

(To report bilateral procedures, report 21010 with modifier 50)

Excision

§ **21015** Radical resection of tumor (eg, malignant neoplasm), soft tissue of face or scalp

(To report excision of skull tumor for osteomyelitis, use 61501)

§ **21025** Excision of bone (eg, for osteomyelitis or bone abscess); mandible

§ **21026** facial bone(s)

§ **21029** Removal by contouring of benign tumor of facial bone (eg, fibrous dysplasia)

§ **21030** Excision of benign tumor or cyst of maxilla or zygoma by enucleation and curettage
➲ *CPT Changes: An Insider's View* 2003

§ **21031** Excision of torus mandibularis

§ **21032** Excision of maxillary torus palatinus

§ **21034** Excision of malignant tumor of maxilla or zygoma

§ **21040** Excision of benign tumor or cyst of mandible, by enucleation and/or curettage
➲ *CPT Changes: An Insider's View* 2003

(21041 has been deleted)

(For enucleation and/or curettage of benign cysts or tumors of mandible not requiring osteotomy, use 21040)

(For excision of benign tumor or cyst of mandible requiring osteotomy, see 21046-21047)

§ **21044** Excision of malignant tumor of mandible;

✿ **21045** radical resection

(For bone graft, use 21215)

§ **21046** Excision of benign tumor or cyst of mandible; requiring intra-oral osteotomy (eg, locally aggressive or destructive lesion(s))
➲ *CPT Changes: An Insider's View* 2003

§ **21047** requiring extra-oral osteotomy and partial mandibulectomy (eg, locally aggressive or destructive lesion(s))
➲ *CPT Changes: An Insider's View* 2003

§ **21048** Excision of benign tumor or cyst of maxilla; requiring intra-oral osteotomy (eg, locally aggressive or destructive lesion(s))
➲ *CPT Changes: An Insider's View* 2003

§ **21049** requiring extra-oral osteotomy and partial maxillectomy (eg, locally aggressive or destructive lesion(s))
➲ *CPT Changes: An Insider's View* 2003

♦§ **21050** Condylectomy, temporomandibular joint (separate procedure)

(For bilateral procedures, report 21050 with modifier 50)

♦§ **21060** Meniscectomy, partial or complete, temporomandibular joint (separate procedure)

(For bilateral procedures, report 21060 with modifier 50)

♦§ **21070** Coronoidectomy (separate procedure)

(For bilateral procedures, report 21070 with modifier 50)

Introduction or Removal

(For application or removal of caliper or tongs, see 20660, 20665.) Codes 21076-21089 describe professional services for the rehabilitation of patients with oral, facial or other anatomical deficiencies by means of prostheses such as an artificial eye, ear, or nose or intraoral obturator to close a cleft. Codes 21076-21089 should only be used when the physician actually designs and prepares the prosthesis (ie, not prepared by an outside laboratory).

§ **21076** Impression and custom preparation; surgical obturator prosthesis

♦§ **21077** orbital prosthesis

§ **21079** interim obturator prosthesis

§ **21080** definitive obturator prosthesis

§ **21081** mandibular resection prosthesis

§ **21082** palatal augmentation prosthesis

§ **21083** palatal lift prosthesis

§ **21084** speech aid prosthesis

§ **21085** oral surgical splint

♦§ **21086** auricular prosthesis

§ **21087** nasal prosthesis

§ **21088** facial prosthesis

§ **21089** Unlisted maxillofacial prosthetic procedure

§ **21100** Application of halo type appliance for maxillofacial fixation, includes removal (separate procedure)

§ **21110** Application of interdental fixation device for conditions other than fracture or dislocation, includes removal

(For removal of interdental fixation by another physician, see 20670-20680)

☆ **21116** Injection procedure for temporomandibular joint arthrography

(For radiological supervision and interpretation, use 70332. Do not report 76003 in addition to 70332)

Repair, Revision, and/or Reconstruction

(For cranioplasty, see 21179, 21180 and 62116, 62120, 62140-62147)

§ **21120** Genioplasty; augmentation (autograft, allograft, prosthetic material)

§ **21121** sliding osteotomy, single piece

§ **21122** sliding osteotomies, two or more osteotomies (eg, wedge excision or bone wedge reversal for asymmetrical chin)

§ **21123** sliding, augmentation with interpositional bone grafts (includes obtaining autografts)

§ **21125** Augmentation, mandibular body or angle; prosthetic material

§ **21127** with bone graft, onlay or interpositional (includes obtaining autograft)

§ **21137** Reduction forehead; contouring only

§ **21138** contouring and application of prosthetic material or bone graft (includes obtaining autograft)

§ **21139** contouring and setback of anterior frontal sinus wall

✿ **21141** Reconstruction midface, LeFort I; single piece, segment movement in any direction (eg, for Long Face Syndrome), without bone graft

✿ **21142** two pieces, segment movement in any direction, without bone graft

✿ **21143** three or more pieces, segment movement in any direction, without bone graft

✿ **21145** single piece, segment movement in any direction, requiring bone grafts (includes obtaining autografts)

✿ **21146** two pieces, segment movement in any direction, requiring bone grafts (includes obtaining autografts) (eg, ungrafted unilateral alveolar cleft)

✿ **21147** three or more pieces, segment movement in any direction, requiring bone grafts (includes obtaining autografts) (eg, ungrafted bilateral alveolar cleft or multiple osteotomies)

✿ **21150** Reconstruction midface, LeFort II; anterior intrusion (eg, Treacher-Collins Syndrome)

✿ **21151** any direction, requiring bone grafts (includes obtaining autografts)

✿ **21154** Reconstruction midface, LeFort III (extracranial), any type, requiring bone grafts (includes obtaining autografts); without LeFort I

✿ **21155** with LeFort I

✿ **21159** Reconstruction midface, LeFort III (extra and intracranial) with forehead advancement (eg, mono bloc), requiring bone grafts (includes obtaining autografts); without LeFort I

✿ **21160** with LeFort I

✿ **21172** Reconstruction superior-lateral orbital rim and lower forehead, advancement or alteration, with or without grafts (includes obtaining autografts)

(For frontal or parietal craniotomy performed for craniosynostosis, use 61556)

✿ **21175** Reconstruction, bifrontal, superior-lateral orbital rims and lower forehead, advancement or alteration (eg, plagiocephaly, trigonocephaly, brachycephaly), with or without grafts (includes obtaining autografts)

(For bifrontal craniotomy performed for craniosynostosis, use 61557)

✿ **21179** Reconstruction, entire or majority of forehead and/or supraorbital rims; with grafts (allograft or prosthetic material)

✿ **21180** with autograft (includes obtaining grafts)

(For extensive craniectomy for multiple suture craniosynostosis, use only 61558 or 61559)

§ **21181** Reconstruction by contouring of benign tumor of cranial bones (eg, fibrous dysplasia), extracranial

Surgery: Musculoskeletal System

✿ 21182 Reconstruction of orbital walls, rims, forehead, nasoethmoid complex following intra- and extracranial excision of benign tumor of cranial bone (eg, fibrous dysplasia), with multiple autografts (includes obtaining grafts); total area of bone grafting less than 40 sq cm

✿ 21183 total area of bone grafting greater than 40 sq cm but less than 80 sq cm

✿ 21184 total area of bone grafting greater than 80 sq cm

(For excision of benign tumor of cranial bones, see 61563, 61564)

✿ 21188 Reconstruction midface, osteotomies (other than LeFort type) and bone grafts (includes obtaining autografts)

✶✿ 21193 Reconstruction of mandibular rami, horizontal, vertical, C, or L osteotomy; without bone graft

✶✿ 21194 with bone graft (includes obtaining graft)

✶✿ 21195 Reconstruction of mandibular rami and/or body, sagittal split; without internal rigid fixation

✶✿ 21196 with internal rigid fixation

§ 21198 Osteotomy, mandible, segmental;

➲ *CPT Changes: An Insider's View* 2001

§ 21199 with genioglossus advancement

➲ *CPT Changes: An Insider's View* 2001

(To report total osteotomy of the maxilla, see 21141-21160)

§ 21206 Osteotomy, maxilla, segmental (eg, Wassmund or Schuchard)

§ 21208 Osteoplasty, facial bones; augmentation (autograft, allograft, or prosthetic implant)

§ 21209 reduction

§ 21210 Graft, bone; nasal, maxillary or malar areas (includes obtaining graft)

(For cleft palate repair, see 42200-42225)

§ 21215 mandible (includes obtaining graft)

§ 21230 Graft; rib cartilage, autogenous, to face, chin, nose or ear (includes obtaining graft)

§ 21235 ear cartilage, autogenous, to nose or ear (includes obtaining graft)

(To report graft augmentation of facial bones, use 21208)

♦§ 21240 Arthroplasty, temporomandibular joint, with or without autograft (includes obtaining graft)

♦§ 21242 Arthroplasty, temporomandibular joint, with allograft

♦§ 21243 Arthroplasty, temporomandibular joint, with prosthetic joint replacement

§ 21244 Reconstruction of mandible, extraoral, with transosteal bone plate (eg, mandibular staple bone plate)

§ 21245 Reconstruction of mandible or maxilla, subperiosteal implant; partial

§ 21246 complete

✿ 21247 Reconstruction of mandibular condyle with bone and cartilage autografts (includes obtaining grafts) (eg, for hemifacial microsomia)

§ 21248 Reconstruction of mandible or maxilla, endosteal implant (eg, blade, cylinder); partial

§ 21249 complete

(To report midface reconstruction, see 21141-21160)

✿ 21255 Reconstruction of zygomatic arch and glenoid fossa with bone and cartilage (includes obtaining autografts)

✿ 21256 Reconstruction of orbit with osteotomies (extracranial) and with bone grafts (includes obtaining autografts) (eg, micro-ophthalmia)

§ 21260 Periorbital osteotomies for orbital hypertelorism, with bone grafts; extracranial approach

§ 21261 combined intra- and extracranial approach

§ 21263 with forehead advancement

§ 21267 Orbital repositioning, periorbital osteotomies, unilateral, with bone grafts; extracranial approach

✿ 21268 combined intra- and extracranial approach

§ 21270 Malar augmentation, prosthetic material

(For malar augmentation with bone graft, use 21210)

§ 21275 Secondary revision of orbitocraniofacial reconstruction

♦§ 21280 Medial canthopexy (separate procedure)

(For medial canthoplasty, use 67950)

♦§ 21282 Lateral canthopexy

§ 21295 Reduction of masseter muscle and bone (eg, for treatment of benign masseteric hypertrophy); extraoral approach

§ 21296 intraoral approach

Other Procedures

§ 21299 Unlisted craniofacial and maxillofacial procedure

Fracture and/or Dislocation

§ 21300 Closed treatment of skull fracture without operation

(For operative repair, see 62000-62010)

§ 21310 Closed treatment of nasal bone fracture without manipulation

§ 21315 Closed treatment of nasal bone fracture; without stabilization

§ 21320 with stabilization

§ 21325 Open treatment of nasal fracture; uncomplicated

§ 21330 complicated, with internal and/or external skeletal fixation

§ 21335 with concomitant open treatment of fractured septum

§ 21336 Open treatment of nasal septal fracture, with or without stabilization

§ 21337 Closed treatment of nasal septal fracture, with or without stabilization

§ 21338 Open treatment of nasoethmoid fracture; without external fixation

§ 21339 with external fixation

§ 21340 Percutaneous treatment of nasoethmoid complex fracture, with splint, wire or headcap fixation, including repair of canthal ligaments and/or the nasolacrimal apparatus

✿ 21343 Open treatment of depressed frontal sinus fracture

✿ 21344 Open treatment of complicated (eg, comminuted or involving posterior wall) frontal sinus fracture, via coronal or multiple approaches

§ 21345 Closed treatment of nasomaxillary complex fracture (LeFort II type), with interdental wire fixation or fixation of denture or splint

✿ 21346 Open treatment of nasomaxillary complex fracture (LeFort II type); with wiring and/or local fixation

✿ 21347 requiring multiple open approaches

✿ 21348 with bone grafting (includes obtaining graft)

§ 21355 Percutaneous treatment of fracture of malar area, including zygomatic arch and malar tripod, with manipulation

§ 21356 Open treatment of depressed zygomatic arch fracture (eg, Gillies approach)

✿ 21360 Open treatment of depressed malar fracture, including zygomatic arch and malar tripod

✿ 21365 Open treatment of complicated (eg, comminuted or involving cranial nerve foramina) fracture(s) of malar area, including zygomatic arch and malar tripod; with internal fixation and multiple surgical approaches

✿ 21366 with bone grafting (includes obtaining graft)

✿ 21385 Open treatment of orbital floor blowout fracture; transantral approach (Caldwell-Luc type operation)

✿ 21386 periorbital approach

✿ 21387 combined approach

§ 21390 periorbital approach, with alloplastic or other implant

➲ *CPT Assistant* Jan 03:14

✿ 21395 periorbital approach with bone graft (includes obtaining graft)

§ 21400 Closed treatment of fracture of orbit, except blowout; without manipulation

§ 21401 with manipulation

§ 21406 Open treatment of fracture of orbit, except blowout; without implant

§ 21407 with implant

✿ 21408 with bone grafting (includes obtaining graft)

§ 21421 Closed treatment of palatal or maxillary fracture (LeFort I type), with interdental wire fixation or fixation of denture or splint

✿ 21422 Open treatment of palatal or maxillary fracture (LeFort I type);

✿ 21423 complicated (comminuted or involving cranial nerve foramina), multiple approaches

✿ 21431 Closed treatment of craniofacial separation (LeFort III type) using interdental wire fixation of denture or splint

✿ 21432 Open treatment of craniofacial separation (LeFort III type); with wiring and/or internal fixation

✿ 21433 complicated (eg, comminuted or involving cranial nerve foramina), multiple surgical approaches

✿ 21435 complicated, utilizing internal and/or external fixation techniques (eg, head cap, halo device, and/or intermaxillary fixation)

(For removal of internal or external fixation device, use 20670)

✿ 21436 complicated, multiple surgical approaches, internal fixation, with bone grafting (includes obtaining graft)

§ 21440 Closed treatment of mandibular or maxillary alveolar ridge fracture (separate procedure)

§ 21445 Open treatment of mandibular or maxillary alveolar ridge fracture (separate procedure)

§ 21450 Closed treatment of mandibular fracture; without manipulation

§ 21451 with manipulation

§ 21452 Percutaneous treatment of mandibular fracture, with external fixation

§ 21453 Closed treatment of mandibular fracture with interdental fixation

§ 21454 Open treatment of mandibular fracture with external fixation

§ 21461 Open treatment of mandibular fracture; without interdental fixation

§ 21462 with interdental fixation

§ 21465 Open treatment of mandibular condylar fracture

§ 21470 Open treatment of complicated mandibular fracture by multiple surgical approaches including internal fixation, interdental fixation, and/or wiring of dentures or splints

♦§ 21480 Closed treatment of temporomandibular dislocation; initial or subsequent

♦§ 21485 complicated (eg, recurrent requiring intermaxillary fixation or splinting), initial or subsequent

♦§ 21490 Open treatment of temporomandibular dislocation

(For interdental wire fixation, use 21497)

§ 21493 Closed treatment of hyoid fracture; without manipulation

§ 21494 with manipulation

✿ 21495 Open treatment of hyoid fracture

(For treatment of fracture of larynx, see 31584-31586)

§ 21497 Interdental wiring, for condition other than fracture

Other Procedures

§ 21499 Unlisted musculoskeletal procedure, head

(For unlisted craniofacial or maxillofacial procedure, use 21299)

Neck (Soft Tissues) and Thorax

(For cervical spine and back, see 21920 et seq)

(For injection of fracture site or trigger point, use 20550)

Incision

(For incision and drainage of abscess or hematoma, superficial, see 10060, 10140)

§ 21501 Incision and drainage, deep abscess or hematoma, soft tissues of neck or thorax;

§ 21502 with partial rib ostectomy

✿ 21510 Incision, deep, with opening of bone cortex (eg, for osteomyelitis or bone abscess), thorax

Excision

(For bone biopsy, see 20220-20251)

§ 21550 Biopsy, soft tissue of neck or thorax

(For needle biopsy of soft tissue, use 20206)

§ 21555 Excision tumor, soft tissue of neck or thorax; subcutaneous

§ 21556 deep, subfascial, intramuscular

§ 21557 Radical resection of tumor (eg, malignant neoplasm), soft tissue of neck or thorax

§ 21600 Excision of rib, partial

(For radical resection of chest wall and rib cage for tumor, use 19260)

(For radical debridement of chest wall and rib cage for injury, see 11040-11044)

§ 21610 Costotransversectomy (separate procedure)

♦✿ 21615 Excision first and/or cervical rib;

♦✿ 21616 with sympathectomy

✿ 21620 Ostectomy of sternum, partial

✿ 21627 Sternal debridement

(For debridement and closure, use 21750)

✿ 21630 Radical resection of sternum;

✿ 21632 with mediastinal lymphadenectomy

Repair, Revision, and/or Reconstruction

(For superficial wound, see **Integumentary System** section under Repair—Simple)

§ 21685 Hyoid myotomy and suspension
➲ *CPT Changes: An Insider's View* 2004

§ 21700 Division of scalenus anticus; without resection of cervical rib

✿ 21705 with resection of cervical rib

§ 21720 Division of sternocleidomastoid for torticollis, open operation; without cast application

(For transection of spinal accessory and cervical nerves, see 63191, 64722)

§ 21725 with cast application

✿ 21740 Reconstructive repair of pectus excavatum or carinatum; open

§ 21742 minimally invasive approach (Nuss procedure), without thoracoscopy
➲ *CPT Changes: An Insider's View* 2003

§ 21743 minimally invasive approach (Nuss procedure), with thoracoscopy
➲ *CPT Changes: An Insider's View* 2003

✿ 21750 Closure of median sternotomy separation with or without debridement (separate procedure)

Fracture and/or Dislocation

§ 21800 Closed treatment of rib fracture, uncomplicated, each

§ 21805 Open treatment of rib fracture without fixation, each

✿ 21810 Treatment of rib fracture requiring external fixation (flail chest)

§ 21820 Closed treatment of sternum fracture

✿ 21825 Open treatment of sternum fracture with or without skeletal fixation

(For sternoclavicular dislocation, see 23520-23532)

Other Procedures

§ 21899 Unlisted procedure, neck or thorax

Back and Flank

Excision

§ 21920 Biopsy, soft tissue of back or flank; superficial

§ 21925 deep

(For needle biopsy of soft tissue, use 20206)

§ 21930 Excision, tumor, soft tissue of back or flank

§ 21935 Radical resection of tumor (eg, malignant neoplasm), soft tissue of back or flank

Spine (Vertebral Column)

Cervical, thoracic, and lumbar spine.

Within the SPINE section, bone grafting procedures are reported separately and in addition to arthrodesis. For bone grafts in other Musculoskeletal sections, see specific code(s) descriptor(s) and/or accompanying guidelines.

To report bone grafts performed after arthrodesis, see codes 20930-20938. Bone graft codes are reported without modifier 51 (multiple procedure). Do not append modifier 62 to bone graft codes 20900-20938.

Example:

Posterior arthrodesis of L5-S1 for degenerative disc disease utilizing morselized autogenous iliac bone graft harvested through a separate fascial incision.

Report as 22612 and 20937.

Within the SPINE section, instrumentation is reported separately and in addition to arthrodesis. To report instrumentation procedures performed with definitive vertebral procedure(s), see codes 22840-22855. Instrumentation procedure codes 22840-22848 and 22851 are reported in addition to the definitive procedure(s) without modifier 51. Modifier 62 may not be appended to the definitive or add-on spinal instrumentation procedure code(s) 22840-22848 and 22850-22852.

Example:

Posterior arthrodesis of L4-S1, utilizing morselized autogenous iliac bone graft harvested through separate fascial incision, and pedicle screw fixation.

Report as 22612, 22614, 22842, and 20937.

Vertebral procedures are sometimes followed by arthrodesis and in addition may include bone grafts and instrumentation.

When arthrodesis is performed in addition to another procedure, the arthrodesis should be reported in addition to the original procedure with modifier 51 (multiple procedures). Examples are after osteotomy, fracture care, vertebral corpectomy and laminectomy. Since bone grafts and instrumentation are never performed without arthrodesis, modifier 51 (multiple procedures) is not used.

Arthrodesis, however, may be performed in the absence of other procedures and therefore when it is combined with another definitive procedure, modifier 51 (multiple procedure) is appropriate.

Example:

Treatment of a burst fracture of L2 by corpec tomy followed by arthrodesis of L1-L3, utilizing anterior instrumentation L1-L3 and structural allograft.

Report as 63090, 22558-51, 22585, 22845, and 20931.

When two surgeons work together as primary surgeons performing distinct part(s) of a single reportable procedure, each surgeon should report his/her distinct operative work by appending modifier 62 to the single definitive procedure code. If additional procedure(s) (including add-on procedure(s)) are performed during the same surgical session, separate code(s) may be reported by each co-surgeon, with modifier 62 appended (see Appendix A).

Example:

A 42-year-old male with a history of posttraumatic degenerative disc disease at L3-4 and L4-5 (internal disc disruption) underwent surgical repair. Surgeon A performed an anterior exposure of the spine with mobilization of the great vessels. Surgeon B performed anterior (minimal) diskectomy and fusion at L3-4 and L4-5 using anterior interbody technique.

Report surgeon A: 22558 append modifier 62, 22585 append modifier 62
Report surgeon B: 22558 append modifier 62, 22585 append modifier 62, 20931

(Do not append modifier 62 to bone graft code 20931)

(For injection procedure for myelography, use 62284)

(For injection procedure for diskography, see 62290, 62291)

(For injection procedure, chemonucleolysis, single or multiple levels, use 62292)

(For injection procedure for facet joints, see 64470-64476, 64622-64627)

(For needle or trocar biopsy, see 20220-20225)

Excision

For the following codes, when two surgeons work together as primary surgeons performing distinct part(s) of partial vertebral body excision, each surgeon should report his/her distinct operative work by appending modifier 62 to the procedure code. In this situation, modifier 62 may be appended to the procedure code(s) 22100-22102, 22110-22114 and, as appropriate, to the associated additional vertebral segment add-on code(s) 22103, 22116 as long as both surgeons continue to work together as primary surgeons.

(For bone biopsy, see 20220-20251)

(To report soft tissue biopsy of back or flank, see 21920-21925)

(For needle biopsy of soft tissue, use 20206)

(To report excision of soft tissue tumor of back or flank, use 21930)

§ **22100** Partial excision of posterior vertebral component (eg, spinous process, lamina or facet) for intrinsic bony lesion, single vertebral segment; cervical

➲ *CPT Assistant* Jan 03:14

§ **22101** thoracic

➲ *CPT Assistant* Jan 03:14

§ **22102** lumbar

➲ *CPT Assistant* Jan 03:14

§+ **22103** each additional segment (List separately in addition to code for primary procedure)

➲ *CPT Assistant* Jan 03:14

(Use 22103 in conjunction with 22100, 22101, 22102)

✿ **22110** Partial excision of vertebral body, for intrinsic bony lesion, without decompression of spinal cord or nerve root(s), single vertebral segment; cervical

✿ **22112** thoracic

✿ **22114** lumbar

✿+ **22116** each additional vertebral segment (List separately in addition to code for primary procedure)

➲ *CPT Assistant* Feb 03: 7

(Use 22116 in conjunction with 22110, 22112, 22114)

(For complete or near complete resection of vertebral body, see vertebral corpectomy, 63081-63091)

(For spinal reconstruction with bone graft (autograft, allograft) and/or methylmethacrylate of cervical vertebral body, use 63081 and 22554 and 20931 or 20938)

(For spinal reconstruction with bone graft (autograft, allograft) and/or methylmethacrylate of thoracic vertebral body, use 63085 or 63087 and 22556 and 20931 or 20938)

(For spinal reconstruction with bone graft (autograft, allograft) and/or methylmethacrylate of lumbar vertebral body, use 63087 or 63090 and 22558 and 20931 or 20938)

(For spinal reconstruction following vertebral body resection, use 63082 or 63086 or 63088 or 63091, and 22585)

(For harvest of bone autograft for vertebral reconstruction, see 20931 or 20938)

(For cervical spinal reconstruction with prosthetic replacement of resected vertebral bodies, see codes 63081 and 22554 and 20931 or 20938 and 22851)

(For thoracic spinal reconstruction with prosthetic replacement of resected vertebral bodies, see codes 63085 or 63087 and 22556 and 20931 or 20938 and 22851)

(For lumbar spinal reconstruction with prosthetic replacement of resected vertebral bodies, see codes 63087 or 63090 and 22558, and 20931 or 20938 and 22851)

(For osteotomy of spine, see 22210-22226)

Osteotomy

To report arthrodesis, see codes 22590-22632. (Report in addition to code(s) for the definitive procedure with modifier 51.)

To report instrumentation procedures, see codes 22840-22855. (Report in addition to code(s) for the definitive procedure(s) without modifier 51.) Do not append modifier 62 to spinal instrumentation codes 22840-22848 and 22850-22852.

To report bone graft procedures, see codes 20930-20938. (Report in addition to code(s) for the definitive procedure(s) without modifier 51.) Do not append modifier 62 to bone graft codes 20900-20938.

For the following codes, when two surgeons work together as primary surgeons performing distinct part(s) of an anterior spine osteotomy, each surgeon should report his/her distinct operative work by appending modifier 62 to the procedure code. In this situation, modifier 62 may be appended to the procedure code(s) 22210-22214, 22220-22224 and, as appropriate, to associated additional segment add-on code(s) 22216, 22226 as long as both surgeons continue to work together as primary surgeons.

✿ **22210** Osteotomy of spine, posterior or posterolateral approach, one vertebral segment; cervical

✿ **22212** thoracic

✿ **22214** lumbar

♦✿+ **22216** each additional vertebral segment (List separately in addition to primary procedure)

(Use 22216 in conjunction with 22210, 22212, 22214)

✿ **22220** Osteotomy of spine, including diskectomy, anterior approach, single vertebral segment; cervical

§ **22222** thoracic

✿ **22224** lumbar

♦✿+ **22226** each additional vertebral segment (List separately in addition to code for primary procedure)

(Use 22226 in conjunction with 22220, 22222, 22224)

(For vertebral corpectomy, see 63081-63091)

Fracture and/or Dislocation

To report arthrodesis, see codes 22590-22632. (Report in addition to code(s) for the definitive procedure with modifier 51.)

To report instrumentation procedures, see codes 22840-22855. (Report in addition to code(s) for the definitive procedure(s) without modifier 51.) Do not append modifier 62 to spinal instrumentation codes 22840-22848 and 22850-22852.

To report bone graft procedures, see codes 20930-20938. (Report in addition to code(s) for the definitive procedure(s) without modifier 51.) Do not append modifier 62 to bone graft codes 20900-20938.

For the following codes, when two surgeons work together as primary surgeons performing distinct part(s) of open fracture and/or dislocation procedure(s), each surgeon should report his/her distinct operative work by appending modifier 62 to the procedure code. In this situation, modifier 62 may be appended to the procedure code(s) 22318-22327 and, as appropriate, the associated additional fracture vertebrae or dislocated segment add-on code 22328 as long as both surgeons continue to work together as primary surgeons.

§ **22305** Closed treatment of vertebral process fracture(s)

§ **22310** Closed treatment of vertebral body fracture(s), without manipulation, requiring and including casting or bracing

§ **22315** Closed treatment of vertebral fracture(s) and/or dislocation(s) requiring casting or bracing, with and including casting and/or bracing, with or without anesthesia, by manipulation or traction

(For spinal subluxation, use 97140)

✿ **22318** Open treatment and/or reduction of odontoid fracture(s) and or dislocation(s) (including os odontoideum), anterior approach, including placement of internal fixation; without grafting

✿ **22319** with grafting

✿ **22325** Open treatment and/or reduction of vertebral fracture(s) and/or dislocation(s), posterior approach, one fractured vertebrae or dislocated segment; lumbar

✿ **22326** cervical

✿ **22327** thoracic

✿+ **22328** each additional fractured vertebrae or dislocated segment (List separately in addition to code for primary procedure)

(Use 22328 in conjunction with 22325, 22326, 22327)

(For treatment of vertebral fracture by the anterior approach, see corpectomy 63081-63091, and appropriate arthrodesis, bone graft and instrument codes)

(For decompression of spine following fracture, see 63001-63091; for arthrodesis of spine following fracture, see 22548-22632)

Manipulation

(For spinal manipulation without anesthesia, use 97140)

§ **22505** Manipulation of spine requiring anesthesia, any region

Vertebral Body, Embolization or Injection

§ **22520** Percutaneous vertebroplasty, one vertebral body, unilateral or bilateral injection; thoracic

§ **22521** lumbar

§+ **22522** each additional thoracic or lumbar vertebral body (List separately in addition to code for primary procedure)

(Use 22522 in conjunction with 22520, 22521 as appropriate)

(For radiological supervision and interpretation, see 76012, 76013)

Lateral Extracavitary Approach Technique

✿ **22532** Arthrodesis, lateral extracavitary technique, including minimal diskectomy to prepare interspace (other than for decompression); thoracic

➔ *CPT Changes: An Insider's View* 2004

✿ **22533** lumbar

➔ *CPT Changes: An Insider's View* 2004

✿+ **22534** thoracic or lumbar, each additional vertebral segment (List separately in addition to code for primary procedure)

➔ *CPT Changes: An Insider's View* 2004

(Use 22534 in conjunction with 22532 and 22533)

Arthrodesis

Arthrodesis may be performed in the absence of other procedures and therefore when it is combined with another definitive procedure (eg, osteotomy, fracture care, vertebral corpectomy or laminectomy), modifier 51 is appropriate. However, arthrodesis codes 22585, 22614, and 22632 are considered add-on procedure codes and should not be used with modifier 51.

►To report instrumentation procedures, see 22840-22855. (Codes 22840-22848, 22851 are reported in conjunction with code(s) for the definitive procedure(s) without modifier 51. When instrumentation reinsertion or removal is reported in conjunction with other definitive procedures including arthrodesis, decompression, and exploration of fusion, append modifier 51 to 22849, 22850, 22852, and 22855.) To report exploration of fusion, use 22830. (When exploration is reported in conjunction with other definitive procedures, including arthrodesis and decompression, append modifier 51 to 22830.) Do not append modifier 62 to spinal instrumentation codes 22840-22848 and 22850-22852.◄

To report bone graft procedures, see codes 20930-20938. (Report in addition to code(s) for the definitive procedure(s) without modifier 51.) Do not append modifier 62 to bone graft codes 20900-20938.

Anterior or Anterolateral Approach Technique

Procedure codes 22554-22558 are for SINGLE interspace; for additional interspaces, use 22585. A vertebral interspace is the non-bony compartment between two adjacent vertebral bodies, which contains the intervertebral disk, and includes the nucleus pulposus, annulus fibrosus, and two cartilagenous endplates.

For the following codes, when two surgeons work together as primary surgeons performing distinct part(s) of an anterior interbody arthrodesis, each surgeon should report his/her distinct operative work by appending modifier 62 to the procedure code. In this situation, modifier 62 may be appended to the procedure code(s) 22548-22558 and, as appropriate, to the associated additional interspace add-on code 22585 as long as both surgeons continue to work together as primary surgeons.

✿ **22548** Arthrodesis, anterior transoral or extraoral technique, clivus-C1-C2 (atlas-axis), with or without excision of odontoid process

(For intervertebral disk excision by laminotomy or laminectomy, see 63020-63042)

✿ **22554** Arthrodesis, anterior interbody technique, including minimal diskectomy to prepare interspace (other than for decompression); cervical below C2

✿ **22556** thoracic

✿ **22558** lumbar

✿+ **22585** each additional interspace (List separately in addition to code for primary procedure)

(Use 22585 in conjunction with 22554, 22556, 22558)

Posterior, Posterolateral or Lateral Transverse Process Technique

To report instrumentation procedures, see codes 22840-22855. (Report in addition to code(s) for the definitive procedure(s) without modifier 51.) Do not append modifier 62 to spinal instrumentation codes 22840-22848 and 22850-22852.

To report bone graft procedures, see codes 20930-20938. (Report in addition to code(s) for the definitive procedure(s) without modifier 51.) Do not append modifier 62 to bone graft codes 20900-20938.

A vertebral segment describes the basic constituent part into which the spine may be divided. It represents a single complete vertebral bone with its associated articular processes and laminae. A vertebral interspace is the non-bony compartment between two adjacent vertebral bodies which contains the intervertebral disk, and includes the nucleus pulposus, annulus fibrosus, and two cartilagenous endplates.

✿ **22590** Arthrodesis, posterior technique, craniocervical (occiput-C2)

✿ **22595** Arthrodesis, posterior technique, atlas-axis (C1-C2)

✿ **22600** Arthrodesis, posterior or posterolateral technique, single level; cervical below C2 segment

✿ **22610** thoracic (with or without lateral transverse technique)

§ **22612** lumbar (with or without lateral transverse technique)
➲ *CPT Assistant* Jan 03:14

§+ **22614** each additional vertebral segment (List separately in addition to code for primary procedure)
➲ *CPT Assistant* Jan 03:15

(Use 22614 in conjunction with 22600, 22610, 22612)

✿ **22630** Arthrodesis, posterior interbody technique, including laminectomy and/or diskectomy to prepare interspace (other than for decompression), single interspace; lumbar

✿+ **22632** each additional interspace (List separately in addition to code for primary procedure)

(Use 22632 in conjunction with 22630)

Spine Deformity (eg, Scoliosis, Kyphosis)

To report instrumentation procedures, see codes 22840-22855. (Report in addition to code(s) for the definitive procedure(s) without modifier 51.) Do not append modifier 62 to spinal instrumentation codes 22840-22848 and 22850-22852.

To report bone graft procedures, see codes 20930-20938. (Report in addition to code(s) for the definitive procedure(s) without modifier 51.) Do not append modifier 62 to bone graft codes 20900-20938.

A vertebral segment describes the basic constituent part into which the spine may be divided. It represents a single complete vertebral bone with its associated articular processes and laminae.

For the following codes, when two surgeons work together as primary surgeons performing distinct part(s) of an arthrodesis for spinal deformity, each surgeon should report his/her distinct operative work by appending modifier 62 to the procedure code. In this situation, modifier 62 may be appended to procedure code(s) 22800-22819 as long as both surgeons continue to work together as primary surgeons.

✿ **22800** Arthrodesis, posterior, for spinal deformity, with or without cast; up to 6 vertebral segments

✿ **22802** 7 to 12 vertebral segments

✿ **22804** 13 or more vertebral segments

✿ **22808** Arthrodesis, anterior, for spinal deformity, with or without cast; 2 to 3 vertebral segments

✿ **22810** 4 to 7 vertebral segments

✿ **22812** 8 or more vertebral segments

✿ **22818** Kyphectomy, circumferential exposure of spine and resection of vertebral segment(s) (including body and posterior elements); single or 2 segments

✿ **22819** 3 or more segments

(To report arthrodesis, see 22800-22804 and add modifier 51)

Exploration

►To report instrumentation procedures, see 22840-22855. (Codes 22840-22848, 22851 are reported in conjunction with code(s) for the definitive procedure(s) without modifier 51. When instrumentation reinsertion or removal is reported in conjunction with other definitive procedures including arthrodesis, decompression, and exploration of fusion, append modifier 51 to 22849, 22850, 22852 and 22855.) To report exploration of fusion, see 22830. (When exploration is reported in conjunction with other definitive procedures, including arthrodesis and decompression, append modifier 51 to 22830.)◄

(To report bone graft procedures, see 20930-20938)

✿ **22830** Exploration of spinal fusion

Spinal Instrumentation

Segmental instrumentation is defined as fixation at each end of the construct and at least one additional interposed bony attachment.

Non-segmental instrumentation is defined as fixation at each end of the construct and may span several vertebral segments without attachment to the intervening segments.

Insertion of spinal instrumentation is reported separately and in addition to arthrodesis. Instrumentation procedure codes 22840-22848, 22851 are reported in addition to the definitive procedure(s) without modifier 51. Do not append modifier 62 to spinal instrumentation codes 22840-22848 and 22850-22852.

To report bone graft procedures, see codes 20930-20938. (Report in addition to code(s) for definitive procedure(s) without modifier 51.) Do not append modifier 62 to bone graft codes 20900-20938.

A vertebral segment describes the basic constituent part into which the spine may be divided. It represents a single complete vertebral bone with its associated articular processes and laminae. A vertebral interspace is the non-bony compartment between two adjacent vertebral bodies, which contains the intervertebral disk, and includes the nucleus pulposus, annulus fibrosus, and two cartilagenous endplates.

►List 22840-22855 separately, in conjunction with code(s) for fracture, dislocation, arthrodesis or exploration of fusion of the spine 22325-22328, 22548-22812, and 22830. Codes 22840-22848, 22851 are reported in conjunction with code(s) for the definitive procedure(s) without modifier 51. Codes 22849, 22850, 22852, and 22855 are subject to modifier 51 if reported with other definitive procedure(s), including arthrodesis, decompression, and exploration of fusion. Code 22849 should not be reported with 22850, 22852, and 22855 at the same spinal levels.◄

✿⊘ **22840** Posterior non-segmental instrumentation (eg, Harrington rod technique, pedicle fixation across one interspace, atlantoaxial transarticular screw fixation, sublaminar wiring at C1, facet screw fixation)

✿⊘ **22841** Internal spinal fixation by wiring of spinous processes

✿⊘ **22842** Posterior segmental instrumentation (eg, pedicle fixation, dual rods with multiple hooks and sublaminar wires); 3 to 6 vertebral segments

✿⊘ **22843** 7 to 12 vertebral segments

✿⊘ **22844** 13 or more vertebral segments

✿⊘ **22845** Anterior instrumentation; 2 to 3 vertebral segments

✿⊘ **22846** 4 to 7 vertebral segments

✿⊘ **22847** 8 or more vertebral segments

✿⊘ **22848** Pelvic fixation (attachment of caudal end of instrumentation to pelvic bony structures) other than sacrum

✿ **22849** Reinsertion of spinal fixation device

✿ **22850** Removal of posterior nonsegmental instrumentation (eg, Harrington rod)

✿⊘ **22851** Application of intervertebral biomechanical device(s) (eg, synthetic cage(s), threaded bone dowel(s), methylmethacrylate) to vertebral defect or interspace

✿ **22852** Removal of posterior segmental instrumentation

✿ **22855** Removal of anterior instrumentation

Other Procedures

§ **22899** Unlisted procedure, spine

Abdomen

Excision

§ **22900** Excision, abdominal wall tumor, subfascial (eg, desmoid)

➲ *CPT Changes: An Insider's View* 2004

Other Procedures

§ **22999** Unlisted procedure, abdomen, musculoskeletal system

Surgery: Musculoskeletal System

Shoulder

Clavicle, scapula, humerus head and neck, sternoclavicular joint, acromioclavicular joint and shoulder joint.

Incision

§ **23000** Removal of subdeltoid calcareous deposits, open
➲ *CPT Changes: An Insider's View* 2002, 2003

(For arthroscopic removal of bursal deposits, use 29999)

◆§ **23020** Capsular contracture release (eg, Sever type procedure)

(For incision and drainage procedures, superficial, see 10040-10160)

§ **23030** Incision and drainage, shoulder area; deep abscess or hematoma

◆§ **23031** infected bursa

◆§ **23035** Incision, bone cortex (eg, osteomyelitis or bone abscess), shoulder area
➲ *CPT Assistant* Jan 03:15

◆§ **23040** Arthrotomy, glenohumeral joint, including exploration, drainage, or removal of foreign body

◆§ **23044** Arthrotomy, acromioclavicular, sternoclavicular joint, including exploration, drainage, or removal of foreign body

Excision

◆§ **23065** Biopsy, soft tissue of shoulder area; superficial

◆§ **23066** deep

(For needle biopsy of soft tissue, use 20206)

◆§ **23075** Excision, soft tissue tumor, shoulder area; subcutaneous

◆§ **23076** deep, subfascial, or intramuscular

◆§ **23077** Radical resection of tumor (eg, malignant neoplasm), soft tissue of shoulder area

◆§ **23100** Arthrotomy, glenohumeral joint, including biopsy

◆§ **23101** Arthrotomy, acromioclavicular joint or sternoclavicular joint, including biopsy and/or excision of torn cartilage

◆§ **23105** Arthrotomy; glenohumeral joint, with synovectomy, with or without biopsy

◆§ **23106** sternoclavicular joint, with synovectomy, with or without biopsy

◆§ **23107** Arthrotomy, glenohumeral joint, with joint exploration, with or without removal of loose or foreign body

§ **23120** Claviculectomy; partial

(For arthroscopic procedure, use 29824)

◆§ **23125** total
➲ *CPT Assistant* Jan 03:15

◆§ **23130** Acromioplasty or acromionectomy, partial, with or without coracoacromial ligament release

◆§ **23140** Excision or curettage of bone cyst or benign tumor of clavicle or scapula;

◆§ **23145** with autograft (includes obtaining graft)

◆§ **23146** with allograft

◆§ **23150** Excision or curettage of bone cyst or benign tumor of proximal humerus;

◆§ **23155** with autograft (includes obtaining graft)

◆§ **23156** with allograft

◆§ **23170** Sequestrectomy (eg, for osteomyelitis or bone abscess), clavicle

◆§ **23172** Sequestrectomy (eg, for osteomyelitis or bone abscess), scapula

◆§ **23174** Sequestrectomy (eg, for osteomyelitis or bone abscess), humeral head to surgical neck

◆§ **23180** Partial excision (craterization, saucerization, or diaphysectomy) bone (eg, osteomyelitis), clavicle

◆§ **23182** Partial excision (craterization, saucerization, or diaphysectomy) bone (eg, osteomyelitis), scapula

◆§ **23184** Partial excision (craterization, saucerization, or diaphysectomy) bone (eg, osteomyelitis), proximal humerus

◆§ **23190** Ostectomy of scapula, partial (eg, superior medial angle)

◆§ **23195** Resection, humeral head
➲ *CPT Assistant* Jan 03:15

(For replacement with implant, use 23470)

◆✿ **23200** Radical resection for tumor; clavicle

◆✿ **23210** scapula

◆✿ **23220** Radical resection of bone tumor, proximal humerus;

◆✿ **23221** with autograft (includes obtaining graft)

◆✿ **23222** with prosthetic replacement

Introduction or Removal

(For arthrocentesis or needling of bursa, use 20610)

(For K-wire or pin insertion or removal, see 20650, 20670, 20680)

◆§ **23330** Removal of foreign body, shoulder; subcutaneous

◆§ **23331** deep (eg, Neer hemiarthroplasty removal)

◆✿ **23332** complicated (eg, total shoulder)

◆☆ **23350** Injection procedure for shoulder arthrography or enhanced CT/MRI shoulder arthrography
➲ *CPT Changes: An Insider's View* 2002

(For radiographic arthrography, radiological supervision and interpretation, use 73040. Fluoroscopy (76003) is inclusive of radiographic arthrography)

(When fluoroscopic guided injection is performed for enhanced CT arthrography, use 23350, 76003, and 73201 or 73202)

(When fluoroscopic guided injection is performed for enhanced MR arthrography, use 23350, 76003, and 73222 or 73223)

(For enhanced CT or enhanced MRI arthrography, use 76003 and either 73201, 73202, 73222 or 73223)

(To report biopsy of the shoulder and joint, see 29805-29826)

Repair, Revision, and/or Reconstruction

§ **23395** Muscle transfer, any type, shoulder or upper arm; single
➲ *CPT Assistant* Jan 03:15

§ **23397** multiple
➲ *CPT Assistant* Jan 03:15

♦§ **23400** Scapulopexy (eg, Sprengels deformity or for paralysis)
➲ *CPT Assistant* Jan 03:15

§ **23405** Tenotomy, shoulder area; single tendon

§ **23406** multiple tendons through same incision

♦§ **23410** Repair of ruptured musculotendinous cuff (eg, rotator cuff) open; acute
➲ *CPT Changes: An Insider's View* 2003

♦§ **23412** chronic

(For arthroscopic procedure, use 29827)

♦§ **23415** Coracoacromial ligament release, with or without acromioplasty

(For arthroscopic procedure, use 29826)

♦§ **23420** Reconstruction of complete shoulder (rotator) cuff avulsion, chronic (includes acromioplasty)

♦§ **23430** Tenodesis of long tendon of biceps

♦§ **23440** Resection or transplantation of long tendon of biceps

♦§ **23450** Capsulorrhaphy, anterior; Putti-Platt procedure or Magnuson type operation

(To report arthroscopic thermal capsulorrhaphy, use 29999)

♦§ **23455** with labral repair (eg, Bankart procedure)

(For arthroscopic procedure, use 29806)

♦§ **23460** Capsulorrhaphy, anterior, any type; with bone block

♦§ **23462** with coracoid process transfer

(To report open thermal capsulorrhaphy, use 23929)

♦§ **23465** Capsulorrhaphy, glenohumeral joint, posterior, with or without bone block

(For sternoclavicular and acromioclavicular reconstruction, see 23530, 23550)

♦§ **23466** Capsulorrhaphy, glenohumeral joint, any type multi-directional instability

♦§ **23470** Arthroplasty, glenohumeral joint; hemiarthroplasty

♦✿ **23472** total shoulder (glenoid and proximal humeral replacement (eg, total shoulder))

(For removal of total shoulder implants, see 23331, 23332)

(For osteotomy, proximal humerus, use 24400)

♦§ **23480** Osteotomy, clavicle, with or without internal fixation;

♦§ **23485** with bone graft for nonunion or malunion (includes obtaining graft and/or necessary fixation)

♦§ **23490** Prophylactic treatment (nailing, pinning, plating or wiring) with or without methylmethacrylate; clavicle

♦§ **23491** proximal humerus

Fracture and/or Dislocation

♦§ **23500** Closed treatment of clavicular fracture; without manipulation

♦§ **23505** with manipulation

♦§ **23515** Open treatment of clavicular fracture, with or without internal or external fixation

♦§ **23520** Closed treatment of sternoclavicular dislocation; without manipulation

♦§ **23525** with manipulation

♦§ **23530** Open treatment of sternoclavicular dislocation, acute or chronic;

♦§ **23532** with fascial graft (includes obtaining graft)

♦§ **23540** Closed treatment of acromioclavicular dislocation; without manipulation

♦§ **23545** with manipulation

♦§ **23550** Open treatment of acromioclavicular dislocation, acute or chronic;

♦§ **23552** with fascial graft (includes obtaining graft)

♦§ **23570** Closed treatment of scapular fracture; without manipulation

♦§ **23575** with manipulation, with or without skeletal traction (with or without shoulder joint involvement)

♦§ **23585** Open treatment of scapular fracture (body, glenoid or acromion) with or without internal fixation

♦§ **23600** Closed treatment of proximal humeral (surgical or anatomical neck) fracture; without manipulation

♦§ **23605** with manipulation, with or without skeletal traction

♦§ **23615** Open treatment of proximal humeral (surgical or anatomical neck) fracture, with or without internal or external fixation, with or without repair of tuberosity(s);

♦§ **23616** with proximal humeral prosthetic replacement

♦§ **23620** Closed treatment of greater humeral tuberosity fracture; without manipulation

♦§ **23625** with manipulation

♦§ **23630** Open treatment of greater humeral tuberosity fracture, with or without internal or external fixation

♦§ **23650** Closed treatment of shoulder dislocation, with manipulation; without anesthesia

♦§ **23655** requiring anesthesia

♦§ **23660** Open treatment of acute shoulder dislocation

(Repairs for recurrent dislocations, see 23450-23466)

♦§ **23665** Closed treatment of shoulder dislocation, with fracture of greater humeral tuberosity, with manipulation

♦§ **23670** Open treatment of shoulder dislocation, with fracture of greater humeral tuberosity, with or without internal or external fixation

♦§ **23675** Closed treatment of shoulder dislocation, with surgical or anatomical neck fracture, with manipulation

♦§ **23680** Open treatment of shoulder dislocation, with surgical or anatomical neck fracture, with or without internal or external fixation

Manipulation

§ **23700** Manipulation under anesthesia, shoulder joint, including application of fixation apparatus (dislocation excluded)

Arthrodesis

♦§ **23800** Arthrodesis, glenohumeral joint;

§ **23802** with autogenous graft (includes obtaining graft)

Amputation

✿ **23900** Interthoracoscapular amputation (forequarter)

✿ **23920** Disarticulation of shoulder;

§ **23921** secondary closure or scar revision

Other Procedures

§ **23929** Unlisted procedure, shoulder

Humerus (Upper Arm) and Elbow

Elbow area includes head and neck of radius and olecranon process.

Incision

(For incision and drainage procedures, superficial, see 10040-10160)

♦§ **23930** Incision and drainage, upper arm or elbow area; deep abscess or hematoma

♦§ **23931** bursa

♦§ **23935** Incision, deep, with opening of bone cortex (eg, for osteomyelitis or bone abscess), humerus or elbow

♦§ **24000** Arthrotomy, elbow, including exploration, drainage, or removal of foreign body

♦§ **24006** Arthrotomy of the elbow, with capsular excision for capsular release (separate procedure)

Excision

♦§ **24065** Biopsy, soft tissue of upper arm or elbow area; superficial

♦§ **24066** deep (subfascial or intramuscular)

(For needle biopsy of soft tissue, use 20206)

♦§ **24075** Excision, tumor, soft tissue of upper arm or elbow area; subcutaneous

➲ *CPT Changes: An Insider's View* 2002

♦§ **24076** deep (subfascial or intramuscular)

♦§ **24077** Radical resection of tumor (eg, malignant neoplasm), soft tissue of upper arm or elbow area

♦§ **24100** Arthrotomy, elbow; with synovial biopsy only

♦§ **24101** with joint exploration, with or without biopsy, with or without removal of loose or foreign body

♦§ **24102** with synovectomy

♦§ **24105** Excision, olecranon bursa

♦§ **24110** Excision or curettage of bone cyst or benign tumor, humerus;

♦§ **24115** with autograft (includes obtaining graft)

♦§ **24116** with allograft

♦§ **24120** Excision or curettage of bone cyst or benign tumor of head or neck of radius or olecranon process;

♦§ **24125** with autograft (includes obtaining graft)

♦§ **24126** with allograft

♦§ **24130** Excision, radial head

(For replacement with implant, use 24366)

♦§ **24134** Sequestrectomy (eg, for osteomyelitis or bone abscess), shaft or distal humerus

♦§ **24136** Sequestrectomy (eg, for osteomyelitis or bone abscess), radial head or neck

♦§ **24138** Sequestrectomy (eg, for osteomyelitis or bone abscess), olecranon process

♦§ **24140** Partial excision (craterization, saucerization, or diaphysectomy) bone (eg, osteomyelitis), humerus

♦§ **24145** Partial excision (craterization, saucerization, or diaphysectomy) bone (eg, osteomyelitis), radial head or neck

♦§ **24147** Partial excision (craterization, saucerization, or diaphysectomy) bone (eg, osteomyelitis), olecranon process

♦§ **24149** Radical resection of capsule, soft tissue, and heterotopic bone, elbow, with contracture release (separate procedure)

(For capsular and soft tissue release only, use 24006)

♦§ **24150** Radical resection for tumor, shaft or distal humerus;
➔ *CPT Assistant* Jan 03:15

♦§ **24151** with autograft (includes obtaining graft)
➔ *CPT Assistant* Jan 03:15

♦§ **24152** Radical resection for tumor, radial head or neck;
➔ *CPT Assistant* Jan 03:15

♦§ **24153** with autograft (includes obtaining graft)
➔ *CPT Assistant* Jan 03:15

♦§ **24155** Resection of elbow joint (arthrectomy)

Introduction or Removal

(For K-wire or pin insertion or removal, see 20650, 20670, 20680)

(For arthrocentesis or needling of bursa or joint, use 20605)

♦§ **24160** Implant removal; elbow joint

♦§ **24164** radial head

♦§ **24200** Removal of foreign body, upper arm or elbow area; subcutaneous

♦§ **24201** deep (subfascial or intramuscular)

♦☆ **24220** Injection procedure for elbow arthrography

(For radiological supervision and interpretation, use 73085. Do not report 76003 in addition to 73085)

(For injection for tennis elbow, use 20550)

Repair, Revision, and/or Reconstruction

♦§ **24300** Manipulation, elbow, under anesthesia
➔ *CPT Changes: An Insider's View* 2002

(For application of external fixation, see 20690 or 20692)

§ **24301** Muscle or tendon transfer, any type, upper arm or elbow, single (excluding 24320-24331)

§ **24305** Tendon lengthening, upper arm or elbow, each tendon

§ **24310** Tenotomy, open, elbow to shoulder, each tendon

§ **24320** Tenoplasty, with muscle transfer, with or without free graft, elbow to shoulder, single (Seddon-Brookes type procedure)

♦§ **24330** Flexor-plasty, elbow (eg, Steindler type advancement);

♦§ **24331** with extensor advancement

♦§ **24332** Tenolysis, triceps
➔ *CPT Changes: An Insider's View* 2002

♦§ **24340** Tenodesis of biceps tendon at elbow (separate procedure)

♦§ **24341** Repair, tendon or muscle, upper arm or elbow, each tendon or muscle, primary or secondary (excludes rotator cuff)

♦§ **24342** Reinsertion of ruptured biceps or triceps tendon, distal, with or without tendon graft

♦§ **24343** Repair lateral collateral ligament, elbow, with local tissue
➔ *CPT Changes: An Insider's View* 2002

♦§ **24344** Reconstruction lateral collateral ligament, elbow, with tendon graft (includes harvesting of graft)
➔ *CPT Changes: An Insider's View* 2002

♦§ **24345** Repair medial collateral ligament, elbow, with local tissue
➔ *CPT Changes: An Insider's View* 2002

♦§ **24346** Reconstruction medial collateral ligament, elbow, with tendon graft (includes harvesting of graft)
➔ *CPT Changes: An Insider's View* 2002

♦§ **24350** Fasciotomy, lateral or medial (eg, tennis elbow or epicondylitis);

♦§ **24351** with extensor origin detachment

♦§ **24352** with annular ligament resection

♦§ **24354** with stripping

♦§ **24356** with partial ostectomy

♦§ **24360** Arthroplasty, elbow; with membrane (eg, fascial)

♦§ **24361** with distal humeral prosthetic replacement

♦§ **24362** with implant and fascia lata ligament reconstruction

♦§ **24363** with distal humerus and proximal ulnar prosthetic replacement (eg, total elbow)

♦§ **24365** Arthroplasty, radial head;

♦§ **24366** with implant

♦§ **24400** Osteotomy, humerus, with or without internal fixation

♦§ **24410** Multiple osteotomies with realignment on intramedullary rod, humeral shaft (Sofield type procedure)

♦§ **24420** Osteoplasty, humerus (eg, shortening or lengthening) (excluding 64876)

♦§ **24430** Repair of nonunion or malunion, humerus; without graft (eg, compression technique)

♦§ **24435** with iliac or other autograft (includes obtaining graft)

(For proximal radius and/or ulna, see 25400-25420)

♦§ **24470** Hemiepiphyseal arrest (eg, cubitus varus or valgus, distal humerus)

♦§ **24495** Decompression fasciotomy, forearm, with brachial artery exploration

♦§ **24498** Prophylactic treatment (nailing, pinning, plating or wiring), with or without methylmethacrylate, humeral shaft

Fracture and/or Dislocation

♦§ 24500 Closed treatment of humeral shaft fracture; without manipulation

♦§ 24505 with manipulation, with or without skeletal traction

♦§ 24515 Open treatment of humeral shaft fracture with plate/screws, with or without cerclage

♦§ 24516 Treatment of humeral shaft fracture, with insertion of intramedullary implant, with or without cerclage and/or locking screws

➔ *CPT Changes: An Insider's View* 2003

♦§ 24530 Closed treatment of supracondylar or transcondylar humeral fracture, with or without intercondylar extension; without manipulation

♦§ 24535 with manipulation, with or without skin or skeletal traction

♦§ 24538 Percutaneous skeletal fixation of supracondylar or transcondylar humeral fracture, with or without intercondylar extension

♦§ 24545 Open treatment of humeral supracondylar or transcondylar fracture, with or without internal or external fixation; without intercondylar extension

♦§ 24546 with intercondylar extension

♦§ 24560 Closed treatment of humeral epicondylar fracture, medial or lateral; without manipulation

♦§ 24565 with manipulation

♦§ 24566 Percutaneous skeletal fixation of humeral epicondylar fracture, medial or lateral, with manipulation

♦§ 24575 Open treatment of humeral epicondylar fracture, medial or lateral, with or without internal or external fixation

♦§ 24576 Closed treatment of humeral condylar fracture, medial or lateral; without manipulation

♦§ 24577 with manipulation

♦§ 24579 Open treatment of humeral condylar fracture, medial or lateral, with or without internal or external fixation

(To report closed treatment of fractures without manipulation, see 24530, 24560, 24576, 24650, 24670)

(To report closed treatment of fractures with manipulation, see 24535, 24565, 24577, 24675)

♦§ 24582 Percutaneous skeletal fixation of humeral condylar fracture, medial or lateral, with manipulation

♦§ 24586 Open treatment of periarticular fracture and/or dislocation of the elbow (fracture distal humerus and proximal ulna and/or proximal radius);

♦§ 24587 with implant arthroplasty

(See also 24361)

♦§ 24600 Treatment of closed elbow dislocation; without anesthesia

♦§ 24605 requiring anesthesia

♦§ 24615 Open treatment of acute or chronic elbow dislocation

➔ *CPT Changes: An Insider's View* 2002

♦§ 24620 Closed treatment of Monteggia type of fracture dislocation at elbow (fracture proximal end of ulna with dislocation of radial head), with manipulation

♦§ 24635 Open treatment of Monteggia type of fracture dislocation at elbow (fracture proximal end of ulna with dislocation of radial head), with or without internal or external fixation

♦§ 24640 Closed treatment of radial head subluxation in child, nursemaid elbow, with manipulation

♦§ 24650 Closed treatment of radial head or neck fracture; without manipulation

♦§ 24655 with manipulation

♦§ 24665 Open treatment of radial head or neck fracture, with or without internal fixation or radial head excision;

♦§ 24666 with radial head prosthetic replacement

♦§ 24670 Closed treatment of ulnar fracture, proximal end (olecranon process); without manipulation

♦§ 24675 with manipulation

♦§ 24685 Open treatment of ulnar fracture proximal end (olecranon process), with or without internal or external fixation

Arthrodesis

♦§ 24800 Arthrodesis, elbow joint; local

♦§ 24802 with autogenous graft (includes obtaining graft)

Amputation

♦✿ 24900 Amputation, arm through humerus; with primary closure

♦✿ 24920 open, circular (guillotine)

♦§ 24925 secondary closure or scar revision

♦✿ 24930 re-amputation

♦✿ 24931 with implant

♦§ 24935 Stump elongation, upper extremity

♦✿ 24940 Cineplasty, upper extremity, complete procedure

Other Procedures

♦§ 24999 Unlisted procedure, humerus or elbow

Forearm and Wrist

Radius, ulna, carpal bones and joints.

Incision

♦§ **25000** Incision, extensor tendon sheath, wrist (eg, deQuervains disease)

(For decompression median nerve or for carpal tunnel syndrome, use 64721)

♦§ **25001** Incision, flexor tendon sheath, wrist (eg, flexor carpi radialis)
➲ *CPT Changes: An Insider's View* 2002

♦§ **25020** Decompression fasciotomy, forearm and/or wrist, flexor OR extensor compartment; without debridement of nonviable muscle and/or nerve
➲ *CPT Changes: An Insider's View* 2002

♦§ **25023** with debridement of nonviable muscle and/or nerve

(For decompression fasciotomy with brachial artery exploration, use 24495)

(For incision and drainage procedures, superficial, see 10060-10160)

(For debridement, see also 11000-11044)

♦§ **25024** Decompression fasciotomy, forearm and/or wrist, flexor AND extensor compartment; without debridement of nonviable muscle and/or nerve
➲ *CPT Changes: An Insider's View* 2002

♦§ **25025** with debridement of nonviable muscle and/or nerve
➲ *CPT Changes: An Insider's View* 2002

♦§ **25028** Incision and drainage, forearm and/or wrist; deep abscess or hematoma

♦§ **25031** bursa

♦§ **25035** Incision, deep, bone cortex, forearm and/or wrist (eg, osteomyelitis or bone abscess)

♦§ **25040** Arthrotomy, radiocarpal or midcarpal joint, with exploration, drainage, or removal of foreign body

Excision

♦§ **25065** Biopsy, soft tissue of forearm and/or wrist; superficial

♦§ **25066** deep (subfascial or intramuscular)

(For needle biopsy of soft tissue, use 20206)

♦§ **25075** Excision, tumor, soft tissue of forearm and/or wrist area; subcutaneous
➲ *CPT Changes: An Insider's View* 2002

♦§ **25076** deep (subfascial or intramuscular)

♦§ **25077** Radical resection of tumor (eg, malignant neoplasm), soft tissue of forearm and/or wrist area

♦§ **25085** Capsulotomy, wrist (eg, contracture)

♦§ **25100** Arthrotomy, wrist joint; with biopsy

♦§ **25101** with joint exploration, with or without biopsy, with or without removal of loose or foreign body

♦§ **25105** with synovectomy

♦§ **25107** Arthrotomy, distal radioulnar joint including repair of triangular cartilage, complex

♦§ **25110** Excision, lesion of tendon sheath, forearm and/or wrist

♦§ **25111** Excision of ganglion, wrist (dorsal or volar); primary

♦§ **25112** recurrent

(For hand or finger, use 26160)

♦§ **25115** Radical excision of bursa, synovia of wrist, or forearm tendon sheaths (eg, tenosynovitis, fungus, Tbc, or other granulomas, rheumatoid arthritis); flexors

♦§ **25116** extensors, with or without transposition of dorsal retinaculum

(For finger synovectomies, use 26145)

♦§ **25118** Synovectomy, extensor tendon sheath, wrist, single compartment;

♦§ **25119** with resection of distal ulna

♦§ **25120** Excision or curettage of bone cyst or benign tumor of radius or ulna (excluding head or neck of radius and olecranon process);

(For head or neck of radius or olecranon process, see 24120-24126)

♦§ **25125** with autograft (includes obtaining graft)

♦§ **25126** with allograft

♦§ **25130** Excision or curettage of bone cyst or benign tumor of carpal bones;

♦§ **25135** with autograft (includes obtaining graft)

♦§ **25136** with allograft

♦§ **25145** Sequestrectomy (eg, for osteomyelitis or bone abscess), forearm and/or wrist

♦§ **25150** Partial excision (craterization, saucerization, or diaphysectomy) of bone (eg, for osteomyelitis); ulna

♦§ **25151** radius

(For head or neck of radius or olecranon process, see 24145, 24147)

♦§ **25170** Radical resection for tumor, radius or ulna
➲ *CPT Assistant* Jan 03:15

§ **25210** Carpectomy; one bone

(For carpectomy with implant, see 25441-25445)

§ **25215** all bones of proximal row

♦§ **25230** Radial styloidectomy (separate procedure)

♦§ **25240** Excision distal ulna partial or complete (eg, Darrach type or matched resection)

(For implant replacement, distal ulna, use 25442)

(For obtaining fascia for interposition, see 20920, 20922)

Introduction or Removal

(For K-wire, pin or rod insertion or removal, see 20650, 20670, 20680)

♦☆ **25246** Injection procedure for wrist arthrography

(For radiological supervision and interpretation, use 73115. Do not report 76003 in addition to 73115)

(For foreign body removal, superficial use 20520)

♦§ **25248** Exploration with removal of deep foreign body, forearm or wrist

♦§ **25250** Removal of wrist prosthesis; (separate procedure)

§ **25251** complicated, including total wrist

♦§ **25259** Manipulation, wrist, under anesthesia

➲ *CPT Changes: An Insider's View* 2002

(For application of external fixation, see 20690 or 20692)

Repair, Revision, and/or Reconstruction

§ **25260** Repair, tendon or muscle, flexor, forearm and/or wrist; primary, single, each tendon or muscle

§ **25263** secondary, single, each tendon or muscle

§ **25265** secondary, with free graft (includes obtaining graft), each tendon or muscle

§ **25270** Repair, tendon or muscle, extensor, forearm and/or wrist; primary, single, each tendon or muscle

§ **25272** secondary, single, each tendon or muscle

§ **25274** secondary, with free graft (includes obtaining graft), each tendon or muscle

➲ *CPT Changes: An Insider's View* 2002

♦§ **25275** Repair, tendon sheath, extensor, forearm and/or wrist, with free graft (includes obtaining graft) (eg, for extensor carpi ulnaris subluxation)

➲ *CPT Changes: An Insider's View* 2002

§ **25280** Lengthening or shortening of flexor or extensor tendon, forearm and/or wrist, single, each tendon

§ **25290** Tenotomy, open, flexor or extensor tendon, forearm and/or wrist, single, each tendon

§ **25295** Tenolysis, flexor or extensor tendon, forearm and/or wrist, single, each tendon

♦§ **25300** Tenodesis at wrist; flexors of fingers

♦§ **25301** extensors of fingers

§ **25310** Tendon transplantation or transfer, flexor or extensor, forearm and/or wrist, single; each tendon

§ **25312** with tendon graft(s) (includes obtaining graft), each tendon

♦§ **25315** Flexor origin slide (eg, for cerebral palsy, Volkmann contracture), forearm and/or wrist;

♦§ **25316** with tendon(s) transfer

♦§ **25320** Capsulorrhaphy or reconstruction, wrist, open (eg, capsulodesis, ligament repair, tendon transfer or graft) (includes synovectomy, capsulotomy and open reduction) for carpal instability

➲ *CPT Changes: An Insider's View* 2003

♦§ **25332** Arthroplasty, wrist, with or without interposition, with or without external or internal fixation

(For obtaining fascia for interposition, see 20920, 20922)

(For prosthetic replacement arthroplasty, see 25441-25446)

♦§ **25335** Centralization of wrist on ulna (eg, radial club hand)

♦§ **25337** Reconstruction for stabilization of unstable distal ulna or distal radioulnar joint, secondary by soft tissue stabilization (eg, tendon transfer, tendon graft or weave, or tenodesis) with or without open reduction of distal radioulnar joint

(For harvesting of fascia lata graft, see 20920, 20922)

♦§ **25350** Osteotomy, radius; distal third

♦§ **25355** middle or proximal third

♦§ **25360** Osteotomy; ulna

♦§ **25365** radius AND ulna

♦§ **25370** Multiple osteotomies, with realignment on intramedullary rod (Sofield type procedure); radius OR ulna

♦§ **25375** radius AND ulna

♦§ **25390** Osteoplasty, radius OR ulna; shortening

➲ *CPT Assistant* Jan 03:15

♦§ **25391** lengthening with autograft

➲ *CPT Assistant* Jan 03:15

♦§ **25392** Osteoplasty, radius AND ulna; shortening (excluding 64876)

➲ *CPT Assistant* Jan 03:15

♦§ **25393** lengthening with autograft

➲ *CPT Assistant* Jan 03:15

♦§ **25394** Osteoplasty, carpal bone, shortening

➲ *CPT Changes: An Insider's View* 2002

♦§ **25400** Repair of nonunion or malunion, radius OR ulna; without graft (eg, compression technique)

♦§ **25405** with autograft (includes obtaining graft)

➲ *CPT Changes: An Insider's View* 2002

♦§ **25415** Repair of nonunion or malunion, radius AND ulna; without graft (eg, compression technique)

♦§ **25420** with autograft (includes obtaining graft)
➲ *CPT Assistant* Jan 03:15; *CPT Changes: An Insider's View* 2002

♦§ **25425** Repair of defect with autograft; radius OR ulna

♦§ **25426** radius AND ulna

♦§ **25430** Insertion of vascular pedicle into carpal bone (eg, Hori procedure)
➲ *CPT Changes: An Insider's View* 2002

♦§ **25431** Repair of nonunion of carpal bone (excluding carpal scaphoid (navicular)) (includes obtaining graft and necessary fixation), each bone
➲ *CPT Changes: An Insider's View* 2002

♦§ **25440** Repair of nonunion, scaphoid carpal (navicular) bone, with or without radial styloidectomy (includes obtaining graft and necessary fixation)
➲ *CPT Changes: An Insider's View* 2002

♦§ **25441** Arthroplasty with prosthetic replacement; distal radius

♦§ **25442** distal ulna

♦§ **25443** scaphoid carpal (navicular)
➲ *CPT Changes: An Insider's View* 2002

♦§ **25444** lunate

♦§ **25445** trapezium

♦§ **25446** distal radius and partial or entire carpus (total wrist)

♦§ **25447** Arthroplasty, interposition, intercarpal or carpometacarpal joints

(For wrist arthroplasty, use 25332)

♦§ **25449** Revision of arthroplasty, including removal of implant, wrist joint

♦§ **25450** Epiphyseal arrest by epiphysiodesis or stapling; distal radius OR ulna

♦§ **25455** distal radius AND ulna

♦§ **25490** Prophylactic treatment (nailing, pinning, plating or wiring) with or without methylmethacrylate; radius

♦§ **25491** ulna

♦§ **25492** radius AND ulna

Fracture and/or Dislocation

♦§ **25500** Closed treatment of radial shaft fracture; without manipulation

♦§ **25505** with manipulation
➲ *CPT Assistant* May 03:15

♦§ **25515** Open treatment of radial shaft fracture, with or without internal or external fixation

♦§ **25520** Closed treatment of radial shaft fracture and closed treatment of dislocation of distal radioulnar joint (Galeazzi fracture/dislocation)

♦§ **25525** Open treatment of radial shaft fracture, with internal and/ or external fixation and closed treatment of dislocation of distal radioulnar joint (Galeazzi fracture/dislocation), with or without percutaneous skeletal fixation

♦§ **25526** Open treatment of radial shaft fracture, with internal and/or external fixation and open treatment, with or without internal or external fixation of distal radioulnar joint (Galeazzi fracture/dislocation), includes repair of triangular fibrocartilage complex

♦§ **25530** Closed treatment of ulnar shaft fracture; without manipulation
➲ *CPT Assistant* Apr 02:14, 16

♦§ **25535** with manipulation

♦§ **25545** Open treatment of ulnar shaft fracture, with or without internal or external fixation

♦§ **25560** Closed treatment of radial and ulnar shaft fractures; without manipulation

♦§ **25565** with manipulation

♦§ **25574** Open treatment of radial AND ulnar shaft fractures, with internal or external fixation; of radius OR ulna

♦§ **25575** of radius AND ulna

♦§ **25600** Closed treatment of distal radial fracture (eg, Colles or Smith type) or epiphyseal separation, with or without fracture of ulnar styloid; without manipulation

♦§ **25605** with manipulation

♦§ **25611** Percutaneous skeletal fixation of distal radial fracture (eg, Colles or Smith type) or epiphyseal separation, with or without fracture of ulnar styloid, requiring manipulation, with or without external fixation

♦§ **25620** Open treatment of distal radial fracture (eg, Colles or Smith type) or epiphyseal separation, with or without fracture of ulnar styloid, with or without internal or external fixation

♦§ **25622** Closed treatment of carpal scaphoid (navicular) fracture; without manipulation

♦§ **25624** with manipulation

♦§ **25628** Open treatment of carpal scaphoid (navicular) fracture, with or without internal or external fixation

♦§ **25630** Closed treatment of carpal bone fracture (excluding carpal scaphoid (navicular)); without manipulation, each bone

♦§ **25635** with manipulation, each bone

♦§ **25645** Open treatment of carpal bone fracture (other than carpal scaphoid (navicular)), each bone
➲ *CPT Changes: An Insider's View* 2002

♦§ **25650** Closed treatment of ulnar styloid fracture

♦§ **25651** Percutaneous skeletal fixation of ulnar styloid fracture
➲ *CPT Changes: An Insider's View* 2002

♦§ **25652** Open treatment of ulnar styloid fracture
➲ *CPT Changes: An Insider's View* 2002

♦§ **25660** Closed treatment of radiocarpal or intercarpal dislocation, one or more bones, with manipulation

♦§ **25670** Open treatment of radiocarpal or intercarpal dislocation, one or more bones

♦§ **25671** Percutaneous skeletal fixation of distal radioulnar dislocation
➲ *CPT Changes: An Insider's View* 2002

♦§ **25675** Closed treatment of distal radioulnar dislocation with manipulation

♦§ **25676** Open treatment of distal radioulnar dislocation, acute or chronic

♦§ **25680** Closed treatment of trans-scaphoperilunar type of fracture dislocation, with manipulation

♦§ **25685** Open treatment of trans-scaphoperilunar type of fracture dislocation

♦§ **25690** Closed treatment of lunate dislocation, with manipulation

♦§ **25695** Open treatment of lunate dislocation

Arthrodesis

♦§ **25800** Arthrodesis, wrist; complete, without bone graft (includes radiocarpal and/or intercarpal and/or carpometacarpal joints)

♦§ **25805** with sliding graft

♦§ **25810** with iliac or other autograft (includes obtaining graft)

♦§ **25820** Arthrodesis, wrist; limited, without bone graft (eg, intercarpal or radiocarpal)

♦§ **25825** with autograft (includes obtaining graft)

♦§ **25830** Arthrodesis, distal radioulnar joint with segmental resection of ulna, with or without bone graft (eg, Sauve-Kapandji procedure)

Amputation

♦✿ **25900** Amputation, forearm, through radius and ulna;

♦✿ **25905** open, circular (guillotine)

♦§ **25907** secondary closure or scar revision

♦✿ **25909** re-amputation

♦✿ **25915** Krukenberg procedure

♦✿ **25920** Disarticulation through wrist;

♦§ **25922** secondary closure or scar revision

♦✿ **25924** re-amputation

♦✿ **25927** Transmetacarpal amputation;

♦§ **25929** secondary closure or scar revision

♦✿ **25931** re-amputation

Other Procedures

♦§ **25999** Unlisted procedure, forearm or wrist

Hand and Fingers

Incision

§ **26010** Drainage of finger abscess; simple
➲ *CPT Assistant* May 03:11

§ **26011** complicated (eg, felon)

§ **26020** Drainage of tendon sheath, digit and/or palm, each

§ **26025** Drainage of palmar bursa; single, bursa

§ **26030** multiple bursa

§ **26034** Incision, bone cortex, hand or finger (eg, osteomyelitis or bone abscess)

§ **26035** Decompression fingers and/or hand, injection injury (eg, grease gun)

§ **26037** Decompressive fasciotomy, hand (excludes 26035)

(For injection injury, use 26035)

♦§ **26040** Fasciotomy, palmar (eg, Dupuytren's contracture); percutaneous

♦§ **26045** open, partial

(For fasciectomy, see 26121-26125)

§ **26055** Tendon sheath incision (eg, for trigger finger)

§ **26060** Tenotomy, percutaneous, single, each digit

♦§ **26070** Arthrotomy, with exploration, drainage, or removal of loose or foreign body; carpometacarpal joint

♦§ **26075** metacarpophalangeal joint, each

§ **26080** interphalangeal joint, each

Excision

♦§ **26100** Arthrotomy with biopsy; carpometacarpal joint, each

♦§ **26105** metacarpophalangeal joint, each

§ **26110** interphalangeal joint, each

§ **26115** Excision, tumor or vascular malformation, soft tissue of hand or finger; subcutaneous
➲ *CPT Changes: An Insider's View* 2002

§ **26116** deep (subfascial or intramuscular)
➲ *CPT Changes: An Insider's View* 2002

§ **26117** Radical resection of tumor (eg, malignant neoplasm), soft tissue of hand or finger

♦§ **26121** Fasciectomy, palm only, with or without Z-plasty, other local tissue rearrangement, or skin grafting (includes obtaining graft)

♦§ **26123** Fasciectomy, partial palmar with release of single digit including proximal interphalangeal joint, with or without Z-plasty, other local tissue rearrangement, or skin grafting (includes obtaining graft);

§✚ **26125** each additional digit (List separately in addition to code for primary procedure)

(Use 26125 in conjunction with 26123)

(For fasciotomy, see 26040, 26045)

♦§ **26130** Synovectomy, carpometacarpal joint

§ **26135** Synovectomy, metacarpophalangeal joint including intrinsic release and extensor hood reconstruction, each digit

§ **26140** Synovectomy, proximal interphalangeal joint, including extensor reconstruction, each interphalangeal joint

§ **26145** Synovectomy, tendon sheath, radical (tenosynovectomy), flexor tendon, palm and/or finger, each tendon

(For tendon sheath synovectomies at wrist, see 25115, 25116)

§ **26160** Excision of lesion of tendon sheath or joint capsule (eg, cyst, mucous cyst, or ganglion), hand or finger
➲ *CPT Changes: An Insider's View* 2002

(For wrist ganglion, see 25111, 25112)

(For trigger digit, use 26055)

§ **26170** Excision of tendon, palm, flexor, single (separate procedure), each

§ **26180** Excision of tendon, finger, flexor (separate procedure), each tendon

♦§ **26185** Sesamoidectomy, thumb or finger (separate procedure)

§ **26200** Excision or curettage of bone cyst or benign tumor of metacarpal;

§ **26205** with autograft (includes obtaining graft)

§ **26210** Excision or curettage of bone cyst or benign tumor of proximal, middle, or distal phalanx of finger;

§ **26215** with autograft (includes obtaining graft)

§ **26230** Partial excision (craterization, saucerization, or diaphysectomy) bone (eg, osteomyelitis); metacarpal

§ **26235** proximal or middle phalanx of finger

§ **26236** distal phalanx of finger

§ **26250** Radical resection, metacarpal (eg, tumor);

§ **26255** with autograft (includes obtaining graft)

§ **26260** Radical resection, proximal or middle phalanx of finger (eg, tumor);

§ **26261** with autograft (includes obtaining graft)

§ **26262** Radical resection, distal phalanx of finger (eg, tumor)

Introduction or Removal

§ **26320** Removal of implant from finger or hand

(For removal of foreign body in hand or finger, see 20520, 20525)

Repair, Revision, and/or Reconstruction

♦§ **26340** Manipulation, finger joint, under anesthesia, each joint
➲ *CPT Changes: An Insider's View* 2002

(For application of external fixation, see 20690 or 20692)

§ **26350** Repair or advancement, flexor tendon, not in zone 2 digital flexor tendon sheath (eg, no man's land); primary or secondary without free graft, each tendon
➲ *CPT Changes: An Insider's View* 2002

§ **26352** secondary with free graft (includes obtaining graft), each tendon

§ **26356** Repair or advancement, flexor tendon, in zone 2 digital flexor tendon sheath (eg, no man's land); primary, without free graft, each tendon
➲ *CPT Changes: An Insider's View* 2002, 2004

§ **26357** secondary, without free graft, each tendon
➲ *CPT Changes: An Insider's View* 2004

§ **26358** secondary, with free graft (includes obtaining graft), each tendon

§ **26370** Repair or advancement of profundus tendon, with intact superficialis tendon; primary, each tendon

§ **26372** secondary with free graft (includes obtaining graft), each tendon

§ **26373** secondary without free graft, each tendon

§ **26390** Excision flexor tendon, with implantation of synthetic rod for delayed tendon graft, hand or finger, each rod
➲ *CPT Changes: An Insider's View* 2002

§ **26392** Removal of synthetic rod and insertion of flexor tendon graft, hand or finger (includes obtaining graft), each rod
➲ *CPT Changes: An Insider's View* 2002

§ **26410** Repair, extensor tendon, hand, primary or secondary; without free graft, each tendon

§ **26412** with free graft (includes obtaining graft), each tendon

§ **26415** Excision of extensor tendon, with implantation of synthetic rod for delayed tendon graft, hand or finger, each rod

§ **26416** Removal of synthetic rod and insertion of extensor tendon graft (includes obtaining graft), hand or finger, each rod
➲ *CPT Changes: An Insider's View* 2002

§ **26418** Repair, extensor tendon, finger, primary or secondary; without free graft, each tendon

§ **26420** with free graft (includes obtaining graft) each tendon

§ **26426** Repair of extensor tendon, central slip, secondary (eg, boutonniere deformity); using local tissue(s), including lateral band(s), each finger
➔ *CPT Changes: An Insider's View* 2002

§ **26428** with free graft (includes obtaining graft), each finger
➔ *CPT Changes: An Insider's View* 2002

§ **26432** Closed treatment of distal extensor tendon insertion, with or without percutaneous pinning (eg, mallet finger)

§ **26433** Repair of extensor tendon, distal insertion, primary or secondary; without graft (eg, mallet finger)

§ **26434** with free graft (includes obtaining graft)

(For tenovaginotomy for trigger finger, use 26055)

§ **26437** Realignment of extensor tendon, hand, each tendon

§ **26440** Tenolysis, flexor tendon; palm OR finger, each tendon
➔ *CPT Changes: An Insider's View* 2003

§ **26442** palm AND finger, each tendon

§ **26445** Tenolysis, extensor tendon, hand OR finger, each tendon
➔ *CPT Changes: An Insider's View* 2002

§ **26449** Tenolysis, complex, extensor tendon, finger, including forearm, each tendon

§ **26450** Tenotomy, flexor, palm, open, each tendon

§ **26455** Tenotomy, flexor, finger, open, each tendon

§ **26460** Tenotomy, extensor, hand or finger, open, each tendon

§ **26471** Tenodesis; of proximal interphalangeal joint, each joint

§ **26474** of distal joint, each joint

§ **26476** Lengthening of tendon, extensor, hand or finger, each tendon

§ **26477** Shortening of tendon, extensor, hand or finger, each tendon

§ **26478** Lengthening of tendon, flexor, hand or finger, each tendon

§ **26479** Shortening of tendon, flexor, hand or finger, each tendon

§ **26480** Transfer or transplant of tendon, carpometacarpal area or dorsum of hand; without free graft, each tendon

§ **26483** with free tendon graft (includes obtaining graft), each tendon

§ **26485** Transfer or transplant of tendon, palmar; without free tendon graft, each tendon

§ **26489** with free tendon graft (includes obtaining graft), each tendon

§ **26490** Opponensplasty; superficialis tendon transfer type, each tendon

§ **26492** tendon transfer with graft (includes obtaining graft), each tendon

§ **26494** hypothenar muscle transfer

§ **26496** other methods

(For thumb fusion in opposition, use 26820)

§ **26497** Transfer of tendon to restore intrinsic function; ring and small finger

§ **26498** all four fingers

§ **26499** Correction claw finger, other methods

§ **26500** Reconstruction of tendon pulley, each tendon; with local tissues (separate procedure)

§ **26502** with tendon or fascial graft (includes obtaining graft) (separate procedure)

§ **26504** with tendon prosthesis (separate procedure)

§ **26508** Release of thenar muscle(s) (eg, thumb contracture)

§ **26510** Cross intrinsic transfer, each tendon
➔ *CPT Changes: An Insider's View* 2002

§ **26516** Capsulodesis, metacarpophalangeal joint; single digit

§ **26517** two digits

§ **26518** three or four digits

§ **26520** Capsulectomy or capsulotomy; metacarpophalangeal joint, each joint

§ **26525** interphalangeal joint, each joint

(To report carpometacarpal joint arthroplasty, use 25447)

§ **26530** Arthroplasty, metacarpophalangeal joint; each joint

§ **26531** with prosthetic implant, each joint

§ **26535** Arthroplasty, interphalangeal joint; each joint

§ **26536** with prosthetic implant, each joint

§ **26540** Repair of collateral ligament, metacarpophalangeal or interphalangeal joint

§ **26541** Reconstruction, collateral ligament, metacarpophalangeal joint, single; with tendon or fascial graft (includes obtaining graft)

§ **26542** with local tissue (eg, adductor advancement)

§ **26545** Reconstruction, collateral ligament, interphalangeal joint, single, including graft, each joint

♦§ **26546** Repair non-union, metacarpal or phalanx, (includes obtaining bone graft with or without external or internal fixation)

§ **26548** Repair and reconstruction, finger, volar plate, interphalangeal joint

§ **26550** Pollicization of a digit

✿ **26551** Transfer, toe-to-hand with microvascular anastomosis; great toe wrap-around with bone graft

(For great toe with web space, use 20973)

✿ **26553** other than great toe, single

✿ **26554** other than great toe, double

(Do not report code 69990 in addition to codes 26551-26554)

§ **26555** Transfer, finger to another position without microvascular anastomosis

✿ **26556** Transfer, free toe joint, with microvascular anastomosis

(Do not report code 69990 in addition to code 26556)

(To report great toe-to-hand transfer, use 20973)

§ **26560** Repair of syndactyly (web finger) each web space; with skin flaps

§ **26561** with skin flaps and grafts

§ **26562** complex (eg, involving bone, nails)

§ **26565** Osteotomy; metacarpal, each

§ **26567** phalanx of finger, each

§ **26568** Osteoplasty, lengthening, metacarpal or phalanx

§ **26580** Repair cleft hand

§ **26587** Reconstruction of polydactylous digit, soft tissue and bone
➔ *CPT Changes: An Insider's View* 2002

(For excision of polydactylous digit, soft tissue only, use 11200)

§ **26590** Repair macrodactylia, each digit
➔ *CPT Changes: An Insider's View* 2002

§ **26591** Repair, intrinsic muscles of hand, each muscle

§ **26593** Release, intrinsic muscles of hand, each muscle

§ **26596** Excision of constricting ring of finger, with multiple Z-plasties

(To report release of scar contracture or graft repairs see 11041-11042, 14040-14041, or 15120, 15240)

Fracture and/or Dislocation

§ **26600** Closed treatment of metacarpal fracture, single; without manipulation, each bone

§ **26605** with manipulation, each bone

§ **26607** Closed treatment of metacarpal fracture, with manipulation, with external fixation, each bone
➔ *CPT Changes: An Insider's View* 2002

§ **26608** Percutaneous skeletal fixation of metacarpal fracture, each bone

§ **26615** Open treatment of metacarpal fracture, single, with or without internal or external fixation, each bone

§ **26641** Closed treatment of carpometacarpal dislocation, thumb, with manipulation

§ **26645** Closed treatment of carpometacarpal fracture dislocation, thumb (Bennett fracture), with manipulation

§ **26650** Percutaneous skeletal fixation of carpometacarpal fracture dislocation, thumb (Bennett fracture), with manipulation, with or without external fixation

§ **26665** Open treatment of carpometacarpal fracture dislocation, thumb (Bennett fracture), with or without internal or external fixation

§ **26670** Closed treatment of carpometacarpal dislocation, other than thumb, with manipulation, each joint; without anesthesia
➔ *CPT Changes: An Insider's View* 2002

§ **26675** requiring anesthesia

§ **26676** Percutaneous skeletal fixation of carpometacarpal dislocation, other than thumb, with manipulation, each joint
➔ *CPT Changes: An Insider's View* 2002

§ **26685** Open treatment of carpometacarpal dislocation, other than thumb; with or without internal or external fixation, each joint
➔ *CPT Changes: An Insider's View* 2002

§ **26686** complex, multiple or delayed reduction

§ **26700** Closed treatment of metacarpophalangeal dislocation, single, with manipulation; without anesthesia

§ **26705** requiring anesthesia

§ **26706** Percutaneous skeletal fixation of metacarpophalangeal dislocation, single, with manipulation

§ **26715** Open treatment of metacarpophalangeal dislocation, single, with or without internal or external fixation

§ **26720** Closed treatment of phalangeal shaft fracture, proximal or middle phalanx, finger or thumb; without manipulation, each

§ **26725** with manipulation, with or without skin or skeletal traction, each

§ **26727** Percutaneous skeletal fixation of unstable phalangeal shaft fracture, proximal or middle phalanx, finger or thumb, with manipulation, each

§ **26735** Open treatment of phalangeal shaft fracture, proximal or middle phalanx, finger or thumb, with or without internal or external fixation, each

§ **26740** Closed treatment of articular fracture, involving metacarpophalangeal or interphalangeal joint; without manipulation, each

§ **26742** with manipulation, each

§ **26746** Open treatment of articular fracture, involving metacarpophalangeal or interphalangeal joint, with or without internal or external fixation, each

§ **26750** Closed treatment of distal phalangeal fracture, finger or thumb; without manipulation, each

§ **26755** with manipulation, each

§ **26756** Percutaneous skeletal fixation of distal phalangeal fracture, finger or thumb, each

§ **26765** Open treatment of distal phalangeal fracture, finger or thumb, with or without internal or external fixation, each

§ **26770** Closed treatment of interphalangeal joint dislocation, single, with manipulation; without anesthesia

§ **26775** requiring anesthesia

§ **26776** Percutaneous skeletal fixation of interphalangeal joint dislocation, single, with manipulation

§ **26785** Open treatment of interphalangeal joint dislocation, with or without internal or external fixation, single

Arthrodesis

§ **26820** Fusion in opposition, thumb, with autogenous graft (includes obtaining graft)

§ **26841** Arthrodesis, carpometacarpal joint, thumb, with or without internal fixation;

§ **26842** with autograft (includes obtaining graft)

§ **26843** Arthrodesis, carpometacarpal joint, digit, other than thumb, each;
➲ *CPT Changes: An Insider's View* 2002

§ **26844** with autograft (includes obtaining graft)

§ **26850** Arthrodesis, metacarpophalangeal joint, with or without internal fixation;

§ **26852** with autograft (includes obtaining graft)

§ **26860** Arthrodesis, interphalangeal joint, with or without internal fixation;

§+ **26861** each additional interphalangeal joint (List separately in addition to code for primary procedure)

(Use 26861 in conjunction with 26860)

§ **26862** with autograft (includes obtaining graft)

§+ **26863** with autograft (includes obtaining graft), each additional joint (List separately in addition to code for primary procedure)

(Use 26863 in conjunction with 26862)

Amputation

(For hand through metacarpal bones, use 25927)

§ **26910** Amputation, metacarpal, with finger or thumb (ray amputation), single, with or without interosseous transfer

(For repositioning, see 26550, 26555)

§ **26951** Amputation, finger or thumb, primary or secondary, any joint or phalanx, single, including neurectomies; with direct closure

§ **26952** with local advancement flaps (V-Y, hood)

(For repair of soft tissue defect requiring split or full thickness graft or other pedicle flaps, see 15050-15758)

Other Procedures

§ **26989** Unlisted procedure, hands or fingers

Pelvis and Hip Joint

Including head and neck of femur.

Incision

(For incision and drainage procedures, superficial, see 10040-10160)

§ **26990** Incision and drainage, pelvis or hip joint area; deep abscess or hematoma

§ **26991** infected bursa

✿ **26992** Incision, bone cortex, pelvis and/or hip joint (eg, osteomyelitis or bone abscess)

♦§ **27000** Tenotomy, adductor of hip, percutaneous (separate procedure)

♦§ **27001** Tenotomy, adductor of hip, open

(To report bilateral procedures, report 27001 with modifier 50)

♦§ **27003** Tenotomy, adductor, subcutaneous, open, with obturator neurectomy

(To report bilateral procedures, report 27003 with modifier 50)

♦✿ **27005** Tenotomy, hip flexor(s), open (separate procedure)

♦✿ **27006** Tenotomy, abductors and/or extensor(s) of hip, open (separate procedure)

♦✿ **27025** Fasciotomy, hip or thigh, any type

(To report bilateral procedures, report 27025 with modifier 50)

♦✿ **27030** Arthrotomy, hip, with drainage (eg, infection)

♦§ **27033** Arthrotomy, hip, including exploration or removal of loose or foreign body

♦§ **27035** Denervation, hip joint, intrapelvic or extrapelvic intra-articular branches of sciatic, femoral, or obturator nerves
➲ *CPT Assistant* Jan 03:15

(For obturator neurectomy, see 64763, 64766)

♦✿ **27036** Capsulectomy or capsulotomy, hip, with or without excision of heterotopic bone, with release of hip flexor muscles (ie, gluteus medius, gluteus minimus, tensor fascia latae, rectus femoris, sartorius, iliopsoas)

Excision

♦§ **27040** Biopsy, soft tissue of pelvis and hip area; superficial

♦§ **27041** deep, subfascial or intramuscular

(For needle biopsy of soft tissue, use 20206)

♦§ **27047** Excision, tumor, pelvis and hip area; subcutaneous tissue

♦§ **27048** deep, subfascial, intramuscular

♦§ **27049** Radical resection of tumor, soft tissue of pelvis and hip area (eg, malignant neoplasm)

♦§ **27050** Arthrotomy, with biopsy; sacroiliac joint

♦§ **27052** hip joint

♦✿ **27054** Arthrotomy with synovectomy, hip joint

♦§ **27060** Excision; ischial bursa

♦§ **27062** trochanteric bursa or calcification

(For arthrocentesis or needling of bursa, use 20610)

♦§ **27065** Excision of bone cyst or benign tumor; superficial (wing of ilium, symphysis pubis, or greater trochanter of femur) with or without autograft

♦§ **27066** deep, with or without autograft

♦§ **27067** with autograft requiring separate incision

♦✿ **27070** Partial excision (craterization, saucerization) (eg, osteomyelitis or bone abscess); superficial (eg, wing of ilium, symphysis pubis, or greater trochanter of femur)

♦✿ **27071** deep (subfascial or intramuscular)

✿ **27075** Radical resection of tumor or infection; wing of ilium, one pubic or ischial ramus or symphysis pubis

✿ **27076** ilium, including acetabulum, both pubic rami, or ischium and acetabulum

✿ **27077** innominate bone, total

✿ **27078** ischial tuberosity and greater trochanter of femur

✿ **27079** ischial tuberosity and greater trochanter of femur, with skin flaps

§ **27080** Coccygectomy, primary

(For pressure (decubitus) ulcer, see 15920, 15922 and 15931-15958)

Introduction or Removal

♦§ **27086** Removal of foreign body, pelvis or hip; subcutaneous tissue

♦§ **27087** deep (subfascial or intramuscular)

♦✿ **27090** Removal of hip prosthesis; (separate procedure)

♦✿ **27091** complicated, including total hip prosthesis, methylmethacrylate with or without insertion of spacer

♦☆ **27093** Injection procedure for hip arthrography; without anesthesia

(For radiological supervision and interpretation, use 73525. Do not report 76003 in addition to 73525)

♦☆ **27095** with anesthesia

(For radiological supervision and interpretation, use 73525. Do not report 76003 in addition to 73525)

♦✣ **27096** Injection procedure for sacroiliac joint, arthrography and/or anesthetic/steroid

➔ *CPT Assistant* Apr 03:8; *CPT Changes: An Insider's View* 2000

(27096 is to be used only with imaging confirmation of intra-articular needle positioning)

(For radiological supervision and interpretation of sacroiliac joint arthrography, use 73542)

(For fluoroscopic guidance without formal arthrography, use 76005)

(Code 27096 is a unilateral procedure. For bilateral procedure, use modifier 50)

Repair, Revision, and/or Reconstruction

♦§ **27097** Release or recession, hamstring, proximal

♦§ **27098** Transfer, adductor to ischium

♦§ **27100** Transfer external oblique muscle to greater trochanter including fascial or tendon extension (graft)

♦§ **27105** Transfer paraspinal muscle to hip (includes fascial or tendon extension graft)

♦§ **27110** Transfer iliopsoas; to greater trochanter of femur

♦§ **27111** to femoral neck

♦✿ **27120** Acetabuloplasty; (eg, Whitman, Colonna, Haygroves, or cup type)

♦✿ **27122** resection, femoral head (eg, Girdlestone procedure)

♦✿ **27125** Hemiarthroplasty, hip, partial (eg, femoral stem prosthesis, bipolar arthroplasty)

(For prosthetic replacement following fracture of the hip, use 27236)

♦✿ **27130** Arthroplasty, acetabular and proximal femoral prosthetic replacement (total hip arthroplasty), with or without autograft or allograft

♦✿ **27132** Conversion of previous hip surgery to total hip arthroplasty, with or without autograft or allograft

♦✿ **27134** Revision of total hip arthroplasty; both components, with or without autograft or allograft

♦✿ **27137** acetabular component only, with or without autograft or allograft

♦✿ **27138** femoral component only, with or without allograft

♦✿ **27140** Osteotomy and transfer of greater trochanter of femur (separate procedure)

♦✿ **27146** Osteotomy, iliac, acetabular or innominate bone;

♦✿ **27147** with open reduction of hip

♦✿ **27151** with femoral osteotomy

♦✿ **27156** with femoral osteotomy and with open reduction of hip

✶✿ **27158** Osteotomy, pelvis, bilateral (eg, congenital malformation)

♦✿ **27161** Osteotomy, femoral neck (separate procedure)

✿ **27165** Osteotomy, intertrochanteric or subtrochanteric including internal or external fixation and/or cast

♦✿ **27170** Bone graft, femoral head, neck, intertrochanteric or subtrochanteric area (includes obtaining bone graft)

♦✿ 27175 Treatment of slipped femoral epiphysis; by traction, without reduction

♦✿ 27176 by single or multiple pinning, in situ

♦✿ 27177 Open treatment of slipped femoral epiphysis; single or multiple pinning or bone graft (includes obtaining graft)

♦✿ 27178 closed manipulation with single or multiple pinning

♦✿ 27179 osteoplasty of femoral neck (Heyman type procedure)

♦✿ 27181 osteotomy and internal fixation

♦✿ 27185 Epiphyseal arrest by epiphysiodesis or stapling, greater trochanter of femur

♦✿ 27187 Prophylactic treatment (nailing, pinning, plating or wiring) with or without methylmethacrylate, femoral neck and proximal femur

Fracture and/or Dislocation

♦§ 27193 Closed treatment of pelvic ring fracture, dislocation, diastasis or subluxation; without manipulation

§ 27194 with manipulation, requiring more than local anesthesia

§ 27200 Closed treatment of coccygeal fracture

§ 27202 Open treatment of coccygeal fracture

✿ 27215 Open treatment of iliac spine(s), tuberosity avulsion, or iliac wing fracture(s) (eg, pelvic fracture(s) which do not disrupt the pelvic ring), with internal fixation

§ 27216 Percutaneous skeletal fixation of posterior pelvic ring fracture and/or dislocation (includes ilium, sacroiliac joint and/or sacrum)

➔ *CPT Assistant* Jan 03:15

✿ 27217 Open treatment of anterior ring fracture and/or dislocation with internal fixation (includes pubic symphysis and/or rami)

✿ 27218 Open treatment of posterior ring fracture and/or dislocation with internal fixation (includes ilium, sacroiliac joint and/or sacrum)

♦§ 27220 Closed treatment of acetabulum (hip socket) fracture(s); without manipulation

♦✿ 27222 with manipulation, with or without skeletal traction

♦✿ 27226 Open treatment of posterior or anterior acetabular wall fracture, with internal fixation

♦✿ 27227 Open treatment of acetabular fracture(s) involving anterior or posterior (one) column, or a fracture running transversely across the acetabulum, with internal fixation

♦✿ 27228 Open treatment of acetabular fracture(s) involving anterior and posterior (two) columns, includes T-fracture and both column fracture with complete articular detachment, or single column or transverse fracture with associated acetabular wall fracture, with internal fixation

♦§ 27230 Closed treatment of femoral fracture, proximal end, neck; without manipulation

♦✿ 27232 with manipulation, with or without skeletal traction

♦§ 27235 Percutaneous skeletal fixation of femoral fracture, proximal end, neck

➔ *CPT Assistant* Jan 03:15; *CPT Changes: An Insider's View* 2003

♦✿ 27236 Open treatment of femoral fracture, proximal end, neck, internal fixation or prosthetic replacement

♦§ 27238 Closed treatment of intertrochanteric, pertrochanteric, or subtrochanteric femoral fracture; without manipulation

♦✿ 27240 with manipulation, with or without skin or skeletal traction

♦✿ 27244 Treatment of intertrochanteric, pertrochanteric, or subtrochanteric femoral fracture; with plate/screw type implant, with or without cerclage

♦✿ 27245 with intramedullary implant, with or without interlocking screws and/or cerclage

♦§ 27246 Closed treatment of greater trochanteric fracture, without manipulation

♦✿ 27248 Open treatment of greater trochanteric fracture, with or without internal or external fixation

♦§ 27250 Closed treatment of hip dislocation, traumatic; without anesthesia

♦§ 27252 requiring anesthesia

♦✿ 27253 Open treatment of hip dislocation, traumatic, without internal fixation

♦✿ 27254 Open treatment of hip dislocation, traumatic, with acetabular wall and femoral head fracture, with or without internal or external fixation

(For treatment of acetabular fracture with fixation, see 27226, 27227)

♦§ 27256 Treatment of spontaneous hip dislocation (developmental, including congenital or pathological), by abduction, splint or traction; without anesthesia, without manipulation

♦§ 27257 with manipulation, requiring anesthesia

♦✿ 27258 Open treatment of spontaneous hip dislocation (developmental, including congenital or pathological), replacement of femoral head in acetabulum (including tenotomy, etc);

♦✿ 27259 with femoral shaft shortening

♦§ 27265 Closed treatment of post hip arthroplasty dislocation; without anesthesia

♦§ 27266 requiring regional or general anesthesia

Manipulation

§ 27275 Manipulation, hip joint, requiring general anesthesia

Arthrodesis

♦✿ 27280 Arthrodesis, sacroiliac joint (including obtaining graft)

(To report bilateral procedures, report 27280 with modifier 50)

✿ **27282** Arthrodesis, symphysis pubis (including obtaining graft)

♦✿ **27284** Arthrodesis, hip joint (including obtaining graft);

♦✿ **27286** with subtrochanteric osteotomy

Amputation

✿ **27290** Interpelviabdominal amputation (hindquarter amputation)

✿ **27295** Disarticulation of hip

Other Procedures

♦§ **27299** Unlisted procedure, pelvis or hip joint

Femur (Thigh Region) and Knee Joint

Including tibial plateaus.

Incision

(For incision and drainage of abscess or hematoma, superficial, see 10040-10160)

♦§ **27301** Incision and drainage, deep abscess, bursa, or hematoma, thigh or knee region

♦✿ **27303** Incision, deep, with opening of bone cortex, femur or knee (eg, osteomyelitis or bone abscess)

♦§ **27305** Fasciotomy, iliotibial (tenotomy), open

(For combined Ober-Yount fasciotomy, use 27025)

♦§ **27306** Tenotomy, percutaneous, adductor or hamstring; single tendon (separate procedure)

♦§ **27307** multiple tendons

♦§ **27310** Arthrotomy, knee, with exploration, drainage, or removal of foreign body (eg, infection)

♦§ **27315** Neurectomy, hamstring muscle

♦§ **27320** Neurectomy, popliteal (gastrocnemius)

Excision

♦§ **27323** Biopsy, soft tissue of thigh or knee area; superficial

♦§ **27324** deep (subfascial or intramuscular)

(For needle biopsy of soft tissue, use 20206)

♦§ **27327** Excision, tumor, thigh or knee area; subcutaneous

♦§ **27328** deep, subfascial, or intramuscular

♦§ **27329** Radical resection of tumor (eg, malignant neoplasm), soft tissue of thigh or knee area

♦§ **27330** Arthrotomy, knee; with synovial biopsy only

♦§ **27331** including joint exploration, biopsy, or removal of loose or foreign bodies

♦§ **27332** Arthrotomy, with excision of semilunar cartilage (meniscectomy) knee; medial OR lateral

♦§ **27333** medial AND lateral

♦§ **27334** Arthrotomy, with synovectomy, knee; anterior OR posterior

♦§ **27335** anterior AND posterior including popliteal area

♦§ **27340** Excision, prepatellar bursa

♦§ **27345** Excision of synovial cyst of popliteal space (eg, Baker's cyst)

♦§ **27347** Excision of lesion of meniscus or capsule (eg, cyst, ganglion), knee

♦§ **27350** Patellectomy or hemipatellectomy

♦§ **27355** Excision or curettage of bone cyst or benign tumor of femur;

♦§ **27356** with allograft

♦§ **27357** with autograft (includes obtaining graft)

♦§+ **27358** with internal fixation (List in addition to code for primary procedure)

(Use 27358 in conjunction with 27355, 27356, or 27357)

♦§ **27360** Partial excision (craterization, saucerization, or diaphysectomy) bone, femur, proximal tibia and/or fibula (eg, osteomyelitis or bone abscess)

♦✿ **27365** Radical resection of tumor, bone, femur or knee

(For radical resection of tumor, soft tissue, use 27329)

Introduction or Removal

♦☆ **27370** Injection procedure for knee arthrography

(For radiological supervision and interpretation, use 73580. Do not report 76003 in addition to 73580)

♦§ **27372** Removal of foreign body, deep, thigh region or knee area

(For removal of knee prosthesis including "total knee," use 27488)

(For surgical arthroscopic knee procedures, see 29870-29887)

Repair, Revision, and/or Reconstruction

♦§ **27380** Suture of infrapatellar tendon; primary

♦§ **27381** secondary reconstruction, including fascial or tendon graft

♦§ **27385** Suture of quadriceps or hamstring muscle rupture; primary

♦§ **27386** secondary reconstruction, including fascial or tendon graft

§ **27390** Tenotomy, open, hamstring, knee to hip; single tendon

§ **27391** multiple tendons, one leg

✶§ **27392** multiple tendons, bilateral

§ **27393** Lengthening of hamstring tendon; single tendon

§ **27394** multiple tendons, one leg

✶§ **27395** multiple tendons, bilateral

§ **27396** Transplant, hamstring tendon to patella; single tendon

§ **27397** multiple tendons

♦§ **27400** Transfer, tendon or muscle, hamstrings to femur (eg, Egger's type procedure)

♦§ **27403** Arthrotomy with meniscus repair, knee

(For arthroscopic repair, use 29882)

♦§ **27405** Repair, primary, torn ligament and/or capsule, knee; collateral

♦§ **27407** cruciate

(For cruciate ligament reconstruction, use 27427)

♦§ **27409** collateral and cruciate ligaments

(For ligament reconstruction, see 27427-27429)

♦§● **27412** Autologous chondrocyte implantation, knee

➲ *CPT Changes: An Insider's View* 2005

►(Do not report 27412 in conjunction with 20926, 27331, 27570)◄

►(For harvesting of chondrocytes, use 29870)◄

♦§● **27415** Osteochondral allograft, knee, open

➲ *CPT Changes: An Insider's View* 2005

►(For arthroscopic implant of osteochondral allograft, use 29867)◄

♦§ **27418** Anterior tibial tubercleplasty (eg, Maquet type procedure)

♦§ **27420** Reconstruction of dislocating patella; (eg, Hauser type procedure)

♦§ **27422** with extensor realignment and/or muscle advancement or release (eg, Campbell, Goldwaite type procedure)

♦§ **27424** with patellectomy

♦§ **27425** Lateral retinacular release, open

➲ *CPT Changes: An Insider's View* 2002, 2003

(For arthroscopic lateral release, use 29873)

♦§ **27427** Ligamentous reconstruction (augmentation), knee; extra-articular

➲ *CPT Changes: An Insider's View* 2000

♦§ **27428** intra-articular (open)

➲ *CPT Changes: An Insider's View* 2000

♦§ **27429** intra-articular (open) and extra-articular

➲ *CPT Changes: An Insider's View* 2000

(For primary repair of ligament(s) performed in conjunction with reconstruction, report 27405, 27407 or 27409 in conjunction with 27427, 27428 or 27429)

♦§ **27430** Quadricepsplasty (eg, Bennett or Thompson type)

♦§ **27435** Capsulotomy, posterior capsular release, knee

♦§ **27437** Arthroplasty, patella; without prosthesis

♦§ **27438** with prosthesis

♦§ **27440** Arthroplasty, knee, tibial plateau;

♦§ **27441** with debridement and partial synovectomy

♦§ **27442** Arthroplasty, femoral condyles or tibial plateau(s), knee;

♦§ **27443** with debridement and partial synovectomy

♦✿ **27445** Arthroplasty, knee, hinge prosthesis (eg, Walldius type)

♦§ **27446** Arthroplasty, knee, condyle and plateau; medial OR lateral compartment

♦✿ **27447** medial AND lateral compartments with or without patella resurfacing (total knee arthroplasty)

(For revision of total knee arthroplasty, use 27487)

(For removal of total knee prosthesis, use 27488)

♦✿ **27448** Osteotomy, femur, shaft or supracondylar; without fixation

(To report bilateral procedures, report 27448 with modifier 50)

♦✿ **27450** with fixation

(To report bilateral procedures, report 27450 with modifier 50)

♦✿ **27454** Osteotomy, multiple, with realignment on intramedullary rod, femoral shaft (eg, Sofield type procedure)

♦✿ **27455** Osteotomy, proximal tibia, including fibular excision or osteotomy (includes correction of genu varus (bowleg) or genu valgus (knock-knee)); before epiphyseal closure

(To report bilateral procedures, report 27455 with modifier 50)

♦✿ **27457** after epiphyseal closure

(To report bilateral procedures, report 27457 with modifier 50)

♦✿ **27465** Osteoplasty, femur; shortening (excluding 64876)

♦✿ **27466** lengthening

♦✿ **27468** combined, lengthening and shortening with femoral segment transfer

♦✿ **27470** Repair, nonunion or malunion, femur, distal to head and neck; without graft (eg, compression technique)

♦✿ **27472** with iliac or other autogenous bone graft (includes obtaining graft)

♦✿ **27475** Arrest, epiphyseal, any method (eg, epiphysiodesis); distal femur

♦✿ **27477** tibia and fibula, proximal

♦✿ **27479** combined distal femur, proximal tibia and fibula

♦✿ **27485** Arrest, hemiepiphyseal, distal femur or proximal tibia or fibula (eg, genu varus or valgus)

♦✿ **27486** Revision of total knee arthroplasty, with or without allograft; one component

♦✿ **27487** femoral and entire tibial component

♦✿ **27488** Removal of prosthesis, including total knee prosthesis, methylmethacrylate with or without insertion of spacer, knee

♦✿ **27495** Prophylactic treatment (nailing, pinning, plating or wiring) with or without methylmethacrylate, femur

♦§ **27496** Decompression fasciotomy, thigh and/or knee, one compartment (flexor or extensor or adductor);

♦§ **27497** with debridement of nonviable muscle and/or nerve

♦§ **27498** Decompression fasciotomy, thigh and/or knee, multiple compartments;

♦§ **27499** with debridement of nonviable muscle and/or nerve

Fracture and/or Dislocation

(For arthroscopic treatment of intercondylar spine(s) and tuberosity fracture(s) of the knee, see 29850, 29851)

(For arthroscopic treatment of tibial fracture, see 29855, 29856)

♦§ **27500** Closed treatment of femoral shaft fracture, without manipulation

♦§ **27501** Closed treatment of supracondylar or transcondylar femoral fracture with or without intercondylar extension, without manipulation

♦§ **27502** Closed treatment of femoral shaft fracture, with manipulation, with or without skin or skeletal traction

♦§ **27503** Closed treatment of supracondylar or transcondylar femoral fracture with or without intercondylar extension, with manipulation, with or without skin or skeletal traction

♦✿ **27506** Open treatment of femoral shaft fracture, with or without external fixation, with insertion of intramedullary implant, with or without cerclage and/or locking screws

♦✿ **27507** Open treatment of femoral shaft fracture with plate/screws, with or without cerclage

♦§ **27508** Closed treatment of femoral fracture, distal end, medial or lateral condyle, without manipulation

♦§ **27509** Percutaneous skeletal fixation of femoral fracture, distal end, medial or lateral condyle, or supracondylar or transcondylar, with or without intercondylar extension, or distal femoral epiphyseal separation

♦§ **27510** Closed treatment of femoral fracture, distal end, medial or lateral condyle, with manipulation

♦✿ **27511** Open treatment of femoral supracondylar or transcondylar fracture without intercondylar extension, with or without internal or external fixation

♦✿ **27513** Open treatment of femoral supracondylar or transcondylar fracture with intercondylar extension, with or without internal or external fixation

♦✿ **27514** Open treatment of femoral fracture, distal end, medial or lateral condyle, with or without internal or external fixation

♦§ **27516** Closed treatment of distal femoral epiphyseal separation; without manipulation

♦§ **27517** with manipulation, with or without skin or skeletal traction

♦✿ **27519** Open treatment of distal femoral epiphyseal separation, with or without internal or external fixation

♦§ **27520** Closed treatment of patellar fracture, without manipulation

♦§ **27524** Open treatment of patellar fracture, with internal fixation and/or partial or complete patellectomy and soft tissue repair

♦§ **27530** Closed treatment of tibial fracture, proximal (plateau); without manipulation

♦§ **27532** with or without manipulation, with skeletal traction

(For arthroscopic treatment, see 29855, 29856)

♦✿ **27535** Open treatment of tibial fracture, proximal (plateau); unicondylar, with or without internal or external fixation

♦✿ **27536** bicondylar, with or without internal fixation

(For arthroscopic treatment, see 29855, 29856)

♦§ **27538** Closed treatment of intercondylar spine(s) and/or tuberosity fracture(s) of knee, with or without manipulation

(For arthroscopic treatment, see 29850, 29851)

♦✿ **27540** Open treatment of intercondylar spine(s) and/or tuberosity fracture(s) of the knee, with or without internal or external fixation

♦§ **27550** Closed treatment of knee dislocation; without anesthesia

♦§ **27552** requiring anesthesia

♦✿ **27556** Open treatment of knee dislocation, with or without internal or external fixation; without primary ligamentous repair or augmentation/reconstruction

♦✿ **27557** with primary ligamentous repair

♦✿ **27558** with primary ligamentous repair, with augmentation/reconstruction

♦§ **27560** Closed treatment of patellar dislocation; without anesthesia

➔ *CPT Assistant* Apr 02:15

(For recurrent dislocation, see 27420-27424)

♦§ **27562** requiring anesthesia

♦§ **27566** Open treatment of patellar dislocation, with or without partial or total patellectomy

Manipulation

§ **27570** Manipulation of knee joint under general anesthesia (includes application of traction or other fixation devices)

Arthrodesis

♦✿ 27580 Arthrodesis, knee, any technique

Amputation

♦✿ 27590 Amputation, thigh, through femur, any level;

♦✿ 27591 immediate fitting technique including first cast

♦✿ 27592 open, circular (guillotine)

♦§ 27594 secondary closure or scar revision

♦✿ 27596 re-amputation

♦✿ 27598 Disarticulation at knee

Other Procedures

♦§ 27599 Unlisted procedure, femur or knee

Leg (Tibia and Fibula) and Ankle Joint

Incision

♦§ 27600 Decompression fasciotomy, leg; anterior and/or lateral compartments only

♦§ 27601 posterior compartment(s) only

♦§ 27602 anterior and/or lateral, and posterior compartment(s)

(For incision and drainage procedures, superficial, see 10040-10160)

(For decompression fasciotomy with debridement, see 27892-27894)

♦§ 27603 Incision and drainage, leg or ankle; deep abscess or hematoma

♦§ 27604 infected bursa

♦§ 27605 Tenotomy, percutaneous, Achilles tendon (separate procedure); local anesthesia

♦§ 27606 general anesthesia

♦§ 27607 Incision (eg, osteomyelitis or bone abscess), leg or ankle

♦§ 27610 Arthrotomy, ankle, including exploration, drainage, or removal of foreign body

♦§ 27612 Arthrotomy, posterior capsular release, ankle, with or without Achilles tendon lengthening

(See also 27685)

Excision

♦§ 27613 Biopsy, soft tissue of leg or ankle area; superficial

♦§ 27614 deep (subfascial or intramuscular)

(For needle biopsy of soft tissue, use 20206)

♦§ 27615 Radical resection of tumor (eg, malignant neoplasm), soft tissue of leg or ankle area

♦§ 27618 Excision, tumor, leg or ankle area; subcutaneous tissue

♦§ 27619 deep (subfascial or intramuscular)

♦§ 27620 Arthrotomy, ankle, with joint exploration, with or without biopsy, with or without removal of loose or foreign body

♦§ 27625 Arthrotomy, with synovectomy, ankle;

♦§ 27626 including tenosynovectomy

♦§ 27630 Excision of lesion of tendon sheath or capsule (eg, cyst or ganglion), leg and/or ankle

♦§ 27635 Excision or curettage of bone cyst or benign tumor, tibia or fibula;

♦§ 27637 with autograft (includes obtaining graft)

♦§ 27638 with allograft

♦§ 27640 Partial excision (craterization, saucerization, or diaphysectomy) bone (eg, osteomyelitis or exostosis); tibia

♦§ 27641 fibula

♦✿ 27645 Radical resection of tumor, bone; tibia

♦✿ 27646 fibula

♦§ 27647 talus or calcaneus

Introduction or Removal

♦☆ 27648 Injection procedure for ankle arthrography

(For radiological supervision and interpretation, use 73615. Do not report 76003 in addition to 73615)

(For ankle arthroscopy, see 29894-29898)

Repair, Revision, and/or Reconstruction

♦§ 27650 Repair, primary, open or percutaneous, ruptured Achilles tendon;

♦§ 27652 with graft (includes obtaining graft)

♦§ 27654 Repair, secondary, Achilles tendon, with or without graft

♦§ 27656 Repair, fascial defect of leg

§ 27658 Repair, flexor tendon, leg; primary, without graft, each tendon

§ 27659 secondary, with or without graft, each tendon

§ 27664 Repair, extensor tendon, leg; primary, without graft, each tendon

§ 27665 secondary, with or without graft, each tendon

♦§ 27675 Repair, dislocating peroneal tendons; without fibular osteotomy

♦§ 27676 with fibular osteotomy

§ 27680 Tenolysis, flexor or extensor tendon, leg and/or ankle; single, each tendon

§ 27681 multiple tendons (through separate incision(s))

§ 27685 Lengthening or shortening of tendon, leg or ankle; single tendon (separate procedure)

§ 27686 multiple tendons (through same incision), each

♦§ 27687 Gastrocnemius recession (eg, Strayer procedure)

(Toe extensors are considered as a group to be a single tendon when transplanted into midfoot)

♦§ 27690 Transfer or transplant of single tendon (with muscle redirection or rerouting); superficial (eg, anterior tibial extensors into midfoot)

♦§ 27691 deep (eg, anterior tibial or posterior tibial through interosseous space, flexor digitorum longus, flexor hallucis longus, or peroneal tendon to midfoot or hindfoot)

♦§+ 27692 each additional tendon (List separately in addition to code for primary procedure)
➔ *CPT Assistant* Feb 03: 8

(Use 27692 in conjunction with 27690, 27691)

♦§ 27695 Repair, primary, disrupted ligament, ankle; collateral

♦§ 27696 both collateral ligaments

♦§ 27698 Repair, secondary, disrupted ligament, ankle, collateral (eg, Watson-Jones procedure)

♦§ 27700 Arthroplasty, ankle;

♦✿ 27702 with implant (total ankle)

♦✿ 27703 revision, total ankle

♦§ 27704 Removal of ankle implant

♦§ 27705 Osteotomy; tibia

♦§ 27707 fibula

♦§ 27709 tibia and fibula

♦✿ 27712 multiple, with realignment on intramedullary rod (eg, Sofield type procedure)

(For osteotomy to correct genu varus (bowleg) or genu valgus (knock-knee), see 27455-27457)

♦✿ 27715 Osteoplasty, tibia and fibula, lengthening or shortening

♦✿ 27720 Repair of nonunion or malunion, tibia; without graft, (eg, compression technique)

♦✿ 27722 with sliding graft

♦✿ 27724 with iliac or other autograft (includes obtaining graft)

♦✿ 27725 by synostosis, with fibula, any method

♦✿ 27727 Repair of congenital pseudarthrosis, tibia

♦§ 27730 Arrest, epiphyseal (epiphysiodesis), open; distal tibia
➔ *CPT Changes: An Insider's View* 2003

♦§ 27732 distal fibula

♦§ 27734 distal tibia and fibula

♦§ 27740 Arrest, epiphyseal (epiphysiodesis), any method, combined, proximal and distal tibia and fibula;

♦§ 27742 and distal femur

(For epiphyseal arrest of proximal tibia and fibula, use 27477)

♦§ 27745 Prophylactic treatment (nailing, pinning, plating or wiring) with or without methylmethacrylate, tibia

Fracture and/or Dislocation

♦§ 27750 Closed treatment of tibial shaft fracture (with or without fibular fracture); without manipulation

♦§ 27752 with manipulation, with or without skeletal traction

♦§ 27756 Percutaneous skeletal fixation of tibial shaft fracture (with or without fibular fracture) (eg, pins or screws)

♦§ 27758 Open treatment of tibial shaft fracture, (with or without fibular fracture) with plate/screws, with or without cerclage

♦§ 27759 Treatment of tibial shaft fracture (with or without fibular fracture) by intramedullary implant, with or without interlocking screws and/or cerclage
➔ *CPT Changes: An Insider's View* 2003

♦§ 27760 Closed treatment of medial malleolus fracture; without manipulation

♦§ 27762 with manipulation, with or without skin or skeletal traction

♦§ 27766 Open treatment of medial malleolus fracture, with or without internal or external fixation

♦§ 27780 Closed treatment of proximal fibula or shaft fracture; without manipulation

♦§ 27781 with manipulation

♦§ 27784 Open treatment of proximal fibula or shaft fracture, with or without internal or external fixation

♦§ 27786 Closed treatment of distal fibular fracture (lateral malleolus); without manipulation

♦§ 27788 with manipulation

♦§ 27792 Open treatment of distal fibular fracture (lateral malleolus), with or without internal or external fixation

(For treatment of tibia and fibula shaft fractures, see 27750-27759)

♦§ 27808 Closed treatment of bimalleolar ankle fracture, (including Potts); without manipulation

♦§ 27810 with manipulation

♦§ 27814 Open treatment of bimalleolar ankle fracture, with or without internal or external fixation

♦§ 27816 Closed treatment of trimalleolar ankle fracture; without manipulation

♦§ 27818 with manipulation

♦§ **27822** Open treatment of trimalleolar ankle fracture, with or without internal or external fixation, medial and/or lateral malleolus; without fixation of posterior lip

♦§ **27823** with fixation of posterior lip

♦§ **27824** Closed treatment of fracture of weight bearing articular portion of distal tibia (eg, pilon or tibial plafond), with or without anesthesia; without manipulation

♦§ **27825** with skeletal traction and/or requiring manipulation

♦§ **27826** Open treatment of fracture of weight bearing articular surface/portion of distal tibia (eg, pilon or tibial plafond), with internal or external fixation; of fibula only

♦§ **27827** of tibia only

♦§ **27828** of both tibia and fibula

♦§ **27829** Open treatment of distal tibiofibular joint (syndesmosis) disruption, with or without internal or external fixation

♦§ **27830** Closed treatment of proximal tibiofibular joint dislocation; without anesthesia

♦§ **27831** requiring anesthesia

♦§ **27832** Open treatment of proximal tibiofibular joint dislocation, with or without internal or external fixation, or with excision of proximal fibula

♦§ **27840** Closed treatment of ankle dislocation; without anesthesia

♦§ **27842** requiring anesthesia, with or without percutaneous skeletal fixation

♦§ **27846** Open treatment of ankle dislocation, with or without percutaneous skeletal fixation; without repair or internal fixation

♦§ **27848** with repair or internal or external fixation

(For surgical or diagnostic arthroscopic procedures, see 29894-29898)

Manipulation

§ **27860** Manipulation of ankle under general anesthesia (includes application of traction or other fixation apparatus)

Arthrodesis

♦§ **27870** Arthrodesis, ankle, open

➔ *CPT Changes: An Insider's View* 2003

(For arthroscopic ankle arthrodesis, use 29899)

♦§ **27871** Arthrodesis, tibiofibular joint, proximal or distal

Amputation

♦✿ **27880** Amputation, leg, through tibia and fibula;

♦✿ **27881** with immediate fitting technique including application of first cast

♦✿ **27882** open, circular (guillotine)

♦§ **27884** secondary closure or scar revision

♦✿ **27886** re-amputation

♦✿ **27888** Amputation, ankle, through malleoli of tibia and fibula (eg, Syme, Pirogoff type procedures), with plastic closure and resection of nerves

♦§ **27889** Ankle disarticulation

Other Procedures

♦§ **27892** Decompression fasciotomy, leg; anterior and/or lateral compartments only, with debridement of nonviable muscle and/or nerve

(For decompression fasciotomy of the leg without debridement, use 27600)

♦§ **27893** posterior compartment(s) only, with debridement of nonviable muscle and/or nerve

(For decompression fasciotomy of the leg without debridement, use 27601)

♦§ **27894** anterior and/or lateral, and posterior compartment(s), with debridement of nonviable muscle and/or nerve

(For decompression fasciotomy of the leg without debridement, use 27602)

♦§ **27899** Unlisted procedure, leg or ankle

Foot and Toes

Incision

(For incision and drainage procedures, superficial, see 10040-10160)

§ **28001** Incision and drainage, bursa, foot

§ **28002** Incision and drainage below fascia, with or without tendon sheath involvement, foot; single bursal space

§ **28003** multiple areas

§ **28005** Incision, bone cortex (eg, osteomyelitis or bone abscess), foot

♦§ **28008** Fasciotomy, foot and/or toe

(See also 28060, 28062, 28250)

§ **28010** Tenotomy, percutaneous, toe; single tendon

§ **28011** multiple tendons

(For open tenotomy, see 28230-28234)

§ **28020** Arthrotomy, including exploration, drainage, or removal of loose or foreign body; intertarsal or tarsometatarsal joint

§ **28022** metatarsophalangeal joint

§ **28024** interphalangeal joint

§ **28030** Neurectomy, intrinsic musculature of foot

§ **28035** Release, tarsal tunnel (posterior tibial nerve decompression)

(For other nerve entrapments, see 64704, 64722)

Excision

♦§ **28043** Excision, tumor, foot; subcutaneous tissue

♦§ **28045** deep, subfascial, intramuscular

♦§ **28046** Radical resection of tumor (eg, malignant neoplasm), soft tissue of foot

♦§ **28050** Arthrotomy with biopsy; intertarsal or tarsometatarsal joint

♦§ **28052** metatarsophalangeal joint

♦§ **28054** interphalangeal joint

♦§ **28060** Fasciectomy, plantar fascia; partial (separate procedure)

§ **28062** radical (separate procedure)

(For plantar fasciotomy, see 28008, 28250)

§ **28070** Synovectomy; intertarsal or tarsometatarsal joint, each

§ **28072** metatarsophalangeal joint, each

§ **28080** Excision, interdigital (Morton) neuroma, single, each

♦§ **28086** Synovectomy, tendon sheath, foot; flexor

♦§ **28088** extensor

♦§ **28090** Excision of lesion, tendon, tendon sheath, or capsule (including synovectomy) (eg, cyst or ganglion); foot

§ **28092** toe(s), each

♦§ **28100** Excision or curettage of bone cyst or benign tumor, talus or calcaneus;

♦§ **28102** with iliac or other autograft (includes obtaining graft)

♦§ **28103** with allograft

§ **28104** Excision or curettage of bone cyst or benign tumor, tarsal or metatarsal, except talus or calcaneus;

➲ *CPT Changes: An Insider's View* 2002

§ **28106** with iliac or other autograft (includes obtaining graft)

§ **28107** with allograft

§ **28108** Excision or curettage of bone cyst or benign tumor, phalanges of foot

(For ostectomy, partial (eg, hallux valgus, Silver type procedure), use 28290)

♦§ **28110** Ostectomy, partial excision, fifth metatarsal head (bunionette) (separate procedure)

♦§ **28111** Ostectomy, complete excision; first metatarsal head

♦§ **28112** other metatarsal head (second, third or fourth)

♦§ **28113** fifth metatarsal head

♦§ **28114** all metatarsal heads, with partial proximal phalangectomy, excluding first metatarsal (eg, Clayton type procedure)

♦§ **28116** Ostectomy, excision of tarsal coalition

♦§ **28118** Ostectomy, calcaneus;

♦§ **28119** for spur, with or without plantar fascial release

♦§ **28120** Partial excision (craterization, saucerization, sequestrectomy, or diaphysectomy) bone (eg, osteomyelitis or bossing); talus or calcaneus

♦§ **28122** tarsal or metatarsal bone, except talus or calcaneus

(For partial excision of talus or calcaneus, use 28120)

(For cheilectomy for hallux rigidus, use 28289)

♦§ **28124** phalanx of toe

§ **28126** Resection, partial or complete, phalangeal base, each toe

♦§ **28130** Talectomy (astragalectomy)

(For calcanectomy, use 28118)

§ **28140** Metatarsectomy

§ **28150** Phalangectomy, toe, each toe

§ **28153** Resection, condyle(s), distal end of phalanx, each toe

§ **28160** Hemiphalangectomy or interphalangeal joint excision, toe, proximal end of phalanx, each

§ **28171** Radical resection of tumor, bone; tarsal (except talus or calcaneus)

§ **28173** metatarsal

§ **28175** phalanx of toe

(For talus or calcaneus, use 27647)

Introduction or Removal

♦§ **28190** Removal of foreign body, foot; subcutaneous

♦§ **28192** deep

♦§ **28193** complicated

Repair, Revision, and/or Reconstruction

§ **28200** Repair, tendon, flexor, foot; primary or secondary, without free graft, each tendon

§ **28202** secondary with free graft, each tendon (includes obtaining graft)

§ **28208** Repair, tendon, extensor, foot; primary or secondary, each tendon

§ **28210** secondary with free graft, each tendon (includes obtaining graft)

§ **28220** Tenolysis, flexor, foot; single tendon

§ **28222** multiple tendons

§ **28225** Tenolysis, extensor, foot; single tendon

§ **28226** multiple tendons

§ **28230** Tenotomy, open, tendon flexor; foot, single or multiple tendon(s) (separate procedure)

§ **28232** toe, single tendon (separate procedure)

§ **28234** Tenotomy, open, extensor, foot or toe, each tendon

(For tendon transfer to midfoot or hindfoot, see 27690, 27691)

♦§ **28238** Reconstruction (advancement), posterior tibial tendon with excision of accessory tarsal navicular bone (eg, Kidner type procedure)

➲ *CPT Changes: An Insider's View* 2002

(For subcutaneous tenotomy, see 28010, 28011)

(For transfer or transplant of tendon with muscle redirection or rerouting, see 27690-27692)

(For extensor hallucis longus transfer with great toe IP fusion (Jones procedure), use 28760)

♦§ **28240** Tenotomy, lengthening, or release, abductor hallucis muscle

♦§ **28250** Division of plantar fascia and muscle (eg, Steindler stripping) (separate procedure)

♦§ **28260** Capsulotomy, midfoot; medial release only (separate procedure)

♦§ **28261** with tendon lengthening

♦§ **28262** extensive, including posterior talotibial capsulotomy and tendon(s) lengthening (eg, resistant clubfoot deformity)

♦§ **28264** Capsulotomy, midtarsal (eg, Heyman type procedure)

♦§ **28270** Capsulotomy; metatarsophalangeal joint, with or without tenorrhaphy, each joint (separate procedure)

♦§ **28272** interphalangeal joint, each joint (separate procedure)

♦§ **28280** Syndactylization, toes (eg, webbing or Kelikian type procedure)

§ **28285** Correction, hammertoe (eg, interphalangeal fusion, partial or total phalangectomy)

§ **28286** Correction, cock-up fifth toe, with plastic skin closure (eg, Ruiz-Mora type procedure)

§ **28288** Ostectomy, partial, exostectomy or condylectomy, metatarsal head, each metatarsal head

♦§ **28289** Hallux rigidus correction with cheilectomy, debridement and capsular release of the first metatarsophalangeal joint

♦§ **28290** Correction, hallux valgus (bunion), with or without sesamoidectomy; simple exostectomy (eg, Silver type procedure)

♦§ **28292** Keller, McBride, or Mayo type procedure

♦§ **28293** resection of joint with implant

♦§ **28294** with tendon transplants (eg, Joplin type procedure)

♦§ **28296** with metatarsal osteotomy (eg, Mitchell, Chevron, or concentric type procedures)

♦§ **28297** Lapidus type procedure

♦§ **28298** by phalanx osteotomy

♦§ **28299** by double osteotomy

➲ *CPT Changes: An Insider's View* 2002

♦§ **28300** Osteotomy; calcaneus (eg, Dwyer or Chambers type procedure), with or without internal fixation

♦§ **28302** talus

♦§ **28304** Osteotomy, tarsal bones, other than calcaneus or talus;

♦§ **28305** with autograft (includes obtaining graft) (eg, Fowler type)

♦§ **28306** Osteotomy, with or without lengthening, shortening or angular correction, metatarsal; first metatarsal

♦§ **28307** first metatarsal with autograft (other than first toe)

♦§ **28308** other than first metatarsal, each

♦§ **28309** multiple (eg, Swanson type cavus foot procedure)

§ **28310** Osteotomy, shortening, angular or rotational correction; proximal phalanx, first toe (separate procedure)

§ **28312** other phalanges, any toe

§ **28313** Reconstruction, angular deformity of toe, soft tissue procedures only (eg, overlapping second toe, fifth toe, curly toes)

♦§ **28315** Sesamoidectomy, first toe (separate procedure)

§ **28320** Repair, nonunion or malunion; tarsal bones

§ **28322** metatarsal, with or without bone graft (includes obtaining graft)

§ **28340** Reconstruction, toe, macrodactyly; soft tissue resection

§ **28341** requiring bone resection

§ **28344** Reconstruction, toe(s); polydactyly

§ **28345** syndactyly, with or without skin graft(s), each web

§ **28360** Reconstruction, cleft foot

Fracture and/or Dislocation

♦§ **28400** Closed treatment of calcaneal fracture; without manipulation

♦§ **28405** with manipulation

♦§ **28406** Percutaneous skeletal fixation of calcaneal fracture, with manipulation

♦§ **28415** Open treatment of calcaneal fracture, with or without internal or external fixation;

♦§ **28420** with primary iliac or other autogenous bone graft (includes obtaining graft)

♦§ **28430** Closed treatment of talus fracture; without manipulation

♦§ **28435** with manipulation

♦§ **28436** Percutaneous skeletal fixation of talus fracture, with manipulation

♦§ **28445** Open treatment of talus fracture, with or without internal or external fixation

§ **28450** Treatment of tarsal bone fracture (except talus and calcaneus); without manipulation, each

§ **28455** with manipulation, each

§ **28456** Percutaneous skeletal fixation of tarsal bone fracture (except talus and calcaneus), with manipulation, each

§ **28465** Open treatment of tarsal bone fracture (except talus and calcaneus), with or without internal or external fixation, each

§ **28470** Closed treatment of metatarsal fracture; without manipulation, each

§ **28475** with manipulation, each

§ **28476** Percutaneous skeletal fixation of metatarsal fracture, with manipulation, each

§ **28485** Open treatment of metatarsal fracture, with or without internal or external fixation, each

§ **28490** Closed treatment of fracture great toe, phalanx or phalanges; without manipulation

§ **28495** with manipulation

§ **28496** Percutaneous skeletal fixation of fracture great toe, phalanx or phalanges, with manipulation

§ **28505** Open treatment of fracture great toe, phalanx or phalanges, with or without internal or external fixation

§ **28510** Closed treatment of fracture, phalanx or phalanges, other than great toe; without manipulation, each

§ **28515** with manipulation, each

§ **28525** Open treatment of fracture, phalanx or phalanges, other than great toe, with or without internal or external fixation, each

§ **28530** Closed treatment of sesamoid fracture

§ **28531** Open treatment of sesamoid fracture, with or without internal fixation

§ **28540** Closed treatment of tarsal bone dislocation, other than talotarsal; without anesthesia

§ **28545** requiring anesthesia

§ **28546** Percutaneous skeletal fixation of tarsal bone dislocation, other than talotarsal, with manipulation

§ **28555** Open treatment of tarsal bone dislocation, with or without internal or external fixation

§ **28570** Closed treatment of talotarsal joint dislocation; without anesthesia

§ **28575** requiring anesthesia

§ **28576** Percutaneous skeletal fixation of talotarsal joint dislocation, with manipulation

§ **28585** Open treatment of talotarsal joint dislocation, with or without internal or external fixation

§ **28600** Closed treatment of tarsometatarsal joint dislocation; without anesthesia

§ **28605** requiring anesthesia

§ **28606** Percutaneous skeletal fixation of tarsometatarsal joint dislocation, with manipulation

§ **28615** Open treatment of tarsometatarsal joint dislocation, with or without internal or external fixation

§ **28630** Closed treatment of metatarsophalangeal joint dislocation; without anesthesia

§ **28635** requiring anesthesia

§ **28636** Percutaneous skeletal fixation of metatarsophalangeal joint dislocation, with manipulation

§ **28645** Open treatment of metatarsophalangeal joint dislocation, with or without internal or external fixation

§ **28660** Closed treatment of interphalangeal joint dislocation; without anesthesia

§ **28665** requiring anesthesia

§ **28666** Percutaneous skeletal fixation of interphalangeal joint dislocation, with manipulation

§ **28675** Open treatment of interphalangeal joint dislocation, with or without internal or external fixation

Arthrodesis

§ **28705** Arthrodesis; pantalar

§ **28715** triple

§ **28725** subtalar

§ **28730** Arthrodesis, midtarsal or tarsometatarsal, multiple or transverse;

§ **28735** with osteotomy (eg, flatfoot correction)

§ **28737** Arthrodesis, with tendon lengthening and advancement, midtarsal, tarsal navicular-cuneiform (eg, Miller type procedure)

➔ *CPT Changes: An Insider's View* 2002

§ **28740** Arthrodesis, midtarsal or tarsometatarsal, single joint

♦§ **28750** Arthrodesis, great toe; metatarsophalangeal joint

♦§ **28755** interphalangeal joint

♦§ **28760** Arthrodesis, with extensor hallucis longus transfer to first metatarsal neck, great toe, interphalangeal joint (eg, Jones type procedure)

(For hammertoe operation or interphalangeal fusion, use 28285)

Surgery: Musculoskeletal System

Amputation

♦✿ **28800** Amputation, foot; midtarsal (eg, Chopart type procedure)

♦✿ **28805** transmetatarsal

§ **28810** Amputation, metatarsal, with toe, single

§ **28820** Amputation, toe; metatarsophalangeal joint

§ **28825** interphalangeal joint

(For amputation of tuft of distal phalanx, use 11752)

Other Procedures

(For extracorporeal shock wave therapy involving musculoskeletal system, or plantar fascia, see Category III codes 0019T, 0020T)

§ **28899** Unlisted procedure, foot or toes

Application of Casts and Strapping

The listed procedures apply when the cast application or strapping is a replacement procedure used during or after the period of follow-up care, or when the cast application or strapping is an initial service performed without a restorative treatment or procedure(s) to stabilize or protect a fracture, injury, or dislocation and/or to afford comfort to a patient. Restorative treatment or procedure(s) rendered by another physician following the application of the initial cast/splint/strap may be reported with a treatment of fracture and/or dislocation code.

A physician who applies the initial cast, strap or splint and also assumes all of the subsequent fracture, dislocation, or injury care cannot use the application of casts and strapping codes as an initial service, since the first cast/splint or strap application is included in the treatment of fracture and/or dislocation codes. (See notes under Musculoskeletal System, page 67. A temporary cast/splint/strap is not considered to be part of the preoperative care, and the use of the modifier 56 is not applicable. Additional evaluation and management services are reportable only if signifi cant identifiable further services are provided at the time of the cast application or strapping.

If cast application or strapping is provided as an initial service (eg, casting of a sprained ankle or knee) in which no other procedure or treatment (eg, surgical repair, reduction of a fracture or joint dislocation) is performed or is expected to be performed by a physician rendering the initial care only, use the casting, strapping and/or supply code (99070) in addition to an evaluation and management code as appropriate.

Listed procedures include removal of cast or strapping.

(For orthotics fitting and training, use 97504)

Body and Upper Extremity

Casts

❖ **29000** Application of halo type body cast (see 20661-20663 for insertion)
➲ *CPT Assistant* Apr 02:13, Mar 03:14, Apr 03:24

❖ **29010** Application of Risser jacket, localizer, body; only
➲ *CPT Assistant* Apr 02:13, Mar 03:14, Apr 03:24

❖ **29015** including head
➲ *CPT Assistant* Apr 02:13, Mar 03:14, Apr 03:24

❖ **29020** Application of turnbuckle jacket, body; only
➲ *CPT Assistant* Apr 02:13, Mar 03:14, Apr 03:24

❖ **29025** including head
➲ *CPT Assistant* Apr 02:13, Mar 03:14, Apr 03:24

❖ **29035** Application of body cast, shoulder to hips;
➲ *CPT Assistant* Apr 02:13, Mar 03:14, Apr 03:24

❖ **29040** including head, Minerva type
➲ *CPT Assistant* Apr 02:13, Mar 03:14, Apr 03:24

❖ **29044** including one thigh
➲ *CPT Assistant* Apr 02:13, Mar 03:14, Apr 03:24

❖ **29046** including both thighs
➲ *CPT Assistant* Apr 02:13, Mar 03:14, Apr 03:24

❖ **29049** Application, cast; figure-of-eight
➲ *CPT Assistant* Apr 02:13, Mar 03:14, Apr 03:24; *CPT Changes: An Insider's View* 2002

❖ **29055** shoulder spica
➲ *CPT Assistant* Apr 02:13, Mar 03:14, Apr 03:24

❖ **29058** plaster Velpeau
➲ *CPT Assistant* Apr 02:13, Mar 03:14, Apr 03:24

♦❖ **29065** shoulder to hand (long arm)
➲ *CPT Assistant* Apr 02:13, Mar 03:14, Apr 03:24

♦❖ **29075** elbow to finger (short arm)
➲ *CPT Assistant* Apr 02:13, Mar 03:14, Apr 03:24

♦❖ **29085** hand and lower forearm (gauntlet)
➲ *CPT Assistant* Apr 02:13, Mar 03:14, Apr 03:24

♦❖ **29086** finger (eg, contracture)
➲ *CPT Assistant* Apr 02:13, Mar 03:14, Apr 03:24; *CPT Changes: An Insider's View* 2002

Splints

♦❖ **29105** Application of long arm splint (shoulder to hand)
➲ *CPT Assistant* Apr 02:13, Mar 03:14, Apr 03:24

♦❖ **29125** Application of short arm splint (forearm to hand); static
➲ *CPT Assistant* Apr 02:13, Mar 03:14, Apr 03:24

♦❖ **29126** dynamic
➲ *CPT Assistant* Apr 02:13, Mar 03:14, Apr 03:24

♦❖ **29130** Application of finger splint; static
➔ *CPT Assistant* Apr 02:13, Mar 03:14, Apr 03:24

♦❖ **29131** dynamic
➔ *CPT Assistant* Apr 02:13, Mar 03:14, Apr 03:24

Strapping—Any Age

❖ **29200** Strapping; thorax
➔ *CPT Assistant* Apr 02:13, Mar 03:14, Apr 03:24

❖ **29220** low back
➔ *CPT Assistant* Apr 02:13, Mar 03:14, Apr 03:24

❖ **29240** shoulder (eg, Velpeau)
➔ *CPT Assistant* Apr 02:13, Mar 03:14, Apr 03:24

♦❖ **29260** elbow or wrist
➔ *CPT Assistant* Apr 02:13, Mar 03:14, Apr 03:24

♦❖ **29280** hand or finger
➔ *CPT Assistant* Apr 02:13, Mar 03:14, Apr 03:24

Lower Extremity

Casts

❖ **29305** Application of hip spica cast; one leg
➔ *CPT Assistant* Apr 02:13, Mar 03:14, Apr 03:24

❖ **29325** one and one-half spica or both legs
➔ *CPT Assistant* Apr 02:13, Mar 03:14, Apr 03:24

(For hip spica (body) cast, including thighs only, use 29046)

♦❖ **29345** Application of long leg cast (thigh to toes);
➔ *CPT Assistant* Apr 02:13, Mar 03:14, Apr 03:24

♦❖ **29355** walker or ambulatory type
➔ *CPT Assistant* Apr 02:13, Mar 03:14, Apr 03:24

♦❖ **29358** Application of long leg cast brace
➔ *CPT Assistant* Apr 02:13, Mar 03:14, Apr 03:24

♦❖ **29365** Application of cylinder cast (thigh to ankle)
➔ *CPT Assistant* Apr 02:13, Mar 03:14, Apr 03:24

♦❖ **29405** Application of short leg cast (below knee to toes);
➔ *CPT Assistant* Apr 02:13, Mar 03:14, 18, Apr 03:24

♦❖ **29425** walking or ambulatory type
➔ *CPT Assistant* Apr 02:13, Mar 03:14, Apr 03:24

♦❖ **29435** Application of patellar tendon bearing (PTB) cast
➔ *CPT Assistant* Apr 02:13, Mar 03:14, Apr 03:24

♦❖ **29440** Adding walker to previously applied cast
➔ *CPT Assistant* Apr 02:13, Mar 03:14, Apr 03:24

♦❖ **29445** Application of rigid total contact leg cast
➔ *CPT Assistant* Apr 02:13, Mar 03:14, Apr 03:24

♦❖ **29450** Application of clubfoot cast with molding or manipulation, long or short leg
➔ *CPT Assistant* Apr 02:13, Mar 03:14, Apr 03:24

(To report bilateral procedure, use 29450 with modifier 50)

Splints

♦❖ **29505** Application of long leg splint (thigh to ankle or toes)
➔ *CPT Assistant* Apr 02:13, Mar 03:14, Apr 03:24

♦❖ **29515** Application of short leg splint (calf to foot)
➔ *CPT Assistant* Apr 02:13, Mar 03:14, 18, 19, Apr 03:24

Strapping—Any Age

❖ **29520** Strapping; hip
➔ *CPT Assistant* Apr 02:13, Mar 03:14, Apr 03:24

❖ **29530** knee
➔ *CPT Assistant* Apr 02:13, Mar 03:14, Apr 03:24

❖ **29540** ankle and/or foot
➔ *CPT Assistant* Apr 02:13, Mar 03:14, 19, Apr 03:24

❖ **29550** toes
➔ *CPT Assistant* Apr 02:13, Mar 03:14, Apr 03:24

♦❖ **29580** Unna boot
➔ *CPT Assistant* Apr 02:13, Mar 03:14, Apr 03:24

❖ **29590** Denis-Browne splint strapping
➔ *CPT Assistant* Apr 02:13, Mar 03:14, Apr 03:24

Removal or Repair

Codes for cast removals should be employed only for casts applied by another physician.

❖ **29700** Removal or bivalving; gauntlet, boot or body cast
➔ *CPT Assistant* Apr 02:13, Mar 03:14, Apr 03:24

♦❖ **29705** full arm or full leg cast
➔ *CPT Assistant* Apr 02:13, Mar 03:14, Apr 03:24

♦❖ **29710** shoulder or hip spica, Minerva, or Risser jacket, etc.
➔ *CPT Assistant* Apr 02:13, Mar 03:14, Apr 03:24

❖ **29715** turnbuckle jacket
➔ *CPT Assistant* Apr 02:13, Mar 03:14, Apr 03:24

❖ **29720** Repair of spica, body cast or jacket
➔ *CPT Assistant* Apr 02:13, Mar 03:14, Apr 03:24

❖ **29730** Windowing of cast
➔ *CPT Assistant* Apr 02:13, Mar 03:14, Apr 03:24

❖ **29740** Wedging of cast (except clubfoot casts)
➔ *CPT Assistant* Apr 02:13, Mar 03:14, Apr 03:24

♦❖ **29750** Wedging of clubfoot cast
➔ *CPT Assistant* Apr 02:13, Mar 03:14, Apr 03:24

(To report bilateral procedure, use 29750 with modifier 50)

Other Procedures

❖ **29799** Unlisted procedure, casting or strapping
➲ *CPT Assistant* Apr 02:13, Mar 03:14, Apr 03:24

Endoscopy/Arthroscopy

Surgical endoscopy/arthroscopy always includes a diagnostic endoscopy/arthroscopy.

When arthroscopy is performed in conjunction with arthrotomy, add modifier 51.

♦§ **29800** Arthroscopy, temporomandibular joint, diagnostic, with or without synovial biopsy (separate procedure)

♦§ **29804** Arthroscopy, temporomandibular joint, surgical

(For open procedure, use 21010)

♦§ **29805** Arthroscopy, shoulder, diagnostic, with or without synovial biopsy (separate procedure)
➲ *CPT Changes: An Insider's View* 2002

(For open procedure, see 23065-23066, 23100-23101)

♦§ **29806** Arthroscopy, shoulder, surgical; capsulorrhaphy
➲ *CPT Changes: An Insider's View* 2002

(For open procedure, see 23450-23466)

(To report thermal capsulorrhaphy, use 29999)

♦§ **29807** repair of SLAP lesion
➲ *CPT Changes: An Insider's View* 2002

♦§ **29819** with removal of loose body or foreign body

(For open procedure, see 23040-23044, 23107)

♦§ **29820** synovectomy, partial

(For open procedure, see 23105)

♦§ **29821** synovectomy, complete

(For open procedure, see 23105)

♦§ **29822** debridement, limited

(For open procedure, see specific open shoulder procedure performed)

♦§ **29823** debridement, extensive

(For open procedure, see specific open shoulder procedure performed)

♦§ **29824** distal claviculectomy including distal articular surface (Mumford procedure)

(For open procedure, use 23120)

♦§ **29825** with lysis and resection of adhesions, with or without manipulation

(For open procedure, see specific open shoulder procedure performed)

♦§ **29826** decompression of subacromial space with partial acromioplasty, with or without coracoacromial release

(For open procedure, use 23130 or 23415)

♦§ **29827** with rotator cuff repair
➲ *CPT Changes: An Insider's View* 2003

(For open or mini-open rotator cuff repair, use 23412)

(When arthroscopic subacromial decompression is performed at the same setting, use 29826 and append modifier 51)

(When arthroscopic distal clavicle resection is performed at the same setting, use 29824 and append modifier 51)

♦§ **29830** Arthroscopy, elbow, diagnostic, with or without synovial biopsy (separate procedure)

♦§ **29834** Arthroscopy, elbow, surgical; with removal of loose body or foreign body

♦§ **29835** synovectomy, partial

♦§ **29836** synovectomy, complete

♦§ **29837** debridement, limited

♦§ **29838** debridement, extensive

♦§ **29840** Arthroscopy, wrist, diagnostic, with or without synovial biopsy (separate procedure)

♦§ **29843** Arthroscopy, wrist, surgical; for infection, lavage and drainage

♦§ **29844** synovectomy, partial

♦§ **29845** synovectomy, complete

♦§ **29846** excision and/or repair of triangular fibrocartilage and/or joint debridement

♦§ **29847** internal fixation for fracture or instability

♦§ **29848** Endoscopy, wrist, surgical, with release of transverse carpal ligament

(For open procedure, use 64721)

♦§ **29850** Arthroscopically aided treatment of intercondylar spine(s) and/or tuberosity fracture(s) of the knee, with or without manipulation; without internal or external fixation (includes arthroscopy)

♦§ **29851** with internal or external fixation (includes arthroscopy)

(For bone graft, use 20900, 20902)

♦§ **29855** Arthroscopically aided treatment of tibial fracture, proximal (plateau); unicondylar, with or without internal or external fixation (includes arthroscopy)

♦§ **29856** bicondylar, with or without internal or external fixation (includes arthroscopy)

(For bone graft, use 20900, 20902)

♦§ **29860** Arthroscopy, hip, diagnostic with or without synovial biopsy (separate procedure)

♦§ **29861** Arthroscopy, hip, surgical; with removal of loose body or foreign body

♦§ **29862** with debridement/shaving of articular cartilage (chondroplasty), abrasion arthroplasty, and/or resection of labrum

♦§ **29863** with synovectomy

♦§● **29866** Arthroscopy, knee, surgical; osteochondral autograft(s) (eg, mosaicplasty) (includes harvesting of the autograft)

➲ *CPT Changes: An Insider's View* 2005

►(Do not report 29866 in conjunction with 29870, 29871, 29874, 29875, 29877, 29884 when performed at the same session and/or 29879, 29885-29887 when performed in the same compartment)◄

♦§● **29867** osteochondral allograft (eg, mosaicplasty)

➲ *CPT Changes: An Insider's View* 2005

►(Do not report 29867 in conjunction with 27570, 29870, 29871, 29874, 29875, 29877, 29884 when performed at the same session and/or 29879, 29885-29887 when performed in the same compartment)◄

►(Do not report 29867 in conjunction with 27415)◄

♦§● **29868** meniscal transplantation (includes arthrotomy for meniscal insertion), medial or lateral

➲ *CPT Changes: An Insider's View* 2005

►(Do not report 29868 in conjunction with 29870, 29871, 29874, 29875, 29880, 29883, 29884 when performed at the same session or 29881, 29882 when performed in the same compartment)◄

♦§ **29870** Arthroscopy, knee, diagnostic, with or without synovial biopsy (separate procedure)

►(For open autologous chondrocyte implantation of the knee, use 27412)◄

♦§ **29871** Arthroscopy, knee, surgical; for infection, lavage and drainage

►(For implantation of osteochondral graft for treatment of articular surface defect, see 27412, 27415, 29866, 29867)◄

♦§ **29873** with lateral release

➲ *CPT Changes: An Insider's View* 2003

(For open lateral release, use 27425)

♦§ **29874** for removal of loose body or foreign body (eg, osteochondritis dissecans fragmentation, chondral fragmentation)

➲ *CPT Assistant* Apr 03:12

♦§ **29875** synovectomy, limited (eg, plica or shelf resection) (separate procedure)

♦§ **29876** synovectomy, major, two or more compartments (eg, medial or lateral)

♦§ **29877** debridement/shaving of articular cartilage (chondroplasty)

➲ *CPT Assistant* Apr 03:12

♦§ **29879** abrasion arthroplasty (includes chondroplasty where necessary) or multiple drilling or microfracture

➲ *CPT Changes: An Insider's View* 2000

♦§ **29880** with meniscectomy (medial AND lateral, including any meniscal shaving)

♦§ **29881** with meniscectomy (medial OR lateral, including any meniscal shaving)

♦§ **29882** with meniscus repair (medial OR lateral)

♦§ **29883** with meniscus repair (medial AND lateral)

►(For meniscal transplantation, medial or lateral, knee, use 29868)◄

♦§ **29884** with lysis of adhesions, with or without manipulation (separate procedure)

♦§ **29885** drilling for osteochondritis dissecans with bone grafting, with or without internal fixation (including debridement of base of lesion)

♦§ **29886** drilling for intact osteochondritis dissecans lesion

♦§ **29887** drilling for intact osteochondritis dissecans lesion with internal fixation

♦§ **29888** Arthroscopically aided anterior cruciate ligament repair/augmentation or reconstruction

♦§ **29889** Arthroscopically aided posterior cruciate ligament repair/augmentation or reconstruction

(Procedures 29888 and 29889 should not be used with reconstruction procedures 27427-27429)

♦§ **29891** Arthroscopy, ankle, surgical, excision of osteochondral defect of talus and/or tibia, including drilling of the defect

♦§ **29892** Arthroscopically aided repair of large osteochondritis dissecans lesion, talar dome fracture, or tibial plafond fracture, with or without internal fixation (includes arthroscopy)

♦§ **29893** Endoscopic plantar fasciotomy

♦§ **29894** Arthroscopy, ankle (tibiotalar and fibulotalar joints), surgical; with removal of loose body or foreign body

♦§ **29895** synovectomy, partial

♦§ **29897** debridement, limited

♦§ **29898** debridement, extensive

♦§ **29899** with ankle arthrodesis

➲ *CPT Changes: An Insider's View* 2003

(For open ankle arthrodesis, use 27870)

♦§ **29900** Arthroscopy, metacarpophalangeal joint, diagnostic, includes synovial biopsy

➲ *CPT Changes: An Insider's View* 2002

(Do not report 29900 with 29901, 29902)

♦§ **29901** Arthroscopy, metacarpophalangeal joint, surgical; with debridement

➲ *CPT Changes: An Insider's View* 2002

♦§ **29902** with reduction of displaced ulnar collateral ligament (eg, Stenar lesion)

➲ *CPT Changes: An Insider's View* 2002

♦§ **29999** Unlisted procedure, arthroscopy

➲ *CPT Changes: An Insider's View* 2002

Respiratory System

Nose

Incision

§ **30000** Drainage abscess or hematoma, nasal, internal approach

(For external approach, see 10060, 10140)

§ **30020** Drainage abscess or hematoma, nasal septum

(For lateral rhinotomy, see specific application (eg, 30118, 30320))

Excision

§ **30100** Biopsy, intranasal

(For biopsy skin of nose, see 11100, 11101)

♦§ **30110** Excision, nasal polyp(s), simple

(30110 would normally be completed in an office setting)

(To report bilateral procedure, use 30110 with modifier 50)

♦§ **30115** Excision, nasal polyp(s), extensive

(30115 would normally require the facilities available in a hospital setting)

(To report bilateral procedure, use 30115 with modifier 50)

§ **30117** Excision or destruction (eg, laser), intranasal lesion; internal approach

➔ *CPT Changes: An Insider's View* 2002

§ **30118** external approach (lateral rhinotomy)

➔ *CPT Changes: An Insider's View* 2002

§ **30120** Excision or surgical planing of skin of nose for rhinophyma

§ **30124** Excision dermoid cyst, nose; simple, skin, subcutaneous

§ **30125** complex, under bone or cartilage

♦§ **30130** Excision turbinate, partial or complete, any method

♦§ **30140** Submucous resection turbinate, partial or complete, any method

(For submucous resection of nasal septum, use 30520)

(For reduction of turbinates, use 30140 with modifier 52)

§ **30150** Rhinectomy; partial

§ **30160** total

(For closure and/or reconstruction, primary or delayed, see **Integumentary System,** 13150-13160, 14060-14300, 15120, 15121, 15260, 15261, 15760, 20900-20912)

Introduction

§ **30200** Injection into turbinate(s), therapeutic

§ **30210** Displacement therapy (Proetz type)

§ **30220** Insertion, nasal septal prosthesis (button)

Removal of Foreign Body

♣ **30300** Removal foreign body, intranasal; office type procedure

§ **30310** requiring general anesthesia

§ **30320** by lateral rhinotomy

Repair

(For obtaining tissues for graft, see 20900-20926, 21210)

§ **30400** Rhinoplasty, primary; lateral and alar cartilages and/or elevation of nasal tip

(For columellar reconstruction, see 13150 et seq)

§ **30410** complete, external parts including bony pyramid, lateral and alar cartilages, and/or elevation of nasal tip

§ **30420** including major septal repair

§ **30430** Rhinoplasty, secondary; minor revision (small amount of nasal tip work)

§ **30435** intermediate revision (bony work with osteotomies)

§ **30450** major revision (nasal tip work and osteotomies)

§ **30460** Rhinoplasty for nasal deformity secondary to congenital cleft lip and/or palate, including columellar lengthening; tip only

§ **30462** tip, septum, osteotomies

§ **30465** Repair of nasal vestibular stenosis (eg, spreader grafting, lateral nasal wall reconstruction)

➔ *CPT Changes: An Insider's View* 2001

(30465 excludes obtaining graft. For graft procedure, see 20900-20926, 21210)

(30465 is used to report a bilateral procedure. For unilateral procedure, use modifier 52)

§ **30520** Septoplasty or submucous resection, with or without cartilage scoring, contouring or replacement with graft

(For submucous resection of turbinates, use 30140)

§ **30540** Repair choanal atresia; intranasal

§ **30545** transpalatine

(Do not report modifier 63 in conjunction with 30540, 30545)

§ **30560** Lysis intranasal synechia

§ **30580** Repair fistula; oromaxillary (combine with 31030 if antrotomy is included)

§ **30600** oronasal

§ **30620** Septal or other intranasal dermatoplasty (does not include obtaining graft)

§ **30630** Repair nasal septal perforations

Destruction

✶§ **30801** Cautery and/or ablation, mucosa of turbinates, unilateral or bilateral, any method, (separate procedure); superficial
➲ *CPT Changes: An Insider's View* 2002

✶§ **30802** intramural

Other Procedures

♦§ **30901** Control nasal hemorrhage, anterior, simple (limited cautery and/or packing) any method

(To report bilateral procedure, use 30901 with modifier 50)

♦§ **30903** Control nasal hemorrhage, anterior, complex (extensive cautery and/or packing) any method

(To report bilateral procedure, use 30903 with modifier 50)

✶§ **30905** Control nasal hemorrhage, posterior, with posterior nasal packs and/or cautery, any method; initial
➲ *CPT Changes: An Insider's View* 2002

✶§ **30906** subsequent

§ **30915** Ligation arteries; ethmoidal

§ **30920** internal maxillary artery, transantral

(For ligation external carotid artery, use 37600)

♦§ **30930** Fracture nasal turbinate(s), therapeutic

§ **30999** Unlisted procedure, nose

Accessory Sinuses

Incision

♦§ **31000** Lavage by cannulation; maxillary sinus (antrum puncture or natural ostium)

(To report bilateral procedure, use 31000 with modifier 50)

♦§ **31002** sphenoid sinus

♦§ **31020** Sinusotomy, maxillary (antrotomy); intranasal

(To report bilateral procedure, use 31020 with modifier 50)

♦§ **31030** radical (Caldwell-Luc) without removal of antrochoanal polyps

(To report bilateral procedure, use 31030 with modifier 50)

♦§ **31032** radical (Caldwell-Luc) with removal of antrochoanal polyps

(To report bilateral procedure, use 31032 with modifier 50)

§ **31040** Pterygomaxillary fossa surgery, any approach

(For transantral ligation of internal maxillary artery, use 30920)

♦§ **31050** Sinusotomy, sphenoid, with or without biopsy;

♦§ **31051** with mucosal stripping or removal of polyp(s)

♦§ **31070** Sinusotomy frontal; external, simple (trephine operation)

(For frontal intranasal sinusotomy, use 31276)

♦§ **31075** transorbital, unilateral (for mucocele or osteoma, Lynch type)

♦§ **31080** obliterative without osteoplastic flap, brow incision (includes ablation)

♦§ **31081** obliterative, without osteoplastic flap, coronal incision (includes ablation)

♦§ **31084** obliterative, with osteoplastic flap, brow incision

♦§ **31085** obliterative, with osteoplastic flap, coronal incision

♦§ **31086** nonobliterative, with osteoplastic flap, brow incision

♦§ **31087** nonobliterative, with osteoplastic flap, coronal incision

♦§ **31090** Sinusotomy, unilateral, three or more paranasal sinuses (frontal, maxillary, ethmoid, sphenoid)

Excision

♦§ **31200** Ethmoidectomy; intranasal, anterior

♦§ **31201** intranasal, total

♦§ **31205** extranasal, total

♦✿ **31225** Maxillectomy; without orbital exenteration

♦✿ **31230** with orbital exenteration (en bloc)

(For orbital exenteration only, see 65110 et seq)

(For skin grafts, see 15120 et seq)

Endoscopy

A surgical sinus endoscopy includes a sinusotomy (when appropriate) and diagnostic endoscopy.

Codes 31231-31294 are used to report unilateral procedures unless otherwise specified.

The codes 31231-31235 for diagnostic evaluation refer to employing a nasal/sinus endoscope to inspect the interior of the nasal cavity and the middle and superior meatus, the turbinates, and the spheno-ethmoid recess. Any time a diagnostic evaluation is performed all these areas would be inspected and a separate code is not reported for each area.

✶§ **31231** Nasal endoscopy, diagnostic, unilateral or bilateral (separate procedure)

♦§ **31233** Nasal/sinus endoscopy, diagnostic with maxillary sinusoscopy (via inferior meatus or canine fossa puncture)

♦§ **31235** Nasal/sinus endoscopy, diagnostic with sphenoid sinusoscopy (via puncture of sphenoidal face or cannulation of ostium)

♦§ **31237** Nasal/sinus endoscopy, surgical; with biopsy, polypectomy or debridement (separate procedure)

♦§ **31238** with control of nasal hemorrhage

♦§ **31239** with dacryocystorhinostomy

♦§ **31240** with concha bullosa resection

(For endoscopic osteomeatal complex (OMC) resection with antrostomy and/or anterior ethmoidectomy, with or without removal of polyp(s), use 31254 and 31256)

(For endoscopic osteomeatal complex (OMC) resection with antrostomy, removal of antral mucosal disease, and/or anterior ethmoidectomy, with or without removal of polyp(s), use 31254 and 31267)

(For endoscopic frontal sinus exploration, osteomeatal complex (OMC) resection and/or anterior ethmoidectomy, with or without removal of polyp(s), use 31254 and 31276)

(For endoscopic frontal sinus exploration, osteomeatal complex (OMC) resection, antrostomy, and/or anterior ethmoidectomy, with or without removal of polyp(s), use 31254, 31256, and 31276)

(For endoscopic nasal diagnostic endoscopy, see 31231-31235)

(For endoscopic osteomeatal complex (OMC) resection, frontal sinus exploration, antrostomy, removal of antral mucosal disease, and/or anterior ethmoidectomy, with or without removal of polyp(s), use 31254, 31267, and 31276)

♦§ **31254** Nasal/sinus endoscopy, surgical; with ethmoidectomy, partial (anterior)

♦§ **31255** with ethmoidectomy, total (anterior and posterior)

♦§ **31256** Nasal/sinus endoscopy, surgical, with maxillary antrostomy;

(For endoscopic anterior and posterior ethmoidectomy (APE) and antrostomy, with or without removal of polyp(s), use 31255 and 31256)

(For endoscopic anterior and posterior ethmoidectomy (APE), antrostomy and removal of antral mucosal disease, with or without removal of polyp(s), use 31255 and 31267)

(For endoscopic anterior and posterior ethmoidectomy (APE), and frontal sinus exploration, with or without removal of polyp(s), use 31255 and 31276)

♦§ **31267** with removal of tissue from maxillary sinus

(For endoscopic anterior and posterior ethmoidectomy (APE), and frontal sinus exploration and antrostomy, with or without removal of polyp(s), use 31255, 31256, and 31276)

(For endoscopic anterior and posterior ethmoidectomy (APE), frontal sinus exploration, antrostomy, and removal of antral mucosal disease, with or without removal of polyp(s), use 31255, 31267, and 31276)

♦§ **31276** Nasal/sinus endoscopy, surgical with frontal sinus exploration, with or without removal of tissue from frontal sinus

(For endoscopic anterior and posterior ethmoidectomy and sphenoidotomy (APS), with or without removal of polyp(s), use 31255, 31287 or 31288)

(For endoscopic anterior and posterior ethmoidectomy and sphenoidotomy (APS), and antrostomy, with or without removal of polyp(s), use 31255, 31256, and 31287 or 31288)

(For endoscopic anterior and posterior ethmoidectomy and sphenoidotomy (APS), antrostomy and removal of antral mucosal disease, with or without removal of polyp(s), use 31255, 31267, and 31287 or 31288)

(For endoscopic anterior and posterior ethmoidectomy and sphenoidotomy (APS), and frontal sinus exploration with or without removal of polyp(s), use 31255, 31287 or 31288, and 31276)

(For endoscopic anterior and posterior ethmoidectomy and sphenoidotomy (APS), with or without removal of polyp(s), with frontal sinus exploration and antrostomy, use 31255, 31256, 31287 or 31288, and 31276)

(For unilateral endoscopy of two or more sinuses, see 31231-31235)

(For endoscopic anterior and posterior ethmoidectomy and sphenoidotomy (APS), frontal sinus exploration, antrostomy and removal of antral mucosal disease, with or without removal of polyp(s), see 31255, 31267, 31287 or 31288 and 31276)

♦§ **31287** Nasal/sinus endoscopy, surgical, with sphenoidotomy;

♦§ **31288** with removal of tissue from the sphenoid sinus

♦✿ **31290** Nasal/sinus endoscopy, surgical, with repair of cerebrospinal fluid leak; ethmoid region

♦✿ **31291** sphenoid region

♦§ **31292** Nasal/sinus endoscopy, surgical; with medial or inferior orbital wall decompression

♦✿ **31293** with medial orbital wall and inferior orbital wall decompression

♦✿ **31294** with optic nerve decompression

Other Procedures

(For hypophysectomy, transantral or transeptal approach, use 61548)

(For transcranial hypophysectomy, use 61546)

§ **31299** Unlisted procedure, accessory sinuses

Surgery: Respiratory System

Larynx

Excision

§ **31300** Laryngotomy (thyrotomy, laryngofissure); with removal of tumor or laryngocele, cordectomy

§ **31320** diagnostic

✿ **31360** Laryngectomy; total, without radical neck dissection

✿ **31365** total, with radical neck dissection

✿ **31367** subtotal supraglottic, without radical neck dissection

✿ **31368** subtotal supraglottic, with radical neck dissection

✿ **31370** Partial laryngectomy (hemilaryngectomy); horizontal

✿ **31375** laterovertical

✿ **31380** anterovertical

✿ **31382** antero-latero-vertical

✿ **31390** Pharyngolaryngectomy, with radical neck dissection; without reconstruction

✿ **31395** with reconstruction

§ **31400** Arytenoidectomy or arytenoidopexy, external approach

(For endoscopic arytenoidectomy, use 31560)

§ **31420** Epiglottidectomy

Introduction

❖⊘ **31500** Intubation, endotracheal, emergency procedure

(For injection procedure for bronchography, see 31656, 31708, 31710)

§ **31502** Tracheotomy tube change prior to establishment of fistula tract

Endoscopy

For endoscopic procedures, code appropriate endoscopy of each anatomic site examined.

§ **31505** Laryngoscopy, indirect; diagnostic (separate procedure)

§ **31510** with biopsy

§ **31511** with removal of foreign body

§ **31512** with removal of lesion

§ **31513** with vocal cord injection

§ **31515** Laryngoscopy direct, with or without tracheoscopy; for aspiration

§ **31520** diagnostic, newborn

(Do not report modifier 63 in conjunction with 31520)

§ **31525** diagnostic, except newborn

§ **31526** diagnostic, with operating microscope

(Do not report code 69990 in addition to code 31526)

§ **31527** with insertion of obturator

§ **31528** with dilation, initial

➲ *CPT Changes: An Insider's View* 2002

§ **31529** with dilation, subsequent

➲ *CPT Changes: An Insider's View* 2002

§ **31530** Laryngoscopy, direct, operative, with foreign body removal;

§ **31531** with operating microscope

(Do not report code 69990 in addition to code 31531)

§ **31535** Laryngoscopy, direct, operative, with biopsy;

§ **31536** with operating microscope

(Do not report code 69990 in addition to code 31536)

§ **31540** Laryngoscopy, direct, operative, with excision of tumor and/or stripping of vocal cords or epiglottis;

§ **31541** with operating microscope

(Do not report code 69990 in addition to code 31541)

§● **31545** Laryngoscopy, direct, operative, with operating microscope or telescope, with submucosal removal of non-neoplastic lesion(s) of vocal cord; reconstruction with local tissue flap(s)

➲ *CPT Changes: An Insider's View* 2005

§● **31546** reconstruction with graft(s) (includes obtaining autograft)

➲ *CPT Changes: An Insider's View* 2005

►(Do not report 31546 in addition to 20926 for graft harvest)◄

►(For reconstruction of vocal cord with allograft, use 31599)◄

►(Do not report 31545 or 31546 in conjunction with 31540, 31541, 69990)◄

§ **31560** Laryngoscopy, direct, operative, with arytenoidectomy;

§ **31561** with operating microscope

(Do not report code 69990 in addition to code 31561)

§ **31570** Laryngoscopy, direct, with injection into vocal cord(s), therapeutic;

§ **31571** with operating microscope

(Do not report code 69990 in addition to code 31571)

§ **31575** Laryngoscopy, flexible fiberoptic; diagnostic

§ **31576** with biopsy

§ **31577** with removal of foreign body

§ **31578** with removal of lesion

(To report flexible fiberoptic endoscopic evaluation of swallowing, see 92612-92613)

(To report flexible fiberoptic endoscopic evaluation with sensory testing, see 92614-92615)

(To report flexible fiberoptic endoscopic evaluation of swallowing with sensory testing, see 92616-92617)

(For flexible fiberoptic laryngoscopy as part of flexible fiberoptic endoscopic evaluation of swallowing and/or laryngeal sensory testing by cine or video recording, see 92612-92617)

§ **31579** Laryngoscopy, flexible or rigid fiberoptic, with stroboscopy

Repair

§ **31580** Laryngoplasty; for laryngeal web, two stage, with keel insertion and removal

§ **31582** for laryngeal stenosis, with graft or core mold, including tracheotomy

➲ *CPT Assistant* Jan 03:16

✿ **31584** with open reduction of fracture

§ **31585** Treatment of closed laryngeal fracture; without manipulation

§ **31586** with closed manipulative reduction

✿ **31587** Laryngoplasty, cricoid split

§ **31588** Laryngoplasty, not otherwise specified (eg, for burns, reconstruction after partial laryngectomy)

§ **31590** Laryngeal reinnervation by neuromuscular pedicle

Destruction

§ **31595** Section recurrent laryngeal nerve, therapeutic (separate procedure), unilateral

Other Procedures

§ **31599** Unlisted procedure, larynx

Trachea and Bronchi

Incision

§ **31600** Tracheostomy, planned (separate procedure);

§ **31601** under two years

§ **31603** Tracheostomy, emergency procedure; transtracheal

§ **31605** cricothyroid membrane

§ **31610** Tracheostomy, fenestration procedure with skin flaps

(For endotracheal intubation, use 31500)

(For tracheal aspiration under direct vision, use 31515)

§ **31611** Construction of tracheoesophageal fistula and subsequent insertion of an alaryngeal speech prosthesis (eg, voice button, Blom-Singer prosthesis)

§ **31612** Tracheal puncture, percutaneous with transtracheal aspiration and/or injection

§ **31613** Tracheostoma revision; simple, without flap rotation

§ **31614** complex, with flap rotation

Endoscopy

For endoscopy procedures, code appropriate endoscopy of each anatomic site examined. Surgical bronchoscopy always includes diagnostic bronchoscopy when performed by the same physician. Codes 31622-31646 include fluoroscopic guidance, when performed.

(For tracheoscopy, see laryngoscopy codes 31515-31578)

§⊙ **31615** Tracheobronchoscopy through established tracheostomy incision

❖⊙+● **31620** Endobronchial ultrasound (EBUS) during bronchoscopic diagnostic or therapeutic intervention(s) (List separately in addition to code for primary procedure(s))

►(Use 31620 in conjunction with 31622-31638)◄

§⊙ **31622** Bronchoscopy, rigid or flexible, with or without fluoroscopic guidance; diagnostic, with or without cell washing (separate procedure)

➲ *CPT Changes: An Insider's View* 2004

§⊙ **31623** with brushing or protected brushings

§⊙ **31624** with bronchial alveolar lavage

§⊙ **31625** with bronchial or endobronchial biopsy(s), single or multiple sites

➲ *CPT Changes: An Insider's View* 2004

§⊙ **31628** with transbronchial lung biopsy(s), single lobe

➲ *CPT Changes: An Insider's View* 2004

(31628 should be reported only once regardless of how many transbronchial lung biopsies are performed in a lobe)

(To report transbronchial lung biopsies performed on additional lobe, use 31632)

§⊙ **31629** with transbronchial needle aspiration biopsy(s), trachea, main stem and/or lobar bronchus(i)

➲ *CPT Changes: An Insider's View* 2004

(31629 should be reported only once for upper airway biopsies regardless of how many transbronchial needle aspiration biopsies are performed in the upper airway or in a lobe)

(To report transbronchial needle aspiration biopsies performed on additional lobe(s), use 31633)

§▲ **31630** with tracheal/bronchial dilation or closed reduction of fracture

➲ *CPT Changes: An Insider's View* 2005

§▲ **31631** with placement of tracheal stent(s) (includes tracheal/bronchial dilation as required)

➲ *CPT Changes: An Insider's View* 2005

►(For placement of bronchial stent, see 31636, 31637)◄

►(For revision of tracheal/bronchial stent, use 31638)◄

Surgery: Respiratory System

§+ **31632** with transbronchial lung biopsy(s), each additional lobe (List separately in addition to code for primary procedure)

➔ *CPT Changes: An Insider's View* 2004

(Use 31632 in conjunction with 31628)

(31632 should be reported only once regardless of how many transbronchial lung biopsies are performed in a lobe)

§+ **31633** with transbronchial needle aspiration biopsy(s), each additional lobe (List separately in addition to code for primary procedure)

➔ *CPT Changes: An Insider's View* 2004

(Use 31633 in conjunction with 31629)

(31633 should be reported only once regardless of how many transbronchial needle aspiration biopsies are performed in the trachea or the additional lobe)

§⊙ **31635** with removal of foreign body

§● **31636** with placement of bronchial stent(s) (includes tracheal/bronchial dilation as required), initial bronchus

➔ *CPT Changes: An Insider's View* 2005

§+● **31637** each additional major bronchus stented (List separately in addition to code for primary procedure)

➔ *CPT Changes: An Insider's View* 2005

►(Use 31637 in conjunction with 31636)◄

§● **31638** with revision of tracheal or bronchial stent inserted at previous session (includes tracheal/bronchial dilation as required)

➔ *CPT Changes: An Insider's View* 2005

§ **31640** with excision of tumor

§ **31641** Bronchoscopy, (rigid or flexible); with destruction of tumor or relief of stenosis by any method other than excision (eg, laser therapy, cryotherapy)

(For bronchoscopic photodynamic therapy, report 31641 in addition to 96570, 96571 as appropriate)

§ **31643** with placement of catheter(s) for intracavitary radioelement application

(For intracavitary radioelement application, see 77761-77763, 77781-77784)

§⊙ **31645** with therapeutic aspiration of tracheobronchial tree, initial (eg, drainage of lung abscess)

§⊙ **31646** with therapeutic aspiration of tracheobronchial tree, subsequent

(For catheter aspiration of tracheobronchial tree at bedside, use 31725)

§⊙ **31656** with injection of contrast material for segmental bronchography (fiberscope only)

(For radiological supervision and interpretation, see 71040, 71060)

Introduction

(For endotracheal intubation, use 31500)

(For tracheal aspiration under direct vision, see 31515)

§ **31700** Catheterization, transglottic (separate procedure)

♦☆ **31708** Instillation of contrast material for laryngography or bronchography, without catheterization

(For radiological supervision and interpretation, see 70373, 71040, 71060)

♦☆ **31710** Catheterization for bronchography, with or without instillation of contrast material

(For bronchoscopic catheterization for bronchography, fiberscope only, use 31656)

(For radiological supervision and interpretation, see 71040, 71060)

♦☆ **31715** Transtracheal injection for bronchography

(For radiological supervision and interpretation, see 71040, 71060)

(For prolonged services, see 99354-99360)

§ **31717** Catheterization with bronchial brush biopsy

§ **31720** Catheter aspiration (separate procedure); nasotracheal

✿⊙ **31725** tracheobronchial with fiberscope, bedside

§ **31730** Transtracheal (percutaneous) introduction of needle wire dilator/stent or indwelling tube for oxygen therapy

Repair

§ **31750** Tracheoplasty; cervical

§ **31755** tracheopharyngeal fistulization, each stage

✿ **31760** intrathoracic

✿ **31766** Carinal reconstruction

✿ **31770** Bronchoplasty; graft repair

✿ **31775** excision stenosis and anastomosis

(For lobectomy and bronchoplasty, use 32501)

✿ **31780** Excision tracheal stenosis and anastomosis; cervical

✿ **31781** cervicothoracic

§ **31785** Excision of tracheal tumor or carcinoma; cervical

➔ *CPT Assistant* Jan 03:16

✿ **31786** thoracic

✿ **31800** Suture of tracheal wound or injury; cervical

✿ **31805** intrathoracic

§ **31820** Surgical closure tracheostomy or fistula; without plastic repair

§ **31825** with plastic repair

(For repair tracheoesophageal fistula, see 43305, 43312)

§ **31830** Revision of tracheostomy scar

Other Procedures

§ **31899** Unlisted procedure, trachea, bronchi

Lungs and Pleura

Incision

§⊘ **32000** Thoracentesis, puncture of pleural cavity for aspiration, initial or subsequent

(If imaging guidance is performed,see 76003, 76360, 76942)

(For total lung lavage, use 32997)

§⊘ **32002** Thoracentesis with insertion of tube with or without water seal (eg, for pneumothorax) (separate procedure)

(If imaging guidance is performed, see 76003, 76360, 76942)

§ **32005** Chemical pleurodesis (eg, for recurrent or persistent pneumothorax)

§⊙● **32019** Insertion of indwelling tunneled pleural catheter with cuff

➔ *CPT Changes: An Insider's View* 2005

►(Do not report 32019 in conjunction with 32000-32005, 32020, 36000, 36410, 62318, 62319, 64450, 64470, 64475)◄

►(If imaging guidance is performed, use 75989)◄

§⊙⊘ **32020** Tube thoracostomy with or without water seal (eg, for abscess, hemothorax, empyema) (separate procedure)

(If imaging guidance is performed, use 75989)

✿ **32035** Thoracostomy; with rib resection for empyema

✿ **32036** with open flap drainage for empyema

✿ **32095** Thoracotomy, limited, for biopsy of lung or pleura

(To report wound exploration due to penetrating trauma without thoractomy, use 20102)

✿ **32100** Thoracotomy, major; with exploration and biopsy

✿ **32110** with control of traumatic hemorrhage and/or repair of lung tear

✿ **32120** for postoperative complications

✿ **32124** with open intrapleural pneumonolysis

✿ **32140** with cyst(s) removal, with or without a pleural procedure

✿ **32141** with excision-plication of bullae, with or without any pleural procedure

(For lung volume reduction, use 32491)

✿ **32150** with removal of intrapleural foreign body or fibrin deposit

✿ **32151** with removal of intrapulmonary foreign body

✿ **32160** with cardiac massage

(For segmental or other resections of lung, see 32480-32525)

✿ **32200** Pneumonostomy; with open drainage of abscess or cyst

§⊙ **32201** with percutaneous drainage of abscess or cyst

➔ *CPT Assistant* Jan 03:16

(For radiological supervision and interpretation, use 75989)

✿ **32215** Pleural scarification for repeat pneumothorax

✿ **32220** Decortication, pulmonary (separate procedure); total

✿ **32225** partial

Excision

✿ **32310** Pleurectomy, parietal (separate procedure)

✿ **32320** Decortication and parietal pleurectomy

§ **32400** Biopsy, pleura; percutaneous needle

(If imaging guidance is performed, see 76003, 76360, 76393, 76942)

(For fine needle aspiration, use 10021 or 10022)

(For evaluation of fine needle aspirate, see 88172, 88173)

✿ **32402** open

§ **32405** Biopsy, lung or mediastinum, percutaneous needle

(For radiological supervision and interpretation, see 76003, 76360, 76393, 76942)

(For fine needle aspiration, use 10022)

(For evaluation of fine needle aspirate, see 88172, 88173)

§ **32420** Pneumocentesis, puncture of lung for aspiration

➔ *CPT Changes: An Insider's View* 2002

✿ **32440** Removal of lung, total pneumonectomy;

✿ **32442** with resection of segment of trachea followed by broncho-tracheal anastomosis (sleeve pneumonectomy)

✿ **32445** extrapleural

(For extrapleural pneumonectomy, with empyemectomy, use 32445 and 32540)

✿ **32480** Removal of lung, other than total pneumonectomy; single lobe (lobectomy)

✿ **32482** two lobes (bilobectomy)

✿ **32484** single segment (segmentectomy)

(For removal of lung with bronchoplasty, use 32501)

✿ **32486** with circumferential resection of segment of bronchus followed by broncho-bronchial anastomosis (sleeve lobectomy)

Surgery: Respiratory System

✿ 32488 all remaining lung following previous removal of a portion of lung (completion pneumonectomy)

(For total or segmental lobectomy, with concomitant decortication, use 32320 and the appropriate removal of lung code)

♦✿ 32491 excision-plication of emphysematous lung(s) (bullous or non-bullous) for lung volume reduction, sternal split or transthoracic approach, with or without any pleural procedure

✿ 32500 wedge resection, single or multiple

♦✿+ 32501 Resection and repair of portion of bronchus (bronchoplasty) when performed at time of lobectomy or segmentectomy (List separately in addition to code for primary procedure)

(Use 32501 in conjunction with 32480, 32482, 32484)

(32501 is to be used when a portion of the bronchus to preserved lung is removed and requires plastic closure to preserve function of that preserved lung. It is not to be used for closure for the proximal end of a resected bronchus)

✿ 32520 Resection of lung; with resection of chest wall

✿ 32522 with reconstruction of chest wall, without prosthesis

✿ 32525 with major reconstruction of chest wall, with prosthesis

✿ 32540 Extrapleural enucleation of empyema (empyemectomy)

(For extrapleural enucleation of empyema (empyemectomy) with lobectomy, use 32540 and the appropriate removal of lung code)

Endoscopy

Surgical thoracoscopy always includes diagnostic thoracoscopy.

For endoscopic procedures, code appropriate endoscopy of each anatomic site examined.

§ 32601 Thoracoscopy, diagnostic (separate procedure); lungs and pleural space, without biopsy

§ 32602 lungs and pleural space, with biopsy

§ 32603 pericardial sac, without biopsy

§ 32604 pericardial sac, with biopsy

§ 32605 mediastinal space, without biopsy

§ 32606 mediastinal space, with biopsy

(Surgical thoracoscopy always includes diagnostic thoracoscopy)

✿ 32650 Thoracoscopy, surgical; with pleurodesis (eg, mechanical or chemical)

✿ 32651 with partial pulmonary decortication

✿ 32652 with total pulmonary decortication, including intrapleural pneumonolysis

✿ 32653 with removal of intrapleural foreign body or fibrin deposit

✿ 32654 with control of traumatic hemorrhage

✿ 32655 with excision-plication of bullae, including any pleural procedure

✿ 32656 with parietal pleurectomy

✿ 32657 with wedge resection of lung, single or multiple

✿ 32658 with removal of clot or foreign body from pericardial sac

✿ 32659 with creation of pericardial window or partial resection of pericardial sac for drainage

✿ 32660 with total pericardiectomy

✿ 32661 with excision of pericardial cyst, tumor, or mass

✿ 32662 with excision of mediastinal cyst, tumor, or mass

✿ 32663 with lobectomy, total or segmental

♦✿ 32664 with thoracic sympathectomy

✿ 32665 with esophagomyotomy (Heller type)

(For exploratory thoracoscopy, and exploratory thoracoscopy with biopsy, see 32601-32606)

Repair

✿ 32800 Repair lung hernia through chest wall

✿ 32810 Closure of chest wall following open flap drainage for empyema (Clagett type procedure)

✿ 32815 Open closure of major bronchial fistula

✿ 32820 Major reconstruction, chest wall (posttraumatic)

Lung Transplantation

►Lung allotransplantation involves three distinct components of physician work:◄

►1) ***Cadaver donor pneumonectomy(s)***, which include(s) harvesting the allograft and cold preservation of the allograft (perfusing with cold preservation solution and cold maintenance) (use 32850).◄

►2) ***Backbench work***:◄

► Preparation of a cadaver donor single lung allograft prior to transplantation, including dissection of the allograft from surrounding soft tissues to prepare the pulmonary venous/atrial cuff, pulmonary artery, and bronchus unilaterally (use 32855).◄

► Preparation of a cadaver donor double lung allograft prior to transplantation, including dissection of the allograft from surrounding soft tissues to prepare the pulmonary venous/atrial cuff, pulmonary artery, and bronchus bilaterally (use 32856).◄

►3) ***Recipient lung allotransplantation***, which includes transplantation of a single or double lung allograft and care of the recipient (see 32851-32854).◄

✿▲ 32850 Donor pneumonectomy (including cold preservation), from cadaver donor

✿ **32851** Lung transplant, single; without cardiopulmonary bypass

✿ **32852** with cardiopulmonary bypass

✶✿ **32853** Lung transplant, double (bilateral sequential or en bloc); without cardiopulmonary bypass

✶✿ **32854** with cardiopulmonary bypass

✿● **32855** Backbench standard preparation of cadaver donor lung allograft prior to transplantation, including dissection of allograft from surrounding soft tissues to prepare pulmonary venous/atrial cuff, pulmonary artery, and bronchus; unilateral

✿● **32856** bilateral

►(For repair or resection procedures on the donor lung, see 32491, 32500, 35216, or 35276)◄

Surgical Collapse Therapy; Thoracoplasty

(See also 32520-32525)

✿ **32900** Resection of ribs, extrapleural, all stages

✿ **32905** Thoracoplasty, Schede type or extrapleural (all stages);

✿ **32906** with closure of bronchopleural fistula

(For open closure of major bronchial fistula, use 32815)

(For resection of first rib for thoracic outlet compression, see 21615, 21616)

✿ **32940** Pneumonolysis, extraperiosteal, including filling or packing procedures

§ **32960** Pneumothorax, therapeutic, intrapleural injection of air

Other Procedures

✿ **32997** Total lung lavage (unilateral)

(For bronchoscopic bronchial alveolar lavage, use 31624)

§ **32999** Unlisted procedure, lungs and pleura

Notes

Cardiovascular System

Selective vascular catheterizations should be coded to include introduction and all lesser order selective catheterizations used in the approach (eg, the description for a selective right middle cerebral artery catheterization includes the introduction and placement catheterization of the right common and internal carotid arteries).

Additional second and/or third order arterial catheterizations within the same family of arteries supplied by a single first order artery should be expressed by 36218 or 36248. Additional first order or higher catheterizations in vascular families supplied by a first order vessel different from a previously selected and coded family should be separately coded using the conventions described above.

(For monitoring, operation of pump and other nonsurgical services, see 99190-99192, 99291, 99292, 99354-99360)

(For other medical or laboratory related services, see appropriate section)

(For radiological supervision and interpretation, see 75600-75978)

Heart and Pericardium

Pericardium

§⊙ **33010** Pericardiocentesis; initial

(For radiological supervision and interpretation, use 76930)

§⊙ **33011** subsequent

(For radiological supervision and interpretation, use 76930)

✿ **33015** Tube pericardiostomy

✿ **33020** Pericardiotomy for removal of clot or foreign body (primary procedure)

✿ **33025** Creation of pericardial window or partial resection for drainage

✿ **33030** Pericardiectomy, subtotal or complete; without cardiopulmonary bypass

✿ **33031** with cardiopulmonary bypass

✿ **33050** Excision of pericardial cyst or tumor

Cardiac Tumor

✿ **33120** Excision of intracardiac tumor, resection with cardiopulmonary bypass

✿ **33130** Resection of external cardiac tumor

Transmyocardial Revascularization

✿ **33140** Transmyocardial laser revascularization, by thoracotomy; (separate procedure)

♦✿+ **33141** performed at the time of other open cardiac procedure(s) (List separately in addition to code for primary procedure)

(Use 33141 in conjunction with 33400-33496, 33510-33536, 33542)

Pacemaker or Pacing Cardioverter-Defibrillator

A pacemaker system includes a pulse generator containing electronics and a battery, and one or more electrodes (leads). Pulse generators are placed in a subcutaneous “pocket” created in either a subclavicular site or underneath the abdominal muscles just below the ribcage. Electrodes may be inserted through a vein (transvenous) or they may be placed on the surface of the heart (epicardial). The epicardial location of electrodes requires a thoracotomy for electrode insertion.

A single chamber pacemaker system includes a pulse generator and one electrode inserted in either the atrium or ventricle. A dual chamber pacemaker system includes a pulse generator and one electrode inserted in the right atrium and one electrode inserted in the right ventricle. In certain circumstances, an additional electrode may be required to achieve pacing of the left ventricle (bi-ventricular pacing). In this event, transvenous (cardiac vein) placement of the electrode should be separately reported using code 33224 or 33225.

Like a pacemaker system, a pacing cardioverter-defibrillator system includes a pulse generator and electrodes, although pacing cardioverter-defibrillators may require multiple leads, even when only a single chamber is being paced. A pacing cardioverter-defibrillator system may be inserted in a single chamber (pacing in the ventricle) or in dual chambers (pacing in atrium and ventricle). These devices use a combination of antitachycardia pacing, low energy cardioversion or defibrillating shocks to treat ventricular tachycardia or ventricular fibrillation.

Pacing cardioverter-defibrillator pulse generators may be implanted in a subcutaneous infraclavicular pocket or in an abdominal pocket. Removal of a pacing cardioverter-defibrillator pulse generator requires opening of the existing subcutaneous pocket and disconnection of the pulse generator from its electrode(s). A thoracotomy (or laparotomy in the case of abdominally placed pulse generators) is not required to remove the pulse generator.

The electrodes (leads) of a pacing cardioverter-defibrillator system are positioned in the heart via the venous system (transvenously), in most circumstances. In certain circumstances, an additional electrode may be required to achieve pacing of the left ventricle (biventricular pacing). In this event, transvenous (cardiac vein) placement of the electrode should be separately reported using code 33224 or 33225.

Electrode positioning on the epicardial surface of the heart requires a thoracotomy (codes 33245-33246). Removal of electrode(s) may first be attempted by transvenous extraction (code 33244). However, if transvenous extraction is unsuccessful, a thoracotomy may be required to remove the electrodes (code 33243).

When the "battery" of a pacemaker or pacing cardioverter-defibrillator is changed, it is actually the pulse generator that is changed. Replacement of a pulse generator should be reported with a code for removal of the pulse generator and another code for insertion of a pulse generator.

Repositioning of a pacemaker electrode, pacing cardioverter-defibrillator electrode(s), or a left ventricular pacing electrode is reported using 33215 or 33226, as appropriate. Replacement of a pacemaker electrode, pacing cardioverter-defibrillator electrode(s), or a left ventricular pacing electrode is reported using 33206-33208, 33210-33213, or 33224, as appropriate.

(For electronic, telephonic analysis of internal pacemaker system, see 93731-93736)

(For radiological supervision and interpretation with insertion of pacemaker, use 71090)

✿ **33200** Insertion of permanent pacemaker with epicardial electrode(s); by thoracotomy

✿ **33201** by xiphoid approach

§⊙ **33206** Insertion or replacement of permanent pacemaker with transvenous electrode(s); atrial

§⊙ **33207** ventricular

§⊙ **33208** atrial and ventricular

(Codes 33206-33208 include subcutaneous insertion of the pulse generator and transvenous placement of electrode(s))

§⊙ **33210** Insertion or replacement of temporary transvenous single chamber cardiac electrode or pacemaker catheter (separate procedure)

§⊙ **33211** Insertion or replacement of temporary transvenous dual chamber pacing electrodes (separate procedure)

§⊙ **33212** Insertion or replacement of pacemaker pulse generator only; single chamber, atrial or ventricular

§⊙ **33213** dual chamber

§⊙ **33214** Upgrade of implanted pacemaker system, conversion of single chamber system to dual chamber system (includes removal of previously placed pulse generator, testing of existing lead, insertion of new lead, insertion of new pulse generator)

§ **33215** Repositioning of previously implanted transvenous pacemaker or pacing cardioverter-defibrillator (right atrial or right ventricular) electrode

➔ *CPT Changes: An Insider's View* 2003

§⊙ **33216** Insertion of a transvenous electrode; single chamber (one electrode) permanent pacemaker or single chamber pacing cardioverter-defibrillator

➔ *CPT Changes: An Insider's View* 2000, 2003

§⊙ **33217** dual chamber (two electrodes) permanent pacemaker or dual chamber pacing cardioverter-defibrillator

➔ *CPT Changes: An Insider's View* 2000

(Do not report 33216-33217 in conjunction with 33214)

§⊙ **33218** Repair of single transvenous electrode for a single chamber, permanent pacemaker or single chamber pacing cardioverter-defibrillator

➔ *CPT Changes: An Insider's View* 2000

(For atrial or ventricular single chamber repair of pacemaker electrode(s) with replacement of pulse generator, see 33212 or 33213 and 33218 or 33220)

§⊙ **33220** Repair of two transvenous electrodes for a dual chamber permanent pacemaker or dual chamber pacing cardioverter-defibrillator

➔ *CPT Changes: An Insider's View* 2000

§⊙ **33222** Revision or relocation of skin pocket for pacemaker

➔ *CPT Changes: An Insider's View* 2000

§⊙ **33223** Revision of skin pocket for single or dual chamber pacing cardioverter-defibrillator

➔ *CPT Changes: An Insider's View* 2000

§ **33224** Insertion of pacing electrode, cardiac venous system, for left ventricular pacing, with attachment to previously placed pacemaker or pacing cardioverter-defibrillator pulse generator (including revision of pocket, removal, insertion and/or replacement of generator)

➔ *CPT Changes: An Insider's View* 2003

❖+ **33225** Insertion of pacing electrode, cardiac venous system, for left ventricular pacing, at time of insertion of pacing cardioverter-defibrillator or pacemaker pulse generator (including upgrade to dual chamber system) (List separately in addition to code for primary procedure)

➔ *CPT Changes: An Insider's View* 2003

(Use 33225 in conjunction with 33206, 33207, 33208, 33212, 33213, 33214, 33216, 33217, 33222, 33233, 33234, 33235, 33240, 33249)

§ **33226** Repositioning of previously implanted cardiac venous system (left ventricular) electrode (including removal, insertion and/or replacement of generator)

➔ *CPT Changes: An Insider's View* 2003

§⊙ **33233** Removal of permanent pacemaker pulse generator

➔ *CPT Changes: An Insider's View* 2000

§⊙ **33234** Removal of transvenous pacemaker electrode(s); single lead system, atrial or ventricular

➔ *CPT Changes: An Insider's View* 2000

§⊙ **33235** dual lead system

➔ *CPT Changes: An Insider's View* 2000

✿ **33236** Removal of permanent epicardial pacemaker and electrodes by thoracotomy; single lead system, atrial or ventricular

✿ **33237** dual lead system

✿ **33238** Removal of permanent transvenous electrode(s) by thoracotomy

✣⊙ **33240** Insertion of single or dual chamber pacing cardioverter-defibrillator pulse generator

➲ *CPT Assistant* Apr 04:7; *CPT Changes: An Insider's View* 2000

§⊙ **33241** Subcutaneous removal of single or dual chamber pacing cardioverter-defibrillator pulse generator

➲ *CPT Assistant* Apr 04:6, 7; *CPT Changes: An Insider's View* 2000

(For removal of electrode(s) by thoracotomy, use 33243 in conjunction with 33241)

(For removal of electrode(s) by transvenous extraction, use 33244 in conjunction with 33241)

(For removal and reinsertion of a pacing cardioverter-defibrillator system (pulse generator and electrodes), report 33241 and 33243 or 33244 and 33249)

(For repair of implantable cardioverter-defibrillator pulse generator and/or leads, see 33218, 33220)

✿ **33243** Removal of single or dual chamber pacing cardioverter-defibrillator electrode(s); by thoracotomy

§⊙ **33244** by transvenous extraction

➲ *CPT Changes: An Insider's View* 2000

(For subcutaneous removal of the pulse generator, use 33241 in conjunction with 33243 or 33244)

✿ **33245** Insertion of epicardial single or dual chamber pacing cardioverter-defibrillator electrodes by thoracotomy;

✿ **33246** with insertion of pulse generator

(For insertion of implantable cardioverter-defibrillator lead(s), without thoracotomy, use 33216)

✣⊙ **33249** Insertion or repositioning of electrode lead(s) for single or dual chamber pacing cardioverter-defibrillator and insertion of pulse generator

➲ *CPT Changes: An Insider's View* 2000

(For removal and reinsertion of a pacing cardioverter-defibrillator system (pulse generator and electrodes), report 33241 and 33243 or 33244 and 33249)

Electrophysiologic Operative Procedures

✿ **33250** Operative ablation of supraventricular arrhythmogenic focus or pathway (eg, Wolff-Parkinson-White, atrioventricular node re-entry), tract(s) and/or focus (foci); without cardiopulmonary bypass

✿ **33251** with cardiopulmonary bypass

✿ **33253** Operative incisions and reconstruction of atria for treatment of atrial fibrillation or atrial flutter (eg, maze procedure)

✿ **33261** Operative ablation of ventricular arrhythmogenic focus with cardiopulmonary bypass

Patient-Activated Event Recorder

❖ **33282** Implantation of patient-activated cardiac event recorder

➲ *CPT Changes: An Insider's View* 2000

(Initial implantation includes programming. For subsequent electronic analysis and/or reprogramming, use 93727)

§ **33284** Removal of an implantable, patient-activated cardiac event recorder

➲ *CPT Changes: An Insider's View* 2000

Wounds of the Heart and Great Vessels

✿ **33300** Repair of cardiac wound; without bypass

✿ **33305** with cardiopulmonary bypass

✿ **33310** Cardiotomy, exploratory (includes removal of foreign body, atrial or ventricular thrombus); without bypass

✿ **33315** with cardiopulmonary bypass

(Do not report removal of thrombus (33310-33315) in conjunction with other cardiac procedures unless a separate incision in the heart is required to remove the atrial or ventricular thrombus)

(If removal of thrombus with coronary bypass (33315) is reported in conjunction with 33120, 33130, 33420-33430, 33460-33468, 33496, 33542, 33545, 33641-33647, 33670, 33681, 33975-33980 which requires a separate heart incision, report 33315 with modifier 59)

✿ **33320** Suture repair of aorta or great vessels; without shunt or cardiopulmonary bypass

✿ **33321** with shunt bypass

✿ **33322** with cardiopulmonary bypass

✿ **33330** Insertion of graft, aorta or great vessels; without shunt, or cardiopulmonary bypass

✿ **33332** with shunt bypass

✿ **33335** with cardiopulmonary bypass

Cardiac Valves

(For multiple valve procedures, see 33400-33478 and add modifier 51 to the secondary valve procedure code)

Aortic Valve

✿ **33400** Valvuloplasty, aortic valve; open, with cardiopulmonary bypass

✿ **33401** open, with inflow occlusion

✿ **33403** using transventricular dilation, with cardiopulmonary bypass

(Do not report modifier 63 in conjunction with 33401, 33403)

✿ **33404** Construction of apical-aortic conduit

Surgery: Cardiovascular System

✿ **33405** Replacement, aortic valve, with cardiopulmonary bypass; with prosthetic valve other than homograft or stentless valve

✿ **33406** with allograft valve (freehand)

(For aortic valve valvotomy, (commissurotomy) with inflow occlusion, use 33401)

(For aortic valve valvotomy, (commissurotomy) with cardiopulmonary bypass, use 33403)

✿ **33410** with stentless tissue valve

✿ **33411** Replacement, aortic valve; with aortic annulus enlargement, noncoronary cusp

✿ **33412** with transventricular aortic annulus enlargement (Konno procedure)

✿ **33413** by translocation of autologous pulmonary valve with allograft replacement of pulmonary valve (Ross procedure)

✿ **33414** Repair of left ventricular outflow tract obstruction by patch enlargement of the outflow tract

✿ **33415** Resection or incision of subvalvular tissue for discrete subvalvular aortic stenosis

✿ **33416** Ventriculomyotomy (-myectomy) for idiopathic hypertrophic subaortic stenosis (eg, asymmetric septal hypertrophy)

✿ **33417** Aortoplasty (gusset) for supravalvular stenosis

Mitral Valve

✿ **33420** Valvotomy, mitral valve; closed heart

✿ **33422** open heart, with cardiopulmonary bypass

✿ **33425** Valvuloplasty, mitral valve, with cardiopulmonary bypass;

✿ **33426** with prosthetic ring

✿ **33427** radical reconstruction, with or without ring

✿ **33430** Replacement, mitral valve, with cardiopulmonary bypass

Tricuspid Valve

✿ **33460** Valvectomy, tricuspid valve, with cardiopulmonary bypass

✿ **33463** Valvuloplasty, tricuspid valve; without ring insertion

✿ **33464** with ring insertion

✿ **33465** Replacement, tricuspid valve, with cardiopulmonary bypass

✿ **33468** Tricuspid valve repositioning and plication for Ebstein anomaly

Pulmonary Valve

✿ **33470** Valvotomy, pulmonary valve, closed heart; transventricular

(Do not report modifier 63 in conjunction with 33470)

✿ **33471** via pulmonary artery

(To report percutaneous valvuloplasty of pulmonary valve, use 92990)

✿ **33472** Valvotomy, pulmonary valve, open heart; with inflow occlusion

(Do not report modifier 63 in conjunction with 33472)

✿ **33474** with cardiopulmonary bypass

✿ **33475** Replacement, pulmonary valve

✿ **33476** Right ventricular resection for infundibular stenosis, with or without commissurotomy

✿ **33478** Outflow tract augmentation (gusset), with or without commissurotomy or infundibular resection

Other Valvular Procedures

✿ **33496** Repair of non-structural prosthetic valve dysfunction with cardiopulmonary bypass (separate procedure)

(For reoperation, use 33530 in addition to 33496)

Coronary Artery Anomalies

Basic procedures include endarterectomy or angioplasty.

✿ **33500** Repair of coronary arteriovenous or arteriocardiac chamber fistula; with cardiopulmonary bypass

✿ **33501** without cardiopulmonary bypass

✿ **33502** Repair of anomalous coronary artery; by ligation

✿ **33503** by graft, without cardiopulmonary bypass

(Do not report modifier 63 in conjunction with 33502, 33503)

✿ **33504** by graft, with cardiopulmonary bypass

✿ **33505** with construction of intrapulmonary artery tunnel (Takeuchi procedure)

✿ **33506** by translocation from pulmonary artery to aorta

(Do not report modifier 63 in conjunction with 33505, 33506)

Endoscopy

Surgical vascular endoscopy always includes diagnostic endoscopy.

♦☆+ **33508** Endoscopy, surgical, including video-assisted harvest of vein(s) for coronary artery bypass procedure (List separately in addition to code for primary procedure)

➲ *CPT Changes: An Insider's View* 2003

(Use 33508 in conjunction with 33510-33523)

(For open harvest of upper extremity vein procedure, use 35500)

Venous Grafting Only for Coronary Artery Bypass

The following codes are used to report coronary artery bypass procedures using venous grafts only. These codes should NOT be used to report the performance of coronary artery bypass procedures using arterial grafts and venous grafts during the same procedure. See 33517-33523 and 33533-33536 for reporting combined arterial-venous grafts.

Procurement of the saphenous vein graft is included in the description of the work for 33510-33516 and should not be reported as a separate service or co-surgery. To report harvesting of an upper extremity vein, use 35500 in addition to the bypass procedure. To report harvesting of a femoropopliteal vein segment, report 35572 in addition to the bypass procedure. When surgical assistant performs graft procurement, add modifier 80 to 33510-33516.

✿ **33510** Coronary artery bypass, vein only; single coronary venous graft

✿ **33511** two coronary venous grafts

✿ **33512** three coronary venous grafts

✿ **33513** four coronary venous grafts

✿ **33514** five coronary venous grafts

✿ **33516** six or more coronary venous grafts

Combined Arterial-Venous Grafting for Coronary Bypass

The following codes are used to report coronary artery bypass procedures using venous grafts and arterial grafts during the same procedure. These codes may NOT be used alone.

To report combined arterial-venous grafts it is necessary to report two codes: 1) the appropriate combined arterial-venous graft code (33517-33523); and 2) the appropriate arterial graft code (33533-33536).

Procurement of the saphenous vein graft is included in the description of the work for 33517-33523 and should not be reported as a separate service or co-surgery. Procurement of the artery for grafting is included in the description of the work for 33533-33536 and should not be reported as a separate service or co-surgery, except when an upper extremity artery (eg, radial artery) is procured. To report harvesting of an upper extremity artery, use 35600 in addition to the bypass procedure. To report harvesting of an upper extremity vein, use 35500 in addition to the bypass procedure. To report harvesting of a femoropopliteal vein segment, report 35572 in addition to the bypass procedure. When surgical assistant performs arterial and/or venous graft procurement, add modifier 80 to 33517-33523, 33533-33536, as appropriate.

✿⊘ **33517** Coronary artery bypass, using venous graft(s) and arterial graft(s); single vein graft (List separately in addition to code for arterial graft)

✿⊘ **33518** two venous grafts (List separately in addition to code for arterial graft)

✿⊘ **33519** three venous grafts (List separately in addition to code for arterial graft)

✿⊘ **33521** four venous grafts (List separately in addition to code for arterial graft)

✿⊘ **33522** five venous grafts (List separately in addition to code for arterial graft)

✿⊘ **33523** six or more venous grafts (List separately in addition to code for arterial graft)

✿+ **33530** Reoperation, coronary artery bypass procedure or valve procedure, more than one month after original operation (List separately in addition to code for primary procedure)

➔ *CPT Assistant* Feb 03:7

(Use 33530 in conjunction with 33400-33496; 33510-33536, 33863)

Arterial Grafting for Coronary Artery Bypass

The following codes are used to report coronary artery bypass procedures using either arterial grafts only or a combination of arterial-venous grafts. The codes include the use of the internal mammary artery, gastroepiploic artery, epigastric artery, radial artery, and arterial conduits procured from other sites.

To report combined arterial-venous grafts it is necessary to report two codes: 1) the appropriate arterial graft code (33533-33536); and 2) the appropriate combined arterial-venous graft code (33517-33523).

Procurement of the artery for grafting is included in the description of the work for 33533-33536 and should not be reported as a separate service or co-surgery, except when an upper extremity artery (eg, radial artery) is procured. To report harvesting of an upper extremity artery, use 35600 in addition to the bypass procedure. To report harvesting of an upper extremity vein, use 35500 in addition to the bypass procedure. To report harvesting of a femoropopliteal vein segment, report 35572 in addition to the bypass procedure. When surgical assistant performs arterial and/or venous graft procurement, add modifier 80 to 33517-33523, 33533-33536, as appropriate.

✿ **33533** Coronary artery bypass, using arterial graft(s); single arterial graft

✿ **33534** two coronary arterial grafts

✿ **33535** three coronary arterial grafts

✿ **33536** four or more coronary arterial grafts

✿ 33542 Myocardial resection (eg, ventricular aneurysmectomy)

✿ 33545 Repair of postinfarction ventricular septal defect, with or without myocardial resection

Coronary Endarterectomy

✿+ 33572 Coronary endarterectomy, open, any method, of left anterior descending, circumflex, or right coronary artery performed in conjunction with coronary artery bypass graft procedure, each vessel (List separately in addition to primary procedure)

(Use 33572 in conjunction with 33510-33516, 33533-33536)

Single Ventricle and Other Complex Cardiac Anomalies

✿ 33600 Closure of atrioventricular valve (mitral or tricuspid) by suture or patch

✿ 33602 Closure of semilunar valve (aortic or pulmonary) by suture or patch

✿ 33606 Anastomosis of pulmonary artery to aorta (Damus-Kaye-Stansel procedure)

✿ 33608 Repair of complex cardiac anomaly other than pulmonary atresia with ventricular septal defect by construction or replacement of conduit from right or left ventricle to pulmonary artery

(For repair of pulmonary atresia with ventricular septal defect, see 33918, 33919, 33920)

✿ 33610 Repair of complex cardiac anomalies (eg, single ventricle with subaortic obstruction) by surgical enlargement of ventricular septal defect

(Do not report modifier 63 in conjunction with 33610)

✿ 33611 Repair of double outlet right ventricle with intraventricular tunnel repair;

(Do not report modifier 63 in conjunction with 33611)

✿ 33612 with repair of right ventricular outflow tract obstruction

✿ 33615 Repair of complex cardiac anomalies (eg, tricuspid atresia) by closure of atrial septal defect and anastomosis of atria or vena cava to pulmonary artery (simple Fontan procedure)

✿ 33617 Repair of complex cardiac anomalies (eg, single ventricle) by modified Fontan procedure

✿ 33619 Repair of single ventricle with aortic outflow obstruction and aortic arch hypoplasia (hypoplastic left heart syndrome) (eg, Norwood procedure)

(Do not report modifier 63 in conjunction with 33619)

Septal Defect

✿ 33641 Repair atrial septal defect, secundum, with cardiopulmonary bypass, with or without patch

✿ 33645 Direct or patch closure, sinus venosus, with or without anomalous pulmonary venous drainage

✿ 33647 Repair of atrial septal defect and ventricular septal defect, with direct or patch closure

(Do not report modifier 63 in conjunction with 33647)

(For repair of tricuspid atresia (eg, Fontan, Gago procedures), use 33615)

✿ 33660 Repair of incomplete or partial atrioventricular canal (ostium primum atrial septal defect), with or without atrioventricular valve repair

✿ 33665 Repair of intermediate or transitional atrioventricular canal, with or without atrioventricular valve repair

✿ 33670 Repair of complete atrioventricular canal, with or without prosthetic valve

(Do not report modifier 63 in conjunction with 33670)

✿ 33681 Closure of ventricular septal defect, with or without patch;

✿ 33684 with pulmonary valvotomy or infundibular resection (acyanotic)

✿ 33688 with removal of pulmonary artery band, with or without gusset

✿ 33690 Banding of pulmonary artery

(Do not report modifier 63 in conjunction with 33690)

✿ 33692 Complete repair tetralogy of Fallot without pulmonary atresia;

✿ 33694 with transannular patch

(Do not report modifier 63 in conjunction with 33694)

(For ligation and takedown of a systemic-to-pulmonary artery shunt, performed in conjunction with a congenital heart procedure; see 33924)

✿ 33697 Complete repair tetralogy of Fallot with pulmonary atresia including construction of conduit from right ventricle to pulmonary artery and closure of ventricular septal defect

(For ligation and takedown of a systemic-to-pulmonary artery shunt, performed in conjunction with a congenital heart procedure; see 33924)

Sinus of Valsalva

✿ 33702 Repair sinus of Valsalva fistula, with cardiopulmonary bypass;

✿ 33710 with repair of ventricular septal defect

✿ 33720 Repair sinus of Valsalva aneurysm, with cardiopulmonary bypass

✿ 33722 Closure of aortico-left ventricular tunnel

Total Anomalous Pulmonary Venous Drainage

✿ **33730** Complete repair of anomalous venous return (supracardiac, intracardiac, or infracardiac types)

(Do not report modifier 63 in conjunction with 33730)

(For partial anomalous return, see atrial septal defect)

✿ **33732** Repair of cor triatriatum or supravalvular mitral ring by resection of left atrial membrane

(Do not report modifier 63 in conjunction with 33732)

Shunting Procedures

✿ **33735** Atrial septectomy or septostomy; closed heart (Blalock-Hanlon type operation)

✿ **33736** open heart with cardiopulmonary bypass

(Do not report modifier 63 in conjunction with 33735, 33736)

✿ **33737** open heart, with inflow occlusion

(For transvenous method cardiac catheterization balloon atrial septectomy or septostomy (Rashkind type), use 92992)

(For blade method cardiac catheterization atrial septectomy or septostomy (Sang-Park septostomy), use 92993)

✿ **33750** Shunt; subclavian to pulmonary artery (Blalock-Taussig type operation)

✿ **33755** ascending aorta to pulmonary artery (Waterston type operation)

✿ **33762** descending aorta to pulmonary artery (Potts-Smith type operation)

(Do not report modifier 63 in conjunction with 33750, 33755, 33762)

✿ **33764** central, with prosthetic graft

✿ **33766** superior vena cava to pulmonary artery for flow to one lung (classical Glenn procedure)

✿ **33767** superior vena cava to pulmonary artery for flow to both lungs (bidirectional Glenn procedure)

Transposition of the Great Vessels

✿ **33770** Repair of transposition of the great arteries with ventricular septal defect and subpulmonary stenosis; without surgical enlargement of ventricular septal defect

✿ **33771** with surgical enlargement of ventricular septal defect

✿ **33774** Repair of transposition of the great arteries, atrial baffle procedure (eg, Mustard or Senning type) with cardiopulmonary bypass;

✿ **33775** with removal of pulmonary band

✿ **33776** with closure of ventricular septal defect

✿ **33777** with repair of subpulmonic obstruction

✿ **33778** Repair of transposition of the great arteries, aortic pulmonary artery reconstruction (eg, Jatene type);

(Do not report modifier 63 in conjunction with 33778)

✿ **33779** with removal of pulmonary band

✿ **33780** with closure of ventricular septal defect

✿ **33781** with repair of subpulmonic obstruction

Truncus Arteriosus

✿ **33786** Total repair, truncus arteriosus (Rastelli type operation)

(Do not report modifier 63 in conjunction with 33786)

✿ **33788** Reimplantation of an anomalous pulmonary artery

(For pulmonary artery band, use 33690)

Aortic Anomalies

✿ **33800** Aortic suspension (aortopexy) for tracheal decompression (eg, for tracheomalacia) (separate procedure)

✿ **33802** Division of aberrant vessel (vascular ring);

✿ **33803** with reanastomosis

✿ **33813** Obliteration of aortopulmonary septal defect; without cardiopulmonary bypass

✿ **33814** with cardiopulmonary bypass

✿ **33820** Repair of patent ductus arteriosus; by ligation

✿ **33822** by division, under 18 years

✿ **33824** by division, 18 years and older

✿ **33840** Excision of coarctation of aorta, with or without associated patent ductus arteriosus; with direct anastomosis

✿ **33845** with graft

✿ **33851** repair using either left subclavian artery or prosthetic material as gusset for enlargement

✿ **33852** Repair of hypoplastic or interrupted aortic arch using autogenous or prosthetic material; without cardiopulmonary bypass

✿ **33853** with cardiopulmonary bypass

(For repair of hypoplastic left heart syndrome (eg, Norwood type), via excision of coarctation of aorta, use 33619)

Thoracic Aortic Aneurysm

✿ 33860 Ascending aorta graft, with cardiopulmonary bypass, with or without valve suspension;

✿ 33861 with coronary reconstruction

✿ 33863 with aortic root replacement using composite prosthesis and coronary reconstruction

(For graft of ascending aorta, with cardiopulmonary bypass and valve replacement, with or without coronary implant or valve suspension; use 33860 or 33861 and 33405 or 33406)

✿ 33870 Transverse arch graft, with cardiopulmonary bypass

✿ 33875 Descending thoracic aorta graft, with or without bypass

✿ 33877 Repair of thoracoabdominal aortic aneurysm with graft, with or without cardiopulmonary bypass

Pulmonary Artery

✿ 33910 Pulmonary artery embolectomy; with cardiopulmonary bypass

✿ 33915 without cardiopulmonary bypass

✿ 33916 Pulmonary endarterectomy, with or without embolectomy, with cardiopulmonary bypass

✿ 33917 Repair of pulmonary artery stenosis by reconstruction with patch or graft

✿ 33918 Repair of pulmonary atresia with ventricular septal defect, by unifocalization of pulmonary arteries; without cardiopulmonary bypass

✿ 33919 with cardiopulmonary bypass

(Do not report modifier 63 in conjunction with 33918, 33919)

✿ 33920 Repair of pulmonary atresia with ventricular septal defect, by construction or replacement of conduit from right or left ventricle to pulmonary artery

(For repair of other complex cardiac anomalies by construction or replacement of right or left ventricle to pulmonary artery conduit, use 33608)

✿ 33922 Transection of pulmonary artery with cardiopulmonary bypass

(Do not report modifier 63 in conjunction with 33922)

✿+ 33924 Ligation and takedown of a systemic-to-pulmonary artery shunt, performed in conjunction with a congenital heart procedure (List separately in addition to code for primary procedure)

(Use 33924 in conjunction with 33470-33475, 33600-33619, 33684-33688, 33692-33697, 33735-33767, 33770-33781, 33786, 33918-33922)

Heart/Lung Transplantation

►Heart with or without lung allotransplantation involves three distinct components of physician work:◄

►1) ***Cadaver donor cardiectomy with or without pneumonectomy***, which includes harvesting the allograft and cold preservation of the allograft (perfusing with cold preservation solution and cold maintenance) (see 33930, 33940).◄

►2) ***Backbench work***:◄

► Preparation of a cadaver donor heart and lung allograft prior to transplantation, including dissection of the allograft from surrounding soft tissues to prepare the aorta, superior vena cava, inferior vena cava, and trachea for implantation (use 33933).◄

► Preparation of a cadaver donor heart allograft prior to transplantation, including dissection of the allograft from surrounding soft tissues to prepare aorta, superior vena cava, inferior vena cava, pulmonary artery, and left atrium for implantation (use 33944).◄

►3) ***Recipient heart with or without lung allotransplantation***, which includes transplantation of allograft and care of the recipient (see 33935, 33945).◄

(For implantation of a total replacement heart system (artificial heart) with recipient cardiectomy or heart replacement system components, see Category III codes 0051T-0053T)

✿▲ 33930 Donor cardiectomy-pneumonectomy (including cold preservation)

✿● 33933 Backbench standard preparation of cadaver donor heart/lung allograft prior to transplantation, including dissection of allograft from surrounding soft tissues to prepare aorta, superior vena cava, inferior vena cava, and trachea for implantation

✿ 33935 Heart-lung transplant with recipient cardiectomy-pneumonectomy

✿▲ 33940 Donor cardiectomy (including cold preservation)

✿● 33944 Backbench standard preparation of cadaver donor heart allograft prior to transplantation, including dissection of allograft from surrounding soft tissues to prepare aorta, superior vena cava, inferior vena cava, pulmonary artery, and left atrium for implantation

►(For repair or resection procedures on the donor heart, see 33300, 33310, 33320, 33400, 33463, 33464, 33510, 33641, 35216, 35276 or 35685)◄

✿ 33945 Heart transplant, with or without recipient cardiectomy

Cardiac Assist

(For percutaneous implantation of extracorporeal ventricular assist device or for removal of percutaneously implanted extracorporeal ventricular assist device, see Category III codes 0048T-0050T)

✿ 33960 Prolonged extracorporeal circulation for cardiopulmonary insufficiency; initial 24 hours

✿+ 33961 each additional 24 hours (List separately in addition to code for primary procedure)

(Do not report modifier 63 in conjunction with 33960, 33961)

(Use 33961 in conjunction with 33960)

(For insertion of cannula for prolonged extracorporeal circulation, use 36822)

✿ 33967 Insertion of intra-aortic balloon assist device, percutaneous

✿ 33968 Removal of intra-aortic balloon assist device, percutaneous

✿ 33970 Insertion of intra-aortic balloon assist device through the femoral artery, open approach

✿ 33971 Removal of intra-aortic balloon assist device including repair of femoral artery, with or without graft

✿ 33973 Insertion of intra-aortic balloon assist device through the ascending aorta

✿ 33974 Removal of intra-aortic balloon assist device from the ascending aorta, including repair of the ascending aorta, with or without graft

⌘✿ 33975 Insertion of ventricular assist device; extracorporeal, single ventricle

✢✿ 33976 extracorporeal, biventricular

⌘✿ 33977 Removal of ventricular assist device; extracorporeal, single ventricle

✢✿ 33978 extracorporeal, biventricular

✿ 33979 Insertion of ventricular assist device, implantable intracorporeal, single ventricle

✿ 33980 Removal of ventricular assist device, implantable intracorporeal, single ventricle

Other Procedures

§ 33999 Unlisted procedure, cardiac surgery

Arteries and Veins

Primary vascular procedure listings include establishing both inflow and outflow by whatever procedures necessary. Also included is that portion of the operative arteriogram performed by the surgeon, as indicated. Sympathectomy, when done, is included in the listed aortic procedures. For unlisted vascular procedure, use 37799.

Embolectomy/Thrombectomy

Arterial, With or Without Catheter

♦✿ 34001 Embolectomy or thrombectomy, with or without catheter; carotid, subclavian or innominate artery, by neck incision

♦✿ 34051 innominate, subclavian artery, by thoracic incision

♦§ 34101 axillary, brachial, innominate, subclavian artery, by arm incision

♦§ 34111 radial or ulnar artery, by arm incision

♦✿ 34151 renal, celiac, mesentery, aortoiliac artery, by abdominal incision

♦§ 34201 femoropopliteal, aortoiliac artery, by leg incision

♦§ 34203 popliteal-tibio-peroneal artery, by leg incision

Venous, Direct or With Catheter

♦✿ 34401 Thrombectomy, direct or with catheter; vena cava, iliac vein, by abdominal incision

♦§ 34421 vena cava, iliac, femoropopliteal vein, by leg incision

♦✿ 34451 vena cava, iliac, femoropopliteal vein, by abdominal and leg incision

♦§ 34471 subclavian vein, by neck incision

♦§ 34490 axillary and subclavian vein, by arm incision

Venous Reconstruction

♦§ 34501 Valvuloplasty, femoral vein

✿ 34502 Reconstruction of vena cava, any method

♦§ 34510 Venous valve transposition, any vein donor

♦§ 34520 Cross-over vein graft to venous system

♦§ 34530 Saphenopopliteal vein anastomosis

Endovascular Repair of Abdominal Aortic Aneurysm

Codes 34800-34826 represent a family of component procedures to report placement of an endovascular graft for abdominal aortic aneurysm repair. These codes describe open femoral or iliac artery exposure, device manipulation and deployment, and closure of the arteriotomy sites. Balloon angioplasty and/or stent deployment within the target treatment zone for the endoprosthesis, either before or after endograft deployment, are not separately reportable. Introduction of guidewires and catheters should be reported separately (eg, 36200, 36245-36248, 36140). Extensive repair or replacement of an artery should be additionally reported (eg, 35226 or 35286).

For fluoroscopic guidance in conjunction with endovascular aneurysm repair, see code 75952 or 75953, as appropriate. Code 75952 includes angiography of the

Surgery: Cardiovascular System

aorta and its branches for diagnostic imaging prior to deployment of the endovascular device (including all routine components of modular devices), fluoroscopic guidance in the delivery of the endovascular components, and intraprocedural arterial angiography (eg, confirm position, detect endoleak, evaluate runoff). Code 75953 includes the analogous services for placement of additional extension prostheses (not for routine components of modular devices).

Other interventional procedures performed at the time of endovascular abdominal aortic aneurysm repair should be additionally reported (eg, renal transluminal angioplasty, arterial embolization, intravascular ultrasound, balloon angioplasty or stenting of native artery(s) outside the endoprosthesis target zone, when done before or after deployment of graft).

✿ **34800** Endovascular repair of infrarenal abdominal aortic aneurysm or dissection; using aorto-aortic tube prosthesis

✿ **34802** using modular bifurcated prosthesis (one docking limb)

✿● **34803** using modular bifurcated prosthesis (two docking limbs)

►(For endovascular repair of abdominal aortic aneurysm or dissection involving visceral vessels using a fenestrated modular bifurcated prosthesis (two docking limbs), use Category III codes 0078T, 0079T)◄

✿ **34804** using unibody bifurcated prosthesis

✿ **34805** using aorto-uniiliac or aorto-unifemoral prosthesis

➔ *CPT Changes: An Insider's View* 2004

✿+ **34808** Endovascular placement of iliac artery occlusion device (List separately in addition to code for primary procedure)

(Use 34808 in conjunction with 34800, 34805, 34813, 34825, 34826)

(For radiological supervision and interpretation, use 75952 in conjunction with ►34800-34808◄)

(For open arterial exposure, report 34812, 34820, 34833, 34834 as appropriate, in addition to ►34800-34808◄)

♦✿ **34812** Open femoral artery exposure for delivery of endovascular prosthesis, by groin incision, unilateral

(For bilateral procedure, use modifier 50)

✿+ **34813** Placement of femoral-femoral prosthetic graft during endovascular aortic aneurysm repair (List separately in addition to code for primary procedure)

(Use 34813 in conjunction with 34812)

(For femoral artery grafting, see 35521, 35533, 35546, 35551-35558, 35566, 35621, 35646, 35651-35661, 35666, 35700)

♦✿ **34820** Open iliac artery exposure for delivery of endovascular prosthesis or iliac occlusion during endovascular therapy, by abdominal or retroperitoneal incision, unilateral

(For bilateral procedure, use modifier 50)

✿ **34825** Placement of proximal or distal extension prosthesis for endovascular repair of infrarenal abdominal aortic or iliac aneurysm, false aneurysm, or dissection; initial vessel

✿+ **34826** each additional vessel (List separately in addition to code for primary procedure)

(Use 34826 in conjunction with 34825)

(Use 34825, 34826 in addition to 34800-34808, 34900 as appropriate)

(For staged procedure, use modifier 58)

(For radiological supervision and interpretation, use 75953)

✿ **34830** Open repair of infrarenal aortic aneurysm or dissection, plus repair of associated arterial trauma, following unsuccessful endovascular repair; tube prosthesis

✿ **34831** aorto-bi-iliac prosthesis

✿ **34832** aorto-bifemoral prosthesis

♦✿ **34833** Open iliac artery exposure with creation of conduit for delivery of infrarenal aortic or iliac endovascular prosthesis, by abdominal or retroperitoneal incision, unilateral

(For bilateral procedure, use modifier 50)

(Do not report 34833 in addition to 34820)

♦✿ **34834** Open brachial artery exposure to assist in the deployment of infrarenal aortic or iliac endovascular prosthesis by arm incision, unilateral

(For bilateral procedure, use modifier 50)

Endovascular Repair of Iliac Aneurysm

Code 34900 represents a procedure to report introduction, positioning, and deployment of an endovascular graft for treatment of aneurysm, pseudoaneurysm, or arteriovenous malformation or trauma of the iliac artery (common, hypogastric, external). All balloon angioplasty and/or stent deployments within the target treatment zone for the endoprosthesis, either before or after endograft deployment, are included in the work of 34900 and are not separately reportable. Open femoral or iliac artery exposure (eg, 34812, 34820), introduction of guidewires and catheters (eg, 36200, 36215-36218), and extensive repair or replacement of an artery (eg, 35206-35286) should be additionally reported.

For fluoroscopic guidance in conjunction with endovascular iliac aneurysm repair, see code 75954. Code 75954 includes angiography of the aorta and iliac arteries for diagnostic imaging prior to deployment of the endovascular device (including all routine components), fluoroscopic guidance in the delivery of the endovascular components, and intraprocedural arterial angiography to confirm appropriate position of the graft, detect endoleaks, and evaluate the status of the runoff vessels (eg, evaluation for dissection, stenosis, thrombosis, distal embolization, or iatrogenic injury).

Other interventional procedures performed at the time of endovascular aortic aneurysm repair should be additionally reported (eg, transluminal angioplasty outside the aneurysm target zone, arterial embolization, intravascular ultrasound).

✿ 34900 Endovascular graft placement for repair of iliac artery (eg, aneurysm, pseudoaneurysm, arteriovenous malformation, trauma)

(For radiological supervision and interpretation, use 75954)

(For placement of extension prosthesis during endovascular iliac artery repair, use 34825)

(For bilateral procedure, use modifier 50)

Direct Repair of Aneurysm or Excision (Partial or Total) and Graft Insertion for Aneurysm, Pseudoaneurysm, Ruptured Aneurysm, and Associated Occlusive Disease

Procedures 35001-►35152◄ include preparation of artery for anastomosis including endarterectomy.

(For direct repairs associated with occlusive disease only, see 35201-35286)

(For intracranial aneurysm, see 61700 et seq)

(For endovascular repair of abdominal aortic aneurysm, see 34800-34826)

(For endovascular repair of iliac artery aneurysm, see 34900)

(For thoracic aortic aneurysm, see 33860-33875)

(For endovascular repair of thoracic aortic aneurysm, see Category III codes 0033T-0034T)

♦✿ 35001 Direct repair of aneurysm, pseudoaneurysm, or excision (partial or total) and graft insertion, with or without patch graft; for aneurysm and associated occlusive disease, carotid, subclavian artery, by neck incision

♦✿ 35002 for ruptured aneurysm, carotid, subclavian artery, by neck incision

♦✿ 35005 for aneurysm, pseudoaneurysm, and associated occlusive disease, vertebral artery

♦§ 35011 for aneurysm and associated occlusive disease, axillary-brachial artery, by arm incision

♦✿ 35013 for ruptured aneurysm, axillary-brachial artery, by arm incision

♦✿ 35021 for aneurysm, pseudoaneurysm, and associated occlusive disease, innominate, subclavian artery, by thoracic incision

♦✿ 35022 for ruptured aneurysm, innominate, subclavian artery, by thoracic incision

♦✿ 35045 for aneurysm, pseudoaneurysm, and associated occlusive disease, radial or ulnar artery

✿ 35081 for aneurysm, pseudoaneurysm, and associated occlusive disease, abdominal aorta

✿ 35082 for ruptured aneurysm, abdominal aorta

♦✿ 35091 for aneurysm, pseudoaneurysm, and associated occlusive disease, abdominal aorta involving visceral vessels (mesenteric, celiac, renal)

♦✿ 35092 for ruptured aneurysm, abdominal aorta involving visceral vessels (mesenteric, celiac, renal)

♦✿ 35102 for aneurysm, pseudoaneurysm, and associated occlusive disease, abdominal aorta involving iliac vessels (common, hypogastric, external)

♦✿ 35103 for ruptured aneurysm, abdominal aorta involving iliac vessels (common, hypogastric, external)

♦✿ 35111 for aneurysm, pseudoaneurysm, and associated occlusive disease, splenic artery

♦✿ 35112 for ruptured aneurysm, splenic artery

♦✿ 35121 for aneurysm, pseudoaneurysm, and associated occlusive disease, hepatic, celiac, renal, or mesenteric artery

♦✿ 35122 for ruptured aneurysm, hepatic, celiac, renal, or mesenteric artery

♦✿ 35131 for aneurysm, pseudoaneurysm, and associated occlusive disease, iliac artery (common, hypogastric, external)

♦✿ 35132 for ruptured aneurysm, iliac artery (common, hypogastric, external)

♦✿ 35141 for aneurysm, pseudoaneurysm, and associated occlusive disease, common femoral artery (profunda femoris, superficial femoral)

♦✿ 35142 for ruptured aneurysm, common femoral artery (profunda femoris, superficial femoral)

♦✿ 35151 for aneurysm, pseudoaneurysm, and associated occlusive disease, popliteal artery

♦✿ 35152 for ruptured aneurysm, popliteal artery

►(35161, 35162 have been deleted. To report, use 37799)◄

Repair Arteriovenous Fistula

§ 35180 Repair, congenital arteriovenous fistula; head and neck

✿ 35182 thorax and abdomen

§ 35184 extremities

§ 35188 Repair, acquired or traumatic arteriovenous fistula; head and neck

✿ 35189 thorax and abdomen

§ 35190 extremities

Surgery: Cardiovascular System

Repair Blood Vessel Other Than for Fistula, With or Without Patch Angioplasty

(For AV fistula repair, see 35180-35190)

♦§ **35201** Repair blood vessel, direct; neck

♦§ **35206** upper extremity

♦§ **35207** hand, finger

♦✿ **35211** intrathoracic, with bypass

♦✿ **35216** intrathoracic, without bypass

♦✿ **35221** intra-abdominal

♦§ **35226** lower extremity

♦§ **35231** Repair blood vessel with vein graft; neck

♦§ **35236** upper extremity

♦✿ **35241** intrathoracic, with bypass

♦✿ **35246** intrathoracic, without bypass

♦✿ **35251** intra-abdominal

♦§ **35256** lower extremity

♦§ **35261** Repair blood vessel with graft other than vein; neck

♦§ **35266** upper extremity

♦✿ **35271** intrathoracic, with bypass

♦✿ **35276** intrathoracic, without bypass

♦✿ **35281** intra-abdominal

♦§ **35286** lower extremity

Thromboendarterectomy

(For coronary artery, see 33510-33536 and 33572)

♦✿ **35301** Thromboendarterectomy, with or without patch graft; carotid, vertebral, subclavian, by neck incision

♦✿ **35311** subclavian, innominate, by thoracic incision

♦§ **35321** axillary-brachial

♦✿ **35331** abdominal aorta

♦✿ **35341** mesenteric, celiac, or renal

♦✿ **35351** iliac

♦✿ **35355** iliofemoral

♦✿ **35361** combined aortoiliac

♦✿ **35363** combined aortoiliofemoral

♦✿ **35371** common femoral

♦✿ **35372** deep (profunda) femoral

♦✿ **35381** femoral and/or popliteal, and/or tibioperoneal

♦✿+ **35390** Reoperation, carotid, thromboendarterectomy, more than one month after original operation (List separately in addition to code for primary procedure)

(Use 35390 in conjunction with 35301)

Angioscopy

✿+ **35400** Angioscopy (non-coronary vessels or grafts) during therapeutic intervention (List separately in addition to code for primary procedure)

Transluminal Angioplasty

If done as part of another operation, use modifier 51 or use modifier 52.

(For radiological supervision and interpretation, see 75962-75968 and 75978)

Open

♦✿ **35450** Transluminal balloon angioplasty, open; renal or other visceral artery

♦✿ **35452** aortic

♦✿ **35454** iliac

♦✿ **35456** femoral-popliteal

♦§ **35458** brachiocephalic trunk or branches, each vessel

♦§ **35459** tibioperoneal trunk and branches

♦§ **35460** venous

Percutaneous

Codes for catheter placement and the radiologic supervision and interpretation should also be reported, in addition to the code(s) for the therapeutic aspect of the procedure.

♦§⊙ **35470** Transluminal balloon angioplasty, percutaneous; tibioperoneal trunk or branches, each vessel

♦§⊙ **35471** renal or visceral artery

♦§⊙ **35472** aortic

♦§⊙ **35473** iliac

♦§⊙ **35474** femoral-popliteal

♦§⊙ **35475** brachiocephalic trunk or branches, each vessel

♦§⊙ **35476** venous

(For radiological supervision and interpretation, use 75978)

Transluminal Atherectomy

If done as part of another operation, use modifier 51 or use modifier 52.

(For radiological supervision and interpretation, see 75992-75996)

Open

✿ 35480 Transluminal peripheral atherectomy, open; renal or other visceral artery

✿ 35481 aortic

✿ 35482 iliac

✿ 35483 femoral-popliteal

§ 35484 brachiocephalic trunk or branches, each vessel

§ 35485 tibioperoneal trunk and branches

Percutaneous

Codes for catheter placement and the radiologic supervision and interpretation should also be reported, in addition to the code(s) for the therapeutic aspect of the procedure.

§ 35490 Transluminal peripheral atherectomy, percutaneous; renal or other visceral artery

§ 35491 aortic

§ 35492 iliac

§ 35493 femoral-popliteal

§ 35494 brachiocephalic trunk or branches, each vessel

§ 35495 tibioperoneal trunk and branches

Bypass Graft

Vein

Procurement of the saphenous vein graft is included in the description of the work for 35501-35587 and should not be reported as a separate service or co-surgery. To report harvesting of an upper extremity vein, use 35500 in addition to the bypass procedure. To report harvesting of a femoropopliteal vein segment, use 35572 in addition to the bypass procedure. To report harvesting and construction of an autogenous composite graft of two segments from two distant locations, report 35682 in addition to the bypass procedure, for autogenous composite of three or more segments from distant sites, report 35683.

♦☆+ 35500 Harvest of upper extremity vein, one segment, for lower extremity or coronary artery bypass procedure (List separately in addition to code for primary procedure)

(Use 35500 in conjunction with 33510-33536, 35556, 35566, 35571, 35583-35587)

(For harvest of more than one vein segment, see 35682, 35683)

(For endoscopic procedure, use 33508)

♦✿ 35501 Bypass graft, with vein; carotid

♦✿ 35506 carotid-subclavian

♦✿ 35507 subclavian-carotid

♦✿ 35508 carotid-vertebral

♦✿ 35509 carotid-carotid

♦✿ 35510 carotid-brachial

♦✿ 35511 subclavian-subclavian

♦✿ 35512 subclavian-brachial

♦✿ 35515 subclavian-vertebral

♦✿ 35516 subclavian-axillary

♦✿ 35518 axillary-axillary

♦✿ 35521 axillary-femoral

(For bypass graft performed with synthetic graft, use 35621)

♦✿ 35522 axillary-brachial

♦✿ 35525 brachial-brachial

♦✿ 35526 aortosubclavian or carotid

(For bypass graft performed with synthetic graft, use 35626)

♦✿ 35531 aortoceliac or aortomesenteric

♦✿ 35533 axillary-femoral-femoral

(For bypass graft performed with synthetic graft, use 35654)

♦✿ 35536 splenorenal

✿ 35541 aortoiliac or bi-iliac

(For bypass graft performed with synthetic graft, use 35641)

♦✿ 35546 aortofemoral or bifemoral

(For bypass graft performed with synthetic graft, use 35646)

⌘✿ 35548 aortoiliofemoral, unilateral

(For bypass graft performed with synthetic graft, use 37799)

✶✿ 35549 aortoiliofemoral, bilateral

(For bypass graft performed with synthetic graft, use 37799)

♦✿ 35551 aortofemoral-popliteal

♦✿ 35556 femoral-popliteal

♦✿ 35558 femoral-femoral

♦✿ 35560 aortorenal

♦✿ 35563 ilioiliac

♦✿ 35565 iliofemoral

♦✿ 35566 femoral-anterior tibial, posterior tibial, peroneal artery or other distal vessels

♦✿ 35571 popliteal-tibial, -peroneal artery or other distal vessels

Surgery: Cardiovascular System

☆+ 35572 Harvest of femoropopliteal vein, one segment, for vascular reconstruction procedure (eg, aortic, vena caval, coronary, peripheral artery) (List separately in addition to code for primary procedure)

➲ *CPT Changes: An Insider's View* 2003

(Use 35572 in conjunction with 33510-33516, 33517-33523, 33533-33536, 34502, 34520, 35001, 35002, 35011-35022, 35102, 35103, 35121-35152, 35231-35256, 35501-35587, ►35879◄-35907)

(For bilateral procedure, use modifier 50)

In-Situ Vein

►(35582 has been deleted)◄

♦✿ 35583 In-situ vein bypass; femoral-popliteal

► (To report aortobifemoral bypass using synthetic conduit, and femoral-popliteal bypass with vein conduit in-situ, use 35646 and 35583. To report aorto(uni)femoral bypass with synthetic conduit, and femoral-popliteal bypass with vein conduit in-situ, use 35647 and 35583. To report aortofemoral bypass using vein conduit, and femoral-popliteal bypass with vein conduit in-situ, use 35546 and 35583)◄

♦✿ 35585 femoral-anterior tibial, posterior tibial, or peroneal artery

♦✿ 35587 popliteal-tibial, peroneal

Other Than Vein

(For arterial transposition and/or reimplantation, see 35691-35695)

♦✿⊘ 35600 Harvest of upper extremity artery, one segment, for coronary artery bypass procedure

♦✿ 35601 Bypass graft, with other than vein; carotid

♦✿ 35606 carotid-subclavian

(For open subclavian to carotid artery transposition performed in conjunction with endovascular thoracic aneurysm repair, use Category III code 0037T)

♦✿ 35612 subclavian-subclavian

♦✿ 35616 subclavian-axillary

♦✿ 35621 axillary-femoral

♦✿ 35623 axillary-popliteal or -tibial

♦✿ 35626 aortosubclavian or carotid

♦✿ 35631 aortoceliac, aortomesenteric, aortorenal

♦✿ 35636 splenorenal (splenic to renal arterial anastomosis)

✿ 35641 aortoiliac or bi-iliac

(For open placement of aorto-bi-iliac prosthesis following unsuccessful endovascular repair, use 34831)

♦✿ 35642 carotid-vertebral

♦✿ 35645 subclavian-vertebral

✿ 35646 aortobifemoral

(For open placement of aortobifemoral prosthesis following unsuccessful endovascular repair, use 34832)

♦✿ 35647 aortofemoral

♦✿ 35650 axillary-axillary

♦✿ 35651 aortofemoral-popliteal

✿ 35654 axillary-femoral-femoral

♦✿ 35656 femoral-popliteal

♦✿ 35661 femoral-femoral

♦✿ 35663 ilioiliac

♦✿ 35665 iliofemoral

♦✿ 35666 femoral-anterior tibial, posterior tibial, or peroneal artery

♦✿ 35671 popliteal-tibial or -peroneal artery

Composite Grafts

Codes 35682-35683 are used to report harvest and anastomosis of multiple vein segments from distant sites for use as arterial bypass graft conduits. These codes are intended for use when the two or more vein segments are harvested from a limb other than that undergoing bypass. Add-on codes 35682 and 35683 may be reported in addition to codes 35556, 35566, 35571, 35583-35587, as appropriate.

♦✿+ 35681 Bypass graft; composite, prosthetic and vein (List separately in addition to code for primary procedure)

(Do not report 35681 in addition to 35682, 35683)

✿+ 35682 autogenous composite, two segments of veins from two locations (List separately in addition to code for primary procedure)

(Do not report 35682 in addition to 35681, 35683)

✿+ 35683 autogenous composite, three or more segments of vein from two or more locations (List separately in addition to code for primary procedure)

(Do not report 35683 in addition to 35681, 35682)

Adjuvant Techniques

Adjuvant (additional) technique(s) may be required at the time a bypass graft is created to improve patency of the lower extremity autogenous or synthetic bypass graft (eg, femoral-popliteal, femoral-tibial, or popliteal-tibial arteries). Code 35685 should be reported in addition to the primary synthetic bypass graft procedure, when an interposition of venous tissue (vein patch or cuff) is placed at the anastomosis between the synthetic bypass conduit and the involved artery (includes harvest).

Surgery: Cardiovascular System

Code 35686 should be reported in addition to the primary bypass graft procedure, when autogenous vein is used to create a fistula between the tibial or peroneal artery and vein at or beyond the distal bypass anastomosis site of the involved artery.

(For composite graft(s), see 35681-35683)

♦§+ **35685** Placement of vein patch or cuff at distal anastomosis of bypass graft, synthetic conduit (List separately in addition to code for primary procedure)

(Use 35685 in conjunction with 35656, 35666, or 35671)

♦§+ **35686** Creation of distal arteriovenous fistula during lower extremity bypass surgery (non-hemodialysis) (List separately in addition to code for primary procedure)

(Use 35686 in conjunction with 35556, 35566, 35571, 35583-35587, 35623, 35656, 35666, 35671)

Arterial Transposition

♦✿ **35691** Transposition and/or reimplantation; vertebral to carotid artery

♦✿ **35693** vertebral to subclavian artery

♦✿ **35694** subclavian to carotid artery

(For open subclavian to carotid artery transposition performed in conjunction with endovascular thoracic aneurysm repair, use Category III code 0037T)

♦✿ **35695** carotid to subclavian artery

✿+ **35697** Reimplantation, visceral artery to infrarenal aortic prosthesis, each artery (List separately in addition to code for primary procedure)

(Do not report 35697 in conjunction with 33877)

Exploration/Revision

♦✿+ **35700** Reoperation, femoral-popliteal or femoral (popliteal)-anterior tibial, posterior tibial, peroneal artery or other distal vessels, more than one month after original operation (List separately in addition to code for primary procedure)

(Use 35700 in conjunction with 35556, 35566, 35571, 35583, 35585, 35587, 35656, 35666, 35671)

♦✿ **35701** Exploration (not followed by surgical repair), with or without lysis of artery; carotid artery

♦✿ **35721** femoral artery

♦✿ **35741** popliteal artery

♦§ **35761** other vessels

✿ **35800** Exploration for postoperative hemorrhage, thrombosis or infection; neck

✿ **35820** chest

✿ **35840** abdomen

§ **35860** extremity

✿ **35870** Repair of graft-enteric fistula

§ **35875** Thrombectomy of arterial or venous graft (other than hemodialysis graft or fistula);

§ **35876** with revision of arterial or venous graft

(For thrombectomy of hemodialysis graft or fistula, see 36831, 36833)

Codes 35879 and 35881 describe open revision of graft-threatening stenoses of lower extremity arterial bypass graft(s) (previously constructed with autogenous vein conduit) using vein patch angioplasty or segmental vein interposition techniques. For thrombectomy with revision of any non-coronary arterial or venous graft, including those of the lower extremity, (other than hemodialysis graft or fistula), use 35876. For direct repair (other than for fistula) of a lower extremity blood vessel (with or without patch angioplasty), use 35226. For repair (other than for fistula) of a lower extremity blood vessel using a vein graft, use 35256.

♦§ **35879** Revision, lower extremity arterial bypass, without thrombectomy, open; with vein patch angioplasty

♦§ **35881** with segmental vein interposition

(For excision of infected graft, see 35901-35907 and appropriate revascularization code)

✿ **35901** Excision of infected graft; neck

§ **35903** extremity

✿ **35905** thorax

✿ **35907** abdomen

Vascular Injection Procedures

Listed services for injection procedures include necessary local anesthesia, introduction of needles or catheter, injection of contrast media with or without automatic power injection, and/or necessary pre- and postinjection care specifically related to the injection procedure.

Catheters, drugs, and contrast media are not included in the listed service for the injection procedures.

Selective vascular catheterization should be coded to include introduction and all lesser order selective catheterization used in the approach (eg, the description for a selective right middle cerebral artery catheterization includes the introduction and placement catheterization of the right common and internal carotid arteries).

Additional second and/or third order arterial catheterization within the same family of arteries or veins supplied by a single first order vessel should be expressed by 36012, 36218 or 36248.

Additional first order or higher catheterization in vascular families supplied by a first order vessel different from a previously selected and coded family should be separately coded using the conventions described above.

(For radiological supervision and interpretation, see **Radiology**)

(For injection procedures in conjunction with cardiac catheterization, see 93541-93545)

(For chemotherapy of malignant disease, see 96400-96549)

Intravenous

An intracatheter is a sheathed combination of needle and short catheter.

♦☆ **36000** Introduction of needle or intracatheter, vein

♦❖ **36002** Injection procedures (eg, thrombin) for percutaneous treatment of extremity pseudoaneurysm

(For imaging guidance, see 76003, 76360, 76393, or 76942)

(For ultrasound guided compression repair of pseudoaneurysms, use 76936)

(Do not report 36002 for vascular sealant of an arteriotomy site)

☆ **36005** Injection procedure for extremity venography (including introduction of needle or intracatheter)

➲ *CPT Changes: An Insider's View* 2002

(For radiological supervision and interpretation, see 75820, 75822)

♦☆ **36010** Introduction of catheter, superior or inferior vena cava

♦☆ **36011** Selective catheter placement, venous system; first order branch (eg, renal vein, jugular vein)

♦☆ **36012** second order, or more selective, branch (eg, left adrenal vein, petrosal sinus)

☆ **36013** Introduction of catheter, right heart or main pulmonary artery

♦☆ **36014** Selective catheter placement, left or right pulmonary artery

♦☆ **36015** Selective catheter placement, segmental or subsegmental pulmonary artery

(For insertion of flow directed catheter (eg, Swan-Ganz), use 93503)

(For venous catheterization for selective organ blood sampling, use 36500)

Intra-Arterial—Intra-Aortic

(For radiological supervision and interpretation, see **Radiology**)

♦☆ **36100** Introduction of needle or intracatheter, carotid or vertebral artery

(For bilateral procedure, report 36100 with modifier 50)

☆ **36120** Introduction of needle or intracatheter; retrograde brachial artery

☆ **36140** extremity artery

☆ **36145** arteriovenous shunt created for dialysis (cannula, fistula, or graft)

(For insertion of arteriovenous cannula, see 36810-36821)

☆ **36160** Introduction of needle or intracatheter, aortic, translumbar

♦☆ **36200** Introduction of catheter, aorta

♦☆ **36215** Selective catheter placement, arterial system; each first order thoracic or brachiocephalic branch, within a vascular family

(For catheter placement for coronary angiography, use 93508)

♦☆ **36216** initial second order thoracic or brachiocephalic branch, within a vascular family

♦☆ **36217** initial third order or more selective thoracic or brachiocephalic branch, within a vascular family

☆+ **36218** additional second order, third order, and beyond, thoracic or brachiocephalic branch, within a vascular family (List in addition to code for initial second or third order vessel as appropriate)

(Use 36218 in conjunction with 36216, 36217)

(For angiography, see 75600-75790)

(For angioplasty, see 35470-35475)

(For transcatheter therapies, see 37200-37208, 61624, 61626)

(When coronary artery, arterial conduit (eg, internal mammary, inferior epigastric or free radical artery) or venous bypass graft angiography is performed in conjunction with cardiac catheterization, see the appropriate cardiac catheterization, injection procedure, and imaging supervision code(s) (93501-93556) in the **Medicine** section of *CPT*. When coronary artery, arterial coronary conduit or venous bypass graft angiography is performed without concomitant left heart cardiac catheterization, use 93508. When internal mammary artery angiography only is performed without a concomitant left heart cardiac catheterization, use 36216 or 36217 as appropriate.)

♦☆ **36245** Selective catheter placement, arterial system; each first order abdominal, pelvic, or lower extremity artery branch, within a vascular family
➲ *CPT Assistant* Apr 03:12

♦☆ **36246** initial second order abdominal, pelvic, or lower extremity artery branch, within a vascular family
➲ *CPT Assistant* Apr 03:12

♦☆ **36247** initial third order or more selective abdominal, pelvic, or lower extremity artery branch, within a vascular family

☆+ **36248** additional second order, third order, and beyond, abdominal, pelvic, or lower extremity artery branch, within a vascular family (List in addition to code for initial second or third order vessel as appropriate)

(Use 36248 in conjunction with 36246, 36247)

§ **36260** Insertion of implantable intra-arterial infusion pump (eg, for chemotherapy of liver)

§ **36261** Revision of implanted intra-arterial infusion pump

§ **36262** Removal of implanted intra-arterial infusion pump

☆ **36299** Unlisted procedure, vascular injection

Venous

Venipuncture, needle or catheter for diagnostic study or intravenous therapy, percutaneous.

☆ **36400** Venipuncture, under age 3 years, necessitating physician's skill, not to be used for routine venipuncture; femoral or jugular vein
➲ *CPT Changes: An Insider's View* 2002, 2004

☆ **36405** scalp vein

☆ **36406** other vein

☆ **36410** Venipuncture, age 3 years or older, necessitating physician's skill (separate procedure), for diagnostic or therapeutic purposes (not to be used for routine venipuncture)
➲ *CPT Changes: An Insider's View* 2004

□ **36415** Collection of venous blood by venipuncture
➲ *CPT Assistant* Apr 03:8

(Do not report modifier 63 in conjunction with 36415)

□ **36416** Collection of capillary blood specimen (eg, finger, heel, ear stick)
➲ *CPT Assistant* Apr 03:8

§ **36420** Venipuncture, cutdown; under age 1 year

(Do not report modifier 63 in conjunction with 36420)

§ **36425** age 1 or over

❖ **36430** Transfusion, blood or blood components
➲ *CPT Assistant* Apr 03:9

❖ **36440** Push transfusion, blood, 2 years or under
➲ *CPT Assistant* Apr 03:9

❖ **36450** Exchange transfusion, blood; newborn
➲ *CPT Assistant* Apr 03:9

(Do not report modifier 63 in conjunction with 36450)

❖ **36455** other than newborn
➲ *CPT Assistant* Apr 03:9

❖ **36460** Transfusion, intrauterine, fetal
➲ *CPT Assistant* Apr 03:9

(Do not report modifier 63 in conjunction with 36460)

(For radiological supervision and interpretation, use 76941)

§ **36468** Single or multiple injections of sclerosing solutions, spider veins (telangiectasia); limb or trunk

§ **36469** face

♦§ **36470** Injection of sclerosing solution; single vein

♦§ **36471** multiple veins, same leg

♦§● **36475** Endovenous ablation therapy of incompetent vein, extremity, inclusive of all imaging guidance and monitoring, percutaneous, radiofrequency; first vein treated
➲ *CPT Changes: An Insider's View* 2005

♦§ +● **36476** second and subsequent veins treated in a single extremity, each through separate access sites (List separately in addition to code for primary procedure)
➲ *CPT Changes: An Insider's View* 2005

►(Use 36476 in conjunction with 36475)◄

►(Do not report 36475, 36476 in conjunction with 36000-36005, 36410, 36425, 36478, 36479, 37204, 75894, 76000-76003, 76937, 76942, 93970, 93971)◄

♦§● **36478** Endovenous ablation therapy of incompetent vein, extremity, inclusive of all imaging guidance and monitoring, percutaneous, laser; first vein treated
➲ *CPT Changes: An Insider's View* 2005

♦§ +● **36479** second and subsequent veins treated in a single extremity, each through separate access sites (List separately in addition to code for primary procedure)
➲ *CPT Changes: An Insider's View* 2005

►(Use 36479 in conjunction with 36478)◄

►(Do not report 36478, 36479 in conjunction with 36000-36005, 36410, 36425, 36475, 36476, 37204, 75894, 76000-76003, 76937, 76942, 93970, 93971)◄

☆ **36481** Percutaneous portal vein catheterization by any method

(For radiological supervision and interpretation, see 75885, 75887)

(36488-36491 have been deleted. To report, see 36555-36556, 36568-36569, 36580, 36584)

(36493 has been deleted. To report, use 36597)

☆ **36500** Venous catheterization for selective organ blood sampling

(For catheterization in superior or inferior vena cava, use 36010)

(For radiological supervision and interpretation, use 75893)

✿ **36510** Catheterization of umbilical vein for diagnosis or therapy, newborn

(Do not report modifier 63 in conjunction with 36510)

❖ **36511** Therapeutic apheresis; for white blood cells

➔ *CPT Changes: An Insider's View* 2003

❖ **36512** for red blood cells

➔ *CPT Changes: An Insider's View* 2003

❖ **36513** for platelets

➔ *CPT Changes: An Insider's View* 2003

❖ **36514** for plasma pheresis

➔ *CPT Changes: An Insider's View* 2003

❖ **36515** with extracorporeal immunoadsorption and plasma reinfusion

➔ *CPT Changes: An Insider's View* 2003

❖ **36516** with extracorporeal selective adsorption or selective filtration and plasma reinfusion

➔ *CPT Changes: An Insider's View* 2003

(For physician evaluation, use modifier 26)

(36520 has been deleted. To report, see 36511-36512)

(36521 has been deleted. To report, use 36515, 36516)

❖ **36522** Photopheresis, extracorporeal

(36530 has been deleted. To report, use 36563)

(36531 has been deleted. To report, see 36575-36576, 36578, 36581-36582, 36584-36585)

(36532 has been deleted. To report, use 36590)

(36533 has been deleted. To report, see 36557-36561, 36565-36566, 36570-36571)

(36534 has been deleted. To report, see 36575-36578, 36581-36583, 36585)

(36535 has been deleted. To report, use 36589)

(36536 has been deleted. To report, use 36595)

(36537 have been deleted. To report, use 36596)

☆ **36540** Collection of blood specimen from a completely implantable venous access device

➔ *CPT Changes: An Insider's View* 2001, 2003

(Do not report 36540 in conjunction with 36415, 36416)

(For collection of venous blood specimen by venipuncture, use 36415)

(For collection of capillary blood specimen, use 36416)

§ **36550** Declotting by thrombolytic agent of implanted vascular access device or catheter

➔ *CPT Changes: An Insider's View* 2000

Central Venous Access Procedures

To qualify as a central venous access catheter or device, the tip of the catheter/device must terminate in the subclavian, brachiocephalic (innominate) or iliac veins, the superior or inferior vena cava, or the right atrium. The venous access device may be either centrally inserted (jugular, subclavian, femoral vein or inferior vena cava catheter entry site) or peripherally inserted (eg, basilic or cephalic vein). The device may be accessed for use either via exposed catheter (external to the skin), via a subcutaneous port or via a subcutaneous pump.

The procedures involving these types of devices fall into five categories:

1) ***Insertion*** (placement of catheter through a newly established venous access)

2) ***Repair*** (fixing device without replacement of either catheter or port/pump, other than pharmacologic or mechanical correction of intracatheter or pericatheter occlusion (see 36595 or 36596))

3) ***Partial replacement*** of only the catheter component associated with a port/pump device, but not entire device

4) ***Complete replacement*** of entire device via same venous access site (complete exchange)

5) ***Removal*** of entire device.

There is no coding distinction between venous access achieved percutaneously versus by cutdown or based on catheter size.

For the repair, partial (catheter only) replacement, complete replacement, or removal of both catheters (placed from separate venous access sites) of a multi-catheter device, with or without subcutaneous ports/pumps, use the appropriate code describing the service with a frequency of two.

If an existing central venous access device is removed and a new one placed via a separate venous access site, appropriate codes for both procedures (removal of old, if code exists, and insertion of new device) should be reported.

When imaging is used for these procedures, either for gaining access to the venous entry site or for manipulating the catheter into final central position, use 76937, 75998.

(For refilling and maintenance of an implantable pump or reservoir for intravenous or intra-arterial drug delivery, use 96530)

Insertion of Central Venous Access Device

§⊙ **36555** Insertion of non-tunneled centrally inserted central venous catheter; under 5 years of age
➔ *CPT Changes: An Insider's View* 2004

(For peripherally inserted non-tunneled central venous catheter, under 5 years of age, use 36568)

§ **36556** age 5 years or older
➔ *CPT Changes: An Insider's View* 2004

(For peripherally inserted non-tunneled central venous catheter, age 5 years or older, use 36569)

♦§⊙ **36557** Insertion of tunneled centrally inserted central venous catheter, without subcutaneous port or pump; under 5 years of age
➔ *CPT Changes: An Insider's View* 2004

♦§⊙ **36558** age 5 years or older
➔ *CPT Changes: An Insider's View* 2004

(For peripherally inserted central venous catheter with port, 5 years or older, use 36571)

♦§⊙ **36560** Insertion of tunneled centrally inserted central venous access device, with subcutaneous port; under 5 years of age
➔ *CPT Changes: An Insider's View* 2004

(For peripherally inserted central venous access device with subcutaneous port, under 5 years of age, use 36570)

♦§⊙ **36561** age 5 years or older
➔ *CPT Changes: An Insider's View* 2004

(For peripherally inserted central venous catheter with subcutaneous port, 5 years or older, use 36571)

§⊙ **36563** Insertion of tunneled centrally inserted central venous access device with subcutaneous pump
➔ *CPT Changes: An Insider's View* 2004

♦§⊙ **36565** Insertion of tunneled centrally inserted central venous access device, requiring two catheters via two separate venous access sites; without subcutaneous port or pump (eg, Tesio type catheter)
➔ *CPT Changes: An Insider's View* 2004

♦§⊙ **36566** with subcutaneous port(s)
➔ *CPT Changes: An Insider's View* 2004

§⊙ **36568** Insertion of peripherally inserted central venous catheter (PICC), without subcutaneous port or pump; under 5 years of age
➔ *CPT Changes: An Insider's View* 2004

(For placement of centrally inserted non-tunneled central venous catheter, without subcutaneous port or pump, under 5 years of age, use 36555)

§ **36569** age 5 years or older
➔ *CPT Changes: An Insider's View* 2004

(For placement of centrally inserted non-tunneled central venous catheter, without subcutaneous port or pump, age 5 years or older, use 36556)

♦§⊙ **36570** Insertion of peripherally inserted central venous access device, with subcutaneous port; under 5 years of age
➔ *CPT Changes: An Insider's View* 2004

(For insertion of tunneled centrally inserted central venous access device with subcutaneous port, under 5 years of age, use 36560)

♦§⊙ **36571** age 5 years or older
➔ *CPT Changes: An Insider's View* 2004

(For insertion of tunneled centrally inserted central venous access device with subcutaneous port, age 5 years or older, use 36561)

Repair of Central Venous Access Device

(For mechanical removal of pericatheter obstructive material, use 36595)

(For mechanical removal of intracatheter obstructive material, use 36596)

§ **36575** Repair of tunneled or non-tunneled central venous access catheter, without subcutaneous port or pump, central or peripheral insertion site
➔ *CPT Changes: An Insider's View* 2004

§⊙ **36576** Repair of central venous access device, with subcutaneous port or pump, central or peripheral insertion site
➔ *CPT Changes: An Insider's View* 2004

Partial Replacement of Central Venous Access Device (Catheter Only)

§⊙ **36578** Replacement, catheter only, of central venous access device, with subcutaneous port or pump, central or peripheral insertion site
➔ *CPT Changes: An Insider's View* 2004

(For complete replacement of entire device through same venous access, use 36582 or 36583)

Complete Replacement of Central Venous Access Device Through Same Venous Access Site

§ **36580** Replacement, complete, of a non-tunneled centrally inserted central venous catheter, without subcutaneous port or pump, through same venous access
➔ *CPT Changes: An Insider's View* 2004

§⊙ **36581** Replacement, complete, of a tunneled centrally inserted central venous catheter, without subcutaneous port or pump, through same venous access
➔ *CPT Changes: An Insider's View* 2004

§⊙ **36582** Replacement, complete, of a tunneled centrally inserted central venous access device, with subcutaneous port, through same venous access
➔ *CPT Changes: An Insider's View* 2004

§⊙ **36583** Replacement, complete, of a tunneled centrally inserted central venous access device, with subcutaneous pump, through same venous access
➔ *CPT Changes: An Insider's View* 2004

§ **36584** Replacement, complete, of a peripherally inserted central venous catheter (PICC), without subcutaneous port or pump, through same venous access
➔ *CPT Changes: An Insider's View* 2004

§⊙ **36585** Replacement, complete, of a peripherally inserted central venous access device, with subcutaneous port, through same venous access
➔ *CPT Changes: An Insider's View* 2004

Removal of Central Venous Access Device

♦§ **36589** Removal of tunneled central venous catheter, without subcutaneous port or pump
➔ *CPT Changes: An Insider's View* 2004

§⊙ **36590** Removal of tunneled central venous access device, with subcutaneous port or pump, central or peripheral insertion
➔ *CPT Changes: An Insider's View* 2004

(Do not report 36589 or 36590 for removal of non-tunneled central venous catheters)

Mechanical Removal of Obstructive Material

§ **36595** Mechanical removal of pericatheter obstructive material (eg, fibrin sheath) from central venous device via separate venous access
➔ *CPT Changes: An Insider's View* 2004

(Do not report 36550 in addition to 36595)

(For venous catheterization, see 36010-36012)

(For radiological supervision and interpretation, use 75901)

§ **36596** Mechanical removal of intraluminal (intracatheter) obstructive material from central venous device through device lumen
➔ *CPT Changes: An Insider's View* 2004

(Do not report 36550 in addition to 36596)

(For venous catheterization, see 36010-36012)

(For radiological supervision and interpretation, use 75902)

Other Central Venous Access Procedures

§ **36597** Repositioning of previously placed central venous catheter under fluoroscopic guidance
➔ *CPT Changes: An Insider's View* 2004

(For fluoroscopic guidance, use 76000)

Arterial

☆ **36600** Arterial puncture, withdrawal of blood for diagnosis

☆⊘ **36620** Arterial catheterization or cannulation for sampling, monitoring or transfusion (separate procedure); percutaneous

☆ **36625** cutdown

§ **36640** Arterial catheterization for prolonged infusion therapy (chemotherapy), cutdown

(See also 96420-96425)

(For arterial catheterization for occlusion therapy, see 75894)

✿⊘ **36660** Catheterization, umbilical artery, newborn, for diagnosis or therapy

(Do not report modifier 63 in conjunction with 36660)

Intraosseous

§ **36680** Placement of needle for intraosseous infusion

Hemodialysis Access, Intervascular Cannulation for Extracorporeal Circulation, or Shunt Insertion

§ **36800** Insertion of cannula for hemodialysis, other purpose (separate procedure); vein to vein

§ **36810** arteriovenous, external (Scribner type)

§ **36815** arteriovenous, external revision, or closure

§● **36818** Arteriovenous anastomosis, open; by upper arm cephalic vein transposition
➔ *CPT Changes: An Insider's View* 2005

►(Do not report 36818 in conjunction with 36819, 36820, 36821, 36830 during a unilateral upper extremity procedure. For bilateral upper extremity open arteriovenous anastomoses performed at the same operative session, use modifier 50 or 59 as appropriate)◄

§ **36819** by upper arm basilic vein transposition
➔ *CPT Changes: An Insider's View* 2000, 2002

►(Do not report 36819 in conjunction with 36818, 36820, 36821, 36830 during a unilateral upper extremity procedure. For bilateral upper extremity open arteriovenous anastomoses performed at the same operative session, use modifier 50 or 59 as appropriate)◄

♦§ **36820** by forearm vein transposition
➔ *CPT Changes: An Insider's View* 2002

§ **36821** direct, any site (eg, Cimino type) (separate procedure)
➔ *CPT Changes: An Insider's View* 2000

✿ **36822** Insertion of cannula(s) for prolonged extracorporeal circulation for cardiopulmonary insufficiency (ECMO) (separate procedure)

(For maintenance of prolonged extracorporeal circulation, see 33960, 33961)

✿ **36823** Insertion of arterial and venous cannula(s) for isolated extracorporeal circulation including regional chemotherapy perfusion to an extremity, with or without hyperthermia, with removal of cannula(s) and repair of arteriotomy and venotomy sites

(36823 includes chemotherapy perfusion supported by a membrane oxygenator/perfusion pump. Do not report 96408-96425 in conjunction with 36823)

§ **36825** Creation of arteriovenous fistula by other than direct arteriovenous anastomosis (separate procedure); autogenous graft

(For direct arteriovenous anastomosis, use 36821)

§ **36830** nonautogenous graft (eg, biological collagen, thermoplastic graft)

➔ *CPT Changes: An Insider's View* 2003

(For direct arteriovenous anastomosis, use 36821)

§ **36831** Thrombectomy, open, arteriovenous fistula without revision, autogenous or nonautogenous dialysis graft (separate procedure)

➔ *CPT Changes: An Insider's View* 2001

§ **36832** Revision, open, arteriovenous fistula; without thrombectomy, autogenous or nonautogenous dialysis graft (separate procedure)

➔ *CPT Changes: An Insider's View* 2000, 2001

§ **36833** with thrombectomy, autogenous or nonautogenous dialysis graft (separate procedure)

§ **36834** Plastic repair of arteriovenous aneurysm (separate procedure)

§ **36835** Insertion of Thomas shunt (separate procedure)

♦§ **36838** Distal revascularization and interval ligation (DRIL), upper extremity hemodialysis access (steal syndrome)

➔ *CPT Changes: An Insider's View* 2004

(Do not report 36838 in conjunction with 35512, 35522, 36832, 37607, 37618)

§ **36860** External cannula declotting (separate procedure); without balloon catheter

§ **36861** with balloon catheter

(If imaging guidance is performed, use 76000)

♦§⊙ **36870** Thrombectomy, percutaneous, arteriovenous fistula, autogenous or nonautogenous graft (includes mechanical thrombus extraction and intra-graft thrombolysis)

➔ *CPT Changes: An Insider's View* 2001

(Do not report 36550 in conjunction with 36870)

(For catheterization, use 36145)

(For radiological supervision and interpretation, use 75790)

Portal Decompression Procedures

✿ **37140** Venous anastomosis, open; portocaval

(For peritoneal-venous shunt, use 49425)

✿ **37145** renoportal

✿ **37160** caval-mesenteric

✿ **37180** splenorenal, proximal

✿ **37181** splenorenal, distal (selective decompression of esophagogastric varices, any technique)

(For percutaneous procedure, use 37182)

✿ **37182** Insertion of transvenous intrahepatic portosystemic shunt(s) (TIPS) (includes venous access, hepatic and portal vein catheterization, portography with hemodynamic evaluation, intrahepatic tract formation/dilatation, stent placement and all associated imaging guidance and documentation)

(Do not report 75885 or 75887 in conjunction with 37182)

(For open procedure, use 37140)

✿ **37183** Revision of transvenous intrahepatic portosystemic shunt(s) (TIPS) (includes venous access, hepatic and portal vein catheterization, portography with hemodynamic evaluation, intrahepatic tract recanulization/dilatation, stent placement and all associated imaging guidance and documentation)

(Do not report 75885 or 75887 in conjunction with 37183)

(For repair of arteriovenous aneurysm, use 36834)

Transcatheter Procedures

Codes for catheter placement and the radiologic supervision and interpretation should also be reported, in addition to the code(s) for the therapeutic aspect of the procedure.

✿ **37195** Thrombolysis, cerebral, by intravenous infusion

§ **37200** Transcatheter biopsy

(For radiological supervision and interpretation, use 75970)

§ **37201** Transcatheter therapy, infusion for thrombolysis other than coronary

(For radiological supervision and interpretation, use 75896)

§ **37202** Transcatheter therapy, infusion other than for thrombolysis, any type (eg, spasmolytic, vasoconstrictive)

(For thrombolysis of coronary vessels, see 92975, 92977)

(For radiological supervision and interpretation, use 75896)

§⊙ **37203** Transcatheter retrieval, percutaneous, of intravascular foreign body (eg, fractured venous or arterial catheter)

(For radiological supervision and interpretation, use 75961)

§ **37204** Transcatheter occlusion or embolization (eg, for tumor destruction, to achieve hemostasis, to occlude a vascular malformation), percutaneous, any method, non-central nervous system, non-head or neck

(See also 61624, 61626)

(For radiological supervision and interpretation, use 75894)

§▲ **37205** Transcatheter placement of an intravascular stent(s), (except coronary, carotid, and vertebral vessel), percutaneous; initial vessel

(For radiological supervision and interpretation, use 75960)

►(For coronary stent placement, see 92980, 92981)◄

§+ **37206** each additional vessel (List separately in addition to code for primary procedure)

(Use 37206 in conjunction with 37205)

(For transcatheter placement of ►intravascular cervical carotid◄ artery stent(s), see ►37215, 37216◄)

►(For transcatheter placement of extracranial vertebral or intrathoracic carotid artery stent(s), see Category III codes 0075T, 0076T)◄

(For radiological supervision and interpretation, use 75960)

♦§ **37207** Transcatheter placement of an intravascular stent(s), (non-coronary vessel), open; initial vessel

♦§+ **37208** each additional vessel (List separately in addition to code for primary procedure)

(Use 37208 in conjunction with 37207)

(For radiological supervision and interpretation, use 75960)

(For catheterizations, see 36215-36248)

(For transcatheter placement of intracoronary stent(s), see 92980, 92981)

§ **37209** Exchange of a previously placed arterial catheter during thrombolytic therapy

(For radiological supervision and interpretation, use 75900)

✿⊙● **37215** Transcatheter placement of intravascular stent(s), cervical carotid artery, percutaneous; with distal embolic protection

➲ *CPT Changes: An Insider's View* 2005

✿⊙● **37216** without distal embolic protection

➲ *CPT Changes: An Insider's View* 2005

►(37215 and 37216 include all ipsilateral selective carotid catheterization, all diagnostic imaging for ipsilateral, cervical and cerebral carotid arteriography, and all related radiological supervision and interpretation. When ipsilateral carotid arteriogram (including imaging and selective catheterization) confirms the need for carotid stenting, 37215 and 37216 are inclusive of these services. If carotid stenting is not indicated, then the appropriate codes for carotid catheterization and imaging should be reported in lieu of 37215 and 37216)◄

►(Do not report 37215, 37216 in conjunction with 75671, 75680)◄

►(For transcatheter placement of extracranial vertebral or intrathoracic carotid artery stent(s), see Category III codes 0075T, 0076T)◄

►(For percutaneous transcatheter placement of intravascular stents other than coronary, carotid, or vertebral, see 37205, 37206)◄

Intravascular Ultrasound Services

Intravascular ultrasound services include all transducer manipulations and repositioning within the specific vessel being examined, both before and after therapeutic intervention (eg, stent placement).

Vascular access for intravascular ultrasound performed during a therapeutic intervention is not reported separately.

❖+ **37250** Intravascular ultrasound (non-coronary vessel) during diagnostic evaluation and/or therapeutic intervention; initial vessel (List separately in addition to code for primary procedure)

➲ *CPT Changes: An Insider's View* 2000

❖+ **37251** each additional vessel (List separately in addition to code for primary procedure)

➲ *CPT Changes: An Insider's View* 2000

(Use 37251 in conjunction with 37250)

(For catheterizations, see 36215-36248)

(For transcatheter therapies, see 37200-37208, 61624, 61626)

(For radiological supervision and interpretation see 75945, 75946)

Endoscopy

Surgical vascular endoscopy always includes diagnostic endoscopy.

♦§ **37500** Vascular endoscopy, surgical, with ligation of perforator veins, subfascial (SEPS)

➲ *CPT Changes: An Insider's View* 2003

(For open procedure, use 37760)

♦§ **37501** Unlisted vascular endoscopy procedure

➲ *CPT Changes: An Insider's View* 2003

Ligation

(For phleborraphy and arteriorraphy, see 35201-35286)

§ 37565 Ligation, internal jugular vein

§ 37600 Ligation; external carotid artery

§ 37605 internal or common carotid artery

§ 37606 internal or common carotid artery, with gradual occlusion, as with Selverstone or Crutchfield clamp

(For transcatheter permanent arterial occlusion or embolization, see 61624-61626)

(For endovascular temporary arterial balloon occlusion, use 61623)

(For ligation treatment of intracranial aneurysm, use 61703)

§ 37607 Ligation or banding of angioaccess arteriovenous fistula

♦§ 37609 Ligation or biopsy, temporal artery

§ 37615 Ligation, major artery (eg, post-traumatic, rupture); neck

✿ 37616 chest

✿ 37617 abdomen

✿ 37618 extremity

§ 37620 Interruption, partial or complete, of inferior vena cava by suture, ligation, plication, clip, extravascular, intravascular (umbrella device)

(For radiological supervision and interpretation, use 75940)

♦§ 37650 Ligation of femoral vein

(For bilateral procedure, report 37650 with modifier 50)

✿ 37660 Ligation of common iliac vein

♦§ 37700 Ligation and division of long saphenous vein at saphenofemoral junction, or distal interruptions

(For bilateral procedure, report 37700 with modifier 50)

♦§ 37720 Ligation and division and complete stripping of long or short saphenous veins

(For bilateral procedure, report 37720 with modifier 50)

♦§ 37730 Ligation and division and complete stripping of long and short saphenous veins

(For bilateral procedure, report 37730 with modifier 50)

♦§ 37735 Ligation and division and complete stripping of long or short saphenous veins with radical excision of ulcer and skin graft and/or interruption of communicating veins of lower leg, with excision of deep fascia

(For bilateral procedure, report 37735 with modifier 50)

§ 37760 Ligation of perforator veins, subfascial, radical (Linton type), with or without skin graft, open

➔ *CPT Changes: An Insider's View* 2003

(For endoscopic procedure, use 37500)

♦§ 37765 Stab phlebectomy of varicose veins, one extremity; 10-20 stab incisions

➔ *CPT Changes: An Insider's View* 2004

(For less than 10 incisions, use 37799)

(For more than 20 incisions, use 37766)

♦§ 37766 more than 20 incisions

➔ *CPT Changes: An Insider's View* 2004

♦§ 37780 Ligation and division of short saphenous vein at saphenopopliteal junction (separate procedure)

(For bilateral procedure, report 37780 with modifier 50)

♦§ 37785 Ligation, division, and/or excision of varicose vein cluster(s), one leg

➔ *CPT Changes: An Insider's View* 2004

(For bilateral procedure, report 37785 with modifier 50)

Other Procedures

✿ 37788 Penile revascularization, artery, with or without vein graft

§ 37790 Penile venous occlusive procedure

§ 37799 Unlisted procedure, vascular surgery

Hemic and Lymphatic Systems

Spleen

Excision

✿ 38100 Splenectomy; total (separate procedure)

✿ 38101 partial (separate procedure)

✿+ 38102 total, en bloc for extensive disease, in conjunction with other procedure (List in addition to code for primary procedure)

Repair

✿ 38115 Repair of ruptured spleen (splenorrhaphy) with or without partial splenectomy

Laparoscopy

Surgical laparoscopy always includes diagnostic laparoscopy. To report a diagnostic laparoscopy (peritoneoscopy) (separate procedure), use 49320.

§ 38120 Laparoscopy, surgical, splenectomy

➔ *CPT Changes: An Insider's View* 2000

§ 38129 Unlisted laparoscopy procedure, spleen

➔ *CPT Changes: An Insider's View* 2000

Introduction

☆ **38200** Injection procedure for splenoportography

(For radiological supervision and interpretation, use 75810)

General

Bone Marrow or Stem Cell Services/Procedures

Codes 38207-38215 describe various steps used to preserve, prepare and purify bone marrow/stem cells prior to transplantation or reinfusion. Each code may be reported only once per day regardless of the quantity of bone marrow/stem cells manipulated.

□ **38204** Management of recipient hematopoietic progenitor cell donor search and cell acquisition
➲ *CPT Assistant* Apr 03:8

❖ **38205** Blood-derived hematopoietic progenitor cell harvesting for transplantation, per collection; allogenic
➲ *CPT Assistant* Apr 03:8; *CPT Changes: An Insider's View* 2003

❖ **38206** autologous
➲ *CPT Assistant* Apr 03:8; *CPT Changes: An Insider's View* 2003

□ **38207** Transplant preparation of hematopoietic progenitor cells; cryopreservation and storage
➲ *CPT Assistant* Apr 03:8

(For diagnostic cryopreservation and storage, see 88240)

□ **38208** thawing of previously frozen harvest, without washing
➲ *CPT Assistant* Apr 03:8; *CPT Changes: An Insider's View* 2004

(For diagnostic thawing and expansion of frozen cells, see 88241)

□ **38209** thawing of previously frozen harvest, with washing
➲ *CPT Assistant* Apr 03:8; *CPT Changes: An Insider's View* 2004

□ **38210** specific cell depletion within harvest, T-cell depletion
➲ *CPT Assistant* Apr 03:8

□ **38211** tumor cell depletion
➲ *CPT Assistant* Apr 03:8

□ **38212** red blood cell removal
➲ *CPT Assistant* Apr 03:8

□ **38213** platelet depletion
➲ *CPT Assistant* Apr 03:8

□ **38214** plasma (volume) depletion
➲ *CPT Assistant* Apr 03:8

□ **38215** cell concentration in plasma, mononuclear, or buffy coat layer
➲ *CPT Assistant* Apr 03:8

(Do not report 38207-38215 in conjunction with ►88182, 88184-88189◄)

♦§ **38220** Bone marrow; aspiration only
➲ *CPT Changes: An Insider's View* 2002, 2003

♦§ **38221** biopsy, needle or trocar
➲ *CPT Changes: An Insider's View* 2002, 2003

(For bone marrow biopsy interpretation, use 88305)

❖ **38230** Bone marrow harvesting for transplantation

(For autologous and allogenic blood-derived peripheral stem cell harvesting for transplantation, see 38205-38206)

(38231 has been deleted. To report, use 38205-38206)

❖ **38240** Bone marrow or blood-derived peripheral stem cell transplantation; allogenic
➲ *CPT Changes: An Insider's View* 2000

❖ **38241** autologous
➲ *CPT Changes: An Insider's View* 2000

❖ **38242** allogeneic donor lymphocyte infusions
➲ *CPT Changes: An Insider's View* 2003

(For bone marrow aspiration, use 38220)

(For modification, treatment, and processing of bone marrow or blood-derived stem cell specimens for transplantation, use 38210-38213)

(For cryopreservation, freezing and storage of blood-derived stem cells for transplantation, use 88240)

(For thawing and expansion of blood-derived stem cells for transplantation, use 88241)

(For compatibility studies, see 86812-86822)

Lymph Nodes and Lymphatic Channels

Incision

§ **38300** Drainage of lymph node abscess or lymphadenitis; simple

§ **38305** extensive

§ **38308** Lymphangiotomy or other operations on lymphatic channels

✿ **38380** Suture and/or ligation of thoracic duct; cervical approach

✿ **38381** thoracic approach

✿ **38382** abdominal approach

Excision

(For injection for sentinel node identification, use 38792)

♦§ **38500** Biopsy or excision of lymph node(s); open, superficial
➲ *CPT Changes: An Insider's View* 2001

(Do not report 38500 with 38700-38780)

♦§ **38505** by needle, superficial (eg, cervical, inguinal, axillary)

(If imaging guidance is performed, see 76360, 76393, 76942)

(For fine needle aspiration, use 10021 or 10022)

(For evaluation of fine needle aspirate, see 88172, 88173)

♦§ **38510** open, deep cervical node(s)
➲ *CPT Changes: An Insider's View* 2001

♦§ **38520** open, deep cervical node(s) with excision scalene fat pad
➲ *CPT Changes: An Insider's View* 2001

♦§ **38525** open, deep axillary node(s)
➲ *CPT Changes: An Insider's View* 2001

♦§ **38530** open, internal mammary node(s)
➲ *CPT Changes: An Insider's View* 2001

(Do not report 38530 with 38720-38746)

(For percutaneous needle biopsy, retroperitoneal lymph node or mass, use 49180. For fine needle aspiration, use 10022)

♦§ **38542** Dissection, deep jugular node(s)

(For radical cervical neck dissection, use 38720)

§ **38550** Excision of cystic hygroma, axillary or cervical; without deep neurovascular dissection

§ **38555** with deep neurovascular dissection

Limited Lymphadenectomy for Staging

✶✿ **38562** Limited lymphadenectomy for staging (separate procedure); pelvic and para-aortic

(When combined with prostatectomy, use 55812 or 55842)

(When combined with insertion of radioactive substance into prostate, use 55862)

✿ **38564** retroperitoneal (aortic and/or splenic)

Laparoscopy

Surgical laparoscopy always includes diagnostic laparoscopy. To report a diagnostic laparoscopy (peritoneoscopy) (separate procedure), use 49320.

§ **38570** Laparoscopy, surgical; with retroperitoneal lymph node sampling (biopsy), single or multiple
➲ *CPT Changes: An Insider's View* 2000

✶§ **38571** with bilateral total pelvic lymphadenectomy
➲ *CPT Changes: An Insider's View* 2000

✶§ **38572** with bilateral total pelvic lymphadenectomy and peri-aortic lymph node sampling (biopsy), single or multiple
➲ *CPT Changes: An Insider's View* 2000

(For drainage of lymphocele to peritoneal cavity, use 49323)

§ **38589** Unlisted laparoscopy procedure, lymphatic system
➲ *CPT Changes: An Insider's View* 2000

Radical Lymphadenectomy (Radical Resection of Lymph Nodes)

(For limited pelvic and retroperitoneal lymphadenectomies, see 38562, 38564)

♦§ **38700** Suprahyoid lymphadenectomy
➲ *CPT Assistant* Jan 03:16

(For bilateral procedure, report 38700 with modifier 50)

♦§ **38720** Cervical lymphadenectomy (complete)

(For bilateral procedure, report 38720 with modifier 50)

♦✿ **38724** Cervical lymphadenectomy (modified radical neck dissection)

§ **38740** Axillary lymphadenectomy; superficial

§ **38745** complete

✿+ **38746** Thoracic lymphadenectomy, regional, including mediastinal and peritracheal nodes (List separately in addition to code for primary procedure)

✿+ **38747** Abdominal lymphadenectomy, regional, including celiac, gastric, portal, peripancreatic, with or without para-aortic and vena caval nodes (List separately in addition to code for primary procedure)

♦§ **38760** Inguinofemoral lymphadenectomy, superficial, including Cloquets node (separate procedure)

(For bilateral procedure, report 38760 with modifier 50

♦✿ **38765** Inguinofemoral lymphadenectomy, superficial, in continuity with pelvic lymphadenectomy, including external iliac, hypogastric, and obturator nodes (separate procedure)

(For bilateral procedure, report 38765 with modifier 50)

♦✿ **38770** Pelvic lymphadenectomy, including external iliac, hypogastric, and obturator nodes (separate procedure)

(For bilateral procedure, report 38770 with modifier 50)

✿ **38780** Retroperitoneal transabdominal lymphadenectomy, extensive, including pelvic, aortic, and renal nodes (separate procedure)

(For excision and repair of lymphedematous skin and subcutaneous tissue, see 15000, 15570-15650)

Introduction

♦☆ **38790** Injection procedure; lymphangiography

(For bilateral procedure, report 38790 with modifier 50)

(For radiological supervision and interpretation, see 75801-75807)

♦☆⊘ **38792** for identification of sentinel node

(For excision of sentinel node, see 38500-38542)

(For nuclear medicine lymphatics and lymph gland imaging, use 78195)

☆ **38794** Cannulation, thoracic duct

Other Procedures

❖ **38999** Unlisted procedure, hemic or lymphatic system

Mediastinum and Diaphragm

Mediastinum

Incision

✿ **39000** Mediastinotomy with exploration, drainage, removal of foreign body, or biopsy; cervical approach

✿ **39010** transthoracic approach, including either transthoracic or median sternotomy

Excision

✿ **39200** Excision of mediastinal cyst

✿ **39220** Excision of mediastinal tumor

(For substernal thyroidectomy, use 60270)

(For thymectomy, use 60520)

Endoscopy

§ **39400** Mediastinoscopy, with or without biopsy

Other Procedures

✿ **39499** Unlisted procedure, mediastinum

Diaphragm

Repair

(For transabdominal repair of diaphragmatic (esophageal hiatal) hernia, see 43324, 43325)

✿ **39501** Repair, laceration of diaphragm, any approach

✿ **39502** Repair, paraesophageal hiatus hernia, transabdominal, with or without fundoplasty, vagotomy, and/or pyloroplasty, except neonatal

✿ **39503** Repair, neonatal diaphragmatic hernia, with or without chest tube insertion and with or without creation of ventral hernia

(Do not report modifier 63 in conjunction with 39503)

✿ **39520** Repair, diaphragmatic hernia (esophageal hiatal); transthoracic

✿ **39530** combined, thoracoabdominal

✿ **39531** combined, thoracoabdominal, with dilation of stricture (with or without gastroplasty)

✿ **39540** Repair, diaphragmatic hernia (other than neonatal), traumatic; acute

✿ **39541** chronic

✿ **39545** Imbrication of diaphragm for eventration, transthoracic or transabdominal, paralytic or nonparalytic

✿ **39560** Resection, diaphragm; with simple repair (eg, primary suture)

✿ **39561** with complex repair (eg, prosthetic material, local muscle flap)

Other Procedures

✿ **39599** Unlisted procedure, diaphragm

Digestive System

Lips

(For procedures on skin of lips, see 10040 et seq)

Excision

§ **40490** Biopsy of lip

§ **40500** Vermilionectomy (lip shave), with mucosal advancement

§ **40510** Excision of lip; transverse wedge excision with primary closure

§ **40520** V-excision with primary direct linear closure

(For excision of mucous lesions, see 40810-40816)

§ **40525** full thickness, reconstruction with local flap (eg, Estlander or fan)

§ **40527** full thickness, reconstruction with cross lip flap (Abbe-Estlander)

§ **40530** Resection of lip, more than one-fourth, without reconstruction

(For reconstruction, see 13131 et seq)

Repair (Cheiloplasty)

§ **40650** Repair lip, full thickness; vermilion only

§ **40652** up to half vertical height

§ **40654** over one-half vertical height, or complex

⌘§ **40700** Plastic repair of cleft lip/nasal deformity; primary, partial or complete, unilateral

✶§ **40701** primary bilateral, one stage procedure

✶§ **40702** primary bilateral, one of two stages

♦§ **40720** secondary, by recreation of defect and reclosure

(For bilateral procedure, report 40720 with modifier 50)

(To report rhinoplasty only for nasal deformity secondary to congenital cleft lip, see 30460, 30462)

(For repair of cleft lip, with cross lip pedicle flap (Abbe-Estlander type), use 40527)

§ **40761** with cross lip pedicle flap (Abbe-Estlander type), including sectioning and inserting of pedicle

(For repair cleft palate, see 42200 et seq)

(For other reconstructive procedures, see 14060, 14061, 15120-15261, 15574, 15576, 15630)

Other Procedures

§ **40799** Unlisted procedure, lips

Vestibule of Mouth

The vestibule is the part of the oral cavity outside the dentoalveolar structures; it includes the mucosal and submucosal tissue of lips and cheeks.

Incision

§ **40800** Drainage of abscess, cyst, hematoma, vestibule of mouth; simple

§ **40801** complicated

♣ **40804** Removal of embedded foreign body, vestibule of mouth; simple

§ **40805** complicated

§ **40806** Incision of labial frenum (frenotomy)

Excision, Destruction

§ **40808** Biopsy, vestibule of mouth

§ **40810** Excision of lesion of mucosa and submucosa, vestibule of mouth; without repair

§ **40812** with simple repair

§ **40814** with complex repair

§ **40816** complex, with excision of underlying muscle

§ **40818** Excision of mucosa of vestibule of mouth as donor graft

§ **40819** Excision of frenum, labial or buccal (frenumectomy, frenulectomy, frenectomy)

§ **40820** Destruction of lesion or scar of vestibule of mouth by physical methods (eg, laser, thermal, cryo, chemical)

Repair

§ **40830** Closure of laceration, vestibule of mouth; 2.5 cm or less

§ **40831** over 2.5 cm or complex

§ **40840** Vestibuloplasty; anterior

§ **40842** posterior, unilateral

⌘§ **40843** posterior, bilateral

§ **40844** entire arch

§ **40845** complex (including ridge extension, muscle repositioning)

(For skin grafts, see 15000 et seq)

Other Procedures

§ **40899** Unlisted procedure, vestibule of mouth

Tongue and Floor of Mouth

Incision

§ **41000** Intraoral incision and drainage of abscess, cyst, or hematoma of tongue or floor of mouth; lingual

§ **41005** sublingual, superficial

§ **41006** sublingual, deep, supramylohyoid

§ **41007** submental space

§ **41008** submandibular space

§ **41009** masticator space

§ **41010** Incision of lingual frenum (frenotomy)

§ **41015** Extraoral incision and drainage of abscess, cyst, or hematoma of floor of mouth; sublingual

§ **41016** submental

§ **41017** submandibular

§ **41018** masticator space

(For frenoplasty, use 41520)

Excision

§ **41100** Biopsy of tongue; anterior two-thirds

§ **41105** posterior one-third

§ **41108** Biopsy of floor of mouth

§ **41110** Excision of lesion of tongue without closure

§ **41112** Excision of lesion of tongue with closure; anterior two-thirds

§ **41113** posterior one-third

§ **41114** with local tongue flap

(List 41114 in addition to code 41112 or 41113)

§ **41115** Excision of lingual frenum (frenectomy)

§ **41116** Excision, lesion of floor of mouth

§ **41120** Glossectomy; less than one-half tongue

✿ **41130** hemiglossectomy

✿ **41135** partial, with unilateral radical neck dissection

✿ **41140** complete or total, with or without tracheostomy, without radical neck dissection

✿ **41145** complete or total, with or without tracheostomy, with unilateral radical neck dissection

✿ **41150** composite procedure with resection floor of mouth and mandibular resection, without radical neck dissection

✿ **41153** composite procedure with resection floor of mouth, with suprahyoid neck dissection

✿ **41155** composite procedure with resection floor of mouth, mandibular resection, and radical neck dissection (Commando type)

Repair

§ **41250** Repair of laceration 2.5 cm or less; floor of mouth and/or anterior two-thirds of tongue

§ **41251** posterior one-third of tongue

§ **41252** Repair of laceration of tongue, floor of mouth, over 2.6 cm or complex

Other Procedures

§ **41500** Fixation of tongue, mechanical, other than suture (eg, K-wire)

§ **41510** Suture of tongue to lip for micrognathia (Douglas type procedure)

§ **41520** Frenoplasty (surgical revision of frenum, eg, with Z-plasty)

(For frenotomy, see 40806, 41010)

§ **41599** Unlisted procedure, tongue, floor of mouth

Dentoalveolar Structures

Incision

§ **41800** Drainage of abscess, cyst, hematoma from dentoalveolar structures

§ **41805** Removal of embedded foreign body from dentoalveolar structures; soft tissues

§ **41806** bone

Excision, Destruction

§ **41820** Gingivectomy, excision gingiva, each quadrant

§ **41821** Operculectomy, excision pericoronal tissues

§ **41822** Excision of fibrous tuberosities, dentoalveolar structures

§ **41823** Excision of osseous tuberosities, dentoalveolar structures

§ **41825** Excision of lesion or tumor (except listed above), dentoalveolar structures; without repair

§ **41826** with simple repair

§ **41827** with complex repair

(For nonexcisional destruction, use 41850)

§ **41828** Excision of hyperplastic alveolar mucosa, each quadrant (specify)

§ **41830** Alveolectomy, including curettage of osteitis or sequestrectomy

§ **41850** Destruction of lesion (except excision), dentoalveolar structures

Other Procedures

§ **41870** Periodontal mucosal grafting

§ **41872** Gingivoplasty, each quadrant (specify)

Surgery: Digestive System

§ **41874** Alveoloplasty, each quadrant (specify)

(For closure of lacerations, see 40830, 40831)

(For segmental osteotomy, use 21206)

(For reduction of fractures, see 21421-21490)

§ **41899** Unlisted procedure, dentoalveolar structures

Palate and Uvula

Incision

§ **42000** Drainage of abscess of palate, uvula

Excision, Destruction

§ **42100** Biopsy of palate, uvula

§ **42104** Excision, lesion of palate, uvula; without closure

§ **42106** with simple primary closure

§ **42107** with local flap closure

(For skin graft, see 14040-14300)

(For mucosal graft, use 40818)

§ **42120** Resection of palate or extensive resection of lesion

(For reconstruction of palate with extraoral tissue, see 14040-14300, 15050, 15120, 15240, 15576)

§ **42140** Uvulectomy, excision of uvula

§ **42145** Palatopharyngoplasty (eg, uvulopalatopharyngoplasty, uvulopharyngoplasty)

(For removal of exostosis of the bony palate, see 21031, 21032)

§ **42160** Destruction of lesion, palate or uvula (thermal, cryo or chemical)

Repair

§ **42180** Repair, laceration of palate; up to 2 cm

§ **42182** over 2 cm or complex

§ **42200** Palatoplasty for cleft palate, soft and/or hard palate only

§ **42205** Palatoplasty for cleft palate, with closure of alveolar ridge; soft tissue only

§ **42210** with bone graft to alveolar ridge (includes obtaining graft)

§ **42215** Palatoplasty for cleft palate; major revision

§ **42220** secondary lengthening procedure

§ **42225** attachment pharyngeal flap

§ **42226** Lengthening of palate, and pharyngeal flap

§ **42227** Lengthening of palate, with island flap

§ **42235** Repair of anterior palate, including vomer flap

(For repair of oronasal fistula, use 30600)

§ **42260** Repair of nasolabial fistula

(For repair of cleft lip, see 40700 et seq)

§ **42280** Maxillary impression for palatal prosthesis

§ **42281** Insertion of pin-retained palatal prosthesis

Other Procedures

§ **42299** Unlisted procedure, palate, uvula

Salivary Gland and Ducts

Incision

§ **42300** Drainage of abscess; parotid, simple

§ **42305** parotid, complicated

§ **42310** Drainage of abscess; submaxillary or sublingual, intraoral

➔ *CPT Changes: An Insider's View* 2003

§ **42320** submaxillary, external

§ **42325** Fistulization of sublingual salivary cyst (ranula);

§ **42326** with prosthesis

§ **42330** Sialolithotomy; submandibular (submaxillary), sublingual or parotid, uncomplicated, intraoral

§ **42335** submandibular (submaxillary), complicated, intraoral

§ **42340** parotid, extraoral or complicated intraoral

Excision

§ **42400** Biopsy of salivary gland; needle

(For fine needle aspiration, see 10021, 10022)

(For evaluation of fine needle aspirate, see 88172, 88173)

(If imaging guidance is performed, see 76003, 76360, 76393, 76942)

§ **42405** incisional

(If imaging guidance is performed, see 76003, 76360, 76393, 76942)

§ **42408** Excision of sublingual salivary cyst (ranula)

§ **42409** Marsupialization of sublingual salivary cyst (ranula)

(For fistulization of sublingual salivary cyst, use 42325)

§ **42410** Excision of parotid tumor or parotid gland; lateral lobe, without nerve dissection

§ **42415** lateral lobe, with dissection and preservation of facial nerve

§ **42420** total, with dissection and preservation of facial nerve

§ **42425** total, en bloc removal with sacrifice of facial nerve

✿ **42426** total, with unilateral radical neck dissection

(For suture or grafting of facial nerve, see 64864, 64865, 69740, 69745)

§ **42440** Excision of submandibular (submaxillary) gland

§ **42450** Excision of sublingual gland

Repair

§ **42500** Plastic repair of salivary duct, sialodochoplasty; primary or simple

§ **42505** secondary or complicated

✶§ **42507** Parotid duct diversion, bilateral (Wilke type procedure);

✶§ **42508** with excision of one submandibular gland

✶§ **42509** with excision of both submandibular glands

✶§ **42510** with ligation of both submandibular (Wharton's) ducts

Other Procedures

☆ **42550** Injection procedure for sialography

(For radiological supervision and interpretation, use 70390)

§ **42600** Closure salivary fistula

§ **42650** Dilation salivary duct

§ **42660** Dilation and catheterization of salivary duct, with or without injection

§ **42665** Ligation salivary duct, intraoral

§ **42699** Unlisted procedure, salivary glands or ducts

Pharynx, Adenoids, and Tonsils

Incision

§ **42700** Incision and drainage abscess; peritonsillar

§ **42720** retropharyngeal or parapharyngeal, intraoral approach

§ **42725** retropharyngeal or parapharyngeal, external approach

Excision, Destruction

§ **42800** Biopsy; oropharynx

§ **42802** hypopharynx

§ **42804** nasopharynx, visible lesion, simple

§ **42806** nasopharynx, survey for unknown primary lesion

(For laryngoscopic biopsy, see 31510, 31535, 31536)

§ **42808** Excision or destruction of lesion of pharynx, any method

♣ **42809** Removal of foreign body from pharynx

§ **42810** Excision branchial cleft cyst or vestige, confined to skin and subcutaneous tissues

§ **42815** Excision branchial cleft cyst, vestige, or fistula, extending beneath subcutaneous tissues and/or into pharynx

§ **42820** Tonsillectomy and adenoidectomy; under age 12

§ **42821** age 12 or over

§ **42825** Tonsillectomy, primary or secondary; under age 12

§ **42826** age 12 or over

§ **42830** Adenoidectomy, primary; under age 12

§ **42831** age 12 or over

§ **42835** Adenoidectomy, secondary; under age 12

§ **42836** age 12 or over

§ **42842** Radical resection of tonsil, tonsillar pillars, and/or retromolar trigone; without closure

➔ *CPT Assistant* Jan 03:16

§ **42844** closure with local flap (eg, tongue, buccal)

✿ **42845** closure with other flap

(For closure with other flap(s), use appropriate number for flap(s))

(When combined with radical neck dissection, use also 38720)

§ **42860** Excision of tonsil tags

§ **42870** Excision or destruction lingual tonsil, any method (separate procedure)

(For resection of the nasopharynx (eg, juvenile angiofibroma) by bicoronal and/or transzygomatic approach, see 61586 and 61600)

§ **42890** Limited pharyngectomy

§ **42892** Resection of lateral pharyngeal wall or pyriform sinus, direct closure by advancement of lateral and posterior pharyngeal walls

(When combined with radical neck dissection, use also 38720)

✿ **42894** Resection of pharyngeal wall requiring closure with myocutaneous flap

(When combined with radical neck dissection, use also 38720)

(For limited pharyngectomy with radical neck dissection, use 38720 with 42890)

Repair

§ **42900** Suture pharynx for wound or injury

§ **42950** Pharyngoplasty (plastic or reconstructive operation on pharynx)

(For pharyngeal flap, use 42225)

✿ **42953** Pharyngoesophageal repair

(For closure with myocutaneous or other flap, use appropriate number in addition)

Other Procedures

§ **42955** Pharyngostomy (fistulization of pharynx, external for feeding)

§ **42960** Control oropharyngeal hemorrhage, primary or secondary (eg, post-tonsillectomy); simple

✿ **42961** complicated, requiring hospitalization

§ **42962** with secondary surgical intervention

§ **42970** Control of nasopharyngeal hemorrhage, primary or secondary (eg, postadenoidectomy); simple, with posterior nasal packs, with or without anterior packs and/or cautery

➲ *CPT Changes: An Insider's View* 2002

✿ **42971** complicated, requiring hospitalization

§ **42972** with secondary surgical intervention

§ **42999** Unlisted procedure, pharynx, adenoids, or tonsils

Esophagus

Incision

(For esophageal intubation with laparotomy, use 43510)

§ **43020** Esophagotomy, cervical approach, with removal of foreign body

§ **43030** Cricopharyngeal myotomy

➲ *CPT Assistant* Jan 03:16

✿ **43045** Esophagotomy, thoracic approach, with removal of foreign body

Excision

(For gastrointestinal reconstruction for previous esophagectomy, see 43360, 43361)

✿ **43100** Excision of lesion, esophagus, with primary repair; cervical approach

✿ **43101** thoracic or abdominal approach

(For wide excision of malignant lesion of cervical esophagus, with total laryngectomy without radical neck dissection, see 43107, 43116, 43124, and 31360)

(For wide excision of malignant lesion of cervical esophagus, with total laryngectomy with radical neck dissection, see 43107, 43116, 43124, and 31365)

✿ **43107** Total or near total esophagectomy, without thoracotomy; with pharyngogastrostomy or cervical esophagogastrostomy, with or without pyloroplasty (transhiatal)

✿ **43108** with colon interposition or small intestine reconstruction, including intestine mobilization, preparation and anastomosis(es)

✿ **43112** Total or near total esophagectomy, with thoracotomy; with pharyngogastrostomy or cervical esophagogastrostomy, with or without pyloroplasty

✿ **43113** with colon interposition or small intestine reconstruction, including intestine mobilization, preparation, and anastomosis(es)

✿ **43116** Partial esophagectomy, cervical, with free intestinal graft, including microvascular anastomosis, obtaining the graft and intestinal reconstruction

(Do not report code 69990 in addition to code 43116)

(Report 43116 with the modifier 52 appended if intestinal or free jejunal graft with microvascular anastomosis is performed by another physician)

(For free jejunal graft with microvascular anastomosis performed by another physician, use 43496)

✿ **43117** Partial esophagectomy, distal two-thirds, with thoracotomy and separate abdominal incision, with or without proximal gastrectomy; with thoracic esophagogastrostomy, with or without pyloroplasty (Ivor Lewis)

✿ **43118** with colon interposition or small intestine reconstruction, including intestine mobilization, preparation, and anastomosis(es)

(For total esophagectomy with gastropharyngostomy, see 43107, 43124)

(For esophagogastrectomy (lower third) and vagotomy, use 43122)

✿ **43121** Partial esophagectomy, distal two-thirds, with thoracotomy only, with or without proximal gastrectomy, with thoracic esophagogastrostomy, with or without pyloroplasty

✿ **43122** Partial esophagectomy, thoracoabdominal or abdominal approach, with or without proximal gastrectomy; with esophagogastrostomy, with or without pyloroplasty

✿ **43123** with colon interposition or small intestine reconstruction, including intestine mobilization, preparation, and anastomosis(es)

✿ **43124** Total or partial esophagectomy, without reconstruction (any approach), with cervical esophagostomy

§ **43130** Diverticulectomy of hypopharynx or esophagus, with or without myotomy; cervical approach

✿ **43135** thoracic approach

Endoscopy

For endoscopic procedures, code appropriate endoscopy of each anatomic site examined.

Surgical endoscopy always includes diagnostic endoscopy.

(For upper gastrointestinal endoscopy with suturing of the esophagogastric junction, use Category III code 0008T)

§⊙ **43200** Esophagoscopy, rigid or flexible; diagnostic, with or without collection of specimen(s) by brushing or washing (separate procedure)

➔ *CPT Assistant* Sep 03:4; *CPT Changes: An Insider's View* 2000

§⊙ **43201** with directed submucosal injection(s), any substance

➔ *CPT Changes: An Insider's View* 2003

(For injection sclerosis of esophageal varices, use 43204)

§⊙ **43202** with biopsy, single or multiple

§⊙ **43204** with injection sclerosis of esophageal varices

§⊙ **43205** with band ligation of esophageal varices

§⊙ **43215** with removal of foreign body

(For radiological supervision and interpretation, use 74235)

§⊙ **43216** with removal of tumor(s), polyp(s), or other lesion(s) by hot biopsy forceps or bipolar cautery

§⊙ **43217** with removal of tumor(s), polyp(s), or other lesion(s) by snare technique

§⊙ **43219** with insertion of plastic tube or stent

§⊙ **43220** with balloon dilation (less than 30 mm diameter)

(If imaging guidance is performed, use 74360)

(For endoscopic dilation with balloon 30 mm diameter or larger, use 43458)

(For dilation without visualization, use 43450-43453)

(For diagnostic fiberoptic esophagogastroscopy, use 43200, 43235)

(For fiberoptic esophagogastroscopy with biopsy or collection of specimen, use 43200, 43202, 43235, 43239)

(For fiberoptic esophagogastroscopy with removal of foreign body, use 43215, 43247)

(For fiberoptic esophagogastroscopy with removal of polyp(s), use 43217, 43251)

§⊙ **43226** with insertion of guide wire followed by dilation over guide wire

(For radiological supervision and interpretation, use 74360)

§⊙ **43227** with control of bleeding (eg, injection, bipolar cautery, unipolar cautery, laser, heater probe, stapler, plasma coagulator)

➔ *CPT Changes: An Insider's View* 2002

§⊙ **43228** with ablation of tumor(s), polyp(s), or other lesion(s), not amenable to removal by hot biopsy forceps, bipolar cautery or snare technique

(For esophagoscopic photodynamic therapy, report 43228 in addition to 96570, 96571 as appropriate)

§⊙ **43231** with endoscopic ultrasound examination

➔ *CPT Changes: An Insider's View* 2001

(Do not report 43231 in conjunction with 76975)

§⊙ **43232** with transendoscopic ultrasound-guided intramural or transmural fine needle aspiration/biopsy(s)

➔ *CPT Changes: An Insider's View* 2001

(Do not report 43232 in conjunction with 76942, 76975)

(For interpretation of specimen, see 88172-88173)

§⊙ **43234** Upper gastrointestinal endoscopy, simple primary examination (eg, with small diameter flexible endoscope) (separate procedure)

§⊙ **43235** Upper gastrointestinal endoscopy including esophagus, stomach, and either the duodenum and/or jejunum as appropriate; diagnostic, with or without collection of specimen(s) by brushing or washing (separate procedure)

➔ *CPT Assistant* Sep 03:3

§⊙ **43236** with directed submucosal injection(s), any substance

➔ *CPT Changes: An Insider's View* 2003

(For injection sclerosis of esophageal and/or gastric varices, use 43243)

§ **43237** with endoscopic ultrasound examination limited to the esophagus

➔ *CPT Changes: An Insider's View* 2004

(Do not report 43237 in conjunction with 76942, 76975)

§ **43238** with transendoscopic ultrasound-guided intramural or transmural fine needle aspiration/biopsy(s), esophagus (includes endoscopic ultrasound examination limited to the esophagus)

➔ *CPT Changes: An Insider's View* 2004

(Do not report 43238 in conjunction with 76942 or 76975)

§⊙ **43239** with biopsy, single or multiple

(For upper gastrointestinal endoscopy with suturing of the esophagogastric junction, use Category III code 0008T)

§⊙ **43240** with transmural drainage of pseudocyst

§⊙ **43241** with transendoscopic intraluminal tube or catheter placement

§⊙ **43242** with transendoscopic ultrasound-guided intramural or transmural fine needle aspiration/biopsy(s) (includes endoscopic ultrasound examination of the esophagus, stomach, and either the duodenum and/or jejunum as appropriate)

(Do not report 43242 in conjunction with 76942, 76975)

(For transendoscopic fine needle aspiration/biopsy limited to esophagus, use 43238)

(For interpretation of specimen, see 88172-88173)

§⊙ **43243** with injection sclerosis of esophageal and/or gastric varices

§⊙ **43244** with band ligation of esophageal and/or gastric varices

§⊙ **43245** with dilation of gastric outlet for obstruction (eg, balloon, guide wire, bougie)

➔ *CPT Changes: An Insider's View* 2002, 2003

(Do not report 43245 in conjunction with 43256)

§⊙ **43246** with directed placement of percutaneous gastrostomy tube

(For radiological supervision and interpretation, use 74350)

§⊙ **43247** with removal of foreign body

(For radiological supervision and interpretation, use 74235)

§⊙ **43248** with insertion of guide wire followed by dilation of esophagus over guide wire

§⊙ **43249** with balloon dilation of esophagus (less than 30 mm diameter)

§⊙ **43250** with removal of tumor(s), polyp(s), or other lesion(s) by hot biopsy forceps or bipolar cautery

§⊙ **43251** with removal of tumor(s), polyp(s), or other lesion(s) by snare technique

§⊙ **43255** with control of bleeding, any method

§⊙ **43256** with transendoscopic stent placement (includes predilation)

➔ *CPT Changes: An Insider's View* 2001

§⊙● **43257** with delivery of thermal energy to the muscle of lower esophageal sphincter and/or gastric cardia, for treatment of gastroesophageal reflux disease

➔ *CPT Changes: An Insider's View* 2005

§⊙ **43258** with ablation of tumor(s), polyp(s), or other lesion(s) not amenable to removal by hot biopsy forceps, bipolar cautery or snare technique

(For injection sclerosis of esophageal varices, use 43204, 43243)

§⊙ **43259** with endoscopic ultrasound examination, including the esophagus, stomach, and either the duodenum and/or jejunum as appropriate

➔ *CPT Changes: An Insider's View* 2004

(Do not report 43259 in conjunction with 76975)

§⊙ **43260** Endoscopic retrograde cholangiopancreatography (ERCP); diagnostic, with or without collection of specimen(s) by brushing or washing (separate procedure)

(For radiological supervision and interpretation, see 74328, 74329, 74330)

§⊙ **43261** with biopsy, single or multiple

(For radiological supervision and interpretation, see 74328, 74329, 74330)

§⊙ **43262** with sphincterotomy/papillotomy

(For radiological supervision and interpretation, see 74328, 74329, 74330)

§⊙ **43263** with pressure measurement of sphincter of Oddi (pancreatic duct or common bile duct)

(For radiological supervision and interpretation, see 74328, 74329, 74330)

§⊙ **43264** with endoscopic retrograde removal of calculus/calculi from biliary and/or pancreatic ducts

➔ *CPT Changes: An Insider's View* 2002

(When done with sphincterotomy, also use 43262)

(For radiological supervision and interpretation, see 74328, 74329, 74330)

§⊙ **43265** with endoscopic retrograde destruction, lithotripsy of calculus/calculi, any method

➔ *CPT Changes: An Insider's View* 2002

(When done with sphincterotomy, also use 43262)

(For radiological supervision and interpretation, see 74328, 74329, 74330)

§⊙ **43267** with endoscopic retrograde insertion of nasobiliary or nasopancreatic drainage tube

(When done with sphincterotomy, also use 43262)

(For radiological supervision and interpretation, see 74328, 74329, 74330)

§⊙ **43268** with endoscopic retrograde insertion of tube or stent into bile or pancreatic duct

(When done with sphincterotomy, also use 43262)

(For radiological supervision and interpretation, see 74328, 74329, 74330)

§⊙ **43269** with endoscopic retrograde removal of foreign body and/or change of tube or stent

(When done with sphincterotomy, also use 43262)

(For radiological supervision and interpretation, see 74328, 74329, 74330)

§⊙ **43271** with endoscopic retrograde balloon dilation of ampulla, biliary and/or pancreatic duct(s)

(When done with sphincterotomy, also use 43262)

(For radiological supervision and interpretation, see 74328, 74329, 74330)

§⊙ **43272** with ablation of tumor(s), polyp(s), or other lesion(s) not amenable to removal by hot biopsy forceps, bipolar cautery or snare technique

(For radiological supervision and interpretation, see 74328, 74329, 74330)

Laparoscopy

Surgical laparoscopy always includes diagnostic laparoscopy. To report a diagnostic laparoscopy (peritoneoscopy) (separate procedure), use 49320.

§ **43280** Laparoscopy, surgical, esophagogastric fundoplasty (eg, Nissen, Toupet procedures)

➔ *CPT Changes: An Insider's View* 2000

(For open approach, use 43324)

§ **43289** Unlisted laparoscopy procedure, esophagus

➔ *CPT Changes: An Insider's View* 2000

Repair

✿ 43300 Esophagoplasty (plastic repair or reconstruction), cervical approach; without repair of tracheoesophageal fistula

✿ 43305 with repair of tracheoesophageal fistula

✿ 43310 Esophagoplasty (plastic repair or reconstruction), thoracic approach; without repair of tracheoesophageal fistula

✿ 43312 with repair of tracheoesophageal fistula

✿ 43313 Esophagoplasty for congenital defect (plastic repair or reconstruction), thoracic approach; without repair of congenital tracheoesophageal fistula

✿ 43314 with repair of congenital tracheoesophageal fistula

(Do not report modifier 63 in conjunction with 43313, 43314)

✿ 43320 Esophagogastrostomy (cardioplasty), with or without vagotomy and pyloroplasty, transabdominal or transthoracic approach

✿ 43324 Esophagogastric fundoplasty (eg, Nissen, Belsey IV, Hill procedures)

(For laparoscopic procedure, use 43280)

✿ 43325 Esophagogastric fundoplasty; with fundic patch (Thal-Nissen procedure)

(For cricopharyngeal myotomy, use 43030)

✿ 43326 with gastroplasty (eg, Collis)

✿ 43330 Esophagomyotomy (Heller type); abdominal approach

✿ 43331 thoracic approach

(For thoracoscopic esophagomyotomy, use 32665)

✿ 43340 Esophagojejunostomy (without total gastrectomy); abdominal approach

✿ 43341 thoracic approach

✿ 43350 Esophagostomy, fistulization of esophagus, external; abdominal approach

✿ 43351 thoracic approach

✿ 43352 cervical approach

✿ 43360 Gastrointestinal reconstruction for previous esophagectomy, for obstructing esophageal lesion or fistula, or for previous esophageal exclusion; with stomach, with or without pyloroplasty

✿ 43361 with colon interposition or small intestine reconstruction, including intestine mobilization, preparation, and anastomosis(es)

✿ 43400 Ligation, direct, esophageal varices

✿ 43401 Transection of esophagus with repair, for esophageal varices

✿ 43405 Ligation or stapling at gastroesophageal junction for pre-existing esophageal perforation

✿ 43410 Suture of esophageal wound or injury; cervical approach

✿ 43415 transthoracic or transabdominal approach

✿ 43420 Closure of esophagostomy or fistula; cervical approach

✿ 43425 transthoracic or transabdominal approach

(For repair of esophageal hiatal hernia, see 39520 et seq)

Manipulation

(For associated esophagogram, use 74220)

§ 43450 Dilation of esophagus, by unguided sound or bougie, single or multiple passes

§⊙ 43453 Dilation of esophagus, over guide wire

(For dilation with direct visualization, use 43220)

(For dilation of esophagus, by balloon or dilator, see 43220, 43458, and 74360)

§⊙ 43456 Dilation of esophagus, by balloon or dilator, retrograde

§⊙ 43458 Dilation of esophagus with balloon (30 mm diameter or larger) for achalasia

(For dilation with balloon less than 30 mm diameter, use 43220)

(For radiological supervision and interpretation, use 74360)

✿ 43460 Esophagogastric tamponade, with balloon (Sengstaaken type)

(For removal of esophageal foreign body by balloon catheter, see 43215, 43247, 74235)

Other Procedures

✿ 43496 Free jejunum transfer with microvascular anastomosis

(Do not report code 69990 in addition to code 43496)

§ 43499 Unlisted procedure, esophagus

Stomach

Incision

✿ 43500 Gastrotomy; with exploration or foreign body removal

✿ 43501 with suture repair of bleeding ulcer

✿ 43502 with suture repair of pre-existing esophagogastric laceration (eg, Mallory-Weiss)

§ 43510 with esophageal dilation and insertion of permanent intraluminal tube (eg, Celestin or Mousseaux-Barbin)

✿ 43520 Pyloromyotomy, cutting of pyloric muscle (Fredet-Ramstedt type operation)

(Do not report modifier 63 in conjunction with 43520)

Excision

§ 43600 Biopsy of stomach; by capsule, tube, peroral (one or more specimens)

✿ 43605 by laparotomy

✿ **43610** Excision, local; ulcer or benign tumor of stomach

✿ **43611** malignant tumor of stomach

✿ **43620** Gastrectomy, total; with esophagoenterostomy

✿ **43621** with Roux-en-Y reconstruction

✿ **43622** with formation of intestinal pouch, any type

✿ **43631** Gastrectomy, partial, distal; with gastroduodenostomy

✿ **43632** with gastrojejunostomy

✿ **43633** with Roux-en-Y reconstruction

✿ **43634** with formation of intestinal pouch

✿+ **43635** Vagotomy when performed with partial distal gastrectomy (List separately in addition to code(s) for primary procedure)

(Use 43635 in conjunction with 43631, 43632, 43633, 43634)

✿ **43638** Gastrectomy, partial, proximal, thoracic or abdominal approach including esophagogastrostomy, with vagotomy;

✿ **43639** with pyloroplasty or pyloromyotomy

(For regional thoracic lymphadenectomy, use 38746)

(For regional abdominal lymphadenectomy, use 38747)

✿ **43640** Vagotomy including pyloroplasty, with or without gastrostomy; truncal or selective

(For pyloroplasty, use 43800)

(For vagotomy, see 64752-64760)

✿ **43641** parietal cell (highly selective)

(For upper gastrointestinal endoscopy, see 43234-43259)

Laparoscopy

Surgical laparoscopy always includes diagnostic laparoscopy. To report a diagnostic laparoscopy (peritoneoscopy) (separate procedure), use 49320.

(For upper gastrointestinal endoscopy including esophagus, stomach, and either the duodenum and/or jejunum, see 43235-43259)

✿● **43644** Laparoscopy, surgical, gastric restrictive procedure; with gastric bypass and Roux-en-Y gastroenterostomy (roux limb 150 cm or less)

►(Do not report 43644 in conjunction with 43846, 49320)◄

►(Esophagogastroduodenoscopy (EGD) performed for a separate condition should be reported with modifier 59)◄

✿● **43645** with gastric bypass and small intestine reconstruction to limit absorption

►(Do not report 43645 in conjunction with 49320, 43847)◄

§ **43651** Laparoscopy, surgical; transection of vagus nerves, truncal
➲ *CPT Changes: An Insider's View* 2000

§ **43652** transection of vagus nerves, selective or highly selective
➲ *CPT Changes: An Insider's View* 2000

§ **43653** gastrostomy, without construction of gastric tube (eg, Stamm procedure) (separate procedure)
➲ *CPT Changes: An Insider's View* 2000

§ **43659** Unlisted laparoscopy procedure, stomach
➲ *CPT Changes: An Insider's View* 2000

Introduction

§ **43750** Percutaneous placement of gastrostomy tube

(For radiological supervision and interpretation, use 74350)

♣ **43752** Naso- or oro-gastric tube placement, requiring physician's skill and fluoroscopic guidance (includes fluoroscopy, image documentation and report)
➲ *CPT Changes: An Insider's View* 2001, 2004

(For enteric tube placement, see 44500, 74340)

(Do not report 43752 in conjunction with critical care codes 99291-99292, neonatal critical care codes 99295-99296, pediatric critical care codes 99293-99294 or low birth weight intensive care service codes 99298-99299)

§ **43760** Change of gastrostomy tube

(For endoscopic placement of gastrostomy tube, use 43246)

(For radiological supervision and interpretation, use 75984)

§ **43761** Repositioning of the gastric feeding tube, any method, through the duodenum for enteric nutrition
➲ *CPT Changes: An Insider's View* 2000

(If imaging guidance is performed, use 75984)

Other Procedures

✿ **43800** Pyloroplasty

(For pyloroplasty and vagotomy, use 43640)

✿ **43810** Gastroduodenostomy

✿ **43820** Gastrojejunostomy; without vagotomy

✿ **43825** with vagotomy, any type

§ **43830** Gastrostomy, open; without construction of gastric tube (eg, Stamm procedure) (separate procedure)
➲ *CPT Changes: An Insider's View* 2000

§ **43831** neonatal, for feeding
➲ *CPT Changes: An Insider's View* 2000

(For change of gastrostomy tube, use 43760)

(Do not report modifier 63 in conjunction with 43831)

✿ **43832** with construction of gastric tube (eg, Janeway procedure)

(For percutaneous endoscopic gastrostomy, use 43246)

✿ **43840** Gastrorrhaphy, suture of perforated duodenal or gastric ulcer, wound, or injury

✿ **43842** Gastric restrictive procedure, without gastric bypass, for morbid obesity; vertical-banded gastroplasty

✿ **43843** other than vertical-banded gastroplasty

✿● **43845** Gastric restrictive procedure with partial gastrectomy, pylorus-preserving duodenoileostomy and ileoileostomy (50 to 100 cm common channel) to limit absorption (biliopancreatic diversion with duodenal switch)

►(Do not report 43845 in conjunction with 43633, 43847, 44130, 49000)◄

✿▲ **43846** Gastric restrictive procedure, with gastric bypass for morbid obesity; with short limb (150 cm or less) Roux-en-Y gastroenterostomy

►(For greater than 150 cm, use 43847)◄

►(For laparoscopic procedure, use 43644)◄

✿ **43847** with small intestine reconstruction to limit absorption

✿ **43848** Revision of gastric restrictive procedure for morbid obesity (separate procedure)

✿ **43850** Revision of gastroduodenal anastomosis (gastroduodenostomy) with reconstruction; without vagotomy

✿ **43855** with vagotomy

✿ **43860** Revision of gastrojejunal anastomosis (gastrojejunostomy) with reconstruction, with or without partial gastrectomy or intestine resection; without vagotomy

✿ **43865** with vagotomy

§ **43870** Closure of gastrostomy, surgical

✿ **43880** Closure of gastrocolic fistula

§ **43999** Unlisted procedure, stomach

Intestines (Except Rectum)

Incision

✿ **44005** Enterolysis (freeing of intestinal adhesion) (separate procedure)

(Do not report 44005 in addition to 45136)

(For laparoscopic approach, use 44200)

✿ **44010** Duodenotomy, for exploration, biopsy(s), or foreign body removal

✿+ **44015** Tube or needle catheter jejunostomy for enteral alimentation, intraoperative, any method (List separately in addition to primary procedure)

✿ **44020** Enterotomy, small intestine, other than duodenum; for exploration, biopsy(s), or foreign body removal

✿ **44021** for decompression (eg, Baker tube)

✿ **44025** Colotomy, for exploration, biopsy(s), or foreign body removal

(For exteriorization of intestine (Mikulicz resection with crushing of spur), see 44602-44605)

✿ **44050** Reduction of volvulus, intussusception, internal hernia, by laparotomy

✿ **44055** Correction of malrotation by lysis of duodenal bands and/or reduction of midgut volvulus (eg, Ladd procedure)

(Do not report modifier 63 in conjunction with 44055)

Excision

►Intestinal allotransplantation involves three distinct components of physician work:◄

►1) ***Cadaver donor enterectomy***, which includes harvesting the intestine graft and cold preservation of the graft (perfusing with cold preservation solution and cold maintenance) (use 44132). ***Living donor enterectomy***, which includes harvesting the intestine graft, cold preservation of the graft (perfusing with cold preservation solution and cold maintenance), and care of the donor (use 44133).◄

►2) ***Backbench work***:◄

► Standard preparation of an intestine allograft prior to transplantation includes mobilization and fashioning of the superior mesenteric artery and vein (see 44715).◄

► Additional reconstruction of an intestine allograft prior to transplantation may include venous and/or arterial anastomosis(es) (see 44720-44721).◄

►3) ***Recipient intestinal allotransplantation with or without recipient enterectomy***, which includes transplantation of allograft and care of the recipient (see 44135, 44136).◄

§ **44100** Biopsy of intestine by capsule, tube, peroral (one or more specimens)

✿ **44110** Excision of one or more lesions of small or large intestine not requiring anastomosis, exteriorization, or fistulization; single enterotomy

✿ **44111** multiple enterotomies

✿ **44120** Enterectomy, resection of small intestine; single resection and anastomosis

(Do not report 44120 in addition to 45136)

✿+ **44121** each additional resection and anastomosis (List separately in addition to code for primary procedure)

(Use 44121 in conjunction with 44120)

✿ **44125** with enterostomy

✿ **44126** Enterectomy, resection of small intestine for congenital atresia, single resection and anastomosis of proximal segment of intestine; without tapering

✿ **44127** with tapering

✿+ **44128** each additional resection and anastomosis (List separately in addition to code for primary procedure)

(Use 44128 in conjunction with 44126, 44127)

(Do not report modifier 63 in conjunction with 44126, 44127, 44128)

✿ **44130** Enteroenterostomy, anastomosis of intestine, with or without cutaneous enterostomy (separate procedure)

✿▲ **44132** Donor enterectomy (including cold preservation), open; from cadaver donor

✿ **44133** partial, from living donor

►(For backbench intestinal graft preparation or reconstruction, see 44715, 44720, 44721)◄

✿ **44135** Intestinal allotransplantation; from cadaver donor

✿ **44136** from living donor

✿● **44137** Removal of transplanted intestinal allograft, complete

►(For partial removal of transplant allograft, see 44120, 44121, 44140)◄

✿+ **44139** Mobilization (take-down) of splenic flexure performed in conjunction with partial colectomy (List separately in addition to primary procedure)

(Use 44139 in conjunction with 44140-44147)

✿ **44140** Colectomy, partial; with anastomosis

(For laparoscopic procedure, use 44204)

✿ **44141** with skin level cecostomy or colostomy

✿ **44143** with end colostomy and closure of distal segment (Hartmann type procedure)

(For laparoscopic procedure, use 44206)

✿ **44144** with resection, with colostomy or ileostomy and creation of mucofistula

✿ **44145** with coloproctostomy (low pelvic anastomosis)

(For laparoscopic procedure, use 44207)

✿ **44146** with coloproctostomy (low pelvic anastomosis), with colostomy

(For laparoscopic procedure, use 44208)

✿ **44147** abdominal and transanal approach

✿ **44150** Colectomy, total, abdominal, without proctectomy; with ileostomy or ileoproctostomy

(For laparoscopic procedure, use 44210)

✿ **44151** with continent ileostomy

✿ **44152** with rectal mucosectomy, ileoanal anastomosis, with or without loop ileostomy

(For laparoscopic procedure, use 44211)

✿ **44153** with rectal mucosectomy, ileoanal anastomosis, creation of ileal reservoir (S or J), with or without loop ileostomy

(For laparoscopic procedure, use 44211)

✿ **44155** Colectomy, total, abdominal, with proctectomy; with ileostomy

(For laparoscopic procedure, use 44212)

✿ **44156** with continent ileostomy

✿ **44160** Colectomy, partial, with removal of terminal ileum with ileocolostomy

(For laparoscopic procedure, use 44205)

Laparoscopy

Surgical laparoscopy always includes diagnostic laparoscopy. To report a diagnostic laparoscopy (peritoneoscopy) (separate procedure), use 49320.

§ **44200** Laparoscopy, surgical; enterolysis (freeing of intestinal adhesion) (separate procedure)
➲ *CPT Changes: An Insider's View* 2000

(For laparoscopy with salpingolysis, ovariolysis, use 58660)

§ **44201** jejunostomy (eg, for decompression or feeding)
➲ *CPT Changes: An Insider's View* 2000

✿ **44202** enterectomy, resection of small intestine, single resection and anastomosis

✿+ **44203** each additional small intestine resection and anastomosis (List separately in addition to code for primary procedure)

(Use 44203 in conjunction with 44202)

(For open procedure, see 44120, 44121)

✿ **44204** colectomy, partial, with anastomosis

(For open procedure, use 44140)

✿ **44205** colectomy, partial, with removal of terminal ileum with ileocolostomy

(For open procedure, use 44160)

§ **44206** colectomy, partial, with end colostomy and closure of distal segment (Hartmann type procedure)

(For open procedure, use 44143)

§ **44207** colectomy, partial, with anastomosis, with coloproctostomy (low pelvic anastomosis)

(For open procedure, use 44145)

§ **44208** colectomy, partial, with anastomosis, with coloproctostomy (low pelvic anastomosis) with colostomy

(For open procedure, use 44146)

(44209 has been deleted. To report, use 44238)

✿ **44210** colectomy, total, abdominal, without proctectomy, with ileostomy or ileoproctostomy

(For open procedure, use 44150)

✿ **44211** colectomy, total, abdominal, with proctectomy, with ileoanal anastomosis, creation of ileal reservoir (S or J), with loop ileostomy, with or without rectal mucosectomy

(For open procedure, see 44152, 44153)

✿ **44212** colectomy, total, abdominal, with proctectomy, with ileostomy

(For open procedure, use 44155)

§ **44238** Unlisted laparoscopy procedure, intestine (except rectum)
➔ *CPT Changes: An Insider's View* 2003

§ **44239** Unlisted laparoscopy procedure, rectum
➔ *CPT Changes: An Insider's View* 2003

Enterostomy—External Fistulization of Intestines

✿ **44300** Enterostomy or cecostomy, tube (eg, for decompression or feeding) (separate procedure)

✿ **44310** Ileostomy or jejunostomy, non-tube (separate procedure)

(Do not report 44310 in addition to 45136)

§ **44312** Revision of ileostomy; simple (release of superficial scar) (separate procedure)

✿ **44314** complicated (reconstruction in-depth) (separate procedure)

✿ **44316** Continent ileostomy (Kock procedure) (separate procedure)

(For fiberoptic evaluation, use 44385)

✿ **44320** Colostomy or skin level cecostomy; (separate procedure)

✿ **44322** with multiple biopsies (eg, for congenital megacolon) (separate procedure)

§ **44340** Revision of colostomy; simple (release of superficial scar) (separate procedure)

✿ **44345** complicated (reconstruction in-depth) (separate procedure)

✿ **44346** with repair of paracolostomy hernia (separate procedure)

Endoscopy, Small Intestine and Stomal

Surgical endoscopy always includes diagnostic endoscopy.

(For upper gastrointestinal endoscopy, see 43234-43258)

§⊙ **44360** Small intestinal endoscopy, enteroscopy beyond second portion of duodenum, not including ileum; diagnostic, with or without collection of specimen(s) by brushing or washing (separate procedure)

§⊙ **44361** with biopsy, single or multiple

§⊙ **44363** with removal of foreign body

§⊙ **44364** with removal of tumor(s), polyp(s), or other lesion(s) by snare technique

§⊙ **44365** with removal of tumor(s), polyp(s), or other lesion(s) by hot biopsy forceps or bipolar cautery

§⊙ **44366** with control of bleeding (eg, injection, bipolar cautery, unipolar cautery, laser, heater probe, stapler, plasma coagulator)
➔ *CPT Changes: An Insider's View* 2002

§⊙ **44369** with ablation of tumor(s), polyp(s), or other lesion(s) not amenable to removal by hot biopsy forceps, bipolar cautery or snare technique

§⊙ **44370** with transendoscopic stent placement (includes predilation)
➔ *CPT Changes: An Insider's View* 2001

§⊙ **44372** with placement of percutaneous jejunostomy tube

§⊙ **44373** with conversion of percutaneous gastrostomy tube to percutaneous jejunostomy tube

(For fiberoptic jejunostomy through stoma, use 43235)

§⊙ **44376** Small intestinal endoscopy, enteroscopy beyond second portion of duodenum, including ileum; diagnostic, with or without collection of specimen(s) by brushing or washing (separate procedure)

§⊙ **44377** with biopsy, single or multiple

§⊙ **44378** with control of bleeding (eg, injection, bipolar cautery, unipolar cautery, laser, heater probe, stapler, plasma coagulator)
➔ *CPT Changes: An Insider's View* 2002

§⊙ **44379** with transendoscopic stent placement (includes predilation)
➔ *CPT Changes: An Insider's View* 2001

§⊙ **44380** Ileoscopy, through stoma; diagnostic, with or without collection of specimen(s) by brushing or washing (separate procedure)

§⊙ **44382** with biopsy, single or multiple

§⊙ **44383** with transendoscopic stent placement (includes predilation)
➔ *CPT Changes: An Insider's View* 2001

§⊙ **44385** Endoscopic evaluation of small intestinal (abdominal or pelvic) pouch; diagnostic, with or without collection of specimen(s) by brushing or washing (separate procedure)

§⊙ **44386** with biopsy, single or multiple

§⊙ **44388** Colonoscopy through stoma; diagnostic, with or without collection of specimen(s) by brushing or washing (separate procedure)

§⊙ **44389** with biopsy, single or multiple

§⊙ **44390** with removal of foreign body

§⊙ **44391** with control of bleeding (eg, injection, bipolar cautery, unipolar cautery, laser, heater probe, stapler, plasma coagulator)

➔ *CPT Changes: An Insider's View* 2002

§⊙ **44392** with removal of tumor(s), polyp(s), or other lesion(s) by hot biopsy forceps or bipolar cautery

§⊙ **44393** with ablation of tumor(s), polyp(s), or other lesion(s) not amenable to removal by hot biopsy forceps, bipolar cautery or snare technique

§⊙ **44394** with removal of tumor(s), polyp(s), or other lesion(s) by snare technique

(For colonoscopy per rectum, see 45330-45385)

§⊙ **44397** with transendoscopic stent placement (includes predilation)

➔ *CPT Changes: An Insider's View* 2001

Introduction

§⊙⊘ **44500** Introduction of long gastrointestinal tube (eg, Miller-Abbott) (separate procedure)

(For radiological supervision and interpretation, use 74340)

(For naso- or oro-gastric tube placement, use 43752)

Repair

✿ **44602** Suture of small intestine (enterorrhaphy) for perforated ulcer, diverticulum, wound, injury or rupture; single perforation

✿ **44603** multiple perforations

✿ **44604** Suture of large intestine (colorrhaphy) for perforated ulcer, diverticulum, wound, injury or rupture (single or multiple perforations); without colostomy

✿ **44605** with colostomy

✿ **44615** Intestinal stricturoplasty (enterotomy and enterorrhaphy) with or without dilation, for intestinal obstruction

✿ **44620** Closure of enterostomy, large or small intestine;

✿ **44625** with resection and anastomosis other than colorectal

✿ **44626** with resection and colorectal anastomosis (eg, closure of Hartmann type procedure)

✿ **44640** Closure of intestinal cutaneous fistula

✿ **44650** Closure of enteroenteric or enterocolic fistula

✿ **44660** Closure of enterovesical fistula; without intestinal or bladder resection

✿ **44661** with intestine and/or bladder resection

(For closure of renocolic fistula, see 50525, 50526)

(For closure of gastrocolic fistula, use 43880)

(For closure of rectovesical fistula, see 45800, 45805)

✿ **44680** Intestinal plication (separate procedure)

Other Procedures

✿ **44700** Exclusion of small intestine from pelvis by mesh or other prosthesis, or native tissue (eg, bladder or omentum)

(For therapeutic radiation clinical treatment, see **Radiation Oncology** section)

☆+ **44701** Intraoperative colonic lavage (List separately in addition to code for primary procedure)

(Use 44701 in conjunction with 44140, 44145, 44150, or 44604 as appropriate)

(Do not report 44701 in conjunction with 44300, 44950-44960)

✿● **44715** Backbench standard preparation of cadaver or living donor intestine allograft prior to transplantation, including mobilization and fashioning of the superior mesenteric artery and vein

✿● **44720** Backbench reconstruction of cadaver or living donor intestine allograft prior to transplantation; venous anastomosis, each

✿● **44721** arterial anastomosis, each

§ **44799** Unlisted procedure, intestine

(For unlisted laparoscopic procedure, intestine except rectum, use 44238)

Meckel's Diverticulum and the Mesentery

Excision

✿ **44800** Excision of Meckel's diverticulum (diverticulectomy) or omphalomesenteric duct

✿ **44820** Excision of lesion of mesentery (separate procedure)

(With intestine resection, see 44120 or 44140 et seq)

Suture

✿ **44850** Suture of mesentery (separate procedure)

(For reduction and repair of internal hernia, use 44050)

Other Procedures

✿ **44899** Unlisted procedure, Meckel's diverticulum and the mesentery

Surgery: Digestive System

Appendix

Incision

✿ 44900 Incision and drainage of appendiceal abscess; open

§⊙ 44901 percutaneous

(For radiological supervision and interpretation, use 75989)

Excision

✿ 44950 Appendectomy;

(Incidental appendectomy during intra-abdominal surgery does not usually warrant a separate identification. If necessary to report, add modifier 52)

✿+ 44955 when done for indicated purpose at time of other major procedure (not as separate procedure) (List separately in addition to code for primary procedure)

✿ 44960 for ruptured appendix with abscess or generalized peritonitis

Laparoscopy

Surgical laparoscopy always includes diagnostic laparoscopy. To report a diagnostic laparoscopy (peritoneoscopy) (separate procedure), use 49320.

§ 44970 Laparoscopy, surgical, appendectomy
➔ *CPT Changes: An Insider's View* 2000

§ 44979 Unlisted laparoscopy procedure, appendix
➔ *CPT Changes: An Insider's View* 2000

Rectum

Incision

§ 45000 Transrectal drainage of pelvic abscess

§ 45005 Incision and drainage of submucosal abscess, rectum

§ 45020 Incision and drainage of deep supralevator, pelvirectal, or retrorectal abscess

(See also 46050, 46060)

Excision

§ 45100 Biopsy of anorectal wall, anal approach (eg, congenital megacolon)

(For endoscopic biopsy, use 45305)

§ 45108 Anorectal myomectomy

✿ 45110 Proctectomy; complete, combined abdominoperineal, with colostomy

✿ 45111 partial resection of rectum, transabdominal approach

✿ 45112 Proctectomy, combined abdominoperineal, pull-through procedure (eg, colo-anal anastomosis)

(For colo-anal anastomosis with colonic reservoir or pouch, use 45119)

✿ 45113 Proctectomy, partial, with rectal mucosectomy, ileoanal anastomosis, creation of ileal reservoir (S or J), with or without loop ileostomy

✿ 45114 Proctectomy, partial, with anastomosis; abdominal and transsacral approach

✿ 45116 transsacral approach only (Kraske type)

✿ 45119 Proctectomy, combined abdominoperineal pull-through procedure (eg, colo-anal anastomosis), with creation of colonic reservoir (eg, J-pouch), with or without proximal diverting ostomy

✿ 45120 Proctectomy, complete (for congenital megacolon), abdominal and perineal approach; with pull-through procedure and anastomosis (eg, Swenson, Duhamel, or Soave type operation)

✿ 45121 with subtotal or total colectomy, with multiple biopsies

✿ 45123 Proctectomy, partial, without anastomosis, perineal approach

✿ 45126 Pelvic exenteration for colorectal malignancy, with proctectomy (with or without colostomy), with removal of bladder and ureteral transplantations, and/or hysterectomy, or cervicectomy, with or without removal of tube(s), with or without removal of ovary(s), or any combination thereof

✿ 45130 Excision of rectal procidentia, with anastomosis; perineal approach

✿ 45135 abdominal and perineal approach

✿ 45136 Excision of ileoanal reservoir with ileostomy

(Do not report 45136 in addition to 44005, 44120, 44310)

§ 45150 Division of stricture of rectum

§ 45160 Excision of rectal tumor by proctotomy, transsacral or transcoccygeal approach

§ 45170 Excision of rectal tumor, transanal approach

Destruction

§ 45190 Destruction of rectal tumor (eg, electrodessication, electrosurgery, laser ablation, laser resection, cryosurgery) transanal approach

Endoscopy

Definitions

Proctosigmoidoscopy is the examination of the rectum and sigmoid colon.

Sigmoidoscopy is the examination of the entire rectum, sigmoid colon and may include examination of a portion of the descending colon.

Colonoscopy is the examination of the entire colon, from the rectum to the cecum, and may include the examination of the terminal ileum.

For an incomplete colonoscopy, with full preparation for a colonoscopy, use a colonoscopy code with the modifier 52 and provide documentation.

Surgical endoscopy always includes diagnostic endoscopy.

§ **45300** Proctosigmoidoscopy, rigid; diagnostic, with or without collection of specimen(s) by brushing or washing (separate procedure)

§⊙ **45303** with dilation (eg, balloon, guide wire, bougie)

(For radiological supervision and interpretation, use 74360)

§⊙ **45305** with biopsy, single or multiple

§⊙ **45307** with removal of foreign body

§⊙ **45308** with removal of single tumor, polyp, or other lesion by hot biopsy forceps or bipolar cautery

§⊙ **45309** with removal of single tumor, polyp, or other lesion by snare technique

§⊙ **45315** with removal of multiple tumors, polyps, or other lesions by hot biopsy forceps, bipolar cautery or snare technique

§⊙ **45317** with control of bleeding (eg, injection, bipolar cautery, unipolar cautery, laser, heater probe, stapler, plasma coagulator)
➲ *CPT Changes: An Insider's View* 2002

§⊙ **45320** with ablation of tumor(s), polyp(s), or other lesion(s) not amenable to removal by hot biopsy forceps, bipolar cautery or snare technique (eg, laser)

§ **45321** with decompression of volvulus

§⊙ **45327** with transendoscopic stent placement (includes predilation)

§ **45330** Sigmoidoscopy, flexible; diagnostic, with or without collection of specimen(s) by brushing or washing (separate procedure)

§ **45331** with biopsy, single or multiple

§⊙ **45332** with removal of foreign body

§⊙ **45333** with removal of tumor(s), polyp(s), or other lesion(s) by hot biopsy forceps or bipolar cautery

§⊙ **45334** with control of bleeding (eg, injection, bipolar cautery, unipolar cautery, laser, heater probe, stapler, plasma coagulator)
➲ *CPT Changes: An Insider's View* 2002

§ **45335** with directed submucosal injection(s), any substance
➲ *CPT Changes: An Insider's View* 2003

§⊙ **45337** with decompression of volvulus, any method

§⊙ **45338** with removal of tumor(s), polyp(s), or other lesion(s) by snare technique

§⊙ **45339** with ablation of tumor(s), polyp(s), or other lesion(s) not amenable to removal by hot biopsy forceps, bipolar cautery or snare technique

§⊙ **45340** with dilation by balloon, 1 or more strictures

(Do not report 45340 in conjunction with 45345)

§⊙ **45341** with endoscopic ultrasound examination
➲ *CPT Changes: An Insider's View* 2001

§⊙ **45342** with transendoscopic ultrasound guided intramural or transmural fine needle aspiration/biopsy(s)
➲ *CPT Changes: An Insider's View* 2001

(Do not report 45341, 45342 in conjunction with 76942)

(Do not report 45341, 45342 in conjunction with 76975)

(For interpretation of specimen, see 88172-88173)

(For transrectal ultrasound utilizing rigid probe device, use 76872)

§⊙ **45345** with transendoscopic stent placement (includes predilation)
➲ *CPT Changes: An Insider's View* 2001

§⊙ **45355** Colonoscopy, rigid or flexible, transabdominal via colotomy, single or multiple

(For fiberoptic colonoscopy beyond 25cm to splenic flexure, see 45330-45345)

§⊙ **45378** Colonoscopy, flexible, proximal to splenic flexure; diagnostic, with or without collection of specimen(s) by brushing or washing, with or without colon decompression (separate procedure)

§⊙ **45379** with removal of foreign body

§⊙ **45380** with biopsy, single or multiple

§⊙ **45381** with directed submucosal injection(s), any substance
➲ *CPT Changes: An Insider's View* 2003

§⊙ **45382** with control of bleeding (eg, injection, bipolar cautery, unipolar cautery, laser, heater probe, stapler, plasma coagulator)
➲ *CPT Changes: An Insider's View* 2002

§⊙ **45383** with ablation of tumor(s), polyp(s), or other lesion(s) not amenable to removal by hot biopsy forceps, bipolar cautery or snare technique

§⊙ **45384** with removal of tumor(s), polyp(s), or other lesion(s) by hot biopsy forceps or bipolar cautery

§⊙ **45385** with removal of tumor(s), polyp(s), or other lesion(s) by snare technique

(For small intestine and stomal endoscopy, see 44360-44393)

§⊙ **45386** with dilation by balloon, 1 or more strictures
➲ *CPT Changes: An Insider's View* 2003

(Do not report 45386 in conjunction with 45387)

§⊙ **45387** with transendoscopic stent placement (includes predilation)
➲ *CPT Changes: An Insider's View* 2001

§⊙● **45391** with endoscopic ultrasound examination
➲ *CPT Changes: An Insider's View* 2005

►(Do not report 45391 in conjunction with 45330, 45341, 45342, 45378, 76872)◄

§⊙● **45392** with transendoscopic ultrasound guided intramural or transmural fine needle aspiration/biopsy(s)
➲ *CPT Changes: An Insider's View* 2005

►(Do not report 45392 in conjunction with 45330, 45341, 45342, 45378, 76872)◄

Repair

§ **45500** Proctoplasty; for stenosis

§ **45505** for prolapse of mucous membrane

§ **45520** Perirectal injection of sclerosing solution for prolapse

✿ **45540** Proctopexy for prolapse; abdominal approach

§ **45541** perineal approach

✿ **45550** Proctopexy combined with sigmoid resection, abdominal approach

§ **45560** Repair of rectocele (separate procedure)

(For repair of rectocele with posterior colporrhaphy, use 57250)

✿ **45562** Exploration, repair, and presacral drainage for rectal injury;

✿ **45563** with colostomy

✿ **45800** Closure of rectovesical fistula;

✿ **45805** with colostomy

✿ **45820** Closure of rectourethral fistula;

✿ **45825** with colostomy

(For rectovaginal fistula closure, see 57300-57308)

Manipulation

§ **45900** Reduction of procidentia (separate procedure) under anesthesia

§ **45905** Dilation of anal sphincter (separate procedure) under anesthesia other than local

§ **45910** Dilation of rectal stricture (separate procedure) under anesthesia other than local

§ **45915** Removal of fecal impaction or foreign body (separate procedure) under anesthesia
➲ *CPT Changes: An Insider's View* 2003

Other Procedures

§ **45999** Unlisted procedure, rectum

(For unlisted laparoscopic procedure, rectum, use 44239)

Anus

Incision

(For subcutaneous fistulotomy, use 46270)

§ **46020** Placement of seton
➲ *CPT Changes: An Insider's View* 2002

(Do not report 46020 in addition to 46060, 46280, 46600)

§ **46030** Removal of anal seton, other marker

§ **46040** Incision and drainage of ischiorectal and/or perirectal abscess (separate procedure)

§ **46045** Incision and drainage of intramural, intramuscular, or submucosal abscess, transanal, under anesthesia

§ **46050** Incision and drainage, perianal abscess, superficial

(See also 45020, 46060)

§ **46060** Incision and drainage of ischiorectal or intramural abscess, with fistulectomy or fistulotomy, submuscular, with or without placement of seton

(Do not report 46060 in addition to 46020)

(See also 45020)

§ **46070** Incision, anal septum (infant)

(For anoplasty, see 46700-46705)

(Do not report modifier 63 in conjunction with 46070)

§ **46080** Sphincterotomy, anal, division of sphincter (separate procedure)

§ **46083** Incision of thrombosed hemorrhoid, external

Excision

§ **46200** Fissurectomy, with or without sphincterotomy

§ **46210** Cryptectomy; single

§ **46211** multiple (separate procedure)

§ **46220** Papillectomy or excision of single tag, anus (separate procedure)

§ **46221** Hemorrhoidectomy, by simple ligature (eg, rubber band)

§ **46230** Excision of external hemorrhoid tags and/or multiple papillae

§ **46250** Hemorrhoidectomy, external, complete

§ **46255** Hemorrhoidectomy, internal and external, simple;

§ **46257** with fissurectomy

§ **46258** with fistulectomy, with or without fissurectomy

§ **46260** Hemorrhoidectomy, internal and external, complex or extensive;

§ **46261** with fissurectomy

§ **46262** with fistulectomy, with or without fissurectomy

►(For injection of hemorrhoids, use 46500; for destruction, see 46934-46936; for ligation, see 46945, 46946; for hemorrhoidopexy, use 46947)◄

§ **46270** Surgical treatment of anal fistula (fistulectomy/fistulotomy); subcutaneous

§ **46275** submuscular

§ **46280** complex or multiple, with or without placement of seton

(Do not report 46280 in addition to 46020)

§ **46285** second stage

§ **46288** Closure of anal fistula with rectal advancement flap

§ **46320** Enucleation or excision of external thrombotic hemorrhoid

Introduction

§ **46500** Injection of sclerosing solution, hemorrhoids

►(For excision of hemorrhoids, see 46250-46262; for destruction, see 46934-46936; for ligation, see 46945, 46946; for hemorrhoidopexy, use 46947)◄

Endoscopy

Surgical endoscopy always includes diagnostic endoscopy.

♣ **46600** Anoscopy; diagnostic, with or without collection of specimen(s) by brushing or washing (separate procedure)

(Do not report 46600 in addition to 46020)

§ **46604** with dilation (eg, balloon, guide wire, bougie)

➔ *CPT Changes: An Insider's View* 2002

§ **46606** with biopsy, single or multiple

§ **46608** with removal of foreign body

§ **46610** with removal of single tumor, polyp, or other lesion by hot biopsy forceps or bipolar cautery

§ **46611** with removal of single tumor, polyp, or other lesion by snare technique

§ **46612** with removal of multiple tumors, polyps, or other lesions by hot biopsy forceps, bipolar cautery or snare technique

§ **46614** with control of bleeding (eg, injection, bipolar cautery, unipolar cautery, laser, heater probe, stapler, plasma coagulator)

➔ *CPT Changes: An Insider's View* 2002

§ **46615** with ablation of tumor(s), polyp(s), or other lesion(s) not amenable to removal by hot biopsy forceps, bipolar cautery or snare technique

Repair

§ **46700** Anoplasty, plastic operation for stricture; adult

✿ **46705** infant

(For simple incision of anal septum, use 46070)

(Do not report modifier 63 in conjunction with 46705)

§ **46706** Repair of anal fistula with fibrin glue

➔ *CPT Changes: An Insider's View* 2003

✿ **46715** Repair of low imperforate anus; with anoperineal fistula (cut-back procedure)

✿ **46716** with transposition of anoperineal or anovestibular fistula

(Do not report modifier 63 in conjunction with 46715, 46716)

✿ **46730** Repair of high imperforate anus without fistula; perineal or sacroperineal approach

✿ **46735** combined transabdominal and sacroperineal approaches

(Do not report modifier 63 in conjunction with 46730, 46735)

✿ **46740** Repair of high imperforate anus with rectourethral or rectovaginal fistula; perineal or sacroperineal approach

✿ **46742** combined transabdominal and sacroperineal approaches

(Do not report modifier 63 in conjunction with 46740, 46742)

✿ **46744** Repair of cloacal anomaly by anorectovaginoplasty and urethroplasty, sacroperineal approach

(Do not report modifier 63 in conjunction with 46744)

✿ **46746** Repair of cloacal anomaly by anorectovaginoplasty and urethroplasty, combined abdominal and sacroperineal approach;

✿ **46748** with vaginal lengthening by intestinal graft or pedicle flaps

§ **46750** Sphincteroplasty, anal, for incontinence or prolapse; adult

✿ **46751** child

§ **46753** Graft (Thiersch operation) for rectal incontinence and/or prolapse

§ **46754** Removal of Thiersch wire or suture, anal canal

§ **46760** Sphincteroplasty, anal, for incontinence, adult; muscle transplant

§ **46761** levator muscle imbrication (Park posterior anal repair)

§ **46762** implantation artificial sphincter

Destruction

§ **46900** Destruction of lesion(s), anus (eg, condyloma, papilloma, molluscum contagiosum, herpetic vesicle), simple; chemical

§ **46910** electrodesiccation

§ **46916** cryosurgery

§ **46917** laser surgery

§ **46922** surgical excision

§ **46924** Destruction of lesion(s), anus (eg, condyloma, papilloma, molluscum contagiosum, herpetic vesicle), extensive (eg, laser surgery, electrosurgery, cryosurgery, chemosurgery)
➔ *CPT Changes: An Insider's View* 2002

§ **46934** Destruction of hemorrhoids, any method; internal

§ **46935** external

§ **46936** internal and external

►(For excision of hemorrhoids, see 46250-46262; for injection, use 46500; for ligation, see 46945, 46946; for hemorrhoidopexy, use 46947)◄

§ **46937** Cryosurgery of rectal tumor; benign

§ **46938** malignant

§ **46940** Curettage or cautery of anal fissure, including dilation of anal sphincter (separate procedure); initial
➔ *CPT Changes: An Insider's View* 2002

§ **46942** subsequent

Suture

§ **46945** Ligation of internal hemorrhoids; single procedure

§ **46946** multiple procedures

§● **46947** Hemorrhoidopexy (eg, for prolapsing internal hemorrhoids) by stapling
➔ *CPT Changes: An Insider's View* 2005

►(For excision of hemorrhoids, see 46250-46262; for injection, use 46500; for destruction, see 46934-46936)◄

Other Procedures

§ **46999** Unlisted procedure, anus

Liver

Incision

§ **47000** Biopsy of liver, needle; percutaneous

(If imaging guidance is performed, see 76003, 76360, 76393, 76942)

☆+ **47001** when done for indicated purpose at time of other major procedure (List separately in addition to code for primary procedure)
➔ *CPT Assistant* Jan 03:16, Feb 03:8

(If imaging guidance is performed, see 76003, 76942)

(For fine needle aspiration in conjunction with 47000, 47001, see 10021, 10022)

(For evaluation of fine needle aspirate in conjunction with 47000, 47001, see 88172, 88173)

✿ **47010** Hepatotomy; for open drainage of abscess or cyst, one or two stages

§⊙ **47011** for percutaneous drainage of abscess or cyst, one or two stages

(For radiological supervision and interpretation, use 75989)

✿ **47015** Laparotomy, with aspiration and/or injection of hepatic parasitic (eg, amoebic or echinococcal) cyst(s) or abscess(es)

Excision

✿ **47100** Biopsy of liver, wedge

✿ **47120** Hepatectomy, resection of liver; partial lobectomy

✿ **47122** trisegmentectomy

✿ **47125** total left lobectomy

✿ **47130** total right lobectomy

►Liver Transplantation◄

►Liver allotransplantation involves three distinct components of physician work:◄

►1) ***Cadaver donor hepatectomy***, which includes harvesting the graft and cold preservation of the graft (perfusing with cold preservation solution and cold maintenance) (use 47133). ***Living donor hepatectomy***, which includes harvesting the graft, cold preservation of the graft (perfusing with cold preservation solution and cold maintenance), and care of the donor (see 47140-47142).◄

►2) ***Backbench work***:◄

- ► Standard preparation of the whole liver graft will include one of the following:◄
- ► Preparation of whole liver graft (including cholecystectomy, if necessary, and dissection and removal of surrounding soft tissues to prepare vena cava, portal vein, hepatic artery, and common bile duct for implantation) (use 47143).◄
- ► Preparation as described for whole liver graft, plus trisegment split into two partial grafts (use 47144).◄
- ► Preparation as described for whole liver graft, plus lobe split into two partial grafts (use 47145).◄
- ► Additional reconstruction of the liver graft may include venous and/or arterial anastomosis(es) (see 47146, 47147).◄

►3) ***Recipient liver allotransplantation***, which includes recipient hepatectomy (partial or whole), transplantation of the allograft (partial or whole), and care of the recipient (see 47135, 47136).◄

✿▲ **47133** Donor hepatectomy (including cold preservation), from cadaver donor

(47134 has been deleted. To report, use 47140)

✿ **47135** Liver allotransplantation; orthotopic, partial or whole, from cadaver or living donor, any age

Surgery: Digestive System

✿ **47136** heterotopic, partial or whole, from cadaver or living donor, any age

✿▲ **47140** Donor hepatectomy (including cold preservation), from living donor; left lateral segment only (segments II and III)

✿ **47141** total left lobectomy (segments II, III and IV)

✿ **47142** total right lobectomy (segments V, VI, VII and VIII)

✿● **47143** Backbench standard preparation of cadaver donor whole liver graft prior to allotransplantation, including cholecystectomy, if necessary, and dissection and removal of surrounding soft tissues to prepare the vena cava, portal vein, hepatic artery, and common bile duct for implantation; without trisegment or lobe split

✿● **47144** with trisegment split of whole liver graft into two partial liver grafts (ie, left lateral segment (segments II and III) and right trisegment (segments I and IV through VIII))

✿● **47145** with lobe split of whole liver graft into two partial liver grafts (ie, left lobe (segments II, III, and IV) and right lobe (segments I and V through VIII))

✿● **47146** Backbench reconstruction of cadaver or living donor liver graft prior to allotransplantation; venous anastomosis, each

✿● **47147** arterial anastomosis, each

►(Do not report 47143-47147 in conjunction with 47120-47125, 47600, 47610)◄

Repair

✿ **47300** Marsupialization of cyst or abscess of liver

✿ **47350** Management of liver hemorrhage; simple suture of liver wound or injury

✿ **47360** complex suture of liver wound or injury, with or without hepatic artery ligation

✿ **47361** exploration of hepatic wound, extensive debridement, coagulation and/or suture, with or without packing of liver

✿ **47362** re-exploration of hepatic wound for removal of packing

Laparoscopy

Surgical laparoscopy always includes diagnostic laparoscopy. To report a diagnostic laparoscopy (peritoneoscopy) (separate procedure), use 49320.

§ **47370** Laparoscopy, surgical, ablation of one or more liver tumor(s); radiofrequency

➔ *CPT Assistant* Feb 03:7; *CPT Changes: An Insider's View* 2002

(For imaging guidance, use 76940)

§ **47371** cryosurgical

➔ *CPT Assistant* Feb 03:7; *CPT Changes: An Insider's View* 2002

(For imaging guidance, use 76940)

§ **47379** Unlisted laparoscopic procedure, liver

➔ *CPT Assistant* Feb 03:7; *CPT Changes: An Insider's View* 2001

Other Procedures

✿ **47380** Ablation, open, of one or more liver tumor(s); radiofrequency

➔ *CPT Assistant* Feb 03:7

(For imaging guidance, use 76940)

✿ **47381** cryosurgical

➔ *CPT Assistant* Feb 03:7

(For imaging guidance, use 76940)

§ **47382** Ablation, one or more liver tumor(s), percutaneous, radiofrequency

➔ *CPT Assistant* Feb 03:7; *CPT Changes: An Insider's View* 2002

(For imaging guidance and monitoring, see code 76362, 76394, or 76940)

§ **47399** Unlisted procedure, liver

Biliary Tract

Incision

✿ **47400** Hepaticotomy or hepaticostomy with exploration, drainage, or removal of calculus

✿ **47420** Choledochotomy or choledochostomy with exploration, drainage, or removal of calculus, with or without cholecystotomy; without transduodenal sphincterotomy or sphincteroplasty

✿ **47425** with transduodenal sphincterotomy or sphincteroplasty

✿ **47460** Transduodenal sphincterotomy or sphincteroplasty, with or without transduodenal extraction of calculus (separate procedure)

✿ **47480** Cholecystotomy or cholecystostomy with exploration, drainage, or removal of calculus (separate procedure)

§ **47490** Percutaneous cholecystostomy

➔ *CPT Assistant* Jan 03:16

(For radiological supervision and interpretation, use 75989)

Introduction

☆ **47500** Injection procedure for percutaneous transhepatic cholangiography

(For radiological supervision and interpretation, use 74320)

☆ **47505** Injection procedure for cholangiography through an existing catheter (eg, percutaneous transhepatic or T-tube)

(For radiological supervision and interpretation, use 74305)

§ 47510 Introduction of percutaneous transhepatic catheter for biliary drainage

(For radiological supervision and interpretation, use 75980)

♦§ 47511 Introduction of percutaneous transhepatic stent for internal and external biliary drainage

(For radiological supervision and interpretation, use 75982)

♦§ 47525 Change of percutaneous biliary drainage catheter

(For radiological supervision and interpretation, use 75984)

§ 47530 Revision and/or reinsertion of transhepatic tube

(For radiological supervision and interpretation, use 75984)

Endoscopy

Surgical endoscopy always includes diagnostic endoscopy.

✿+ 47550 Biliary endoscopy, intraoperative (choledochoscopy) (List separately in addition to code for primary procedure)

§ 47552 Biliary endoscopy, percutaneous via T-tube or other tract; diagnostic, with or without collection of specimen(s) by brushing and/or washing (separate procedure)

§ 47553 with biopsy, single or multiple

§ 47554 with removal of calculus/calculi
➔ *CPT Changes: An Insider's View* 2002

§ 47555 with dilation of biliary duct stricture(s) without stent

(For ERCP, see 43260-43272, 74363)

(If imaging guidance is performed, see 74363, 75982)

§ 47556 with dilation of biliary duct stricture(s) with stent

(If imaging guidance is performed, see 74363, 75982)

Laparoscopy

Surgical laparoscopy always includes diagnostic laparoscopy. To report a diagnostic laparoscopy (peritoneoscopy) (separate procedure), use 49320.

§ 47560 Laparoscopy, surgical; with guided transhepatic cholangiography, without biopsy
➔ *CPT Changes: An Insider's View* 2002

§ 47561 with guided transhepatic cholangiography with biopsy
➔ *CPT Changes: An Insider's View* 2002

§ 47562 cholecystectomy
➔ *CPT Assistant* May 03:9; *CPT Changes: An Insider's View* 2000

§ 47563 cholecystectomy with cholangiography
➔ *CPT Changes: An Insider's View* 2000

§ 47564 cholecystectomy with exploration of common duct
➔ *CPT Changes: An Insider's View* 2000

✿ 47570 cholecystoenterostomy

§ 47579 Unlisted laparoscopy procedure, biliary tract
➔ *CPT Changes: An Insider's View* 2000

Excision

✿ 47600 Cholecystectomy;

✿ 47605 with cholangiography

(For laparoscopic approach, see 47562-47564)

✿ 47610 Cholecystectomy with exploration of common duct;

(For cholecystectomy with exploration of common duct with biliary endoscopy, use 47610 with 47550)

✿ 47612 with choledochoenterostomy

✿ 47620 with transduodenal sphincterotomy or sphincteroplasty, with or without cholangiography

§ 47630 Biliary duct stone extraction, percutaneous via T-tube tract, basket, or snare (eg, Burhenne technique)

(For radiological supervision and interpretation, use 74327)

✿ 47700 Exploration for congenital atresia of bile ducts, without repair, with or without liver biopsy, with or without cholangiography

(Do not report modifier 63 in conjunction with 47700)

✿ 47701 Portoenterostomy (eg, Kasai procedure)

(Do not report modifier 63 in conjunction with 47701)

✿ 47711 Excision of bile duct tumor, with or without primary repair of bile duct; extrahepatic

✿ 47712 intrahepatic

(For anastomosis, see 47760-47800)

✿ 47715 Excision of choledochal cyst

✿ 47716 Anastomosis, choledochal cyst, without excision

Repair

✿ 47720 Cholecystoenterostomy; direct

(For laparoscopic approach, use 47570)

✿ 47721 with gastroenterostomy

✿ 47740 Roux-en-Y

✿ 47741 Roux-en-Y with gastroenterostomy

✿ 47760 Anastomosis, of extrahepatic biliary ducts and gastrointestinal tract

✿ 47765 Anastomosis, of intrahepatic ducts and gastrointestinal tract

✿ 47780 Anastomosis, Roux-en-Y, of extrahepatic biliary ducts and gastrointestinal tract

✿ **47785** Anastomosis, Roux-en-Y, of intrahepatic biliary ducts and gastrointestinal tract

✿ **47800** Reconstruction, plastic, of extrahepatic biliary ducts with end-to-end anastomosis

✿ **47801** Placement of choledochal stent

✿ **47802** U-tube hepaticoenterostomy

✿ **47900** Suture of extrahepatic biliary duct for pre-existing injury (separate procedure)

Other Procedures

§ **47999** Unlisted procedure, biliary tract

Pancreas

(For peroral pancreatic endoscopic procedures, see 43260-43272)

Incision

✿ **48000** Placement of drains, peripancreatic, for acute pancreatitis;

✿ **48001** with cholecystostomy, gastrostomy, and jejunostomy

✿ **48005** Resection or debridement of pancreas and peripancreatic tissue for acute necrotizing pancreatitis

✿ **48020** Removal of pancreatic calculus

Excision

✿ **48100** Biopsy of pancreas, open (eg, fine needle aspiration, needle core biopsy, wedge biopsy)

§ **48102** Biopsy of pancreas, percutaneous needle

(For radiological supervision and interpretation, see 76003, 76360, 76393, 76942)

(For fine needle aspiration, use 10022)

(For evaluation of fine needle aspirate, see 88172, 88173)

✿ **48120** Excision of lesion of pancreas (eg, cyst, adenoma)

✿ **48140** Pancreatectomy, distal subtotal, with or without splenectomy; without pancreaticojejunostomy

✿ **48145** with pancreaticojejunostomy

✿ **48146** Pancreatectomy, distal, near-total with preservation of duodenum (Child-type procedure)

✿ **48148** Excision of ampulla of Vater

✿ **48150** Pancreatectomy, proximal subtotal with total duodenectomy, partial gastrectomy, choledochoenterostomy and gastrojejunostomy (Whipple-type procedure); with pancreatojejunostomy

✿ **48152** without pancreatojejunostomy

✿ **48153** Pancreatectomy, proximal subtotal with near-total duodenectomy, choledochoenterostomy and duodenojejunostomy (pylorus-sparing, Whipple-type procedure); with pancreatojejunostomy

✿ **48154** without pancreatojejunostomy

✿ **48155** Pancreatectomy, total

□ **48160** Pancreatectomy, total or subtotal, with autologous transplantation of pancreas or pancreatic islet cells

✿ **48180** Pancreaticojejunostomy, side-to-side anastomosis (Puestow-type operation)

Introduction

✿+ **48400** Injection procedure for intraoperative pancreatography (List separately in addition to code for primary procedure)

(For radiological supervision and interpretation, see 74300-74305)

Repair

✿ **48500** Marsupialization of pancreatic cyst

✿ **48510** External drainage, pseudocyst of pancreas; open

§⊙ **48511** percutaneous

(For radiological supervision and interpretation, use 75989)

✿ **48520** Internal anastomosis of pancreatic cyst to gastrointestinal tract; direct

✿ **48540** Roux-en-Y

✿ **48545** Pancreatorrhaphy for injury

✿ **48547** Duodenal exclusion with gastrojejunostomy for pancreatic injury

Pancreas Transplantation

►Pancreas allotransplantation involves three distinct components of physician work:◄

►1) ***Cadaver donor pancreatectomy***, which includes harvesting the pancreas graft, with or without duodenal segment, and cold preservation of the graft (perfusing with cold preservation solution and cold maintenance) (use 48550).◄

►2) ***Backbench work:***◄

► Standard preparation of a cadaver donor pancreas allograft prior to transplantation includes dissection of the allograft from surrounding soft tissues, splenectomy, duodenotomy, ligation of bile duct, ligation of mesenteric vessels, and Y-graft arterial anastomoses from the iliac artery to the superior mesenteric artery and to the splenic artery (use 48551).◄

► Additional reconstruction of a cadaver donor pancreas allograft prior to transplantation may include venous anastomosis(es) (use 48552).◄

Surgery: Digestive System

►3) ***Recipient pancreas allotransplantation***, which includes transplantation of allograft, and care of the recipient (use 48554).◄

□▲ **48550** Donor pancreatectomy (including cold preservation), with or without duodenal segment for transplantation

✿● **48551** Backbench standard preparation of cadaver donor pancreas allograft prior to transplantation, including dissection of allograft from surrounding soft tissues, splenectomy, duodenotomy, ligation of bile duct, ligation of mesenteric vessels, and Y-graft arterial anastomoses from iliac artery to superior mesenteric artery and to splenic artery

✿● **48552** Backbench reconstruction of cadaver donor pancreas allograft prior to transplantation, venous anastomosis, each

►(Do not report 48551 and 48552 in conjunction with 35531, 35563, 35685, 38100-38102, 44010, 44820, 44850, 47460, 47505-47525, 47550-47556, 48100-48120, 48545)◄

□ **48554** Transplantation of pancreatic allograft

✿ **48556** Removal of transplanted pancreatic allograft

Other Procedures

§ **48999** Unlisted procedure, pancreas

Abdomen, Peritoneum, and Omentum

Incision

✿ **49000** Exploratory laparotomy, exploratory celiotomy with or without biopsy(s) (separate procedure)

(To report wound exploration due to penetrating trauma without laparotomy, use 20102)

✿ **49002** Reopening of recent laparotomy

(To report re-exploration of hepatic wound for removal of packing, use 47362)

✿ **49010** Exploration, retroperitoneal area with or without biopsy(s) (separate procedure)

(To report wound exploration due to penetrating trauma without laparotomy, use 20102)

✿ **49020** Drainage of peritoneal abscess or localized peritonitis, exclusive of appendiceal abscess; open

(For appendiceal abscess, use 44900)

§⊙ **49021** percutaneous

(For radiological supervision and interpretation, use 75989)

✿ **49040** Drainage of subdiaphragmatic or subphrenic abscess; open

§⊙ **49041** percutaneous

(For radiological supervision and interpretation, use 75989)

✿ **49060** Drainage of retroperitoneal abscess; open

§⊙ **49061** percutaneous

(For laparoscopic drainage, use 49323)

(For radiological supervision and interpretation, use 75989)

✿ **49062** Drainage of extraperitoneal lymphocele to peritoneal cavity, open

§ **49080** Peritoneocentesis, abdominal paracentesis, or peritoneal lavage (diagnostic or therapeutic); initial

§ **49081** subsequent

(If imaging guidance is performed, see 76360, 76942)

§ **49085** Removal of peritoneal foreign body from peritoneal cavity

(For lysis of intestinal adhesions, use 44005)

Excision, Destruction

§ **49180** Biopsy, abdominal or retroperitoneal mass, percutaneous needle

(If imaging guidance is performed, see 76003, 76360, 76393, 76942)

(For fine needle aspiration, use 10021 or 10022)

(For evaluation of fine needle aspirate, see 88172, 88173)

§ **49200** Excision or destruction, open, intra-abdominal or retroperitoneal tumors or cysts or endometriomas;

✿ **49201** extensive

✿ **49215** Excision of presacral or sacrococcygeal tumor

(Do not report modifier 63 in conjunction with 49215)

✿ **49220** Staging laparotomy for Hodgkins disease or lymphoma (includes splenectomy, needle or open biopsies of both liver lobes, possibly also removal of abdominal nodes, abdominal node and/or bone marrow biopsies, ovarian repositioning)

§ **49250** Umbilectomy, omphalectomy, excision of umbilicus (separate procedure)

✿ **49255** Omentectomy, epiploectomy, resection of omentum (separate procedure)

Laparoscopy

Surgical laparoscopy always includes diagnostic laparoscopy. To report a diagnostic laparoscopy (peritoneoscopy), (separate procedure), use 49320.

For laparoscopic fulguration or excision of lesions of the ovary, pelvic viscera, or peritoneal surface use 58662.

§ **49320** Laparoscopy, abdomen, peritoneum, and omentum, diagnostic, with or without collection of specimen(s) by brushing or washing (separate procedure)

➲ *CPT Changes: An Insider's View* 2000, 2001

§ **49321** Laparoscopy, surgical; with biopsy (single or multiple)
➲ *CPT Changes: An Insider's View* 2000, 2001

§ **49322** with aspiration of cavity or cyst (eg, ovarian cyst) (single or multiple)
➲ *CPT Changes: An Insider's View* 2000

§ **49323** with drainage of lymphocele to peritoneal cavity
➲ *CPT Changes: An Insider's View* 2000

(For percutaneous or open drainage, see 49060, 49061)

§ **49329** Unlisted laparoscopy procedure, abdomen, peritoneum and omentum
➲ *CPT Changes: An Insider's View* 2000

Introduction, Revision, and/or Removal

☆ **49400** Injection of air or contrast into peritoneal cavity (separate procedure)

(For radiological supervision and interpretation, use 74190)

§ **49419** Insertion of intraperitoneal cannula or catheter, with subcutaneous reservoir, permanent (ie, totally implantable)
➲ *CPT Changes: An Insider's View* 2003

(For removal, use 49422)

§ **49420** Insertion of intraperitoneal cannula or catheter for drainage or dialysis; temporary

§ **49421** permanent

§ **49422** Removal of permanent intraperitoneal cannula or catheter

(For removal of a temporary catheter/cannula, use appropriate E/M code)

§ **49423** Exchange of previously placed abscess or cyst drainage catheter under radiological guidance (separate procedure)

(For radiological supervision and interpretation, use 75984)

☆ **49424** Contrast injection for assessment of abscess or cyst via previously placed drainage catheter or tube (separate procedure)
➲ *CPT Changes: An Insider's View* 2002

(For radiological supervision and interpretation, use 76080)

✿ **49425** Insertion of peritoneal-venous shunt

§ **49426** Revision of peritoneal-venous shunt

(For shunt patency test, use 78291)

☆ **49427** Injection procedure (eg, contrast media) for evaluation of previously placed peritoneal-venous shunt

(For radiological supervision and interpretation, see 75809, 78291)

✿ **49428** Ligation of peritoneal-venous shunt

§ **49429** Removal of peritoneal-venous shunt

Repair

Hernioplasty, Herniorrhaphy, Herniotomy

The hernia repair codes in this section are categorized primarily by the type of hernia (inguinal, femoral, incisional, etc.).

Some types of hernias are further categorized as "initial" or "recurrent" based on whether or not the hernia has required previous repair(s).

Additional variables accounted for by some of the codes include patient age and clinical presentation (reducible vs. incarcerated or strangulated).

With the exception of the incisional hernia repairs (see 49560-49566) the use of mesh or other prostheses is not separately reported.

The excision/repair of strangulated organs or structures such as testicle(s), intestine, ovaries are reported by using the appropriate code for the excision/repair (eg, 44120, 54520, and 58940) in addition to the appropriate code for the repair of the strangulated hernia.

(For reduction and repair of intra-abdominal hernia, use 44050)

(For debridement of abdominal wall, see 11042, 11043)

(Codes 49491-49651 are unilateral procedures. To report bilateral procedures, report modifier 50 with the appropriate procedure code)

♦§ **49491** Repair, initial inguinal hernia, preterm infant (less than 37 weeks gestation at birth), performed from birth up to 50 weeks postconception age, with or without hydrocelectomy; reducible
➲ *CPT Changes: An Insider's View* 2002

♦§ **49492** incarcerated or strangulated
➲ *CPT Changes: An Insider's View* 2002

(Do not report modifier 63 in conjunction with 49491, 49492)

(Postconception age equals gestational age at birth plus age of infant in weeks at the time of the hernia repair. Initial inguinal hernia repairs that are performed on preterm infants who are over 50 weeks postconception age and under age 6 months at the time of surgery, should be reported using codes 49495, 49496)

♦§ **49495** Repair, initial inguinal hernia, full term infant under age 6 months, or preterm infant over 50 weeks postconception age and under age 6 months at the time of surgery, with or without hydrocelectomy; reducible
➲ *CPT Changes: An Insider's View* 2002

♦§ **49496** incarcerated or strangulated
➲ *CPT Changes: An Insider's View* 2002

(Do not report modifier 63 in conjunction with 49495, 49496)

Surgery: Digestive System

(Postconception age equals gestational age at birth plus age in weeks at the time of the hernia repair. Initial inguinal hernia repairs that are performed on preterm infants who are under or up to 50 weeks postconception age but under 6 months of age since birth, should be reported using codes 49491, 49492. Inguinal hernia repairs on infants age 6 months to under 5 years should be reported using codes 49500-49501)

♦§ **49500** Repair initial inguinal hernia, age 6 months to under 5 years, with or without hydrocelectomy; reducible
➔ *CPT Changes: An Insider's View* 2002

♦§ **49501** incarcerated or strangulated
➔ *CPT Changes: An Insider's View* 2002

♦§ **49505** Repair initial inguinal hernia, age 5 years or over; reducible

♦§ **49507** incarcerated or strangulated

(For inguinal hernia repair, with simple orchiectomy, see 49505 or 49507 and 54520)

(For inguinal hernia repair, with excision of hydrocele or spermatocele, see 49505 or 49507 and 54840 or 55040)

♦§ **49520** Repair recurrent inguinal hernia, any age; reducible

♦§ **49521** incarcerated or strangulated

♦§ **49525** Repair inguinal hernia, sliding, any age

(For incarcerated or strangulated inguinal hernia repair, see 49496, 49501, 49507, 49521)

♦§ **49540** Repair lumbar hernia

♦§ **49550** Repair initial femoral hernia, any age; reducible

♦§ **49553** incarcerated or strangulated

♦§ **49555** Repair recurrent femoral hernia; reducible

♦§ **49557** incarcerated or strangulated

♦§ **49560** Repair initial incisional or ventral hernia; reducible

♦§ **49561** incarcerated or strangulated

♦§ **49565** Repair recurrent incisional or ventral hernia; reducible

♦§ **49566** incarcerated or strangulated

♦§+ **49568** Implantation of mesh or other prosthesis for incisional or ventral hernia repair (List separately in addition to code for the incisional or ventral hernia repair)

♦§ **49570** Repair epigastric hernia (eg, preperitoneal fat); reducible (separate procedure)

♦§ **49572** incarcerated or strangulated

§ **49580** Repair umbilical hernia, under age 5 years; reducible

§ **49582** incarcerated or strangulated

§ **49585** Repair umbilical hernia, age 5 years or over; reducible

§ **49587** incarcerated or strangulated

♦§ **49590** Repair spigelian hernia

§ **49600** Repair of small omphalocele, with primary closure

(Do not report modifier 63 in conjunction with 49600)

✿ **49605** Repair of large omphalocele or gastroschisis; with or without prosthesis

✿ **49606** with removal of prosthesis, final reduction and closure, in operating room

(Do not report modifier 63 in conjunction with 49605, 49606)

✿ **49610** Repair of omphalocele (Gross type operation); first stage

✿ **49611** second stage

(Do not report modifier 63 in conjunction with 49610, 49611)

(For diaphragmatic or hiatal hernia repair, see 39502-39541)

(For surgical repair of omentum, use 49999)

Laparoscopy

Surgical laparoscopy always includes diagnostic laparoscopy. To report a diagnostic laparoscopy (peritoneoscopy) (separate procedure), use 49320.

♦§ **49650** Laparoscopy, surgical; repair initial inguinal hernia
➔ *CPT Changes: An Insider's View* 2000

♦§ **49651** repair recurrent inguinal hernia

§ **49659** Unlisted laparoscopy procedure, hernioplasty, herniorrhaphy, herniotomy
➔ *CPT Changes: An Insider's View* 2000

Suture

✿ **49900** Suture, secondary, of abdominal wall for evisceration or dehiscence

(For suture of ruptured diaphragm, see 39540, 39541)

(For debridement of abdominal wall, see 11042, 11043)

Other Procedures

✿ **49904** Omental flap, extra-abdominal (eg, for reconstruction of sternal and chest wall defects)

(Code 49904 includes harvest and transfer. If a second surgeon harvests the omental flap, then the two surgeons should code 49904 as co-surgeons, using modifier 62)

✿+ **49905** Omental flap, intra-abdominal (List separately in addition to code for primary procedure)

(Do not report 49905 in conjunction with 44700)

✿ **49906** Free omental flap with microvascular anastomosis

(Do not report code 69990 in addition to 49906)

§ **49999** Unlisted procedure, abdomen, peritoneum and omentum

Urinary System

(For provision of chemotherapeutic agents, use 96545 in addition to code for primary procedure)

Kidney

Incision

(For retroperitoneal exploration, abscess, tumor, or cyst, see 49010, 49060, 49200, 49201)

✿ **50010** Renal exploration, not necessitating other specific procedures

(For laparoscopic ablation of renal mass lesion(s), use 50542)

§ **50020** Drainage of perirenal or renal abscess; open

§⊙ **50021** percutaneous

(For radiological supervision and interpretation, use 75989)

✿ **50040** Nephrostomy, nephrotomy with drainage

✿ **50045** Nephrotomy, with exploration

(For renal endoscopy performed in conjunction with this procedure, see 50570-50580)

✿ **50060** Nephrolithotomy; removal of calculus

✿ **50065** secondary surgical operation for calculus

✿ **50070** complicated by congenital kidney abnormality

✿ **50075** removal of large staghorn calculus filling renal pelvis and calyces (including anatrophic pyelolithotomy)

§ **50080** Percutaneous nephrostolithotomy or pyelostolithotomy, with or without dilation, endoscopy, lithotripsy, stenting, or basket extraction; up to 2 cm

§ **50081** over 2 cm

(For establishment of nephrostomy without nephrostolithotomy, see 50040, 50395, 52334)

(For fluoroscopic guidance, see 76000, 76001)

✿ **50100** Transection or repositioning of aberrant renal vessels (separate procedure)

✿ **50120** Pyelotomy; with exploration

(For renal endoscopy performed in conjunction with this procedure, see 50570-50580)

✿ **50125** with drainage, pyelostomy

✿ **50130** with removal of calculus (pyelolithotomy, pelviolithotomy, including coagulum pyelolithotomy)

✿ **50135** complicated (eg, secondary operation, congenital kidney abnormality)

(For supply of anticarcinogenic agents, use 99070 in addition to code for primary procedure)

Excision

(For excision of retroperitoneal tumor or cyst, see 49200, 49201)

(For laparoscopic ablation of renal mass lesion(s), use 50542)

§ **50200** Renal biopsy; percutaneous, by trocar or needle

(For radiological supervision and interpretation, see 76003, 76360, 76393, 76942)

(For fine needle aspiration, use 10022)

(For evaluation of fine needle aspirate, see 88172, 88173)

✿ **50205** by surgical exposure of kidney

✿ **50220** Nephrectomy, including partial ureterectomy, any open approach including rib resection;

✿ **50225** complicated because of previous surgery on same kidney

✿ **50230** radical, with regional lymphadenectomy and/or vena caval thrombectomy

(When vena caval resection with reconstruction is necessary, use 37799)

✿ **50234** Nephrectomy with total ureterectomy and bladder cuff; through same incision

✿ **50236** through separate incision

✿ **50240** Nephrectomy, partial

(For laparoscopic partial nephrectomy, use 50543)

✿ **50280** Excision or unroofing of cyst(s) of kidney

(For laparoscopic ablation of renal cysts, use 50541)

✿ **50290** Excision of perinephric cyst

Renal Transplantation

►Renal *auto*transplantation includes reimplantation of the autograft as the primary procedure, along with secondary extra-corporeal procedure(s) (eg, partial nephrectomy, nephrolithotomy) reported with modifier 51 (see 50380 and applicable secondary procedure(s)).◄

►Renal *allo*transplantation involves three distinct components of physician work:◄

►1) ***Cadaver donor nephrectomy, unilateral or bilateral***, which includes harvesting the graft(s) and cold preservation of the graft(s) (perfusing with cold preservation solution and cold maintenance) (use 50300). ***Living donor nephrectomy***, which includes harvesting the graft, cold preservation of the graft (perfusing with cold preservation solution and cold maintenance), and care of the donor (see 50320, 50547).◄

►2) ***Backbench work***:◄

► Standard preparation of a cadaver donor renal allograft prior to transplantation including dissection and removal of perinephric fat, diaphragmatic and

Surgery: Urinary System

retroperitoneal attachments; excision of adrenal gland; and preparation of ureter(s), renal vein(s), and renal artery(s), ligating branches, as necessary (use 50323).◄

- ► Standard preparation of a living donor renal allograft (open or laparoscopic) prior to transplantation including dissection and removal of perinephric fat and preparation of ureter(s), renal vein(s), and renal artery(s), ligating branches, as necessary (use 50325).◄
- ► Additional reconstruction of a cadaver or living donor renal allograft prior to transplantation may include venous, arterial, and/or ureteral anastomosis(es) necessary for implantation (see 50327-50329).◄

►3) ***Recipient renal allotransplantation***, which includes transplantation of the allograft (with or without recipient nephrectomy) and care of the recipient (see 50360, 50365).◄

(For dialysis, see 90935-90999)

(For laparoscopic donor nephrectomy, use 50547)

(For laparoscopic drainage of lymphocele to peritoneal cavity, use 49323)

✿▲ **50300** Donor nephrectomy (including cold preservation); from cadaver donor, unilateral or bilateral

♦✿▲ **50320** open, from living donor

✿● **50323** Backbench standard preparation of cadaver donor renal allograft prior to transplantation, including dissection and removal of perinephric fat, diaphragmatic and retroperitoneal attachments, excision of adrenal gland, and preparation of ureter(s), renal vein(s), and renal artery(s), ligating branches, as necessary

►(Do not report 50323 in conjunction with 60540, 60545)◄

✿● **50325** Backbench standard preparation of living donor renal allograft (open or laparoscopic) prior to transplantation, including dissection and removal of perinephric fat and preparation of ureter(s), renal vein(s), and renal artery(s), ligating branches, as necessary

✿● **50327** Backbench reconstruction of cadaver or living donor renal allograft prior to transplantation; venous anastomosis, each

✿● **50328** arterial anastomosis, each

✿● **50329** ureteral anastomosis, each

♦✿ **50340** Recipient nephrectomy (separate procedure)

(For bilateral procedure, report 50340 with modifier 50)

✿▲ **50360** Renal allotransplantation, implantation of graft; without recipient nephrectomy

♦✿ **50365** with recipient nephrectomy

(For bilateral procedure, report 50365 with modifier 50)

✿ **50370** Removal of transplanted renal allograft

✿ **50380** Renal autotransplantation, reimplantation of kidney

(For ►renal autotransplantation◄ extra-corporeal ►(bench)◄ surgery, use autotransplantation as the primary procedure and report secondary procedure►(s)◄ (eg, partial nephrectomy, nephrolithotomy) ►with◄ modifier 51)

Introduction

♦§ **50390** Aspiration and/or injection of renal cyst or pelvis by needle, percutaneous

(For radiological supervision and interpretation, see 74425, 74470, 76003, 76360, 76393, 76942)

(For evaluation of fine needle aspirate, see 88172, 88173)

§● **50391** Instillation(s) of therapeutic agent into renal pelvis and/or ureter through established nephrostomy, pyelostomy or ureterostomy tube (eg, anticarcinogenic or antifungal agent)

➔ *CPT Changes: An Insider's View* 2005

♦§ **50392** Introduction of intracatheter or catheter into renal pelvis for drainage and/or injection, percutaneous

(For radiological supervision and interpretation, see 74475, 76360, 76942)

♦§ **50393** Introduction of ureteral catheter or stent into ureter through renal pelvis for drainage and/or injection, percutaneous

(For radiological supervision and interpretation, see 74480, 76003, 76360, 76942)

♦☆ **50394** Injection procedure for pyelography (as nephrostogram, pyelostogram, antegrade pyeloureterograms) through nephrostomy or pyelostomy tube, or indwelling ureteral catheter

(For radiological supervision and interpretation, use 74425)

♦§ **50395** Introduction of guide into renal pelvis and/or ureter with dilation to establish nephrostomy tract, percutaneous

(For radiological supervision and interpretation, see 74475, 74480, 74485)

(For nephrostolithotomy, see 50080, 50081)

(For retrograde percutaneous nephrostomy, use 52334)

(For endoscopic surgery, see 50551-50561)

♦§ **50396** Manometric studies through nephrostomy or pyelostomy tube, or indwelling ureteral catheter

(For radiological supervision and interpretation, see 74425, 74475, 74480)

♦§ **50398** Change of nephrostomy or pyelostomy tube

(For radiological supervision and interpretation, use 75984)

Repair

✿ **50400** Pyeloplasty (Foley Y-pyeloplasty), plastic operation on renal pelvis, with or without plastic operation on ureter, nephropexy, nephrostomy, pyelostomy, or ureteral splinting; simple

✿ **50405** complicated (congenital kidney abnormality, secondary pyeloplasty, solitary kidney, calycoplasty)

(For laparoscopic approach, use 50544)

✿ **50500** Nephrorrhaphy, suture of kidney wound or injury

✿ **50520** Closure of nephrocutaneous or pyelocutaneous fistula

✿ **50525** Closure of nephrovisceral fistula (eg, renocolic), including visceral repair; abdominal approach

✿ **50526** thoracic approach

✶✿ **50540** Symphysiotomy for horseshoe kidney with or without pyeloplasty and/or other plastic procedure, unilateral or bilateral (one operation)

Laparoscopy

Surgical laparoscopy always includes diagnostic laparoscopy. To report a diagnostic laparoscopy (peritoneoscopy) (separate procedure), use 49320.

§ **50541** Laparoscopy, surgical; ablation of renal cysts
➔ *CPT Changes: An Insider's View* 2000

§ **50542** ablation of renal mass lesion(s)
➔ *CPT Changes: An Insider's View* 2003

(For open procedure, see 50220-50240)

§ **50543** partial nephrectomy
➔ *CPT Changes: An Insider's View* 2003

(For open procedure, use 50240)

§ **50544** pyeloplasty

♦✿ **50545** radical nephrectomy (includes removal of Gerota's fascia and surrounding fatty tissue, removal of regional lymph nodes, and adrenalectomy)

(For open procedure, use 50230)

✿ **50546** nephrectomy, including partial ureterectomy

♦✿▲ **50547** donor nephrectomy (including cold preservation), from living donor

(For open procedure, use 50320)

►(For backbench renal allograft standard preparation prior to transplantation, use 50325)◄

►(For backbench renal allograft reconstruction prior to transplantation, see 50327-50329)◄

✿ **50548** nephrectomy with total ureterectomy

(For open procedure, see 50234, 50236)

♦§ **50549** Unlisted laparoscopy procedure, renal

(For laparoscopic drainage of lymphocele to peritoneal cavity, use 49323)

Endoscopy

(For supplies and materials, use 99070)

♦§ **50551** Renal endoscopy through established nephrostomy or pyelostomy, with or without irrigation, instillation, or ureteropyelography, exclusive of radiologic service;

♦§ **50553** with ureteral catheterization, with or without dilation of ureter

♦§ **50555** with biopsy

♦§ **50557** with fulguration and/or incision, with or without biopsy

►(50559 has been deleted)◄

♦§ **50561** with removal of foreign body or calculus

§ **50562** with resection of tumor
➔ *CPT Changes: An Insider's View* 2003

(When procedures 50570-50580 provide a significant identifiable service, they may be added to 50045 and 50120)

♦§ **50570** Renal endoscopy through nephrotomy or pyelotomy, with or without irrigation, instillation, or ureteropyelography, exclusive of radiologic service;

(For nephrotomy, use 50045)

(For pyelotomy, use 50120)

♦§ **50572** with ureteral catheterization, with or without dilation of ureter

♦§ **50574** with biopsy

♦§ **50575** with endopyelotomy (includes cystoscopy, ureteroscopy, dilation of ureter and ureteral pelvic junction, incision of ureteral pelvic junction and insertion of endopyelotomy stent)

♦§ **50576** with fulguration and/or incision, with or without biopsy

►(50578 has been deleted)◄

♦✿ **50580** with removal of foreign body or calculus

Other Procedures

♦§ **50590** Lithotripsy, extracorporeal shock wave

Ureter

Incision

♦✿ **50600** Ureterotomy with exploration or drainage (separate procedure)

(For ureteral endoscopy performed in conjunction with this procedure, see 50970-50980)

♦✿ **50605** Ureterotomy for insertion of indwelling stent, all types

♦✿ 50610 Ureterolithotomy; upper one-third of ureter

♦✿ 50620 middle one-third of ureter

♦✿ 50630 lower one-third of ureter

(For laparoscopic approach, use 50945)

(For transvesical ureterolithotomy, use 51060)

(For cystotomy with stone basket extraction of ureteral calculus, use 51065)

(For endoscopic extraction or manipulation of ureteral calculus, see 50080, 50081, 50561, 50961, 50980, 52320-52330, 52352, 52353)

Excision

(For ureterocele, see 51535, 52300)

✿ 50650 Ureterectomy, with bladder cuff (separate procedure)

✿ 50660 Ureterectomy, total, ectopic ureter, combination abdominal, vaginal and/or perineal approach

Introduction

♦☆ 50684 Injection procedure for ureterography or ureteropyelography through ureterostomy or indwelling ureteral catheter

(For radiological supervision and interpretation, use 74425)

§ 50686 Manometric studies through ureterostomy or indwelling ureteral catheter

§ 50688 Change of ureterostomy tube

(If imaging guidance is performed, use 75984)

☆ 50690 Injection procedure for visualization of ileal conduit and/or ureteropyelography, exclusive of radiologic service

(For radiological supervision and interpretation, use 74425)

Repair

✿ 50700 Ureteroplasty, plastic operation on ureter (eg, stricture)

♦✿ 50715 Ureterolysis, with or without repositioning of ureter for retroperitoneal fibrosis

(For bilateral procedure, report 50715 with modifier 50)

✿ 50722 Ureterolysis for ovarian vein syndrome

✿ 50725 Ureterolysis for retrocaval ureter, with reanastomosis of upper urinary tract or vena cava

✿ 50727 Revision of urinary-cutaneous anastomosis (any type urostomy);

✿ 50728 with repair of fascial defect and hernia

✿ 50740 Ureteropyelostomy, anastomosis of ureter and renal pelvis

✿ 50750 Ureterocalycostomy, anastomosis of ureter to renal calyx

✿ 50760 Ureteroureterostomy

✿ 50770 Transureteroureterostomy, anastomosis of ureter to contralateral ureter

(Codes 50780-50785 include minor procedures to prevent vesicoureteral reflux)

♦✿ 50780 Ureteroneocystostomy; anastomosis of single ureter to bladder

(For bilateral procedure, report 50780 with modifier 50)

(When combined with cystourethroplasty or vesical neck revision, use 51820)

♦✿ 50782 anastomosis of duplicated ureter to bladder

♦✿ 50783 with extensive ureteral tailoring

♦✿ 50785 with vesico-psoas hitch or bladder flap

(For bilateral procedure, report 50785 with modifier 50)

♦✿ 50800 Ureteroenterostomy, direct anastomosis of ureter to intestine

(For bilateral procedure, report 50800 with modifier 50)

✿ 50810 Ureterosigmoidostomy, with creation of sigmoid bladder and establishment of abdominal or perineal colostomy, including intestine anastomosis

♦✿ 50815 Ureterocolon conduit, including intestine anastomosis

(For bilateral procedure, report 50815 with modifier 50)

♦✿ 50820 Ureteroileal conduit (ileal bladder), including intestine anastomosis (Bricker operation)

(For bilateral procedure, report 50820 with modifier 50)

(For combination of 50800-50820 with cystectomy, see 51580-51595)

✿ 50825 Continent diversion, including intestine anastomosis using any segment of small and/or large intestine (Kock pouch or Camey enterocystoplasty)

✿ 50830 Urinary undiversion (eg, taking down of ureteroileal conduit, ureterosigmoidostomy or ureteroenterostomy with ureteroureterostomy or ureteroneocystostomy)

♦✿ 50840 Replacement of all or part of ureter by intestine segment, including intestine anastomosis

(For bilateral procedure, report 50840 with modifier 50)

✿ 50845 Cutaneous appendico-vesicostomy

♦✿ 50860 Ureterostomy, transplantation of ureter to skin

(For bilateral procedure, report 50860 with modifier 50)

✿ 50900 Ureterorrhaphy, suture of ureter (separate procedure)

✿ 50920 Closure of ureterocutaneous fistula

✿ 50930 Closure of ureterovisceral fistula (including visceral repair)

♦✿ 50940 Deligation of ureter

(For ureteroplasty, ureterolysis, see 50700-50860)

Laparoscopy

Surgical laparoscopy always includes diagnostic laparoscopy. To report a diagnostic laparoscopy (peritoneoscopy) (separate procedure), use 49320.

♦§ **50945** Laparoscopy, surgical; ureterolithotomy
➲ *CPT Changes: An Insider's View* 2000

♦§ **50947** ureteroneocystostomy with cystoscopy and ureteral stent placement
➲ *CPT Changes: An Insider's View* 2001

♦§ **50948** ureteroneocystostomy without cystoscopy and ureteral stent placement
➲ *CPT Changes: An Insider's View* 2001

(For open ureteroneocystostomy, see 50780-50785)

♦§ **50949** Unlisted laparoscopy procedure, ureter
➲ *CPT Changes: An Insider's View* 2001

Endoscopy

♦§ **50951** Ureteral endoscopy through established ureterostomy, with or without irrigation, instillation, or ureteropyelography, exclusive of radiologic service;

♦§ **50953** with ureteral catheterization, with or without dilation of ureter

♦§ **50955** with biopsy

♦§ **50957** with fulguration and/or incision, with or without biopsy

►(50959 has been deleted)◄

♦§ **50961** with removal of foreign body or calculus

(When procedures 50970-50980 provide a significant identifiable service, they may be added to 50600)

♦§ **50970** Ureteral endoscopy through ureterotomy, with or without irrigation, instillation, or ureteropyelography, exclusive of radiologic service;

(For ureterotomy, use 50600)

♦§ **50972** with ureteral catheterization, with or without dilation of ureter

♦§ **50974** with biopsy

♦§ **50976** with fulguration and/or incision, with or without biopsy

►(50978 has been deleted)◄

♦§ **50980** with removal of foreign body or calculus

Bladder

Incision

§ **51000** Aspiration of bladder by needle

§ **51005** Aspiration of bladder; by trocar or intracatheter

§ **51010** with insertion of suprapubic catheter

(If imaging guidance is performed, see 76003, 76360, 76942)

§ **51020** Cystotomy or cystostomy; with fulguration and/or insertion of radioactive material

§ **51030** with cryosurgical destruction of intravesical lesion

§ **51040** Cystostomy, cystotomy with drainage

§ **51045** Cystotomy, with insertion of ureteral catheter or stent (separate procedure)

§ **51050** Cystolithotomy, cystotomy with removal of calculus, without vesical neck resection

✿ **51060** Transvesical ureterolithotomy

§ **51065** Cystotomy, with calculus basket extraction and/or ultrasonic or electrohydraulic fragmentation of ureteral calculus

§ **51080** Drainage of perivesical or prevesical space abscess

Excision

§ **51500** Excision of urachal cyst or sinus, with or without umbilical hernia repair

§ **51520** Cystotomy; for simple excision of vesical neck (separate procedure)

✿ **51525** for excision of bladder diverticulum, single or multiple (separate procedure)

✿ **51530** for excision of bladder tumor

(For transurethral resection, see 52234-52240, 52305)

♦✿ **51535** Cystotomy for excision, incision, or repair of ureterocele

(For bilateral procedure, report 51535 with modifier 50)

(For transurethral excision, use 52300)

✿ **51550** Cystectomy, partial; simple

✿ **51555** complicated (eg, postradiation, previous surgery, difficult location)

✿ **51565** Cystectomy, partial, with reimplantation of ureter(s) into bladder (ureteroneocystostomy)

✿ **51570** Cystectomy, complete; (separate procedure)

+✿ **51575** with bilateral pelvic lymphadenectomy, including external iliac, hypogastric, and obturator nodes

✿ **51580** Cystectomy, complete, with ureterosigmoidostomy or ureterocutaneous transplantations;

+✿ **51585** with bilateral pelvic lymphadenectomy, including external iliac, hypogastric, and obturator nodes

✿ 51590 Cystectomy, complete, with ureteroileal conduit or sigmoid bladder, including intestine anastomosis;

+✿ 51595 with bilateral pelvic lymphadenectomy, including external iliac, hypogastric, and obturator nodes

✿ 51596 Cystectomy, complete, with continent diversion, any open technique, using any segment of small and/or large intestine to construct neobladder

✿ 51597 Pelvic exenteration, complete, for vesical, prostatic or urethral malignancy, with removal of bladder and ureteral transplantations, with or without hysterectomy and/or abdominoperineal resection of rectum and colon and colostomy, or any combination thereof

(For pelvic exenteration for gynecologic malignancy, use 58240)

Introduction

☆ 51600 Injection procedure for cystography or voiding urethrocystography

(For radiological supervision and interpretation, see 74430, 74455)

☆ 51605 Injection procedure and placement of chain for contrast and/or chain urethrocystography

(For radiological supervision and interpretation, use 74430)

☆ 51610 Injection procedure for retrograde urethrocystography

(For radiological supervision and interpretation, use 74450)

§ 51700 Bladder irrigation, simple, lavage and/or instillation

(Codes 51701-51702 are reported only when performed independently. Do not report 51701-51702 when catheter insertion is an inclusive component of another procedure.)

☆ 51701 Insertion of non-indwelling bladder catheter (eg, straight catheterization for residual urine)

➔ *CPT Changes: An Insider's View* 2003

☆ 51702 Insertion of temporary indwelling bladder catheter; simple (eg, Foley)

➔ *CPT Changes: An Insider's View* 2003

☆ 51703 complicated (eg, altered anatomy, fractured catheter/balloon)

➔ *CPT Changes: An Insider's View* 2003

§ 51705 Change of cystostomy tube; simple

§ 51710 complicated

(If imaging guidance is performed, use 75984)

§ 51715 Endoscopic injection of implant material into the submucosal tissues of the urethra and/or bladder neck

§ 51720 Bladder instillation of anticarcinogenic agent (including detention time)

Urodynamics

The following section (51725-51797) lists procedures that may be used separately or in many and varied combinations.

When multiple procedures are performed in the same investigative session, modifier 51 should be employed.

All procedures in this section imply that these services are performed by, or are under the direct supervision of, a physician and that all instruments, equipment, fluids, gases, probes, catheters, technician's fees, medications, gloves, trays, tubing and other sterile supplies be provided by the physician. When the physician only interprets the results and/or operates the equipment, a professional component, modifier 26, should be used to identify physicians' services.

§ 51725 Simple cystometrogram (CMG) (eg, spinal manometer)

§ 51726 Complex cystometrogram (eg, calibrated electronic equipment)

§ 51736 Simple uroflowmetry (UFR) (eg, stop-watch flow rate, mechanical uroflowmeter)

§ 51741 Complex uroflowmetry (eg, calibrated electronic equipment)

§ 51772 Urethral pressure profile studies (UPP) (urethral closure pressure profile), any technique

§ 51784 Electromyography studies (EMG) of anal or urethral sphincter, other than needle, any technique

§ 51785 Needle electromyography studies (EMG) of anal or urethral sphincter, any technique

§ 51792 Stimulus evoked response (eg, measurement of bulbocavernosus reflex latency time)

§ 51795 Voiding pressure studies (VP); bladder voiding pressure, any technique

§ 51797 intra-abdominal voiding pressure (AP) (rectal, gastric, intraperitoneal)

♣ 51798 Measurement of post-voiding residual urine and/or bladder capacity by ultrasound, non-imaging

➔ *CPT Changes: An Insider's View* 2003

Repair

✿ 51800 Cystoplasty or cystourethroplasty, plastic operation on bladder and/or vesical neck (anterior Y-plasty, vesical fundus resection), any procedure, with or without wedge resection of posterior vesical neck

✶✿ 51820 Cystourethroplasty with unilateral or bilateral ureteroneocystostomy

✿ 51840 Anterior vesicourethropexy, or urethropexy (eg, Marshall-Marchetti-Krantz, Burch); simple

✿ 51841 complicated (eg, secondary repair)

(For urethropexy (Pereyra type), use 57289)

✿ **51845** Abdomino-vaginal vesical neck suspension, with or without endoscopic control (eg, Stamey, Raz, modified Pereyra)

✿ **51860** Cystorrhaphy, suture of bladder wound, injury or rupture; simple

✿ **51865** complicated

§ **51880** Closure of cystostomy (separate procedure)

✿ **51900** Closure of vesicovaginal fistula, abdominal approach

(For vaginal approach, see 57320-57330)

✿ **51920** Closure of vesicouterine fistula;

✿ **51925** with hysterectomy

(For closure of vesicoenteric fistula, see 44660, 44661)

(For closure of rectovesical fistula, see 45800-45805)

✿ **51940** Closure, exstrophy of bladder

(See also 54390)

✿ **51960** Enterocystoplasty, including intestinal anastomosis

✿ **51980** Cutaneous vesicostomy

Laparoscopy

Surgical laparoscopy always includes diagnostic laparoscopy. To report a diagnostic laparoscopy (peritoneoscopy) (separate procedure), use 49320.

§ **51990** Laparoscopy, surgical; urethral suspension for stress incontinence

➔ *CPT Changes: An Insider's View* 2000

§ **51992** sling operation for stress incontinence (eg, fascia or synthetic)

➔ *CPT Changes: An Insider's View* 2000

(For open sling operation for stress incontinence, use 57288)

(For reversal or removal of sling operation for stress incontinence, use 57287)

Endoscopy—Cystoscopy, Urethroscopy, Cystourethroscopy

Endoscopic descriptions are listed so that the main procedure can be identified without having to list all the minor related functions performed at the same time. For example: meatotomy, urethral calibration and/or dilation, urethro-scopy, and cystoscopy prior to a transurethral resection of prostate; ureteral catheterization following extraction of ureteral calculus; internal urethrotomy and bladder neck fulguration when performing a cystourethroscopy for the female urethral syndrome. When the secondary procedure requires significant additional time and effort, it may be identified by the addition of modifier 22.

For example: urethrotomy performed for a documented pre-existing stricture or bladder neck contracture.

§ **52000** Cystourethroscopy (separate procedure)

§ **52001** Cystourethroscopy with irrigation and evacuation of multiple obstructing clots

➔ *CPT Changes: An Insider's View* 2002, 2003

(Do not report 52001 in addition to 52000)

§ **52005** Cystourethroscopy, with ureteral catheterization, with or without irrigation, instillation, or ureteropyelography, exclusive of radiologic service;

♦§ **52007** with brush biopsy of ureter and/or renal pelvis

§ **52010** Cystourethroscopy, with ejaculatory duct catheterization, with or without irrigation, instillation, or duct radiography, exclusive of radiologic service

(For radiological supervision and interpretation, use 74440)

Transurethral Surgery

Urethra and Bladder

§ **52204** Cystourethroscopy, with biopsy

§ **52214** Cystourethroscopy, with fulguration (including cryosurgery or laser surgery) of trigone, bladder neck, prostatic fossa, urethra, or periurethral glands

§ **52224** Cystourethroscopy, with fulguration (including cryosurgery or laser surgery) or treatment of MINOR (less than 0.5 cm) lesion(s) with or without biopsy

§▲ **52234** Cystourethroscopy, with fulguration (including cryosurgery or laser surgery) and/or resection of; SMALL bladder tumor(s) (0.5 up to 2.0 cm)

➔ *CPT Changes: An Insider's View* 2005

§ **52235** MEDIUM bladder tumor(s) (2.0 to 5.0 cm)

§ **52240** LARGE bladder tumor(s)

§ **52250** Cystourethroscopy with insertion of radioactive substance, with or without biopsy or fulguration

§ **52260** Cystourethroscopy, with dilation of bladder for interstitial cystitis; general or conduction (spinal) anesthesia

§ **52265** local anesthesia

§ **52270** Cystourethroscopy, with internal urethrotomy; female

§ **52275** male

§ **52276** Cystourethroscopy with direct vision internal urethrotomy

§ **52277** Cystourethroscopy, with resection of external sphincter (sphincterotomy)

§ **52281** Cystourethroscopy, with calibration and/or dilation of urethral stricture or stenosis, with or without meatotomy, with or without injection procedure for cystography, male or female

§ **52282** Cystourethroscopy, with insertion of urethral stent

§ **52283** Cystourethroscopy, with steroid injection into stricture

§ **52285** Cystourethroscopy for treatment of the female urethral syndrome with any or all of the following: urethral meatotomy, urethral dilation, internal urethrotomy, lysis of urethrovaginal septal fibrosis, lateral incisions of the bladder neck, and fulguration of polyp(s) of urethra, bladder neck, and/or trigone

✶§ **52290** Cystourethroscopy; with ureteral meatotomy, unilateral or bilateral

✶§ **52300** with resection or fulguration of orthotopic ureterocele(s), unilateral or bilateral

✶§ **52301** with resection or fulguration of ectopic ureterocele(s), unilateral or bilateral

§ **52305** with incision or resection of orifice of bladder diverticulum, single or multiple

§ **52310** Cystourethroscopy, with removal of foreign body, calculus, or ureteral stent from urethra or bladder (separate procedure); simple

§ **52315** complicated

§ **52317** Litholapaxy: crushing or fragmentation of calculus by any means in bladder and removal of fragments; simple or small (less than 2.5 cm)

§ **52318** complicated or large (over 2.5 cm)

Ureter and Pelvis

Surgical cystourethroscopy always includes diagnostic cystourethroscopy. To report a diagnostic cystourethroscopy, use 52351.

Do not report 52351 in conjunction with 52341-52346, 52352-52355.

The insertion and removal of a temporary stent during diagnostic or therapeutic cystourethroscopic intervention(s) is included in 52320-52355 and should not be reported separately.

To report insertion of a self-retaining, indwelling stent performed during cystourethroscopic diagnostic or therapeutic intervention(s), report 52332, in addition to primary procedure(s) performed, and append modifier 51. 52332 is used to report a unilateral procedure unless otherwise specified.

For bilateral insertion of self-retaining, indwelling ureteral stents, use code 52332, and append modifier 50.

To report cystourethroscopic removal of a self-retaining, indwelling ureteral stent, see 52310, 52315, and append modifier 58.

♦§ **52320** Cystourethroscopy (including ureteral catheterization); with removal of ureteral calculus

♦§ **52325** with fragmentation of ureteral calculus (eg, ultrasonic or electro-hydraulic technique)

♦§ **52327** with subureteric injection of implant material

♦§ **52330** with manipulation, without removal of ureteral calculus

♦§ **52332** Cystourethroscopy, with insertion of indwelling ureteral stent (eg, Gibbons or double-J type)

♦§ **52334** Cystourethroscopy with insertion of ureteral guide wire through kidney to establish a percutaneous nephrostomy, retrograde

(For percutaneous nephrostolithotomy, see 50080, 50081; for establishment of nephrostomy tract only, use 50395)

(For cystourethroscopy, with ureteroscopy and/or pyeloscopy, see 52351-52355)

(For cystourethroscopy with incision, fulguration, or resection of congenital posterior urethral valves or obstructive hypertrophic mucosal folds, use 52400)

♦§ **52341** Cystourethroscopy; with treatment of ureteral stricture (eg, balloon dilation, laser, electrocautery, and incision)
➲ *CPT Changes: An Insider's View* 2001

♦§ **52342** with treatment of ureteropelvic junction stricture (eg, balloon dilation, laser, electrocautery, and incision)
➲ *CPT Changes: An Insider's View* 2001

♦§ **52343** with treatment of intra-renal stricture (eg, balloon dilation, laser, electrocautery, and incision)
➲ *CPT Changes: An Insider's View* 2001

♦§ **52344** Cystourethroscopy with ureteroscopy; with treatment of ureteral stricture (eg, balloon dilation, laser, electrocautery, and incision)
➲ *CPT Changes: An Insider's View* 2001

§ **52345** with treatment of ureteropelvic junction stricture (eg, balloon dilation, laser, electrocautery, and incision)
➲ *CPT Changes: An Insider's View* 2001

§ **52346** with treatment of intra-renal stricture (eg, balloon dilation, laser, electrocautery, and incision)
➲ *CPT Changes: An Insider's View* 2001

►(52347 has been deleted)◄

►(For transurethral resection or incision of ejaculatory ducts, use 52402)◄

§ **52351** Cystourethroscopy, with ureteroscopy and/or pyeloscopy; diagnostic
➲ *CPT Changes: An Insider's View* 2001

(For radiological supervision and interpretation, use 74485)

(Do not report 52351 in conjunction with 52341-52346, 52352-52355)

♦§ **52352** with removal or manipulation of calculus (ureteral catheterization is included)
➲ *CPT Changes: An Insider's View* 2001

♦§ **52353** with lithotripsy (ureteral catheterization is included)
➲ *CPT Changes: An Insider's View* 2001

♦§ **52354** with biopsy and/or fulguration of ureteral or renal pelvic lesion
➲ *CPT Changes: An Insider's View* 2001, 2003

♦§ **52355** with resection of ureteral or renal pelvic tumor
➲ *CPT Changes: An Insider's View* 2001, 2003

Vesical Neck and Prostate

§ **52400** Cystourethroscopy with incision, fulguration, or resection of congenital posterior urethral valves, or congenital obstructive hypertrophic mucosal folds
➲ *CPT Changes: An Insider's View* 2001

§● **52402** Cystourethroscopy with transurethral resection or incision of ejaculatory ducts
➲ *CPT Changes: An Insider's View* 2005

§ **52450** Transurethral incision of prostate

§ **52500** Transurethral resection of bladder neck (separate procedure)

§ **52510** Transurethral balloon dilation of the prostatic urethra
➲ *CPT Changes: An Insider's View* 2002

§ **52601** Transurethral electrosurgical resection of prostate, including control of postoperative bleeding, complete (vasectomy, meatotomy, cystourethroscopy, urethral calibration and/or dilation, and internal urethrotomy are included)

(For other approaches, see 55801-55845)

§ **52606** Transurethral fulguration for postoperative bleeding occurring after the usual follow-up time

§ **52612** Transurethral resection of prostate; first stage of two-stage resection (partial resection)

§ **52614** second stage of two-stage resection (resection completed)

§ **52620** Transurethral resection; of residual obstructive tissue after 90 days postoperative

§ **52630** of regrowth of obstructive tissue longer than one year postoperative

§ **52640** of postoperative bladder neck contracture

§ **52647** Non-contact laser coagulation of prostate, including control of postoperative bleeding, complete (vasectomy, meatotomy, cystourethroscopy, urethral calibration and/or dilation, and internal urethrotomy are included)

§ **52648** Contact laser vaporization with or without transurethral resection of prostate, including control of postoperative bleeding, complete (vasectomy, meatotomy, cystourethroscopy, urethral calibration and/or dilation, and internal urethrotomy are included)

§ **52700** Transurethral drainage of prostatic abscess

(For litholapaxy, use 52317, 52318)

Urethra

(For endoscopy, see cystoscopy, urethroscopy, cystourethroscopy, 52000-52700)

(For injection procedure for urethrocystography, see 51600-51610)

Incision

§ **53000** Urethrotomy or urethrostomy, external (separate procedure); pendulous urethra

§ **53010** perineal urethra, external

§ **53020** Meatotomy, cutting of meatus (separate procedure); except infant

§ **53025** infant

(Do not report modifier 63 in conjunction with 53025)

§ **53040** Drainage of deep periurethral abscess

(For subcutaneous abscess, see 10060, 10061)

§ **53060** Drainage of Skene's gland abscess or cyst

§ **53080** Drainage of perineal urinary extravasation; uncomplicated (separate procedure)

§ **53085** complicated

Excision

§ **53200** Biopsy of urethra

§ **53210** Urethrectomy, total, including cystostomy; female

§ **53215** male

§ **53220** Excision or fulguration of carcinoma of urethra

§ **53230** Excision of urethral diverticulum (separate procedure); female

§ **53235** male

§ **53240** Marsupialization of urethral diverticulum, male or female

§ **53250** Excision of bulbourethral gland (Cowper's gland)

§ **53260** Excision or fulguration; urethral polyp(s), distal urethra

(For endoscopic approach, see 52214, 52224)

§ **53265** urethral caruncle

§ **53270** Skene's glands

§ **53275** urethral prolapse

Repair

(For hypospadias, see 54300-54352)

§ **53400** Urethroplasty; first stage, for fistula, diverticulum, or stricture (eg, Johannsen type)

§ **53405** second stage (formation of urethra), including urinary diversion

§ **53410** Urethroplasty, one-stage reconstruction of male anterior urethra

✿ **53415** Urethroplasty, transpubic or perineal, one stage, for reconstruction or repair of prostatic or membranous urethra

§ **53420** Urethroplasty, two-stage reconstruction or repair of prostatic or membranous urethra; first stage

§ **53425** second stage

§ **53430** Urethroplasty, reconstruction of female urethra

§ **53431** Urethroplasty with tubularization of posterior urethra and/or lower bladder for incontinence (eg, Tenago, Leadbetter procedure)
➲ *CPT Changes: An Insider's View* 2002

❖ **53440** Sling operation for correction of male urinary incontinence (eg, fascia or synthetic)
➲ *CPT Changes: An Insider's View* 2003

§ **53442** Removal or revision of sling for male urinary incontinence (eg, fascia or synthetic)
➲ *CPT Changes: An Insider's View* 2003

❖ **53444** Insertion of tandem cuff (dual cuff)
➲ *CPT Changes: An Insider's View* 2002

❖ **53445** Insertion of inflatable urethral/bladder neck sphincter, including placement of pump, reservoir, and cuff
➲ *CPT Changes: An Insider's View* 2002

§ **53446** Removal of inflatable urethral/bladder neck sphincter, including pump, reservoir, and cuff
➲ *CPT Changes: An Insider's View* 2002

❖ **53447** Removal and replacement of inflatable urethral/bladder neck sphincter including pump, reservoir, and cuff at the same operative session
➲ *CPT Changes: An Insider's View* 2002

✿ **53448** Removal and replacement of inflatable urethral/bladder neck sphincter including pump, reservoir, and cuff through an infected field at the same operative session including irrigation and debridement of infected tissue

(Do not report 11040-11043 in addition to 53448)

§ **53449** Repair of inflatable urethral/bladder neck sphincter, including pump, reservoir, and cuff
➲ *CPT Changes: An Insider's View* 2002

§ **53450** Urethromeatoplasty, with mucosal advancement

(For meatotomy, see 53020, 53025)

§ **53460** Urethromeatoplasty, with partial excision of distal urethral segment (Richardson type procedure)

§ **53500** Urethrolysis, transvaginal, secondary, open, including cystourethroscopy (eg, postsurgical obstruction, scarring)
➲ *CPT Changes: An Insider's View* 2004

(For urethrolysis by retropubic approach, use 53899)

(Do not report 53500 in conjunction with 52000)

§ **53502** Urethrorrhaphy, suture of urethral wound or injury, female

§ **53505** Urethrorrhaphy, suture of urethral wound or injury; penile

§ **53510** perineal

§ **53515** prostatomembranous

§ **53520** Closure of urethrostomy or urethrocutaneous fistula, male (separate procedure)

(For closure of urethrovaginal fistula, use 57310)

(For closure of urethrorectal fistula, see 45820, 45825)

Manipulation

(For radiological supervision and interpretation, use 74485)

§ **53600** Dilation of urethral stricture by passage of sound or urethral dilator, male; initial

§ **53601** subsequent

§ **53605** Dilation of urethral stricture or vesical neck by passage of sound or urethral dilator, male, general or conduction (spinal) anesthesia

§ **53620** Dilation of urethral stricture by passage of filiform and follower, male; initial

§ **53621** subsequent

§ **53660** Dilation of female urethra including suppository and/or instillation; initial

§ **53661** subsequent

§ **53665** Dilation of female urethra, general or conduction (spinal) anesthesia

(For urethral catheterization, see 51701-51703)

(53670 has been deleted. To report, see 51701, 51702)

(53675 has been deleted. To report, use 51703)

Other Procedures

(For two or three glass urinalysis, use 81020)

§ **53850** Transurethral destruction of prostate tissue; by microwave thermotherapy

§ **53852** by radiofrequency thermotherapy

§ **53853** by water-induced thermotherapy
➲ *CPT Changes: An Insider's View* 2002

§ **53899** Unlisted procedure, urinary system

Male Genital System

Penis

Incision

►(For abdominal perineal gangrene debridement, see 11004-11006)◄

§ **54000** Slitting of prepuce, dorsal or lateral (separate procedure); newborn

(Do not report modifier 63 in conjunction with 54000)

§ **54001** except newborn

§ **54015** Incision and drainage of penis, deep

(For skin and subcutaneous abscess, see 10060-10160)

Destruction

§ **54050** Destruction of lesion(s), penis (eg, condyloma, papilloma, molluscum contagiosum, herpetic vesicle), simple; chemical

§ **54055** electrodesiccation

§ **54056** cryosurgery

§ **54057** laser surgery

§ **54060** surgical excision

§ **54065** Destruction of lesion(s), penis (eg, condyloma, papilloma, molluscum contagiosum, herpetic vesicle), extensive (eg, laser surgery, electrosurgery, cryosurgery, chemosurgery)
➔ *CPT Changes: An Insider's View* 2002

(For destruction or excision of other lesions, see **Integumentary System**)

Excision

§ **54100** Biopsy of penis; (separate procedure)
➔ *CPT Changes: An Insider's View* 2000

§ **54105** deep structures

§ **54110** Excision of penile plaque (Peyronie disease);

§ **54111** with graft to 5 cm in length

§ **54112** with graft greater than 5 cm in length

§ **54115** Removal foreign body from deep penile tissue (eg, plastic implant)

§ **54120** Amputation of penis; partial

✿ **54125** complete

✶✿ **54130** Amputation of penis, radical; with bilateral inguinofemoral lymphadenectomy

✶✿ **54135** in continuity with bilateral pelvic lymphadenectomy, including external iliac, hypogastric and obturator nodes

(For lymphadenectomy (separate procedure), see 38760-38770)

§ **54150** Circumcision, using clamp or other device; newborn

(Do not report modifier 63 in conjunction with 54150)

§ **54152** except newborn

§ **54160** Circumcision, surgical excision other than clamp, device or dorsal slit; newborn

(Do not report modifier 63 in conjunction with 54160)

§ **54161** except newborn

§ **54162** Lysis or excision of penile post-circumcision adhesions
➔ *CPT Changes: An Insider's View* 2002

§ **54163** Repair incomplete circumcision
➔ *CPT Changes: An Insider's View* 2002

§ **54164** Frenulotomy of penis
➔ *CPT Changes: An Insider's View* 2002

(Do not report 54164 with circumcision codes 54150-54161, 54162, 54163)

Introduction

§ **54200** Injection procedure for Peyronie disease;

§ **54205** with surgical exposure of plaque

§ **54220** Irrigation of corpora cavernosa for priapism

☆ **54230** Injection procedure for corpora cavernosography

(For radiological supervision and interpretation, use 74445)

§ **54231** Dynamic cavernosometry, including intracavernosal injection of vasoactive drugs (eg, papaverine, phentolamine)

§ **54235** Injection of corpora cavernosa with pharmacologic agent(s) (eg, papaverine, phentolamine)

§ **54240** Penile plethysmography

§ **54250** Nocturnal penile tumescence and/or rigidity test

Repair

(For other urethroplasties, see 53400-53430)

(For penile revascularization, use 37788)

§ **54300** Plastic operation of penis for straightening of chordee (eg, hypospadias), with or without mobilization of urethra

§ **54304** Plastic operation on penis for correction of chordee or for first stage hypospadias repair with or without transplantation of prepuce and/or skin flaps

§ **54308** Urethroplasty for second stage hypospadias repair (including urinary diversion); less than 3 cm

§ **54312** greater than 3 cm

§ **54316** Urethroplasty for second stage hypospadias repair (including urinary diversion) with free skin graft obtained from site other than genitalia

§ **54318** Urethroplasty for third stage hypospadias repair to release penis from scrotum (eg, third stage Cecil repair)

§ **54322** One stage distal hypospadias repair (with or without chordee or circumcision); with simple meatal advancement (eg, Magpi, V-flap)

§ **54324** with urethroplasty by local skin flaps (eg, flip-flap, prepucial flap)

§ **54326** with urethroplasty by local skin flaps and mobilization of urethra

§ **54328** with extensive dissection to correct chordee and urethroplasty with local skin flaps, skin graft patch, and/or island flap

(For urethroplasty and straightening of chordee, use 54308)

✿ **54332** One stage proximal penile or penoscrotal hypospadias repair requiring extensive dissection to correct chordee and urethroplasty by use of skin graft tube and/or island flap

✿ **54336** One stage perineal hypospadias repair requiring extensive dissection to correct chordee and urethroplasty by use of skin graft tube and/or island flap

§ **54340** Repair of hypospadias complications (ie, fistula, stricture, diverticula); by closure, incision, or excision, simple

§ **54344** requiring mobilization of skin flaps and urethroplasty with flap or patch graft

§ **54348** requiring extensive dissection and urethroplasty with flap, patch or tubed graft (includes urinary diversion)

§ **54352** Repair of hypospadias cripple requiring extensive dissection and excision of previously constructed structures including re-release of chordee and reconstruction of urethra and penis by use of local skin as grafts and island flaps and skin brought in as flaps or grafts

§ **54360** Plastic operation on penis to correct angulation

§ **54380** Plastic operation on penis for epispadias distal to external sphincter;

§ **54385** with incontinence

✿ **54390** with exstrophy of bladder

❖ **54400** Insertion of penile prosthesis; non-inflatable (semi-rigid)

❖ **54401** inflatable (self-contained)

(For removal or replacement of penile prosthesis, see 54415, 54416)

❖ **54405** Insertion of multi-component, inflatable penile prosthesis, including placement of pump, cylinders, and reservoir

➲ *CPT Changes: An Insider's View* 2002

(For reduced services, report 54405 with modifier 52)

§ **54406** Removal of all components of a multi-component, inflatable penile prosthesis without replacement of prosthesis

➲ *CPT Changes: An Insider's View* 2002

(For reduced services, report 54406 with modifier 52)

§ **54408** Repair of component(s) of a multi-component, inflatable penile prosthesis

➲ *CPT Changes: An Insider's View* 2002

❖ **54410** Removal and replacement of all component(s) of a multi-component, inflatable penile prosthesis at the same operative session

➲ *CPT Changes: An Insider's View* 2002

✿ **54411** Removal and replacement of all components of a multi-component inflatable penile prosthesis through an infected field at the same operative session, including irrigation and debridement of infected tissue

(For reduced services, report 54411 with modifier 52)

(Do not report 11040-11043 in addition to 54411)

§ **54415** Removal of non-inflatable (semi-rigid) or inflatable (self-contained) penile prosthesis, without replacement of prosthesis

➲ *CPT Changes: An Insider's View* 2002

❖ **54416** Removal and replacement of non-inflatable (semi-rigid) or inflatable (self-contained) penile prosthesis at the same operative session

➲ *CPT Changes: An Insider's View* 2002

✿ **54417** Removal and replacement of non-inflatable (semi-rigid) or inflatable (self-contained) penile prosthesis through an infected field at the same operative session, including irrigation and debridement of infected tissue

(Do not report 11040-11043 in addition to 54417)

§ **54420** Corpora cavernosa-saphenous vein shunt (priapism operation), unilateral or bilateral

✶✿ **54430** Corpora cavernosa-corpus spongiosum shunt (priapism operation), unilateral or bilateral

§ **54435** Corpora cavernosa-glans penis fistulization (eg, biopsy needle, Winter procedure, rongeur, or punch) for priapism

§ **54440** Plastic operation of penis for injury

Manipulation

§ **54450** Foreskin manipulation including lysis of preputial adhesions and stretching

Testis

Excision

►(For abdominal perineal gangrene debridement, see 11004-11006)◄

♦§ **54500** Biopsy of testis, needle (separate procedure)

(For fine needle aspiration, see 10021, 10022)

(For evaluation of fine needle aspirate, see 88172, 88173)

♦§ **54505** Biopsy of testis, incisional (separate procedure)

(For bilateral procedure, report 54505 with modifier 50)

(When combined with vasogram, seminal vesiculogram, or epididymogram, use 55300)

♦§ **54512** Excision of extraparenchymal lesion of testis
➔ *CPT Changes: An Insider's View* 2001

♦§ **54520** Orchiectomy, simple (including subcapsular), with or without testicular prosthesis, scrotal or inguinal approach

(For bilateral procedure, report 54520 with modifier 50)

♦§ **54522** Orchiectomy, partial

♦§ **54530** Orchiectomy, radical, for tumor; inguinal approach

♦✿ **54535** with abdominal exploration

(For orchiectomy with repair of hernia, see 49505 or 49507 and 54520)

(For radical retroperitoneal lymphadenectomy, use 38780)

♦§ **54550** Exploration for undescended testis (inguinal or scrotal area)

(For bilateral procedure, report 54550 with modifier 50)

♦✿ **54560** Exploration for undescended testis with abdominal exploration

(For bilateral procedure, report 54560 with modifier 50)

Repair

♦§ **54600** Reduction of torsion of testis, surgical, with or without fixation of contralateral testis

♦§ **54620** Fixation of contralateral testis (separate procedure)

♦§ **54640** Orchiopexy, inguinal approach, with or without hernia repair

(For bilateral procedure, report 54640 with modifier 50

(For inguinal hernia repair performed in conjunction with inguinal orchiopexy, see 49495-49525)

♦✿ **54650** Orchiopexy, abdominal approach, for intra-abdominal testis (eg, Fowler-Stephens)

(For laparoscopic approach, use 54692)

♦§ **54660** Insertion of testicular prosthesis (separate procedure)

(For bilateral procedure, report 54660 with modifier 50)

♦§ **54670** Suture or repair of testicular injury

♦§ **54680** Transplantation of testis(es) to thigh (because of scrotal destruction)

Laparoscopy

Surgical laparoscopy always includes diagnostic laparoscopy. To report a diagnostic laparoscopy (peritoneoscopy) (separate procedure), use 49320.

♦§ **54690** Laparoscopy, surgical; orchiectomy
➔ *CPT Changes: An Insider's View* 2000

♦§ **54692** orchiopexy for intra-abdominal testis
➔ *CPT Changes: An Insider's View* 2000

§ **54699** Unlisted laparoscopy procedure, testis
➔ *CPT Changes: An Insider's View* 2000

Epididymis

Incision

§ **54700** Incision and drainage of epididymis, testis and/or scrotal space (eg, abscess or hematoma)

Excision

§ **54800** Biopsy of epididymis, needle

(For fine needle aspiration, see 10021, 10022)

(For evaluation of fine needle aspirate, see 88172, 88173)

§ **54820** Exploration of epididymis, with or without biopsy

§ **54830** Excision of local lesion of epididymis

§ **54840** Excision of spermatocele, with or without epididymectomy

⌘§ **54860** Epididymectomy; unilateral

✶§ **54861** bilateral

Repair

⌘§ **54900** Epididymovasostomy, anastomosis of epididymis to vas deferens; unilateral

✶§ **54901** bilateral

(For operating microscope, use 69990)

Tunica Vaginalis

Incision

§ **55000** Puncture aspiration of hydrocele, tunica vaginalis, with or without injection of medication

Excision

⌘§ **55040** Excision of hydrocele; unilateral

✶§ **55041** bilateral

(With hernia repair, see 49495-49501)

Repair

♦§ **55060** Repair of tunica vaginalis hydrocele (Bottle type)

Scrotum

Incision

§ **55100** Drainage of scrotal wall abscess

(See also 54700)

§ **55110** Scrotal exploration

§ **55120** Removal of foreign body in scrotum

Excision

(For excision of local lesion of skin of scrotum, see **Integumentary System**)

§ **55150** Resection of scrotum

Repair

§ **55175** Scrotoplasty; simple

§ **55180** complicated

Vas Deferens

Incision

✶§ **55200** Vasotomy, cannulization with or without incision of vas, unilateral or bilateral (separate procedure)

Excision

✶§ **55250** Vasectomy, unilateral or bilateral (separate procedure), including postoperative semen examination(s)

Introduction

✶☆ **55300** Vasotomy for vasograms, seminal vesiculograms, or epididymograms, unilateral or bilateral

(For radiological supervision and interpretation, use 74440)

(When combined with biopsy of testis, see 54505 and use modifier 51)

Repair

♦§ **55400** Vasovasostomy, vasovasorrhaphy

(For bilateral procedure, report 55400 with modifier 50)

(For operating microscope, use 69990)

Suture

✶§ **55450** Ligation (percutaneous) of vas deferens, unilateral or bilateral (separate procedure)

Spermatic Cord

Excision

§ **55500** Excision of hydrocele of spermatic cord, unilateral (separate procedure)

§ **55520** Excision of lesion of spermatic cord (separate procedure)

♦§ **55530** Excision of varicocele or ligation of spermatic veins for varicocele; (separate procedure)

♦§ **55535** abdominal approach

♦§ **55540** with hernia repair

Laparoscopy

Surgical laparoscopy always includes diagnostic laparoscopy. To report a diagnostic laparoscopy (peritoneoscopy) (separate procedure), use 49320.

♦§ **55550** Laparoscopy, surgical, with ligation of spermatic veins for varicocele

➔ *CPT Changes: An Insider's View* 2000

♦§ **55559** Unlisted laparoscopy procedure, spermatic cord

➔ *CPT Changes: An Insider's View* 2000

Seminal Vesicles

Incision

♦✿ **55600** Vesiculotomy;

(For bilateral procedure, report 55600 with modifier 50)

♦✿ **55605** complicated

Excision

♦✿ **55650** Vesiculectomy, any approach

(For bilateral procedure, report 55650 with modifier 50)

§ **55680** Excision of Mullerian duct cyst

(For injection procedure, see 52010, 55300)

Prostate

Incision

§ **55700** Biopsy, prostate; needle or punch, single or multiple, any approach

(If imaging guidance is performed, use 76942)

(For fine needle aspiration, see 10021, 10022)

(For evaluation of fine needle aspirate, see 88172, 88173)

§ **55705** incisional, any approach

§ **55720** Prostatotomy, external drainage of prostatic abscess, any approach; simple

§ **55725** complicated

(For transurethral drainage, use 52700)

Excision

(For transurethral removal of prostate, see 52601-52640)

(For transurethral destruction of prostate, see 53850-53852)

(For limited pelvic lymphadenectomy for staging (separate procedure), use 38562)

(For independent node dissection, see 38770-38780)

✿ **55801** Prostatectomy, perineal, subtotal (including control of postoperative bleeding, vasectomy, meatotomy, urethral calibration and/or dilation, and internal urethrotomy)

✿ **55810** Prostatectomy, perineal radical;

✿ **55812** with lymph node biopsy(s) (limited pelvic lymphadenectomy)

✶✿ **55815** with bilateral pelvic lymphadenectomy, including external iliac, hypogastric and obturator nodes

(If 55815 is carried out on separate days, use 38770 with modifier 50 and 55810)

✿ **55821** Prostatectomy (including control of postoperative bleeding, vasectomy, meatotomy, urethral calibration and/or dilation, and internal urethrotomy); suprapubic, subtotal, one or two stages

✿ **55831** retropubic, subtotal

✿ **55840** Prostatectomy, retropubic radical, with or without nerve sparing;

✿ **55842** with lymph node biopsy(s) (limited pelvic lymphadenectomy)

✶✿ **55845** with bilateral pelvic lymphadenectomy, including external iliac, hypogastric, and obturator nodes

(If 55845 is carried out on separate days, use 38770 with modifier 50 and 55840)

(For laparoscopic retropubic radical prostatectomy, use 55866)

§ **55859** Transperineal placement of needles or catheters into prostate for interstitial radioelement application, with or without cystoscopy

➲ *CPT Assistant* Apr 03: 7, Apr 04:7

(For interstitial radioelement application, see 77776-►77784◄)

(For ultrasonic guidance for interstitial radioelement application, use 76965)

§ **55860** Exposure of prostate, any approach, for insertion of radioactive substance;

(For application of interstitial radioelement, see 77776-77778)

✿ **55862** with lymph node biopsy(s) (limited pelvic lymphadenectomy)

✶✿ **55865** with bilateral pelvic lymphadenectomy, including external iliac, hypogastric and obturator nodes

Laparoscopy

Surgical laparoscopy always includes diagnostic laparoscopy. To report a diagnostic laparoscopy (peritoneoscopy) (separate procedure), use 49320.

✿ **55866** Laparoscopy, surgical prostatectomy, retropubic radical, including nerve sparing

(For open procedure, use 55840)

Other Procedures

(For artificial insemination, see 58321, 58322)

§ **55870** Electroejaculation

§ **55873** Cryosurgical ablation of the prostate (includes ultrasonic guidance for interstitial cryosurgical probe placement)

➲ *CPT Changes: An Insider's View* 2001

§ **55899** Unlisted procedure, male genital system

Intersex Surgery

☐ **55970** Intersex surgery; male to female

☐ **55980** female to male

Notes

Female Genital System

(For pelvic laparotomy, use 49000)

(For excision or destruction of endometriomas, open method, see 49200, 49201)

(For paracentesis, see 49080, 49081)

(For secondary closure of abdominal wall evisceration or disruption, use 49900)

(For fulguration or excision of lesions, laparoscopic approach, use 58662)

(For chemotherapy, see 96400-96549)

Vulva, Perineum and Introitus

Definitions

The following definitions apply to the vulvectomy codes (56620-56640).

A ***simple*** procedure is the removal of skin and superficial subcutaneous tissues.

A ***radical*** procedure is the removal of skin and deep subcutaneous tissue.

A ***partial*** procedure is the removal of less than 80% of the vulvar area.

A ***complete*** procedure is the removal of greater than 80% of the vulvar area.

Incision

(For incision and drainage of sebaceous cyst, furuncle, or abscess, see 10040, 10060, 10061)

§ **56405** Incision and drainage of vulva or perineal abscess

§ **56420** Incision and drainage of Bartholin's gland abscess

(For incision and drainage of Skene's gland abscess or cyst, use 53060)

§ **56440** Marsupialization of Bartholin's gland cyst

§ **56441** Lysis of labial adhesions

Destruction

§ **56501** Destruction of lesion(s), vulva; simple (eg, laser surgery, electrosurgery, cryosurgery, chemosurgery)

➔ *CPT Changes: An Insider's View* 2002

§ **56515** extensive (eg, laser surgery, electrosurgery, cryosurgery, chemosurgery)

➔ *CPT Changes: An Insider's View* 2002

(For destruction of Skene's gland cyst or abscess, use 53270)

(For cautery destruction of urethral caruncle, use 53265)

Excision

§ **56605** Biopsy of vulva or perineum (separate procedure); one lesion

§+ **56606** each separate additional lesion (List separately in addition to code for primary procedure)

(Use 56606 in conjunction with 56605)

(For excision of local lesion, see 11420-11426, 11620-11626)

§ **56620** Vulvectomy simple; partial

§ **56625** complete

(For skin graft, see 15000 et seq)

✿ **56630** Vulvectomy, radical, partial;

(For skin graft, if used, see 15000, 15120, 15121, 15240, 15241)

⌘✿ **56631** with unilateral inguinofemoral lymphadenectomy

✶✿ **56632** with bilateral inguinofemoral lymphadenectomy

✿ **56633** Vulvectomy, radical, complete;

⌘✿ **56634** with unilateral inguinofemoral lymphadenectomy

✶✿ **56637** with bilateral inguinofemoral lymphadenectomy

♦✿ **56640** Vulvectomy, radical, complete, with inguinofemoral, iliac, and pelvic lymphadenectomy

(For bilateral procedure, report 56640 with modifier 50)

(For lymphadenectomy, see 38760-38780)

§ **56700** Partial hymenectomy or revision of hymenal ring

§ **56720** Hymenotomy, simple incision

§ **56740** Excision of Bartholin's gland or cyst

(For excision of Skene's gland, use 53270)

(For excision of urethral caruncle, use 53265)

(For excision or fulguration of urethral carcinoma, use 53220)

(For excision or marsupialization of urethral diverticulum, see 53230, 53240)

Repair

(For repair of urethra for mucosal prolapse, use 53275)

§ **56800** Plastic repair of introitus

§ **56805** Clitoroplasty for intersex state

§ **56810** Perineoplasty, repair of perineum, nonobstetrical (separate procedure)

(See also 56800)

(For repair of wounds to genitalia, see 12001-12007, 12041-12047, 13131-13133)

(For repair of recent injury of vagina and perineum, nonobstetrical, use 57210)

(For anal sphincteroplasty, see 46750, 46751)

(For episiorrhaphy, episioperineorrhaphy for recent injury of vulva and/or perineum, nonobstetrical, use 57210)

Endoscopy

§ **56820** Colposcopy of the vulva;
➔ *CPT Changes: An Insider's View* 2003

§ **56821** with biopsy(s)
➔ *CPT Changes: An Insider's View* 2003

(For colposcopic examinations/procedures involving the vagina, see 57420, 57421; cervix, see 57452-57461)

Vagina

Incision

§ **57000** Colpotomy; with exploration

§ **57010** with drainage of pelvic abscess

§ **57020** Colpocentesis (separate procedure)

§ **57022** Incision and drainage of vaginal hematoma; obstetrical/postpartum
➔ *CPT Changes: An Insider's View* 2001, 2002

§ **57023** non-obstetrical (eg, post-trauma, spontaneous bleeding)
➔ *CPT Changes: An Insider's View* 2001

Destruction

§ **57061** Destruction of vaginal lesion(s); simple (eg, laser surgery, electrosurgery, cryosurgery, chemosurgery)
➔ *CPT Changes: An Insider's View* 2002

§ **57065** extensive (eg, laser surgery, electrosurgery, cryosurgery, chemosurgery)
➔ *CPT Changes: An Insider's View* 2002

Excision

§ **57100** Biopsy of vaginal mucosa; simple (separate procedure)

§ **57105** extensive, requiring suture (including cysts)

§ **57106** Vaginectomy, partial removal of vaginal wall;

§ **57107** with removal of paravaginal tissue (radical vaginectomy)

✶§ **57109** with removal of paravaginal tissue (radical vaginectomy) with bilateral total pelvic lymphadenectomy and para-aortic lymph node sampling (biopsy)

✿ **57110** Vaginectomy, complete removal of vaginal wall;

✶✿ **57111** with removal of paravaginal tissue (radical vaginectomy)

✶✿ **57112** with removal of paravaginal tissue (radical vaginectomy) with bilateral total pelvic lymphadenectomy and para-aortic lymph node sampling (biopsy)

§ **57120** Colpocleisis (Le Fort type)

§ **57130** Excision of vaginal septum

§ **57135** Excision of vaginal cyst or tumor

Introduction

§ **57150** Irrigation of vagina and/or application of medicament for treatment of bacterial, parasitic, or fungoid disease

§ **57155** Insertion of uterine tandems and/or vaginal ovoids for clinical brachytherapy
➔ *CPT Changes: An Insider's View* 2002

(For insertion of radioelement sources or ribbons, see 77761-77763, 77781-77784)

§ **57160** Fitting and insertion of pessary or other intravaginal support device

§ **57170** Diaphragm or cervical cap fitting with instructions

§ **57180** Introduction of any hemostatic agent or pack for spontaneous or traumatic nonobstetrical vaginal hemorrhage (separate procedure)

Repair

(For urethral suspension, Marshall-Marchetti-Krantz type, abdominal approach, see 51840, 51841)

(For laparoscopic suspension, use 51990)

§ **57200** Colporrhaphy, suture of injury of vagina (nonobstetrical)

§ **57210** Colpoperineorrhaphy, suture of injury of vagina and/or perineum (nonobstetrical)

§ **57220** Plastic operation on urethral sphincter, vaginal approach (eg, Kelly urethral plication)

§ **57230** Plastic repair of urethrocele

§ **57240** Anterior colporrhaphy, repair of cystocele with or without repair of urethrocele

§ **57250** Posterior colporrhaphy, repair of rectocele with or without perineorrhaphy

(For repair of rectocele (separate procedure) without posterior colporrhaphy, use 45560)

§ **57260** Combined anteroposterior colporrhaphy;

§ **57265** with enterocele repair

♦§+● **57267** Insertion of mesh or other prosthesis for repair of pelvic floor defect, each site (anterior, posterior compartment), vaginal approach (List separately in addition to code for primary procedure)

➔ *CPT Changes: An Insider's View* 2005

►(Use 57267 in addition to 45560, 57240-57265)◄

§ **57268** Repair of enterocele, vaginal approach (separate procedure)

✿ **57270** Repair of enterocele, abdominal approach (separate procedure)

✿ **57280** Colpopexy, abdominal approach

✿▲ **57282** Colpopexy, vaginal; extra-peritoneal approach (sacrospinous, iliococcygeus)

✿● **57283** intra-peritoneal approach (uterosacral, levator myorrhaphy)

§ **57284** Paravaginal defect repair (including repair of cystocele, stress urinary incontinence, and/or incomplete vaginal prolapse)

§ **57287** Removal or revision of sling for stress incontinence (eg, fascia or synthetic)

➔ *CPT Changes: An Insider's View* 2001

§ **57288** Sling operation for stress incontinence (eg, fascia or synthetic)

➔ *CPT Changes: An Insider's View* 2000

(For laparoscopic approach, use 51992)

§ **57289** Pereyra procedure, including anterior colporrhaphy

§ **57291** Construction of artificial vagina; without graft

✿ **57292** with graft

§ **57300** Closure of rectovaginal fistula; vaginal or transanal approach

✿ **57305** abdominal approach

✿ **57307** abdominal approach, with concomitant colostomy

✿ **57308** transperineal approach, with perineal body reconstruction, with or without levator plication

§ **57310** Closure of urethrovaginal fistula;

✿ **57311** with bulbocavernosus transplant

§ **57320** Closure of vesicovaginal fistula; vaginal approach

(For concomitant cystostomy, see 51005-51040)

§ **57330** transvesical and vaginal approach

(For abdominal approach, use 51900)

✿ **57335** Vaginoplasty for intersex state

Manipulation

§ **57400** Dilation of vagina under anesthesia

§ **57410** Pelvic examination under anesthesia

§ **57415** Removal of impacted vaginal foreign body (separate procedure) under anesthesia

(For removal without anesthesia of an impacted vaginal foreign body, use the appropriate E/M code)

Endoscopy

(For speculoscopy, see Category III codes 0031T, 0032T)

§ **57420** Colposcopy of the entire vagina, with cervix if present;

➔ *CPT Changes: An Insider's View* 2003

§ **57421** with biopsy(s)

➔ *CPT Changes: An Insider's View* 2003

(For colposcopic visualization of cervix and adjacent upper vagina, use 57452)

(When reporting colposcopies of multiple sites, use modifier 51 as appropriate. For colposcopic examinations/procedures involving the vulva, see 56820, 56821; cervix, see 57452-57461)

(57450, 57451 have been deleted)

§ **57425** Laparoscopy, surgical, colpopexy (suspension of vaginal apex)

➔ *CPT Changes: An Insider's View* 2004

Cervix Uteri

(For cervicography, see Category III code 0003T)

Endoscopy

(For colposcopic examinations/procedures involving the vulva, see 56820, 56821; vagina, see 57420, 57421)

§ **57452** Colposcopy of the cervix including upper/adjacent vagina;

➔ *CPT Changes: An Insider's View* 2003

(Do not report 57452 in addition to 57454-57461)

§ **57454** with biopsy(s) of the cervix and endocervical curettage

➔ *CPT Changes: An Insider's View* 2003

§ **57455** with biopsy(s) of the cervix

➔ *CPT Changes: An Insider's View* 2003

§ **57456** with endocervical curettage

➔ *CPT Changes: An Insider's View* 2003

§ **57460** with loop electrode biopsy(s) of the cervix

➔ *CPT Changes: An Insider's View* 2003

§ **57461** with loop electrode conization of the cervix

➔ *CPT Changes: An Insider's View* 2003

(Do not report 57456 in addition to 57461)

Excision

(For radical surgical procedures, see 58200-58240)

§ **57500** Biopsy, single or multiple, or local excision of lesion, with or without fulguration (separate procedure)

§ **57505** Endocervical curettage (not done as part of a dilation and curettage)

§ **57510** Cautery of cervix; electro or thermal

➲ *CPT Changes: An Insider's View* 2002

§ **57511** cryocautery, initial or repeat

§ **57513** laser ablation

§ **57520** Conization of cervix, with or without fulguration, with or without dilation and curettage, with or without repair; cold knife or laser

(See also 58120)

§ **57522** loop electrode excision

§ **57530** Trachelectomy (cervicectomy), amputation of cervix (separate procedure)

✶✿ **57531** Radical trachelectomy, with bilateral total pelvic lymphadenectomy and para-aortic lymph node sampling biopsy, with or without removal of tube(s), with or without removal of ovary(s)

(For radical abdominal hysterectomy, use 58210)

✿ **57540** Excision of cervical stump, abdominal approach;

✿ **57545** with pelvic floor repair

§ **57550** Excision of cervical stump, vaginal approach;

§ **57555** with anterior and/or posterior repair

§ **57556** with repair of enterocele

(For insertion of intrauterine device, use 58300)

(For insertion of any hemostatic agent or pack for control of spontaneous non-obstetrical hemorrhage, see 57180)

Repair

§ **57700** Cerclage of uterine cervix, nonobstetrical

§ **57720** Trachelorrhaphy, plastic repair of uterine cervix, vaginal approach

Manipulation

§ **57800** Dilation of cervical canal, instrumental (separate procedure)

§ **57820** Dilation and curettage of cervical stump

Corpus Uteri

Excision

§ **58100** Endometrial sampling (biopsy) with or without endocervical sampling (biopsy), without cervical dilation, any method (separate procedure)

(For endocervical curettage only, use 57505)

§ **58120** Dilation and curettage, diagnostic and/or therapeutic (nonobstetrical)

(For postpartum hemorrhage, use 59160)

✿ **58140** Myomectomy, excision of fibroid tumor(s) of uterus, 1 to 4 intramural myoma(s) with total weight of 250 grams or less and/or removal of surface myomas; abdominal approach

§ **58145** vaginal approach

✿ **58146** Myomectomy, excision of fibroid tumor(s) of uterus, 5 or more intramural myomas and/or intramural myomas with total weight greater than 250 grams, abdominal approach

(Do not report 58146 in addition to 58140-58145, 58150-58240)

✿ **58150** Total abdominal hysterectomy (corpus and cervix), with or without removal of tube(s), with or without removal of ovary(s);

✿ **58152** with colpo-urethrocystopexy (eg, Marshall-Marchetti-Krantz, Burch)

(For urethrocystopexy without hysterectomy, see 51840, 51841)

✿ **58180** Supracervical abdominal hysterectomy (subtotal hysterectomy), with or without removal of tube(s), with or without removal of ovary(s)

✿ **58200** Total abdominal hysterectomy, including partial vaginectomy, with para-aortic and pelvic lymph node sampling, with or without removal of tube(s), with or without removal of ovary(s)

✶✿ **58210** Radical abdominal hysterectomy, with bilateral total pelvic lymphadenectomy and para-aortic lymph node sampling (biopsy), with or without removal of tube(s), with or without removal of ovary(s)

(For radical hysterectomy with ovarian transposition, use also 58825)

✿ **58240** Pelvic exenteration for gynecologic malignancy, with total abdominal hysterectomy or cervicectomy, with or without removal of tube(s), with or without removal of ovary(s), with removal of bladder and ureteral transplantations, and/or abdominoperineal resection of rectum and colon and colostomy, or any combination thereof

(For pelvic exenteration for lower urinary tract or male genital malignancy, use 51597)

✿ **58260** Vaginal hysterectomy, for uterus 250 grams or less;

✿ **58262** with removal of tube(s), and/or ovary(s)

✿ **58263** with removal of tube(s), and/or ovary(s), with repair of enterocele

►(Do not report 58263 in addition to 57283)◄

✿ **58267** with colpo-urethrocystopexy (Marshall-Marchetti-Krantz type, Pereyra type) with or without endoscopic control

✿ **58270** with repair of enterocele

(For repair of enterocele with removal of tubes and/or ovaries, use 58263)

✿ **58275** Vaginal hysterectomy, with total or partial vaginectomy;

✿ **58280** with repair of enterocele

✿ **58285** Vaginal hysterectomy, radical (Schauta type operation)

✿ **58290** Vaginal hysterectomy, for uterus greater than 250 grams;

✿ **58291** with removal of tube(s) and/or ovary(s)

✿ **58292** with removal of tube(s) and/or ovary(s), with repair of enterocele

✿ **58293** with colpo-urethrocystopexy (Marshall-Marchetti-Krantz type, Pereyra type) with or without endoscopic control

✿ **58294** with repair of enterocele

Introduction

(For insertion/removal of implantable contraceptive capsules, see 11975, 11976, 11977)

□ **58300** Insertion of intrauterine device (IUD)

§ **58301** Removal of intrauterine device (IUD)

§ **58321** Artificial insemination; intra-cervical

§ **58322** intra-uterine

§ **58323** Sperm washing for artificial insemination

☆ **58340** Catheterization and introduction of saline or contrast material for saline infusion sonohysterography (SIS) or hysterosalpingography

➔ *CPT Changes: An Insider's View* 2004

(For radiological supervision and interpretation of saline infusion sonohysterography, use 76831)

(For radiological supervision and interpretation of hysterosalpingography, use 74740)

♦§ **58345** Transcervical introduction of fallopian tube catheter for diagnosis and/or re-establishing patency (any method), with or without hysterosalpingography

(For radiological supervision and interpretation, use 74742)

§ **58346** Insertion of Heyman capsules for clinical brachytherapy

➔ *CPT Changes: An Insider's View* 2002

(For insertion of radioelement sources or ribbons, see 77761-77763, 77781-77784)

§ **58350** Chromotubation of oviduct, including materials

(For materials supplied by physician, use 99070)

♦§ **58353** Endometrial ablation, thermal, without hysteroscopic guidance

➔ *CPT Changes: An Insider's View* 2001

(For hysteroscopic procedure, use 58563)

♦§● **58356** Endometrial cryoablation with ultrasonic guidance, including endometrial curettage, when performed

➔ *CPT Changes: An Insider's View* 2005

►(Do not report 58356 in conjunction with 58100, 58120, 58340, 76700, 76856)◄

Repair

✿ **58400** Uterine suspension, with or without shortening of round ligaments, with or without shortening of sacrouterine ligaments; (separate procedure)

✿ **58410** with presacral sympathectomy

(For anastomosis of tubes to uterus, use 58752)

✿ **58520** Hysterorrhaphy, repair of ruptured uterus (nonobstetrical)

✿ **58540** Hysteroplasty, repair of uterine anomaly (Strassman type)

(For closure of vesicouterine fistula, use 51920)

Laparoscopy/Hysteroscopy

Surgical laparoscopy always includes diagnostic laparoscopy. To report a diagnostic laparoscopy (peritoneoscopy) (separate procedure), use 49320. To report a diagnostic hysteroscopy (separate procedure), use 58555.

§ **58545** Laparoscopy, surgical, myomectomy, excision; 1 to 4 intramural myomas with total weight of 250 grams or less and/or removal of surface myomas

➔ *CPT Changes: An Insider's View* 2003

§ **58546** 5 or more intramural myomas and/or intramural myomas with total weight greater than 250 grams

➔ *CPT Changes: An Insider's View* 2003

§ **58550** Laparoscopy surgical, with vaginal hysterectomy, for uterus 250 grams or less;

➔ *CPT Changes: An Insider's View* 2000, 2003

(58551 has been deleted. To report see 58545, 58546)

§ **58552** with removal of tube(s) and/or ovary(s)

➔ *CPT Changes: An Insider's View* 2003

§ **58553** Laparoscopy, surgical, with vaginal hysterectomy, for uterus greater than 250 grams;

➔ *CPT Changes: An Insider's View* 2003

§ **58554** with removal of tube(s) and/or ovary(s)

➔ *CPT Changes: An Insider's View* 2003

§ **58555** Hysteroscopy, diagnostic (separate procedure)

➔ *CPT Changes: An Insider's View* 2003

§ **58558** Hysteroscopy, surgical; with sampling (biopsy) of endometrium and/or polypectomy, with or without D & C
➲ *CPT Assistant* Jan 03:7; *CPT Changes: An Insider's View* 2000

§ **58559** with lysis of intrauterine adhesions (any method)
➲ *CPT Changes: An Insider's View* 2000

§ **58560** with division or resection of intrauterine septum (any method)
➲ *CPT Changes: An Insider's View* 2000

§ **58561** with removal of leiomyomata
➲ *CPT Assistant* Jan 03:7; *CPT Changes: An Insider's View* 2000

§ **58562** with removal of impacted foreign body
➲ *CPT Changes: An Insider's View* 2000

§ **58563** with endometrial ablation (eg, endometrial resection, electrosurgical ablation, thermoablation)
➲ *CPT Assistant* Jan 03:7; *CPT Changes: An Insider's View* 2000, 2002

✶§● **58565** with bilateral fallopian tube cannulation to induce occlusion by placement of permanent implants
➲ *CPT Changes: An Insider's View* 2005

►(Do not report 58565 in conjunction with 58555 or 57800)◄

►(For unilateral procedure, use modifier 52)◄

♦§ **58578** Unlisted laparoscopy procedure, uterus
➲ *CPT Changes: An Insider's View* 2000

♦§ **58579** Unlisted hysteroscopy procedure, uterus
➲ *CPT Changes: An Insider's View* 2000

Oviduct/Ovary

Incision

✶§ **58600** Ligation or transection of fallopian tube(s), abdominal or vaginal approach, unilateral or bilateral
➲ *CPT Changes: An Insider's View* 2000

✶✿ **58605** Ligation or transection of fallopian tube(s), abdominal or vaginal approach, postpartum, unilateral or bilateral, during same hospitalization (separate procedure)

(For laparoscopic procedures, use 58670, 58671)

✿+ **58611** Ligation or transection of fallopian tube(s) when done at the time of cesarean delivery or intra-abdominal surgery (not a separate procedure) (List separately in addition to code for primary procedure)

§ **58615** Occlusion of fallopian tube(s) by device (eg, band, clip, Falope ring) vaginal or suprapubic approach
➲ *CPT Changes: An Insider's View* 2000

(For laparoscopic approach, use 58671)

(For lysis of adnexal adhesions, use 58740)

Laparoscopy

Surgical laparoscopy always includes diagnostic laparoscopy. To report a diagnostic laparoscopy (peritoneoscopy) (separate procedure), use 49320.

(For laparoscopic biopsy of the ovary or fallopian tube, use 49321)

§ **58660** Laparoscopy, surgical; with lysis of adhesions (salpingolysis, ovariolysis) (separate procedure)
➲ *CPT Changes: An Insider's View* 2000

§ **58661** with removal of adnexal structures (partial or total oophorectomy and/or salpingectomy)
➲ *CPT Changes: An Insider's View* 2000

§ **58662** with fulguration or excision of lesions of the ovary, pelvic viscera, or peritoneal surface by any method
➲ *CPT Changes: An Insider's View* 2000

§ **58670** with fulguration of oviducts (with or without transection)
➲ *CPT Changes: An Insider's View* 2000

§ **58671** with occlusion of oviducts by device (eg, band, clip, or Falope ring)
➲ *CPT Changes: An Insider's View* 2000

♦§ **58672** with fimbrioplasty
➲ *CPT Changes: An Insider's View* 2000

♦§ **58673** with salpingostomy (salpingoneostomy)
➲ *CPT Changes: An Insider's View* 2000

(Codes 58672 and 58673 are used to report unilateral procedures. For bilateral procedure, use modifier 50)

♦§ **58679** Unlisted laparoscopy procedure, oviduct, ovary
➲ *CPT Changes: An Insider's View* 2000

Excision

✶✿ **58700** Salpingectomy, complete or partial, unilateral or bilateral (separate procedure)

✶✿ **58720** Salpingo-oophorectomy, complete or partial, unilateral or bilateral (separate procedure)

Repair

✿ **58740** Lysis of adhesions (salpingolysis, ovariolysis)

(For laparoscopic approach, use 58660)

(For excision or destruction of endometriomas, open method, see 49200, 49201)

(For fulguration or excision of lesions, laparoscopic approach, use 58662)

✿ **58750** Tubotubal anastomosis

✿ **58752** Tubouterine implantation

♦✿ **58760** Fimbrioplasty

(For laparoscopic approach, use 58672)

♦§ **58770** Salpingostomy (salpingoneostomy)

(For laparoscopic approach, use 58673)

Ovary

Incision

✶§ **58800** Drainage of ovarian cyst(s), unilateral or bilateral, (separate procedure); vaginal approach

✶✿ **58805** abdominal approach

§ **58820** Drainage of ovarian abscess; vaginal approach, open

✿ **58822** abdominal approach

§⊙ **58823** Drainage of pelvic abscess, transvaginal or transrectal approach, percutaneous (eg, ovarian, pericolic)

(For radiological supervision and interpretation, use 75989)

✿ **58825** Transposition, ovary(s)

Excision

✶§ **58900** Biopsy of ovary, unilateral or bilateral (separate procedure)

➔ *CPT Assistant* May 03:13; *CPT Changes: An Insider's View* 2000

(For laparoscopic biopsy of the ovary or fallopian tube, use 49321)

✶§ **58920** Wedge resection or bisection of ovary, unilateral or bilateral

✶§ **58925** Ovarian cystectomy, unilateral or bilateral

✶✿ **58940** Oophorectomy, partial or total, unilateral or bilateral;

(For oophorectomy with concomitant debulking for ovarian malignancy, use 58952)

✿ **58943** for ovarian, tubal or primary peritoneal malignancy, with para-aortic and pelvic lymph node biopsies, peritoneal washings, peritoneal biopsies, diaphragmatic assessments, with or without salpingectomy(s), with or without omentectomy

✶✿ **58950** Resection of ovarian, tubal or primary peritoneal malignancy with bilateral salpingo-oophorectomy and omentectomy;

✶✿ **58951** with total abdominal hysterectomy, pelvic and limited para-aortic lymphadenectomy

✶✿ **58952** with radical dissection for debulking (ie, radical excision or destruction, intra-abdominal or retroperitoneal tumors)

✶✿ **58953** Bilateral salpingo-oophorectomy with omentectomy, total abdominal hysterectomy and radical dissection for debulking;

✶✿ **58954** with pelvic lymphadenectomy and limited para-aortic lymphadenectomy

✶✿● **58956** Bilateral salpingo-oophorectomy with total omentectomy, total abdominal hysterectomy for malignancy

►(Do not report 58956 in conjunction with 49255, 58150, 58180, 58262, 58263, 58550, 58661, 58700, 58720, 58900, 58925, 58940)◄

✿ **58960** Laparotomy, for staging or restaging of ovarian, tubal or primary peritoneal malignancy (second look), with or without omentectomy, peritoneal washing, biopsy of abdominal and pelvic peritoneum, diaphragmatic assessment with pelvic and limited para-aortic lymphadenectomy

In Vitro Fertilization

§ **58970** Follicle puncture for oocyte retrieval, any method

(For radiological supervision and interpretation, use 76948)

§ **58974** Embryo transfer, intrauterine

§ **58976** Gamete, zygote, or embryo intrafallopian transfer, any method

(For laparoscopic adnexal procedures, see 58660-58673)

Other Procedures

§ **58999** Unlisted procedure, female genital system (nonobstetrical)

Maternity Care and Delivery

The services normally provided in uncomplicated maternity cases include antepartum care, delivery, and postpartum care.

Antepartum care includes the initial and subsequent history, physical examinations, recording of weight, blood pressures, fetal heart tones, routine chemical urinalysis, and monthly visits up to 28 weeks gestation, biweekly visits to 36 weeks gestation, and weekly visits until delivery. Any other visits or services within this time period should be coded separately.

Delivery services include admission to the hospital, the admission history and physical examination, management of uncomplicated labor, vaginal delivery (with or without episiotomy, with or without forceps), or cesarean delivery. Medical problems complicating labor and delivery management may require additional resources and should be identified by utilizing the codes in the **Medicine** and **Evaluation and Management Services** section in addition to codes for maternity care.

Postpartum care includes hospital and office visits following vaginal or cesarean section delivery.

For medical complications of pregnancy (eg, cardiac problems, neurological problems, diabetes, hypertension, toxemia, hyperemesis, pre-term labor, premature rupture of membranes), see services in the **Medicine** and **Evaluation and Management Services** section.

For surgical complications of pregnancy (eg, appendectomy, hernia, ovarian cyst, Bartholin cyst), see services in the **Surgery** section.

If a physician provides all or part of the antepartum and/or postpartum patient care but does not perform delivery due to termination of pregnancy by abortion or referral to another physician for delivery, see the antepartum and postpartum care codes 59425-59426 and 59430.

(For circumcision of newborn, see 54150, 54160)

Antepartum Services

(For insertion of transcervical or transvaginal fetal oximetry sensor, use Category III code 0021T)

§ **59000** Amniocentesis; diagnostic

(For radiological supervision and interpretation, use 76946)

§ **59001** therapeutic amniotic fluid reduction (includes ultrasound guidance)

➔ *CPT Changes: An Insider's View* 2002

§ **59012** Cordocentesis (intrauterine), any method

(For radiological supervision and interpretation, use 76941)

§ **59015** Chorionic villus sampling, any method

(For radiological supervision and interpretation, use 76945)

§ **59020** Fetal contraction stress test

§ **59025** Fetal non-stress test

§ **59030** Fetal scalp blood sampling

(For repeat fetal scalp blood sampling, use 59030 and see modifiers 76 and 77)

□ **59050** Fetal monitoring during labor by consulting physician (ie, non-attending physician) with written report; supervision and interpretation

✣ **59051** interpretation only

§ **59070** Transabdominal amnioinfusion, including ultrasound guidance

➔ *CPT Changes: An Insider's View* 2004

§ **59072** Fetal umbilical cord occlusion, including ultrasound guidance

➔ *CPT Changes: An Insider's View* 2004

§ **59074** Fetal fluid drainage (eg, vesicocentesis, thoracocentesis, paracentesis), including ultrasound guidance

➔ *CPT Changes: An Insider's View* 2004

§ **59076** Fetal shunt placement, including ultrasound guidance

➔ *CPT Changes: An Insider's View* 2004

(For unlisted fetal invasive procedure, use 59897)

Excision

✿ **59100** Hysterotomy, abdominal (eg, for hydatidiform mole, abortion)

(When tubal ligation is performed at the same time as hysterotomy, use 58611 in addition to 59100)

✿ **59120** Surgical treatment of ectopic pregnancy; tubal or ovarian, requiring salpingectomy and/or oophorectomy, abdominal or vaginal approach

✿ **59121** tubal or ovarian, without salpingectomy and/or oophorectomy

✿ **59130** abdominal pregnancy

✿ **59135** interstitial, uterine pregnancy requiring total hysterectomy

✿ **59136** interstitial, uterine pregnancy with partial resection of uterus

✿ **59140** cervical, with evacuation

§ **59150** Laparoscopic treatment of ectopic pregnancy; without salpingectomy and/or oophorectomy

§ **59151** with salpingectomy and/or oophorectomy

§ **59160** Curettage, postpartum

Introduction

(For intrauterine fetal transfusion, use 36460)

(For introduction of hypertonic solution and/or prostaglandins to initiate labor, see 59850-59857)

§ **59200** Insertion of cervical dilator (eg, laminaria, prostaglandin) (separate procedure)

Repair

(For tracheloplasty, use 57700)

§ **59300** Episiotomy or vaginal repair, by other than attending physician

§ **59320** Cerclage of cervix, during pregnancy; vaginal

✿ **59325** abdominal

✿ **59350** Hysterorrhaphy of ruptured uterus

Vaginal Delivery, Antepartum and Postpartum Care

(For insertion of transcervical or transvaginal fetal oximetry sensor, use Category III code 0021T)

✣ **59400** Routine obstetric care including antepartum care, vaginal delivery (with or without episiotomy, and/or forceps) and postpartum care

§ **59409** Vaginal delivery only (with or without episiotomy and/or forceps);

✣ **59410** including postpartum care

Surgery: Male/Female Genital System

§ **59412** External cephalic version, with or without tocolysis

(Use 59412 in addition to code(s) for delivery)

§ **59414** Delivery of placenta (separate procedure)

(For antepartum care only, see 59425, 59426 or appropriate E/M code(s))

(For 1-3 antepartum care visits, see appropriate E/M code(s))

✣ **59425** Antepartum care only; 4-6 visits

✣ **59426** 7 or more visits

✣ **59430** Postpartum care only (separate procedure)

Cesarean Delivery

(For insertion of transcervical or transvaginal fetal oximetry sensor, use Category III code 0021T)

(For standby attendance for infant, use 99360)

(For low cervical Cesarean section, see 59510, 59515, 59525)

☐ **59510** Routine obstetric care including antepartum care, cesarean delivery, and postpartum care

✿ **59514** Cesarean delivery only;

☐ **59515** including postpartum care

(For classic Cesarean section, see 59510, 59515, 59525)

✿+ **59525** Subtotal or total hysterectomy after cesarean delivery (List separately in addition to code for primary procedure)

(Use 59525 in conjunction with 59510, 59514, 59515, 59618, 59620, 59622)

(For extraperitoneal Cesarean section, or Cesarean section with subtotal or total hysterectomy, see 59510, 59515, 59525)

Delivery After Previous Cesarean Delivery

Patients who have had a previous cesarean delivery and now present with the expectation of a vaginal delivery are coded using codes 59610-59622. If the patient has a successful vaginal delivery after a previous cesarean delivery (VBAC), use codes 59610-59614. If the attempt is unsuccessful and another cesarean delivery is carried out, use codes 59618-59622. To report elective cesarean deliveries use code 59510, 59514 or 59515.

(For insertion of transcervical or transvaginal fetal oximetry sensor, use Category III code 0021T)

☐ **59610** Routine obstetric care including antepartum care, vaginal delivery (with or without episiotomy, and/or forceps) and postpartum care, after previous cesarean delivery

§ **59612** Vaginal delivery only, after previous cesarean delivery (with or without episiotomy and/or forceps);

☐ **59614** including postpartum care

☐ **59618** Routine obstetric care including antepartum care, cesarean delivery, and postpartum care, following attempted vaginal delivery after previous cesarean delivery

✿ **59620** Cesarean delivery only, following attempted vaginal delivery after previous cesarean delivery;

☐ **59622** including postpartum care

Abortion

(For medical treatment of spontaneous complete abortion, any trimester, use E/M codes 99201-99233)

(For surgical treatment of spontaneous abortion, use 59812)

§ **59812** Treatment of incomplete abortion, any trimester, completed surgically

§ **59820** Treatment of missed abortion, completed surgically; first trimester

§ **59821** second trimester

✿ **59830** Treatment of septic abortion, completed surgically

§ **59840** Induced abortion, by dilation and curettage

§ **59841** Induced abortion, by dilation and evacuation

✿ **59850** Induced abortion, by one or more intra-amniotic injections (amniocentesis-injections), including hospital admission and visits, delivery of fetus and secundines;

✿ **59851** with dilation and curettage and/or evacuation

✿ **59852** with hysterotomy (failed intra-amniotic injection)

(For insertion of cervical dilator, use 59200)

✿ **59855** Induced abortion, by one or more vaginal suppositories (eg, prostaglandin) with or without cervical dilation (eg, laminaria), including hospital admission and visits, delivery of fetus and secundines;

✿ **59856** with dilation and curettage and/or evacuation

✿ **59857** with hysterotomy (failed medical evacuation)

Other Procedures

§ **59866** Multifetal pregnancy reduction(s) (MPR)

§ **59870** Uterine evacuation and curettage for hydatidiform mole

§ **59871** Removal of cerclage suture under anesthesia (other than local)

§ **59897** Unlisted fetal invasive procedure, including ultrasound guidance

➲ *CPT Changes: An Insider's View* 2004

§ **59898** Unlisted laparoscopy procedure, maternity care and delivery

➲ *CPT Changes: An Insider's View* 2000

§ **59899** Unlisted procedure, maternity care and delivery

Notes

Endocrine System

(For pituitary and pineal surgery, see **Nervous System**)

Thyroid Gland

Incision

§ **60000** Incision and drainage of thyroglossal duct cyst, infected

➲ *CPT Changes: An Insider's View* 2002

Excision

§ **60001** Aspiration and/or injection, thyroid cyst

(For fine needle aspiration, see 10021, 10022)

(If imaging guidance is performed, see 76360, 76942)

§ **60100** Biopsy thyroid, percutaneous core needle

(If imaging guidance is performed, see 76003, 76360, 76393, 76942)

(For fine needle aspiration, use 10021 or 10022)

(For evaluation of fine needle aspirate, see 88172, 88173)

§ **60200** Excision of cyst or adenoma of thyroid, or transection of isthmus

⌘§ **60210** Partial thyroid lobectomy, unilateral; with or without isthmusectomy

✶§ **60212** with contralateral subtotal lobectomy, including isthmusectomy

⌘§ **60220** Total thyroid lobectomy, unilateral; with or without isthmusectomy

✶§ **60225** with contralateral subtotal lobectomy, including isthmusectomy

§ **60240** Thyroidectomy, total or complete

(For thyroidectomy, subtotal or partial, use 60271)

§ **60252** Thyroidectomy, total or subtotal for malignancy; with limited neck dissection

✿ **60254** with radical neck dissection

✶§ **60260** Thyroidectomy, removal of all remaining thyroid tissue following previous removal of a portion of thyroid

(For bilateral procedure, report 60260 with modifier 50)

✿ **60270** Thyroidectomy, including substernal thyroid; sternal split or transthoracic approach

✿ **60271** cervical approach

§ **60280** Excision of thyroglossal duct cyst or sinus;

§ **60281** recurrent

(For thyroid ultrasonography, use 76536)

Parathyroid, Thymus, Adrenal Glands, Pancreas, and Carotid Body

Excision

(For pituitary and pineal surgery, see **Nervous System**)

§ **60500** Parathyroidectomy or exploration of parathyroid(s);

✿ **60502** re-exploration

✿ **60505** with mediastinal exploration, sternal split or transthoracic approach

§✚ **60512** Parathyroid autotransplantation (List separately in addition to code for primary procedure)

(Use 60512 in conjunction with 60500, 60502, 60505, 60212, 60225, 60240, 60252, 60254, 60260, 60270, 60271)

✿ **60520** Thymectomy, partial or total; transcervical approach (separate procedure)

✿ **60521** sternal split or transthoracic approach, without radical mediastinal dissection (separate procedure)

✿ **60522** sternal split or transthoracic approach, with radical mediastinal dissection (separate procedure)

♦✿ **60540** Adrenalectomy, partial or complete, or exploration of adrenal gland with or without biopsy, transabdominal, lumbar or dorsal (separate procedure);

✿ **60545** with excision of adjacent retroperitoneal tumor

►(Do not report 60540, 60545 in conjunction with 50323)◄

(For bilateral procedure, report 60540 with modifier 50)

(For excision of remote or disseminated pheochromocytoma, see 49200, 49201)

(For laparoscopic approach, use 60650)

✿ **60600** Excision of carotid body tumor; without excision of carotid artery

✿ **60605** with excision of carotid artery

Laparoscopy

Surgical laparoscopy always includes diagnostic laparoscopy. To report a diagnostic laparoscopy (peritoneoscopy) (separate procedure), use 49320.

♦✿ **60650** Laparoscopy, surgical, with adrenalectomy, partial or complete, or exploration of adrenal gland with or without biopsy, transabdominal, lumbar or dorsal

♦§ **60659** Unlisted laparoscopy procedure, endocrine system

➲ *CPT Changes: An Insider's View* 2000

Other Procedures

§ **60699** Unlisted procedure, endocrine system

Notes

Nervous System

Skull, Meninges, and Brain

(For injection procedure for cerebral angiography, see 36100-36218)

(For injection procedure for ventriculography, see 61026, 61120)

(For injection procedure for pneumoencephalography, use 61055)

Injection, Drainage, or Aspiration

✶§ **61000** Subdural tap through fontanelle, or suture, infant, unilateral or bilateral; initial

✶§ **61001** subsequent taps

§ **61020** Ventricular puncture through previous burr hole, fontanelle, suture, or implanted ventricular catheter/reservoir; without injection

§ **61026** with injection of medication or other substance for diagnosis or treatment

➔ *CPT Changes: An Insider's View* 2002

§ **61050** Cisternal or lateral cervical (C1-C2) puncture; without injection (separate procedure)

§ **61055** with injection of medication or other substance for diagnosis or treatment (eg, C1-C2)

➔ *CPT Changes: An Insider's View* 2002

(For radiological supervision and interpretation, see **Radiology**)

§ **61070** Puncture of shunt tubing or reservoir for aspiration or injection procedure

(For radiological supervision and interpretation, use 75809)

Twist Drill, Burr Hole(s), or Trephine

✿ **61105** Twist drill hole for subdural or ventricular puncture;

✿⊘ **61107** for implanting ventricular catheter or pressure recording device

(For intracranial neuroendoscopic ventricular catheter placement, use 62160)

►(For twist drill or burr hole performed to place thermal perfusion probe, use Category III code 0077T)◄

✿ **61108** for evacuation and/or drainage of subdural hematoma

✿ **61120** Burr hole(s) for ventricular puncture (including injection of gas, contrast media, dye, or radioactive material)

✿ **61140** Burr hole(s) or trephine; with biopsy of brain or intracranial lesion

✿ **61150** with drainage of brain abscess or cyst

✿ **61151** with subsequent tapping (aspiration) of intracranial abscess or cyst

♦✿ **61154** Burr hole(s) with evacuation and/or drainage of hematoma, extradural or subdural

(For bilateral procedure, report 61154 with modifier 50)

✿ **61156** Burr hole(s); with aspiration of hematoma or cyst, intracerebral

✿⊘ **61210** for implanting ventricular catheter, reservoir, EEG electrode(s) or pressure recording device (separate procedure)

(For intracranial neuroendoscopic ventricular catheter placement, use 62160)

§ **61215** Insertion of subcutaneous reservoir, pump or continuous infusion system for connection to ventricular catheter

(For refilling and maintenance of an implantable infusion pump for spinal or brain drug therapy, use 95990)

(For chemotherapy, use 96450)

♦✿ **61250** Burr hole(s) or trephine, supratentorial, exploratory, not followed by other surgery

(For bilateral procedure, report 61250 with modifier 50)

✶✿ **61253** Burr hole(s) or trephine, infratentorial, unilateral or bilateral

(If burr hole(s) or trephine are followed by craniotomy at same operative session, use 61304-61321; do not use 61250 or 61253)

Craniectomy or Craniotomy

✿ **61304** Craniectomy or craniotomy, exploratory; supratentorial

✿ **61305** infratentorial (posterior fossa)

✿ **61312** Craniectomy or craniotomy for evacuation of hematoma, supratentorial; extradural or subdural

✿ **61313** intracerebral

✿ **61314** Craniectomy or craniotomy for evacuation of hematoma, infratentorial; extradural or subdural

✿ **61315** intracerebellar

✿+ **61316** Incision and subcutaneous placement of cranial bone graft (List separately in addition to code for primary procedure)

(Use 61316 in conjunction with 61304, 61312, 61313, 61322, 61323, 61340, 61570, 61571, 61680-61705)

✿ **61320** Craniectomy or craniotomy, drainage of intracranial abscess; supratentorial

✿ **61321** infratentorial

✿ **61322** Craniectomy or craniotomy, decompressive, with or without duraplasty, for treatment of intracranial hypertension, without evacuation of associated intraparenchymal hematoma; without lobectomy

(Do not report 61313 in addition to 61322)

(For subtemporal decompression, use 61340)

✿ **61323** with lobectomy

(Do not report 61313 in addition to 61323)

(For subtemporal decompression, use 61340)

♦§ **61330** Decompression of orbit only, transcranial approach

(For bilateral procedure, report 61330 with modifier 50)

✿ **61332** Exploration of orbit (transcranial approach); with biopsy

✿ **61333** with removal of lesion

✿ **61334** with removal of foreign body

♦✿ **61340** Subtemporal cranial decompression (pseudotumor cerebri, slit ventricle syndrome)

(For bilateral procedure, report 61340 with modifier 50)

(For decompressive craniotomy or craniectomy for intracranial hypertension, without hematoma evacuation, see 61322, 61323)

✿ **61343** Craniectomy, suboccipital with cervical laminectomy for decompression of medulla and spinal cord, with or without dural graft (eg, Arnold-Chiari malformation)

✿ **61345** Other cranial decompression, posterior fossa

(For orbital decompression by lateral wall approach, Kroenlein type, use 67445)

✿ **61440** Craniotomy for section of tentorium cerebelli (separate procedure)

✿ **61450** Craniectomy, subtemporal, for section, compression, or decompression of sensory root of gasserian ganglion

✿ **61458** Craniectomy, suboccipital; for exploration or decompression of cranial nerves

✿ **61460** for section of one or more cranial nerves

✿ **61470** for medullary tractotomy

✿ **61480** for mesencephalic tractotomy or pedunculotomy

♦✿ **61490** Craniotomy for lobotomy, including cingulotomy

(For bilateral procedure, report 61490 with modifier 50)

✿ **61500** Craniectomy; with excision of tumor or other bone lesion of skull

✿ **61501** for osteomyelitis

✿ **61510** Craniectomy, trephination, bone flap craniotomy; for excision of brain tumor, supratentorial, except meningioma

✿ **61512** for excision of meningioma, supratentorial

✿ **61514** for excision of brain abscess, supratentorial

✿ **61516** for excision or fenestration of cyst, supratentorial

(For excision of pituitary tumor or craniopharyngioma, see 61545, 61546, 61548)

✿+ **61517** Implantation of brain intracavitary chemotherapy agent (List separately in addition to code for primary procedure)

(Use 61517 only in conjunction with 61510 or 61518)

(Do not report 61517 for brachytherapy insertion. For intracavitary insertion of radioelement sources or ribbons, see 77781-77784)

✿ **61518** Craniectomy for excision of brain tumor, infratentorial or posterior fossa; except meningioma, cerebellopontine angle tumor, or midline tumor at base of skull

✿ **61519** meningioma

✿ **61520** cerebellopontine angle tumor

✿ **61521** midline tumor at base of skull

✿ **61522** Craniectomy, infratentorial or posterior fossa; for excision of brain abscess

✿ **61524** for excision or fenestration of cyst

✿ **61526** Craniectomy, bone flap craniotomy, transtemporal (mastoid) for excision of cerebellopontine angle tumor;

✿ **61530** combined with middle/posterior fossa craniotomy/craniectomy

✿ **61531** Subdural implantation of strip electrodes through one or more burr or trephine hole(s) for long term seizure monitoring

(For stereotactic implantation of electrodes, use 61760)

(For craniotomy for excision of intracranial arteriovenous malformation, see 61680-61692)

✿ **61533** Craniotomy with elevation of bone flap; for subdural implantation of an electrode array, for long term seizure monitoring

(For continuous EEG monitoring, see 95950-95954)

✿ **61534** for excision of epileptogenic focus without electrocorticography during surgery

✿ **61535** for removal of epidural or subdural electrode array, without excision of cerebral tissue (separate procedure)

✿ **61536** for excision of cerebral epileptogenic focus, with electrocorticography during surgery (includes removal of electrode array)

✿ **61537** for lobectomy, temporal lobe, without electrocorticography during surgery

✿ **61538** for lobectomy, temporal lobe, with electrocorticography during surgery

✿ **61539** for lobectomy, other than temporal lobe, partial or total, with electrocorticography during surgery

✿ **61540** for lobectomy, other than temporal lobe, partial or total, without electrocorticography during surgery

✿ **61541** for transection of corpus callosum

✿ **61542** for total hemispherectomy

✿ **61543** for partial or subtotal (functional) hemispherectomy

✿ **61544** for excision or coagulation of choroid plexus

✿ **61545** for excision of craniopharyngioma

(For craniotomy for selective amygdalohippocampectomy, use 61566)

(For craniotomy for multiple subpial transections during surgery, use 61567)

✿ **61546** Craniotomy for hypophysectomy or excision of pituitary tumor, intracranial approach

✿ **61548** Hypophysectomy or excision of pituitary tumor, transnasal or transseptal approach, nonstereotactic

(Do not report code 69990 in addition to code 61548)

✿ **61550** Craniectomy for craniosynostosis; single cranial suture

✿ **61552** multiple cranial sutures

(For cranial reconstruction for orbital hypertelorism, see 21260-21263)

(For reconstruction, see 21172-21180)

✿ **61556** Craniotomy for craniosynostosis; frontal or parietal bone flap

✿ **61557** bifrontal bone flap

✿ **61558** Extensive craniectomy for multiple cranial suture craniosynostosis (eg, cloverleaf skull); not requiring bone grafts

✿ **61559** recontouring with multiple osteotomies and bone autografts (eg, barrel-stave procedure) (includes obtaining grafts)

(For reconstruction, see 21172-21180)

✿ **61563** Excision, intra and extracranial, benign tumor of cranial bone (eg, fibrous dysplasia); without optic nerve decompression

✿ **61564** with optic nerve decompression

(For reconstruction, see 21181-21183)

✿ **61566** Craniotomy with elevation of bone flap; for selective amygdalohippocampectomy

✿ **61567** for multiple subpial transections, with electrocorticography during surgery

✿ **61570** Craniectomy or craniotomy; with excision of foreign body from brain

✿ **61571** with treatment of penetrating wound of brain

(For sequestrectomy for osteomyelitis, use 61501)

✿ **61575** Transoral approach to skull base, brain stem or upper spinal cord for biopsy, decompression or excision of lesion;

✿ **61576** requiring splitting of tongue and/or mandible (including tracheostomy)

(For arthrodesis, use 22548)

Surgery of Skull Base

The surgical management of lesions involving the skull base (base of anterior, middle, and posterior cranial fossae) often requires the skills of several surgeons of different surgical specialties working together or in tandem during the operative session. These operations are usually not staged because of the need for definitive closure of dura, subcutaneous tissues, and skin to avoid serious infections such as osteomyelitis and/or meningitis.

The procedures are categorized according to: 1) ***approach procedure*** necessary to obtain adequate exposure to the lesion (pathologic entity), 2) ***definitive procedure(s)*** necessary to biopsy, excise or otherwise treat the lesion, and 3) ***repair/reconstruction*** of the defect present following the definitive procedure(s).

The ***approach procedure*** is described according to anatomical area involved, ie, anterior cranial fossa, middle cranial fossa, posterior cranial fossa, and brain stem or upper spinal cord.

The ***definitive procedure(s)*** describes the repair, biopsy, resection, or excision of various lesions of the skull base and, when appropriate, primary closure of the dura, mucous membranes, and skin.

The ***repair/reconstruction procedure(s)*** is reported separately if extensive dural grafting, cranioplasty, local or regional myocutaneous pedicle flaps, or extensive skin grafts are required.

For primary closure, see the appropriate codes, ie, 15732, 15756-15758.

When one surgeon performs the approach procedure, another surgeon performs the definitive procedure, and another surgeon performs the repair/reconstruction procedure, each surgeon reports only the code for the specific procedure performed.

If one surgeon performs more than one procedure (ie, approach procedure and definitive procedure), then both codes are reported, adding modifier 51 to the secondary, additional procedure(s).

Approach Procedures

Anterior Cranial Fossa

♦✿ **61580** Craniofacial approach to anterior cranial fossa; extradural, including lateral rhinotomy, ethmoidectomy, sphenoidectomy, without maxillectomy or orbital exenteration

♦✿ **61581** extradural, including lateral rhinotomy, orbital exenteration, ethmoidectomy, sphenoidectomy and/or maxillectomy

✿ 61582 extradural, including unilateral or bifrontal craniotomy, elevation of frontal lobe(s), osteotomy of base of anterior cranial fossa

✿ 61583 intradural, including unilateral or bifrontal craniotomy, elevation or resection of frontal lobe, osteotomy of base of anterior cranial fossa

♦✿ 61584 Orbitocranial approach to anterior cranial fossa, extradural, including supraorbital ridge osteotomy and elevation of frontal and/or temporal lobe(s); without orbital exenteration

♦✿ 61585 with orbital exenteration

✿ 61586 Bicoronal, transzygomatic and/or LeFort I osteotomy approach to anterior cranial fossa with or without internal fixation, without bone graft

Middle Cranial Fossa

♦✿ 61590 Infratemporal pre-auricular approach to middle cranial fossa (parapharyngeal space, infratemporal and midline skull base, nasopharynx), with or without disarticulation of the mandible, including parotidectomy, craniotomy, decompression and/or mobilization of the facial nerve and/or petrous carotid artery

♦✿ 61591 Infratemporal post-auricular approach to middle cranial fossa (internal auditory meatus, petrous apex, tentorium, cavernous sinus, parasellar area, infratemporal fossa) including mastoidectomy, resection of sigmoid sinus, with or without decompression and/or mobilization of contents of auditory canal or petrous carotid artery

♦✿ 61592 Orbitocranial zygomatic approach to middle cranial fossa (cavernous sinus and carotid artery, clivus, basilar artery or petrous apex) including osteotomy of zygoma, craniotomy, extra- or intradural elevation of temporal lobe

Posterior Cranial Fossa

♦✿ 61595 Transtemporal approach to posterior cranial fossa, jugular foramen or midline skull base, including mastoidectomy, decompression of sigmoid sinus and/or facial nerve, with or without mobilization

♦✿ 61596 Transcochlear approach to posterior cranial fossa, jugular foramen or midline skull base, including labyrinthectomy, decompression, with or without mobilization of facial nerve and/or petrous carotid artery

♦✿ 61597 Transcondylar (far lateral) approach to posterior cranial fossa, jugular foramen or midline skull base, including occipital condylectomy, mastoidectomy, resection of C1-C3 vertebral body(s), decompression of vertebral artery, with or without mobilization

✿ 61598 Transpetrosal approach to posterior cranial fossa, clivus or foramen magnum, including ligation of superior petrosal sinus and/or sigmoid sinus

Definitive Procedures

Base of Anterior Cranial Fossa

✿ 61600 Resection or excision of neoplastic, vascular or infectious lesion of base of anterior cranial fossa; extradural

✿ 61601 intradural, including dural repair, with or without graft

Base of Middle Cranial Fossa

✿ 61605 Resection or excision of neoplastic, vascular or infectious lesion of infratemporal fossa, parapharyngeal space, petrous apex; extradural

✿ 61606 intradural, including dural repair, with or without graft

✿ 61607 Resection or excision of neoplastic, vascular or infectious lesion of parasellar area, cavernous sinus, clivus or midline skull base; extradural

✿ 61608 intradural, including dural repair, with or without graft

Codes 61609-61612 are reported in addition to code(s) for primary procedure(s) 61605-61608. Report only one transection or ligation of carotid artery code per operative session.

♦✿+ 61609 Transection or ligation, carotid artery in cavernous sinus; without repair (List separately in addition to code for primary procedure)

♦✿+ 61610 with repair by anastomosis or graft (List separately in addition to code for primary procedure)

♦✿+ 61611 Transection or ligation, carotid artery in petrous canal; without repair (List separately in addition to code for primary procedure)

♦✿+ 61612 with repair by anastomosis or graft (List separately in addition to code for primary procedure)

♦✿ 61613 Obliteration of carotid aneurysm, arteriovenous malformation, or carotid-cavernous fistula by dissection within cavernous sinus

Base of Posterior Cranial Fossa

✿ 61615 Resection or excision of neoplastic, vascular or infectious lesion of base of posterior cranial fossa, jugular foramen, foramen magnum, or C1-C3 vertebral bodies; extradural

✿ 61616 intradural, including dural repair, with or without graft

Repair and/or Reconstruction of Surgical Defects of Skull Base

✿ 61618 Secondary repair of dura for cerebrospinal fluid leak, anterior, middle or posterior cranial fossa following surgery of the skull base; by free tissue graft (eg, pericranium, fascia, tensor fascia lata, adipose tissue, homologous or synthetic grafts)

✿ 61619 by local or regionalized vascularized pedicle flap or myocutaneous flap (including galea, temporalis, frontalis or occipitalis muscle)

Endovascular Therapy

§ **61623** Endovascular temporary balloon arterial occlusion, head or neck (extracranial/intracranial) including selective catheterization of vessel to be occluded, positioning and inflation of occlusion balloon, concomitant neurological monitoring, and radiologic supervision and interpretation of all angiography required for balloon occlusion and to exclude vascular injury post occlusion

(If selective catheterization and angiography of arteries other than artery to be occluded is performed, use appropriate catheterization and radiologic supervision and interpretation codes)

(If complete diagnostic angiography of the artery to be occluded is performed immediately prior to temporary occlusion, use appropriate radiologic supervision and interpretation codes only)

✿ **61624** Transcatheter permanent occlusion or embolization (eg, for tumor destruction, to achieve hemostasis, to occlude a vascular malformation), percutaneous, any method; central nervous system (intracranial, spinal cord)

(See also 37204)

(For radiological supervision and interpretation, use 75894)

§ **61626** non-central nervous system, head or neck (extracranial, brachiocephalic branch)

(See also 37204)

(For radiological supervision and interpretation, use 75894)

Surgery for Aneurysm, Arteriovenous Malformation or Vascular Disease

Includes craniotomy when appropriate for procedure.

✿ **61680** Surgery of intracranial arteriovenous malformation; supratentorial, simple

✿ **61682** supratentorial, complex

✿ **61684** infratentorial, simple

✿ **61686** infratentorial, complex

✿ **61690** dural, simple

✿ **61692** dural, complex

✿ **61697** Surgery of complex intracranial aneurysm, intracranial approach; carotid circulation

✿ **61698** vertebrobasilar circulation

(61697, 61698 involve aneurysms that are larger than 15 mm or with calcification of the aneurysm neck, or with incorporation of normal vessels into the aneurysm neck, or a procedure requiring temporary vessel occlusion, trapping or cardiopulmonary bypass to successfully treat the aneurysm)

✿ **61700** Surgery of simple intracranial aneurysm, intracranial approach; carotid circulation

✿ **61702** vertebrobasilar circulation

✿ **61703** Surgery of intracranial aneurysm, cervical approach by application of occluding clamp to cervical carotid artery (Selverstone-Crutchfield type)

(For cervical approach for direct ligation of carotid artery, see 37600-37606)

✿ **61705** Surgery of aneurysm, vascular malformation or carotid-cavernous fistula; by intracranial and cervical occlusion of carotid artery

✿ **61708** by intracranial electrothrombosis

(For ligation or gradual occlusion of internal/common carotid artery, see 37605, 37606)

✿ **61710** by intra-arterial embolization, injection procedure, or balloon catheter

✿ **61711** Anastomosis, arterial, extracranial-intracranial (eg, middle cerebral/cortical) arteries

(For carotid or vertebral thromboendarterectomy, use 35301)

(Use 69990 when the surgical microscope is employed for the microsurgical procedure. Do not use 69990 for visualization with magnifying loupes or corrected vision)

Stereotaxis

✿ **61720** Creation of lesion by stereotactic method, including burr hole(s) and localizing and recording techniques, single or multiple stages; globus pallidus or thalamus

✿ **61735** subcortical structure(s) other than globus pallidus or thalamus

✿ **61750** Stereotactic biopsy, aspiration, or excision, including burr hole(s), for intracranial lesion;

✿ **61751** with computed tomography and/or magnetic resonance guidance

(For radiological supervision and interpretation of computerized tomography, see 70450, 70460, or 70470 as appropriate)

(For radiological supervision and interpretation of magnetic resonance imaging, see 70551, 70552, or 70553 as appropriate)

✿ **61760** Stereotactic implantation of depth electrodes into the cerebrum for long term seizure monitoring

✿ **61770** Stereotactic localization, including burr hole(s), with insertion of catheter(s) or probe(s) for placement of radiation source

§ **61790** Creation of lesion by stereotactic method, percutaneous, by neurolytic agent (eg, alcohol, thermal, electrical, radiofrequency); gasserian ganglion

§ **61791** trigeminal medullary tract

□ **61793** Stereotactic radiosurgery (particle beam, gamma ray or linear accelerator), one or more sessions

(For intensity modulated beam delivery plan and treatment, see 77301, 77418)

❖+ **61795** Stereotactic computer assisted volumetric (navigational) procedure, intracranial, extracranial, or spinal (List separately in addition to code for primary procedure)

➔ *CPT Changes: An Insider's View* 2000

Neurostimulators (Intracranial)

Codes 61850-61888 apply to both simple and complex neurostimulators. For initial or subsequent electronic analysis and programming of neurostimulator pulse generators, see codes 95970-95975.

Microelectrode recording, when performed by the operating surgeon in association with implantation of neurostimulator electrode arrays, is an inclusive service and should not be reported separately. If another physician participates in neurophysiological mapping during a deep brain stimulator implantation procedure, this service may be reported by the other physician with codes 95961-95962.

✿ **61850** Twist drill or burr hole(s) for implantation of neurostimulator electrodes, cortical

✿ **61860** Craniectomy or craniotomy for implantation of neurostimulator electrodes, cerebral, cortical

(61862 has been deleted. To report, see 61867, 61868)

♦✿ **61863** Twist drill, burr hole, craniotomy, or craniectomy with stereotactic implantation of neurostimulator electrode array in subcortical site (eg, thalamus, globus pallidus, subthalamic nucleus, periventricular, periaqueductal gray), without use of intraoperative microelectrode recording; first array

♦✿+ **61864** each additional array (List separately in addition to primary procedure)

(Use 61864 in conjunction with 61863)

(61865 has been deleted. To report, use 61867, 61868)

♦✿ **61867** Twist drill, burr hole, craniotomy, or craniectomy with stereotactic implantation of neurostimulator electrode array in subcortical site (eg, thalamus, globus pallidus, subthalamic nucleus, periventricular, periaqueductal gray), with use of intraoperative microelectrode recording; first array

♦✿+ **61868** each additional array (List separately in addition to primary procedure)

(Use 61868 in conjunction with 61867)

✿ **61870** Craniectomy for implantation of neurostimulator electrodes, cerebellar; cortical

✿ **61875** subcortical

♦§ **61880** Revision or removal of intracranial neurostimulator electrodes

♦❖▲ **61885** Insertion or replacement of cranial neurostimulator pulse generator or receiver, direct or inductive coupling; with connection to a single electrode array

➔ *CPT Assistant* Sep 03:5; *CPT Changes: An Insider's View* 2000, 2005

§ **61886** with connection to two or more electrode arrays

➔ *CPT Assistant* Sep 03:6; *CPT Changes: An Insider's View* 2000

(For open placement of cranial nerve (eg, vagal, trigeminal) neurostimulator electrode(s), use 64573)

(For percutaneous placement of cranial nerve (eg, vagal, trigeminal) neurostimulator electrode(s), use 64553)

(For revision or removal of cranial nerve (eg, vagal, trigeminal) neurostimulator electrode(s), use 64585)

♦§ **61888** Revision or removal of cranial neurostimulator pulse generator or receiver

►(Do not report 61888 in conjunction with 61885 or 61886 for the same pulse generator)◄

Repair

✿ **62000** Elevation of depressed skull fracture; simple, extradural

✿ **62005** compound or comminuted, extradural

✿ **62010** with repair of dura and/or debridement of brain

✿ **62100** Craniotomy for repair of dural/cerebrospinal fluid leak, including surgery for rhinorrhea/otorrhea

(For repair of spinal dural/CSF leak, see 63707, 63709)

✿ **62115** Reduction of craniomegalic skull (eg, treated hydrocephalus); not requiring bone grafts or cranioplasty

✿ **62116** with simple cranioplasty

✿ **62117** requiring craniotomy and reconstruction with or without bone graft (includes obtaining grafts)

✿ **62120** Repair of encephalocele, skull vault, including cranioplasty

✿ **62121** Craniotomy for repair of encephalocele, skull base

✿ **62140** Cranioplasty for skull defect; up to 5 cm diameter

✿ **62141** larger than 5 cm diameter

✿ **62142** Removal of bone flap or prosthetic plate of skull

✿ **62143** Replacement of bone flap or prosthetic plate of skull

✿ **62145** Cranioplasty for skull defect with reparative brain surgery

✿ **62146** Cranioplasty with autograft (includes obtaining bone grafts); up to 5 cm diameter

✿ **62147** larger than 5 cm diameter

✿+ **62148** Incision and retrieval of subcutaneous cranial bone graft for cranioplasty (List separately in addition to code for primary procedure)

(Use 62148 in conjunction with 62140-62147)

Neuroendoscopy

Surgical endoscopy always includes diagnostic endoscopy.

✿+ **62160** Neuroendoscopy, intracranial, for placement or replacement of ventricular catheter and attachment to shunt system or external drainage (List separately in addition to code for primary procedure)

(Use 62160 only in conjunction with 61107, 61210, 62220, 62223, 62225, or 62230)

✿ **62161** Neuroendoscopy, intracranial; with dissection of adhesions, fenestration of septum pellucidum or intraventricular cysts (including placement, replacement, or removal of ventricular catheter)

✿ **62162** with fenestration or excision of colloid cyst, including placement of external ventricular catheter for drainage

✿ **62163** with retrieval of foreign body

✿ **62164** with excision of brain tumor, including placement of external ventricular catheter for drainage

✿ **62165** with excision of pituitary tumor, transnasal or trans-sphenoidal approach

Cerebrospinal Fluid (CSF) Shunt

✿ **62180** Ventriculocisternostomy (Torkildsen type operation)

✿ **62190** Creation of shunt; subarachnoid/subdural-atrial, -jugular, -auricular

✿ **62192** subarachnoid/subdural-peritoneal, -pleural, other terminus

§ **62194** Replacement or irrigation, subarachnoid/subdural catheter

✿ **62200** Ventriculocisternostomy, third ventricle;

✿ **62201** stereotactic, neuroendoscopic method

(For intracranial neuroendoscopic procedures, see 62161-62165)

✿ **62220** Creation of shunt; ventriculo-atrial, -jugular, -auricular

(For intracranial neuroendoscopic ventricular catheter placement, use 62160)

✿ **62223** ventriculo-peritoneal, -pleural, other terminus

(For intracranial neuroendoscopic ventricular catheter placement, use 62160)

§ **62225** Replacement or irrigation, ventricular catheter

(For intracranial neuroendoscopic ventricular catheter placement, use 62160)

§ **62230** Replacement or revision of cerebrospinal fluid shunt, obstructed valve, or distal catheter in shunt system

➲ *CPT Changes: An Insider's View* 2002

(For intracranial neuroendoscopic ventricular catheter placement, use 62160)

❖ **62252** Reprogramming of programmable cerebrospinal shunt

✿ **62256** Removal of complete cerebrospinal fluid shunt system; without replacement

✿ **62258** with replacement by similar or other shunt at same operation

(For percutaneous irrigation or aspiration of shunt reservoir, use 61070)

(For reprogramming of programmable CSF shunt, use 62252)

Spine and Spinal Cord

(For application of caliper or tongs, use 20660)

(For treatment of fracture or dislocation of spine, see 22305-22327)

Injection, Drainage, or Aspiration

Injection of contrast during fluoroscopic guidance and localization is an inclusive component of codes 62263-62264, 62270-62273, 62280-62282, 62310-62319, 0027T. Fluoroscopic guidance and localization is reported by code 76005, unless a formal contrast study (myelography, epidurography, or arthrography) is performed, in which case the use of fluoroscopy is included in the supervision and interpretation codes.

For radiologic supervision and interpretation of epidurography, use 72275. Code 72275 is only to be used when an epidurogram is performed, images documented, and a formal radiologic report is issued.

Code 62263 describes a catheter-based treatment involving targeted injection of various substances (eg, hypertonic saline, steroid, anesthetic) via an indwelling epidural catheter. Code 62263 includes percutaneous insertion and removal of an epidural catheter (remaining in place over a several-day period), for the administration of multiple injections of a neurolytic agent(s) performed during serial treatment sessions (ie, spanning two or more treatment days). If required, adhesions or scarring may also be lysed by mechanical means. Code 62263 is NOT reported for each adhesiolysis treatment, but should be reported ONCE to describe the entire series of injections/infusions spanning two or more treatment days. For endoscopic lysis of adhesions, use 0027T.

Code 62264 describes multiple adhesiolysis treatment sessions performed on the same day. Adhesions or scarring may be lysed by injections of neurolytic agent(s). If required, adhesions or scarring may also be lysed mechanically using a percutaneously-deployed catheter.

Codes 62263 and 62264 include the procedure of injections of contrast for epidurography (72275) and fluoroscopic guidance and localization (76005) during initial or subsequent sessions.

Surgery: Nervous System

(Report 01996 for daily hospital management of continuous epidural or subarachnoid drug administration performed in conjunction with 62318-62319)

(For endoscopic lysis of epidural adhesions, use Category III code 0027T)

§ **62263** Percutaneous lysis of epidural adhesions using solution injection (eg, hypertonic saline, enzyme) or mechanical means (eg, catheter) including radiologic localization (includes contrast when administered), multiple adhesiolysis sessions; 2 or more days
➔ *CPT Changes: An Insider's View* 2000, 2003

(62263 includes codes 76005 and 72275)

§ **62264** 1 day
➔ *CPT Changes: An Insider's View* 2003

(Do not report 62264 with 62263)

(62264 includes codes 76005 and 72275)

§ **62268** Percutaneous aspiration, spinal cord cyst or syrinx

(For radiological supervision and interpretation, see 76003, 76360, 76942)

§ **62269** Biopsy of spinal cord, percutaneous needle

(For radiological supervision and interpretation, see 76003, 76360, 76942)

(For fine needle aspiration, see 10021, 10022)

(For evaluation of fine needle aspirate, see 88172, 88173)

§ **62270** Spinal puncture, lumbar, diagnostic
➔ *CPT Changes: An Insider's View* 2000, 2002

§ **62272** Spinal puncture, therapeutic, for drainage of cerebrospinal fluid (by needle or catheter)
➔ *CPT Changes: An Insider's View* 2000

§ **62273** Injection, epidural, of blood or clot patch
➔ *CPT Changes: An Insider's View* 2000

(For injection of diagnostic or therapeutic substance(s), see 62310, 62311, 62318, 62319)

§ **62280** Injection/infusion of neurolytic substance (eg, alcohol, phenol, iced saline solutions), with or without other therapeutic substance; subarachnoid
➔ *CPT Changes: An Insider's View* 2000

§ **62281** epidural, cervical or thoracic
➔ *CPT Changes: An Insider's View* 2000

§ **62282** epidural, lumbar, sacral (caudal)
➔ *CPT Changes: An Insider's View* 2000

☆⊘ **62284** Injection procedure for myelography and/or computed tomography, spinal (other than C1-C2 and posterior fossa)
➔ *CPT Changes: An Insider's View* 2003

(For injection procedure at C1-C2, use 61055)

(For radiological supervision and interpretation, see **Radiology**)

§ **62287** Aspiration or decompression procedure, percutaneous, of nucleus pulposus of intervertebral disk, any method, single or multiple levels, lumbar (eg, manual or automated percutaneous diskectomy, percutaneous laser diskectomy)
➔ *CPT Changes: An Insider's View* 2000

(For fluoroscopic guidance, use 76003)

(For injection of non-neurolytic diagnostic or therapeutic substance(s), see 62310, 62311)

☆ **62290** Injection procedure for diskography, each level; lumbar
➔ *CPT Changes: An Insider's View* 2000

☆ **62291** cervical or thoracic
➔ *CPT Changes: An Insider's View* 2000

(For radiological supervision and interpretation, see 72285, 72295)

§ **62292** Injection procedure for chemonucleolysis, including diskography, intervertebral disk, single or multiple levels, lumbar

§ **62294** Injection procedure, arterial, for occlusion of arteriovenous malformation, spinal

§ **62310** Injection, single (not via indwelling catheter), not including neurolytic substances, with or without contrast (for either localization or epidurography), of diagnostic or therapeutic substance(s) (including anesthetic, antispasmodic, opioid, steroid, other solution), epidural or subarachnoid; cervical or thoracic
➔ *CPT Changes: An Insider's View* 2000

§ **62311** lumbar, sacral (caudal)
➔ *CPT Changes: An Insider's View* 2000

§ **62318** Injection, including catheter placement, continuous infusion or intermittent bolus, not including neurolytic substances, with or without contrast (for either localization or epidurography), of diagnostic or therapeutic substance(s) (including anesthetic, antispasmodic, opioid, steroid, other solution), epidural or subarachnoid; cervical or thoracic
➔ *CPT Changes: An Insider's View* 2000

§ **62319** lumbar, sacral (caudal)
➔ *CPT Changes: An Insider's View* 2000

(For transforaminal epidural injection, see 64479-64484)

(Report 01996 for daily hospital management of continuous epidural or subarachnoid drug administration performed in conjunction with 62318-62319)

Catheter Implantation

(For percutaneous placement of intrathecal or epidural catheter, see codes 62270-62273, 62280-62284, 62310-62319)

§ **62350** Implantation, revision or repositioning of tunneled intrathecal or epidural catheter, for long-term medication administration via an external pump or implantable reservoir/infusion pump; without laminectomy
➔ *CPT Changes: An Insider's View* 2000

§ **62351** with laminectomy
➔ *CPT Changes: An Insider's View* 2000

(For refilling and maintenance of an implantable infusion pump for spinal or brain drug therapy, use 95990)

§ **62355** Removal of previously implanted intrathecal or epidural catheter

Reservoir/Pump Implantation

§ **62360** Implantation or replacement of device for intrathecal or epidural drug infusion; subcutaneous reservoir

§ **62361** non-programmable pump

§ **62362** programmable pump, including preparation of pump, with or without programming

§ **62365** Removal of subcutaneous reservoir or pump, previously implanted for intrathecal or epidural infusion

❖ **62367** Electronic analysis of programmable, implanted pump for intrathecal or epidural drug infusion (includes evaluation of reservoir status, alarm status, drug prescription status); without reprogramming

❖ **62368** with reprogramming

(For refilling and maintenance of an implantable infusion pump for spinal or brain drug therapy, use 95990-95991)

Posterior Extradural Laminotomy or Laminectomy for Exploration/ Decompression of Neural Elements or Excision of Herniated Intervertebral Disks

(When 63001-63048 are followed by arthrodesis, see 22590-22614)

§ **63001** Laminectomy with exploration and/or decompression of spinal cord and/or cauda equina, without facetectomy, foraminotomy or diskectomy, (eg, spinal stenosis), one or two vertebral segments; cervical

§ **63003** thoracic

§ **63005** lumbar, except for spondylolisthesis

§ **63011** sacral

§ **63012** Laminectomy with removal of abnormal facets and/or pars inter-articularis with decompression of cauda equina and nerve roots for spondylolisthesis, lumbar (Gill type procedure)

§ **63015** Laminectomy with exploration and/or decompression of spinal cord and/or cauda equina, without facetectomy, foraminotomy or diskectomy, (eg, spinal stenosis), more than 2 vertebral segments; cervical

§ **63016** thoracic

§ **63017** lumbar

♦§ **63020** Laminotomy (hemilaminectomy), with decompression of nerve root(s), including partial facetectomy, foraminotomy and/or excision of herniated intervertebral disk; one interspace, cervical
➔ *CPT Changes: An Insider's View* 2000

(For bilateral procedure, report 63020 with modifier 50)

♦§ **63030** one interspace, lumbar (including open or endoscopically-assisted approach)
➔ *CPT Changes: An Insider's View* 2000

(For bilateral procedure, report 63030 with modifier 50)

♦§+ **63035** each additional interspace, cervical or lumbar (List separately in addition to code for primary procedure)
➔ *CPT Changes: An Insider's View* 2000

(Use 63035 in conjunction with 63020-63030)

(For bilateral procedure, report 63035 with modifier 50)

♦§ **63040** Laminotomy (hemilaminectomy), with decompression of nerve root(s), including partial facetectomy, foraminotomy and/or excision of herniated intervertebral disk, reexploration, single interspace; cervical
➔ *CPT Changes: An Insider's View* 2000

(For bilateral procedure, report 63040 with modifier 50)

♦§ **63042** lumbar

(For bilateral procedure, report 63042 with modifier 50)

♦✿+ **63043** each additional cervical interspace (List separately in addition to code for primary procedure)

(Use 63043 in conjunction with 63040)

(For bilateral procedure, report 63043 with modifier 50)

♦✿+ **63044** each additional lumbar interspace (List separately in addition to code for primary procedure)

(Use 63044 in conjunction with 63042)

(For bilateral procedure, report 63044 with modifier 50)

✶§ **63045** Laminectomy, facetectomy and foraminotomy (unilateral or bilateral with decompression of spinal cord, cauda equina and/or nerve root(s), (eg, spinal or lateral recess stenosis)), single vertebral segment; cervical

✶§ **63046** thoracic

✶§ **63047** lumbar

✶§+ **63048** each additional segment, cervical, thoracic, or lumbar (List separately in addition to code for primary procedure)

(Use 63048 in conjunction with 63045-63047)

Surgery: Nervous System

✿● **63050** Laminoplasty, cervical, with decompression of the spinal cord, two or more vertebral segments;

➲ *CPT Changes: An Insider's View* 2005

✿● **63051** with reconstruction of the posterior bony elements (including the application of bridging bone graft and non-segmental fixation devices (eg, wire, suture, mini-plates), when performed)

➲ *CPT Changes: An Insider's View* 2005

►(Do not report 63050 or 63051 in conjunction with 22600, 22614, 22840-22842, 63001, 63015, 63045, 63048, 63295 for the same vertebral segment(s))◄

Transpedicular or Costovertebral Approach for Posterolateral Extradural Exploration/Decompression

§ **63055** Transpedicular approach with decompression of spinal cord, equina and/or nerve root(s) (eg, herniated intervertebral disk), single segment; thoracic

➲ *CPT Changes: An Insider's View* 2000

§ **63056** lumbar (including transfacet, or lateral extraforaminal approach) (eg, far lateral herniated intervertebral disk)

➲ *CPT Changes: An Insider's View* 2000

§+ **63057** each additional segment, thoracic or lumbar (List separately in addition to code for primary procedure)

➲ *CPT Changes: An Insider's View* 2000

(Use 63057 in conjunction with 63055, 63056)

§ **63064** Costovertebral approach with decompression of spinal cord or nerve root(s), (eg, herniated intervertebral disk), thoracic; single segment

§+ **63066** each additional segment (List separately in addition to code for primary procedure)

(Use 63066 in conjunction with 63064)

(For excision of thoracic intraspinal lesions by laminectomy, see 63266, 63271, 63276, 63281, 63286)

Anterior or Anterolateral Approach for Extradural Exploration/Decompression

For the following codes, when two surgeons work together as primary surgeons performing distinct part(s) of spinal cord exploration/decompression operation, each surgeon should report his/her distinct operative work by appending modifier 62 to the procedure code (and any associated add-on codes for that procedure code as long as both surgeons continue to work together as primary surgeons). In this situation, modifier 62 may be appended to the definitive procedure code(s) 63075, 63077, 63081, 63085, 63087, 63090 and, as appropriate, to associated additional interspace add-on code(s) 63076, 63078 or additional segment add-on code(s) 63082, 63086, 63088, 63091 as long as both surgeons continue to work together as primary surgeons.

✿ **63075** Diskectomy, anterior, with decompression of spinal cord and/or nerve root(s), including osteophytectomy; cervical, single interspace

✿+ **63076** cervical, each additional interspace (List separately in addition to code for primary procedure)

(Use 63076 in conjunction with 63075)

✿ **63077** thoracic, single interspace

✿+ **63078** thoracic, each additional interspace (List separately in addition to code for primary procedure)

(Use 63078 in conjunction with 63077)

(Do not report code 69990 in addition to codes 63075-63078)

✿ **63081** Vertebral corpectomy (vertebral body resection), partial or complete, anterior approach with decompression of spinal cord and/or nerve root(s); cervical, single segment

✿+ **63082** cervical, each additional segment (List separately in addition to code for primary procedure)

(Use 63082 in conjunction with 63081)

(For transoral approach, see 61575, 61576)

✿ **63085** Vertebral corpectomy (vertebral body resection), partial or complete, transthoracic approach with decompression of spinal cord and/or nerve root(s); thoracic, single segment

✿+ **63086** thoracic, each additional segment (List separately in addition to code for primary procedure)

(Use 63086 in conjunction with 63085)

✿ **63087** Vertebral corpectomy (vertebral body resection), partial or complete, combined thoracolumbar approach with decompression of spinal cord, cauda equina or nerve root(s), lower thoracic or lumbar; single segment

✿+ **63088** each additional segment (List separately in addition to code for primary procedure)

(Use 63088 in conjunction with 63087)

✿ **63090** Vertebral corpectomy (vertebral body resection), partial or complete, transperitoneal or retroperitoneal approach with decompression of spinal cord, cauda equina or nerve root(s), lower thoracic, lumbar, or sacral; single segment

✿+ **63091** each additional segment (List separately in addition to code for primary procedure)

(Use 63091 in conjunction with 63090)

(Procedures 63081-63091 include diskectomy above and/or below vertebral segment)

(If followed by arthrodesis, see 22548-22812)

(For reconstruction of spine, use appropriate vertebral corpectomy codes 63081-63091, bone graft codes 20930-20938, arthrodesis codes 22548-22812, and spinal instrumentation codes 22840-22855)

Lateral Extracavitary Approach for Extradural Exploration/Decompression

✿ **63101** Vertebral corpectomy (vertebral body resection), partial or complete, lateral extracavitary approach with decompression of spinal cord and/or nerve root(s) (eg, for tumor or retropulsed bone fragments); thoracic, single segment

✿ **63102** lumbar, single segment

✿+ **63103** thoracic or lumbar, each additional segment (List separately in addition to code for primary procedure)

(Use 63103 in conjunction with 63101 and 63102)

Incision

✿ **63170** Laminectomy with myelotomy (eg, Bischof or DREZ type), cervical, thoracic, or thoracolumbar

✿ **63172** Laminectomy with drainage of intramedullary cyst/syrinx; to subarachnoid space

✿ **63173** to peritoneal or pleural space

✿ **63180** Laminectomy and section of dentate ligaments, with or without dural graft, cervical; one or two segments

✿ **63182** more than two segments

✿ **63185** Laminectomy with rhizotomy; one or two segments

✿ **63190** more than two segments

♦✿ **63191** Laminectomy with section of spinal accessory nerve

(For bilateral procedure, report 63191 with modifier 50)

(For resection of sternocleidomastoid muscle, use 21720)

✿ **63194** Laminectomy with cordotomy, with section of one spinothalamic tract, one stage; cervical

✿ **63195** thoracic

✿ **63196** Laminectomy with cordotomy, with section of both spinothalamic tracts, one stage; cervical

✿ **63197** thoracic

✿ **63198** Laminectomy with cordotomy with section of both spinothalamic tracts, two stages within 14 days; cervical

✿ **63199** thoracic

✿ **63200** Laminectomy, with release of tethered spinal cord, lumbar

Excision by Laminectomy of Lesion Other Than Herniated Disk

✿ **63250** Laminectomy for excision or occlusion of arteriovenous malformation of spinal cord; cervical

✿ **63251** thoracic

✿ **63252** thoracolumbar

✿ **63265** Laminectomy for excision or evacuation of intraspinal lesion other than neoplasm, extradural; cervical

✿ **63266** thoracic

✿ **63267** lumbar

✿ **63268** sacral

✿ **63270** Laminectomy for excision of intraspinal lesion other than neoplasm, intradural; cervical

✿ **63271** thoracic

✿ **63272** lumbar

✿ **63273** sacral

✿ **63275** Laminectomy for biopsy/excision of intraspinal neoplasm; extradural, cervical

✿ **63276** extradural, thoracic

✿ **63277** extradural, lumbar

✿ **63278** extradural, sacral

✿ **63280** intradural, extramedullary, cervical

✿ **63281** intradural, extramedullary, thoracic

✿ **63282** intradural, extramedullary, lumbar

✿ **63283** intradural, sacral

✿ **63285** intradural, intramedullary, cervical

✿ **63286** intradural, intramedullary, thoracic

✿ **63287** intradural, intramedullary, thoracolumbar

✿ **63290** combined extradural-intradural lesion, any level

(For drainage of intramedullary cyst/syrinx, use 63172, 63173)

★✿ +● **63295** Osteoplastic reconstruction of dorsal spinal elements, following primary intraspinal procedure (List separately in addition to code for primary procedure)

➔ *CPT Changes: An Insider's View* 2005

►(Use 63295 in conjunction with 63172, 63173, 63185, 63190, 63200-63290)◄

►(Do not report 63295 in conjunction with 22590-22614, 22840-22844, 63050, 63051 for the same vertebral segment(s))◄

Excision, Anterior or Anterolateral Approach, Intraspinal Lesion

For the following codes, when two surgeons work together as primary surgeons performing distinct part(s) of an anterior approach for an intraspinal excision, each surgeon should report his/her distinct operative work by appending modifier 62 to the single definitive procedure code. In this situation, modifier 62 may be appended to the definitive procedure code(s) 63300-63307 and, as appropriate, to the associated additional segment add-on code 63308 as long as both surgeons continue to work together as primary surgeons.

(For arthrodesis, see 22548-22585)

(For reconstruction of spine, see 20930-20938)

✿ 63300 Vertebral corpectomy (vertebral body resection), partial or complete, for excision of intraspinal lesion, single segment; extradural, cervical

✿ 63301 extradural, thoracic by transthoracic approach

✿ 63302 extradural, thoracic by thoracolumbar approach

✿ 63303 extradural, lumbar or sacral by transperitoneal or retroperitoneal approach

✿ 63304 intradural, cervical

✿ 63305 intradural, thoracic by transthoracic approach

✿ 63306 intradural, thoracic by thoracolumbar approach

✿ 63307 intradural, lumbar or sacral by transperitoneal or retroperitoneal approach

✿+ 63308 each additional segment (List separately in addition to codes for single segment)

(Use 63308 in conjunction with 63300-63307)

Stereotaxis

§ 63600 Creation of lesion of spinal cord by stereotactic method, percutaneous, any modality (including stimulation and/or recording)

§ 63610 Stereotactic stimulation of spinal cord, percutaneous, separate procedure not followed by other surgery

§ 63615 Stereotactic biopsy, aspiration, or excision of lesion, spinal cord

Neurostimulators (Spinal)

Codes 63650-63688 apply to both simple and complex neurostimulators. For initial or subsequent electronic analysis and programming of neurostimulator pulse generators, see codes 95970-95975.

Codes 63650, 63655, and 63660 describe the operative placement, revision, or removal of the spinal neurostimulator system components to provide spinal electrical stimulation. A neurostimulator system includes an implanted neurostimulator, external controller, extension, and collection of contacts. Multiple contacts or electrodes (4 or more) provide the actual electrical stimulation in the epidural space.

For percutaneously placed neurostimulator systems (63650, 63660), the contacts are on a catheter-like lead. An array defines the collection of contacts that are on one catheter.

For systems placed via an open surgical exposure (63655, 63660), the contacts are on a plate or paddle-shaped surface.

❖ 63650 Percutaneous implantation of neurostimulator electrode array, epidural

❖ 63655 Laminectomy for implantation of neurostimulator electrodes, plate/paddle, epidural

§ 63660 Revision or removal of spinal neurostimulator electrode percutaneous array(s) or plate/paddle(s)

§▲ 63685 Insertion or replacement of spinal neurostimulator pulse generator or receiver, direct or inductive coupling

➲ *CPT Changes: An Insider's View* 2005

►(Do not report 63685 in conjunction with 63688 for the same pulse generator or receiver)◄

§ 63688 Revision or removal of implanted spinal neurostimulator pulse generator or receiver

(For electronic analysis of implanted neurostimulator pulse generator system, see 95970-95975)

Repair

✿ 63700 Repair of meningocele; less than 5 cm diameter

✿ 63702 larger than 5 cm diameter

(Do not use modifier 63 in conjunction with 63700, 63702)

✿ 63704 Repair of myelomeningocele; less than 5 cm diameter

✿ 63706 larger than 5 cm diameter

(Do not use modifier 63 in conjunction with 63704, 63706)

(For complex skin closure, see **Integumentary System**)

✿ 63707 Repair of dural/cerebrospinal fluid leak, not requiring laminectomy

✿ 63709 Repair of dural/cerebrospinal fluid leak or pseudomeningocele, with laminectomy

✿ 63710 Dural graft, spinal

(For laminectomy and section of dentate ligaments, with or without dural graft, cervical, see 63180, 63182)

Shunt, Spinal CSF

✿ 63740 Creation of shunt, lumbar, subarachnoid-peritoneal, -pleural, or other; including laminectomy

§ 63741 percutaneous, not requiring laminectomy

§ 63744 Replacement, irrigation or revision of lumbosubarachnoid shunt

§ 63746 Removal of entire lumbosubarachnoid shunt system without replacement

(For insertion of subarachnoid catheter with reservoir and/or pump for intermittent or continuous infusion of drug including laminectomy, see 62351 and 62360, 62361 or 62362)

(For insertion or replacement of subarachnoid or epidural catheter, with reservoir and/or pump for drug infusion without laminectomy, see 62350 and 62360, 62361 or 62362)

Extracranial Nerves, Peripheral Nerves, and Autonomic Nervous System

(For intracranial surgery on cranial nerves, see 61450, 61460, 61790)

Introduction/Injection of Anesthetic Agent (Nerve Block), Diagnostic or Therapeutic

Somatic Nerves

§ **64400** Injection, anesthetic agent; trigeminal nerve, any division or branch
➲ *CPT Changes: An Insider's View* 2000

§ **64402** facial nerve

§ **64405** greater occipital nerve

§ **64408** vagus nerve

§ **64410** phrenic nerve

§ **64412** spinal accessory nerve

§ **64413** cervical plexus

§ **64415** brachial plexus, single
➲ *CPT Changes: An Insider's View* 2003

§ **64416** brachial plexus, continuous infusion by catheter (including catheter placement) including daily management for anesthetic agent administration
➲ *CPT Changes: An Insider's View* 2003

(Do not report 01996 in addition to 64416)

§ **64417** axillary nerve

§ **64418** suprascapular nerve

§ **64420** intercostal nerve, single

§ **64421** intercostal nerves, multiple, regional block

§ **64425** ilioinguinal, iliohypogastric nerves

§ **64430** pudendal nerve

§ **64435** paracervical (uterine) nerve

§ **64445** sciatic nerve, single
➲ *CPT Changes: An Insider's View* 2003

§ **64446** sciatic nerve, continuous infusion by catheter, (including catheter placement) including daily management for anesthetic agent administration
➲ *CPT Changes: An Insider's View* 2003

(Do not report 01996 in addition to 64446)

§ **64447** femoral nerve, single
➲ *CPT Changes: An Insider's View* 2003

(Do not report 01996 in addition to 64447)

§ **64448** femoral nerve, continuous infusion by catheter (including catheter placement) including daily management for anesthetic agent administration
➲ *CPT Changes: An Insider's View* 2003

(Do not report 01996 in addition to 64448)

§ **64449** lumbar plexus, posterior approach, continuous infusion by catheter (including catheter placement) including daily management for anesthetic agent administration
➲ *CPT Changes: An Insider's View* 2004

(Do not report 01996 in conjunction with 64449)

§ **64450** other peripheral nerve or branch
➲ *CPT Changes: An Insider's View* 2000

(For phenol destruction, see 64622-64627)

(For subarachnoid or subdural injection, see 62280, 62310-62319)

(For epidural or caudal injection, see 62273, 62281-62282, 62310-62319)

(Codes 64470-64484 are unilateral procedures. For bilateral procedures, use modifier 50)

(For fluoroscopic guidance and localization for needle placement and injection in conjunction with 64470-64484, use code 76005)

♦§ **64470** Injection, anesthetic agent and/or steroid, paravertebral facet joint or facet joint nerve; cervical or thoracic, single level
➲ *CPT Changes: An Insider's View* 2000

♦§+ **64472** cervical or thoracic, each additional level (List separately in addition to code for primary procedure)
➲ *CPT Changes: An Insider's View* 2000

(Use 64472 in conjunction with 64470)

♦§ **64475** lumbar or sacral, single level
➲ *CPT Changes: An Insider's View* 2000

♦§+ **64476** lumbar or sacral, each additional level (List separately in addition to code for primary procedure)
➲ *CPT Changes: An Insider's View* 2000

(Use 64476 in conjunction with 64475)

♦§ **64479** Injection, anesthetic agent and/or steroid, transforaminal epidural; cervical or thoracic, single level
➲ *CPT Changes: An Insider's View* 2000

♦§+ **64480** cervical or thoracic, each additional level (List separately in addition to code for primary procedure)
➲ *CPT Changes: An Insider's View* 2000

(Use 64480 in conjunction with 64479)

♦§ **64483** lumbar or sacral, single level
➲ *CPT Changes: An Insider's View* 2000

♦§+ **64484** lumbar or sacral, each additional level (List separately in addition to code for primary procedure)
➲ *CPT Changes: An Insider's View* 2000

(Use 64484 in conjunction with 64483)

Sympathetic Nerves

§ **64505** Injection, anesthetic agent; sphenopalatine ganglion

§ **64508** carotid sinus (separate procedure)

§ **64510** stellate ganglion (cervical sympathetic)

§ **64517** superior hypogastric plexus
➲ *CPT Changes: An Insider's View* 2004

§ **64520** lumbar or thoracic (paravertebral sympathetic)

§ **64530** celiac plexus, with or without radiologic monitoring

Neurostimulators (Peripheral Nerve)

Codes 64553-64595 apply to both simple and complex neurostimulators. For initial or subsequent electronic analysis and programming of neurostimulator pulse generators, see codes 95970-95975.

♠ **64550** Application of surface (transcutaneous) neurostimulator

❖ **64553** Percutaneous implantation of neurostimulator electrodes; cranial nerve
➲ *CPT Changes: An Insider's View* 2000

(For open placement of cranial nerve (eg, vagal, trigeminal) neurostimulator pulse generator or receiver, see 61885, 61886, as appropriate)

❖ **64555** peripheral nerve (excludes sacral nerve)
➲ *CPT Changes: An Insider's View* 2002

❖ **64560** autonomic nerve

❖ **64561** sacral nerve (transforaminal placement)
➲ *CPT Changes: An Insider's View* 2002

❖ **64565** neuromuscular

❖ **64573** Incision for implantation of neurostimulator electrodes; cranial nerve
➲ *CPT Changes: An Insider's View* 2000

(For opcn placement of cranial nerve (eg, vagal, trigeminal) neurostimulator pulse generator or receiver, see 61885, 61886, as appropriate)

(For revision or removal of cranial nerve (eg, vagal, trigeminal) neurostimulator pulse generator or receiver, use 61888)

❖ **64575** peripheral nerve (excludes sacral nerve)
➲ *CPT Changes: An Insider's View* 2002

❖ **64577** autonomic nerve

❖ **64580** neuromuscular

❖ **64581** sacral nerve (transforaminal placement)
➲ *CPT Changes: An Insider's View* 2002

§ **64585** Revision or removal of peripheral neurostimulator electrodes

§▲ **64590** Insertion or replacement of peripheral neurostimulator pulse generator or receiver, direct or inductive coupling
➲ *CPT Changes: An Insider's View* 2002, 2005

►(Do not report 64590 in conjunction with 64595)◄

§ **64595** Revision or removal of peripheral neurostimulator pulse generator or receiver

Destruction by Neurolytic Agent (eg, Chemical, Thermal, Electrical or Radiofrequency)

(Codes 64600-64681 include the injection of other therapeutic agents (eg, corticosteroids).

Somatic Nerves

✶§ **64600** Destruction by neurolytic agent, trigeminal nerve; supraorbital, infraorbital, mental, or inferior alveolar branch

§ **64605** second and third division branches at foramen ovale

§ **64610** second and third division branches at foramen ovale under radiologic monitoring

♦§ **64612** Chemodenervation of muscle(s); muscle(s) innervated by facial nerve (eg, for blepharospasm, hemifacial spasm)
➲ *CPT Changes: An Insider's View* 2000, 2001

§ **64613** cervical spinal muscle(s) (eg, for spasmodic torticollis)
➲ *CPT Changes: An Insider's View* 2001

♦§ **64614** extremity(s) and/or trunk muscle(s) (eg, for dystonia, cerebral palsy, multiple sclerosis)
➲ *CPT Changes: An Insider's View* 2001

(For chemodenervation for strabismus involving the extraocular muscles, use 67345)

§ **64620** Destruction by neurolytic agent, intercostal nerve
➲ *CPT Changes: An Insider's View* 2000

(For fluoroscopic guidance and localization for needle placement and neurolysis in conjunction with 64622-64627, use 76005)

♦§ **64622** Destruction by neurolytic agent, paravertebral facet joint nerve; lumbar or sacral, single level
➲ *CPT Changes: An Insider's View* 2000

(For bilateral procedure, report 64622 with modifier 50)

♦§+ **64623** lumbar or sacral, each additional level (List separately in addition to code for primary procedure)
➲ *CPT Changes: An Insider's View* 2000

(Use 64623 in conjunction with 64622)

(For bilateral procedure, report 64623 with modifier 50)

♦§ **64626** cervical or thoracic, single level
➔ *CPT Changes: An Insider's View* 2000

(For bilateral procedure, report 64626 with modifier 50)

♦§+ **64627** cervical or thoracic, each additional level (List separately in addition to code for primary procedure)
➔ *CPT Changes: An Insider's View* 2000

(Use 64627 in conjunction with 64626)

(For bilateral procedure, report 64627 with modifier 50)

§ **64630** Destruction by neurolytic agent; pudendal nerve
➔ *CPT Changes: An Insider's View* 2001

§ **64640** other peripheral nerve or branch

Sympathetic Nerves

§ **64680** Destruction by neurolytic agent, with or without radiologic monitoring; celiac plexus
➔ *CPT Changes: An Insider's View* 2004

§ **64681** superior hypogastric plexus
➔ *CPT Changes: An Insider's View* 2004

Neuroplasty (Exploration, Neurolysis or Nerve Decompression)

Neuroplasty is the decompression or freeing of intact nerve from scar tissue, including external neurolysis and/or transposition.

(For internal neurolysis requiring use of operating microscope, use 64727)

(For facial nerve decompression, use 69720)

§ **64702** Neuroplasty; digital, one or both, same digit

§ **64704** nerve of hand or foot

§ **64708** Neuroplasty, major peripheral nerve, arm or leg; other than specified

§ **64712** sciatic nerve

§ **64713** brachial plexus

§ **64714** lumbar plexus

§ **64716** Neuroplasty and/or transposition; cranial nerve (specify)

§ **64718** ulnar nerve at elbow

§ **64719** ulnar nerve at wrist

♦§ **64721** median nerve at carpal tunnel

(For arthroscopic procedure, use 29848)

§ **64722** Decompression; unspecified nerve(s) (specify)

§ **64726** plantar digital nerve

§+ **64727** Internal neurolysis, requiring use of operating microscope (List separately in addition to code for neuroplasty) (Neuroplasty includes external neurolysis)

(Do not report code 69990 in addition to code 64727)

Transection or Avulsion

(For stereotactic lesion of gasserian ganglion, use 61790)

§ **64732** Transection or avulsion of; supraorbital nerve

§ **64734** infraorbital nerve

§ **64736** mental nerve

§ **64738** inferior alveolar nerve by osteotomy

§ **64740** lingual nerve

§ **64742** facial nerve, differential or complete

♦§ **64744** greater occipital nerve

§ **64746** phrenic nerve

(For section of recurrent laryngeal nerve, use 31595)

✿ **64752** vagus nerve (vagotomy), transthoracic

✿ **64755** vagus nerves limited to proximal stomach (selective proximal vagotomy, proximal gastric vagotomy, parietal cell vagotomy, supra- or highly selective vagotomy)

(For laparoscopic approach, use 43652)

✿ **64760** vagus nerve (vagotomy), abdominal

(For laparoscopic approach, use 43651)

♦§ **64761** pudendal nerve

(For bilateral procedure, report 64761 with modifier 50)

♦✿ **64763** Transection or avulsion of obturator nerve, extrapelvic, with or without adductor tenotomy

(For bilateral procedure, report 64763 with modifier 50)

♦✿ **64766** Transection or avulsion of obturator nerve, intrapelvic, with or without adductor tenotomy

(For bilateral procedure, report 64766 with modifier 50)

§ **64771** Transection or avulsion of other cranial nerve, extradural

§ **64772** Transection or avulsion of other spinal nerve, extradural

(For excision of tender scar, skin and subcutaneous tissue, with or without tiny neuroma, see 11400-11446, 13100-13153)

Excision

Somatic Nerves

(For Morton neurectomy, use 28080)

§ **64774** Excision of neuroma; cutaneous nerve, surgically identifiable

§ **64776** digital nerve, one or both, same digit

§+ **64778** digital nerve, each additional digit (List separately in addition to code for primary procedure)

(Use 64778 in conjunction with 64776)

§ **64782** hand or foot, except digital nerve

§+ 64783 hand or foot, each additional nerve, except same digit (List separately in addition to code for primary procedure)

(Use 64783 in conjunction with 64782)

§ 64784 major peripheral nerve, except sciatic

§ 64786 sciatic nerve

§+ 64787 Implantation of nerve end into bone or muscle (List separately in addition to neuroma excision)

(Use 64787 in conjunction with 64774-64786)

§ 64788 Excision of neurofibroma or neurolemmoma; cutaneous nerve

§ 64790 major peripheral nerve

§ 64792 extensive (including malignant type)

§ 64795 Biopsy of nerve

Sympathetic Nerves

♦§ 64802 Sympathectomy, cervical

(For bilateral procedure, report 64802 with modifier 50)

♦✿ 64804 Sympathectomy, cervicothoracic

(For bilateral procedure, report 64804 with modifier 50)

♦✿ 64809 Sympathectomy, thoracolumbar

(For bilateral procedure, report 64809 with modifier 50)

♦✿ 64818 Sympathectomy, lumbar

(For bilateral procedure, report 64818 with modifier 50)

§ 64820 Sympathectomy; digital arteries, each digit
➲ *CPT Assistant* Jan 03:16; *CPT Changes: An Insider's View* 2002

(Do not report 69990 in addition to code 64820)

♦§ 64821 radial artery
➲ *CPT Changes: An Insider's View* 2002

(Do not report 69990 in addition to code 64821)

♦§ 64822 ulnar artery
➲ *CPT Changes: An Insider's View* 2002

(Do not report 69990 in addition to code 64822)

♦§ 64823 superficial palmar arch
➲ *CPT Changes: An Insider's View* 2002

(Do not report 69990 in addition to code 64823)

Neurorrhaphy

§ 64831 Suture of digital nerve, hand or foot; one nerve

§+ 64832 each additional digital nerve (List separately in addition to code for primary procedure)

(Use 64832 in conjunction with 64831)

§ 64834 Suture of one nerve, hand or foot; common sensory nerve

§ 64835 median motor thenar

§ 64836 ulnar motor

§+ 64837 Suture of each additional nerve, hand or foot (List separately in addition to code for primary procedure)

(Use 64837 in conjunction with 64834-64836)

§ 64840 Suture of posterior tibial nerve

§ 64856 Suture of major peripheral nerve, arm or leg, except sciatic; including transposition

§ 64857 without transposition

§ 64858 Suture of sciatic nerve

§+ 64859 Suture of each additional major peripheral nerve (List separately in addition to code for primary procedure)

(Use 64859 in conjunction with 64856, 64857)

§ 64861 Suture of; brachial plexus

§ 64862 lumbar plexus

§ 64864 Suture of facial nerve; extracranial

§ 64865 infratemporal, with or without grafting

✿ 64866 Anastomosis; facial-spinal accessory

✿ 64868 facial-hypoglossal

§ 64870 facial-phrenic

§+ 64872 Suture of nerve; requiring secondary or delayed suture (List separately in addition to code for primary neurorrhaphy)

(Use 64872 in conjunction with 64831-64865)

§+ 64874 requiring extensive mobilization, or transposition of nerve (List separately in addition to code for nerve suture)

(Use 64874 in conjunction with 64831-64865)

§+ 64876 requiring shortening of bone of extremity (List separately in addition to code for nerve suture)

(Use 64876 in conjunction with 64831-64865)

Neurorrhaphy With Nerve Graft

§ 64885 Nerve graft (includes obtaining graft), head or neck; up to 4 cm in length

§ 64886 more than 4 cm length

§ 64890 Nerve graft (includes obtaining graft), single strand, hand or foot; up to 4 cm length

§ 64891 more than 4 cm length

§ 64892 Nerve graft (includes obtaining graft), single strand, arm or leg; up to 4 cm length

§ 64893 more than 4 cm length

§ **64895** Nerve graft (includes obtaining graft), multiple strands (cable), hand or foot; up to 4 cm length

§ **64896** more than 4 cm length

§ **64897** Nerve graft (includes obtaining graft), multiple strands (cable), arm or leg; up to 4 cm length

§ **64898** more than 4 cm length

§+ **64901** Nerve graft, each additional nerve; single strand (List separately in addition to code for primary procedure)

(Use 64901 in conjunction with 64885-64893)

§+ **64902** multiple strands (cable) (List separately in addition to code for primary procedure)

(Use 64902 in conjunction with 64885, 64886, 64895-64898)

§ **64905** Nerve pedicle transfer; first stage

§ **64907** second stage

Other Procedures

§ **64999** Unlisted procedure, nervous system

Notes

Eye and Ocular Adnexa

(For diagnostic and treatment ophthalmological services, see **Medicine, Ophthalmology,** and 92002 et seq)

(Do not report code 69990 in addition to codes 65091-68850)

Eyeball

Removal of Eye

♦§ **65091** Evisceration of ocular contents; without implant

♦§ **65093** with implant

♦§ **65101** Enucleation of eye; without implant

♦§ **65103** with implant, muscles not attached to implant

♦§ **65105** with implant, muscles attached to implant

(For conjunctivoplasty after enucleation, see 68320 et seq)

♦§ **65110** Exenteration of orbit (does not include skin graft), removal of orbital contents; only

♦§ **65112** with therapeutic removal of bone

♦§ **65114** with muscle or myocutaneous flap

(For skin graft to orbit (split skin), see 15120, 15121; free, full thickness, see 15260, 15261)

(For eyelid repair involving more than skin, see 67930 et seq)

Secondary Implant(s) Procedures

An ocular implant is an implant inside muscular cone; an orbital implant is an implant outside muscular cone.

♦§ **65125** Modification of ocular implant with placement or replacement of pegs (eg, drilling receptacle for prosthesis appendage) (separate procedure)

♦§ **65130** Insertion of ocular implant secondary; after evisceration, in scleral shell

♦§ **65135** after enucleation, muscles not attached to implant

♦§ **65140** after enucleation, muscles attached to implant

♦§ **65150** Reinsertion of ocular implant; with or without conjunctival graft

♦§ **65155** with use of foreign material for reinforcement and/or attachment of muscles to implant

♦§ **65175** Removal of ocular implant

(For orbital implant (implant outside muscle cone) insertion, use 67550; removal, use 67560)

Removal of Foreign Body

(For removal of implanted material: ocular implant, use 65175; anterior segment implant, use 65920; posterior segment implant, use 67120; orbital implant, use 67560)

(For diagnostic x-ray for foreign body, use 70030)

(For diagnostic echography for foreign body, use 76529)

(For removal of foreign body from orbit: frontal approach, use 67413; lateral approach, use 67430; transcranial approach, use 61334)

(For removal of foreign body from eyelid, embedded, use 67938)

(For removal of foreign body from lacrimal system, use 68530)

♦❖ **65205** Removal of foreign body, external eye; conjunctival superficial

♦❖ **65210** conjunctival embedded (includes concretions), subconjunctival, or scleral nonperforating

♦❖ **65220** corneal, without slit lamp

♦❖ **65222** corneal, with slit lamp

(For repair of corneal laceration with foreign body, use 65275)

♦§ **65235** Removal of foreign body, intraocular; from anterior chamber of eye or lens

➔ *CPT Changes: An Insider's View* 2002

(For removal of implanted material from anterior segment, use 65920)

♦§ **65260** from posterior segment, magnetic extraction, anterior or posterior route

♦§ **65265** from posterior segment, nonmagnetic extraction

(For removal of implanted material from posterior segment, use 67120)

Repair of Laceration

(For fracture of orbit, see 21385 et seq)

(For repair of wound of eyelid, skin, linear, simple, see 12011-12018; intermediate, layered closure, see 12051-12057; linear, complex, see 13150-13160; other, see 67930, 67935)

(For repair of wound of lacrimal system, use 68700)

(For repair of operative wound, use 66250)

♦§ **65270** Repair of laceration; conjunctiva, with or without nonperforating laceration sclera, direct closure

♦§ **65272** conjunctiva, by mobilization and rearrangement, without hospitalization

♦✿ **65273** conjunctiva, by mobilization and rearrangement, with hospitalization

♦§ **65275** cornea, nonperforating, with or without removal foreign body

♦§ 65280 cornea and/or sclera, perforating, not involving uveal tissue

♦§ 65285 cornea and/or sclera, perforating, with reposition or resection of uveal tissue

♦§ 65286 application of tissue glue, wounds of cornea and/or sclera

(Repair of laceration includes use of conjunctival flap and restoration of anterior chamber, by air or saline injection when indicated)

(For repair of iris or ciliary body, use 66680)

♦§ 65290 Repair of wound, extraocular muscle, tendon and/or Tenon's capsule

Anterior Segment

Cornea

Excision

♦§ 65400 Excision of lesion, cornea (keratectomy, lamellar, partial), except pterygium

♦§ 65410 Biopsy of cornea

♦§ 65420 Excision or transposition of pterygium; without graft

♦§ 65426 with graft

Removal or Destruction

♦❖ 65430 Scraping of cornea, diagnostic, for smear and/or culture

♦§ 65435 Removal of corneal epithelium; with or without chemocauterization (abrasion, curettage)

♦§ 65436 with application of chelating agent (eg, EDTA)

♦❖ 65450 Destruction of lesion of cornea by cryotherapy, photocoagulation or thermocauterization

♦§ 65600 Multiple punctures of anterior cornea (eg, for corneal erosion, tattoo)

Keratoplasty

Corneal transplant includes use of fresh or preserved grafts, and preparation of donor material.

(Keratoplasty excludes refractive keratoplasty procedures, 65760, 65765, and 65767)

♦§ 65710 Keratoplasty (corneal transplant); lamellar

♦§ 65730 penetrating (except in aphakia)

♦§ 65750 penetrating (in aphakia)

♦§ 65755 penetrating (in pseudophakia)

Other Procedures

☐ 65760 Keratomileusis

☐ 65765 Keratophakia

☐ 65767 Epikeratoplasty

♦§ 65770 Keratoprosthesis

☐ 65771 Radial keratotomy

♦§ 65772 Corneal relaxing incision for correction of surgically induced astigmatism

♦§ 65775 Corneal wedge resection for correction of surgically induced astigmatism

(For fitting of contact lens for treatment of disease, use 92070)

(For unlisted procedures on cornea, use 66999)

♦§ 65780 Ocular surface reconstruction; amniotic membrane transplantation

➔ *CPT Changes: An Insider's View* 2004

♦§ 65781 limbal stem cell allograft (eg, cadaveric or living donor)

➔ *CPT Changes: An Insider's View* 2004

♦§ 65782 limbal conjunctival autograft (includes obtaining graft)

➔ *CPT Changes: An Insider's View* 2004

(For harvesting conjunctival allograft, living donor, use 68371)

Anterior Chamber

Incision

♦§ 65800 Paracentesis of anterior chamber of eye (separate procedure); with diagnostic aspiration of aqueous

♦§ 65805 with therapeutic release of aqueous

♦§ 65810 with removal of vitreous and/or discission of anterior hyaloid membrane, with or without air injection

♦§ 65815 with removal of blood, with or without irrigation and/or air injection

(For injection, see 66020-66030)

(For removal of blood clot, use 65930)

♦§ 65820 Goniotomy

(Do not report modifier 63 in conjunction with 65820)

♦§ 65850 Trabeculotomy ab externo

♦§ 65855 Trabeculoplasty by laser surgery, one or more sessions (defined treatment series)

(If re-treatment is necessary after several months because of disease progression, a new treatment or treatment series should be reported with a modifier, if necessary, to indicate lesser or greater complexity)

(For trabeculectomy, use 66170)

♦§ 65860 Severing adhesions of anterior segment, laser technique (separate procedure)

Other Procedures

♦§ 65865 Severing adhesions of anterior segment of eye, incisional technique (with or without injection of air or liquid) (separate procedure); goniosynechiae

(For trabeculoplasty by laser surgery, use 65855)

♦§ 65870 anterior synechiae, except goniosynechiae

♦§ 65875 posterior synechiae

♦§ 65880 corneovitreal adhesions

(For laser surgery, use 66821)

♦§ 65900 Removal of epithelial downgrowth, anterior chamber of eye
➲ *CPT Changes: An Insider's View* 2002

♦§ 65920 Removal of implanted material, anterior segment of eye
➲ *CPT Changes: An Insider's View* 2002

♦§ 65930 Removal of blood clot, anterior segment of eye
➲ *CPT Changes: An Insider's View* 2002

♦§ 66020 Injection, anterior chamber of eye (separate procedure); air or liquid
➲ *CPT Changes: An Insider's View* 2002

♦§ 66030 medication

(For unlisted procedures on anterior segment, use 66999)

Anterior Sclera

Excision

(For removal of intraocular foreign body, use 65235)

(For operations on posterior sclera, use 67250, 67255)

♦§ 66130 Excision of lesion, sclera

♦§ 66150 Fistulization of sclera for glaucoma; trephination with iridectomy

♦§ 66155 thermocauterization with iridectomy

♦§ 66160 sclerectomy with punch or scissors, with iridectomy

♦§ 66165 iridencleisis or iridotasis

♦§ 66170 trabeculectomy ab externo in absence of previous surgery

(For trabeculotomy ab externo, use 65850)

(For repair of operative wound, use 66250)

♦§ 66172 trabeculectomy ab externo with scarring from previous ocular surgery or trauma (includes injection of antifibrotic agents)

♦§ 66180 Aqueous shunt to extraocular reservoir (eg, Molteno, Schocket, Denver-Krupin)

♦§ 66185 Revision of aqueous shunt to extraocular reservoir

(For removal of implanted shunt, use 67120)

Repair or Revision

(For scleral procedures in retinal surgery, see 67101 et seq)

♦§ 66220 Repair of scleral staphyloma; without graft

♦§ 66225 with graft

(For scleral reinforcement, see 67250, 67255)

♦§ 66250 Revision or repair of operative wound of anterior segment, any type, early or late, major or minor procedure

(For unlisted procedures on anterior sclera, use 66999)

Iris, Ciliary Body

Incision

♦§ 66500 Iridotomy by stab incision (separate procedure); except transfixion

♦§ 66505 with transfixion as for iris bombe

(For iridotomy by photocoagulation, use 66761)

Excision

♦§ 66600 Iridectomy, with corneoscleral or corneal section; for removal of lesion

♦§ 66605 with cyclectomy

♦§ 66625 peripheral for glaucoma (separate procedure)

♦§ 66630 sector for glaucoma (separate procedure)

♦§ 66635 optical (separate procedure)

(For coreoplasty by photocoagulation, use 66762)

Repair

♦§ **66680** Repair of iris, ciliary body (as for iridodialysis)

(For reposition or resection of uveal tissue with perforating wound of cornea or sclera, use 65285)

♦§ **66682** Suture of iris, ciliary body (separate procedure) with retrieval of suture through small incision (eg, McCannel suture)

Destruction

♦§ **66700** Ciliary body destruction; diathermy

♦§▲ **66710** cyclophotocoagulation, transscleral
➲ *CPT Changes: An Insider's View* 2005

♦§● **66711** cyclophotocoagulation, endoscopic
➲ *CPT Changes: An Insider's View* 2005

►(Do not report 66711 in conjunction with 66990)◄

♦§⊙ **66720** cryotherapy

♦§ **66740** cyclodialysis

♦§ **66761** Iridotomy/iridectomy by laser surgery (eg, for glaucoma) (one or more sessions)

♦§ **66762** Iridoplasty by photocoagulation (one or more sessions) (eg, for improvement of vision, for widening of anterior chamber angle)

♦§ **66770** Destruction of cyst or lesion iris or ciliary body (nonexcisional procedure)

(For excision lesion iris, ciliary body, see 66600, 66605; for removal of epithelial downgrowth, use 65900)

(For unlisted procedures on iris, ciliary body, use 66999)

Lens

Incision

♦§ **66820** Discission of secondary membranous cataract (opacified posterior lens capsule and/or anterior hyaloid); stab incision technique (Ziegler or Wheeler knife)

♦§ **66821** laser surgery (eg, YAG laser) (one or more stages)

♦§ **66825** Repositioning of intraocular lens prosthesis, requiring an incision (separate procedure)

Removal Cataract

Lateral canthotomy, iridectomy, iridotomy, anterior capsulotomy, posterior capsulotomy, the use of viscoelastic agents, enzymatic zonulysis, use of other pharmacologic agents, and subconjunctival or sub-tenon injections are included as part of the code for the extraction of lens.

♦§ **66830** Removal of secondary membranous cataract (opacified posterior lens capsule and/or anterior hyaloid) with corneo-scleral section, with or without iridectomy (iridocapsulotomy, iridocapsulectomy)

♦§ **66840** Removal of lens material; aspiration technique, one or more stages

♦§ **66850** phacofragmentation technique (mechanical or ultrasonic) (eg, phacoemulsification), with aspiration

♦§ **66852** pars plana approach, with or without vitrectomy

♦§ **66920** intracapsular

♦§ **66930** intracapsular, for dislocated lens

♦§ **66940** extracapsular (other than 66840, 66850, 66852)

(For removal of intralenticular foreign body without lens extraction, use 65235)

(For repair of operative wound, use 66250)

♦§ **66982** Extracapsular cataract removal with insertion of intraocular lens prosthesis (one stage procedure), manual or mechanical technique (eg, irrigation and aspiration or phacoemulsification), complex, requiring devices or techniques not generally used in routine cataract surgery (eg, iris expansion device, suture support for intraocular lens, or primary posterior capsulorrhexis) or performed on patients in the amblyogenic developmental stage
➲ *CPT Changes: An Insider's View* 2001, 2002

♦§ **66983** Intracapsular cataract extraction with insertion of intraocular lens prosthesis (one stage procedure)

♦§ **66984** Extracapsular cataract removal with insertion of intraocular lens prosthesis (one stage procedure), manual or mechanical technique (eg, irrigation and aspiration or phacoemulsification)

(For complex extracapsular cataract removal, use 66982)

♦§ **66985** Insertion of intraocular lens prosthesis (secondary implant), not associated with concurrent cataract removal

(To code implant at time of concurrent cataract surgery, see 66982, 66983, 66984)

(For intraocular lens prosthesis supplied by physician, use 99070)

(For ultrasonic determination of intraocular lens power, use 76519)

(For removal of implanted material from anterior segment, use 65920)

(For secondary fixation (separate procedure), use 66682)

♦§ **66986** Exchange of intraocular lens

♦☆+ **66990** Use of ophthalmic endoscope (List separately in addition to code for primary procedure)
➲ *CPT Changes: An Insider's View* 2003

(66990 may be used only with codes 65820, 65875, 65920, 66985, 66986, 67038, 67039, 67040)

Other Procedures

§ **66999** Unlisted procedure, anterior segment of eye

Posterior Segment

Vitreous

♦§ **67005** Removal of vitreous, anterior approach (open sky technique or limbal incision); partial removal

♦§ **67010** subtotal removal with mechanical vitrectomy

(For removal of vitreous by paracentesis of anterior chamber, use 65810)

(For removal of corneovitreal adhesions, use 65880)

♦§ **67015** Aspiration or release of vitreous, subretinal or choroidal fluid, pars plana approach (posterior sclerotomy)

♦§ **67025** Injection of vitreous substitute, pars plana or limbal approach, (fluid-gas exchange), with or without aspiration (separate procedure)

♦§ **67027** Implantation of intravitreal drug delivery system (eg, ganciclovir implant), includes concomitant removal of vitreous

(For removal, use 67121)

♦§ **67028** Intravitreal injection of a pharmacologic agent (separate procedure)

♦§ **67030** Discission of vitreous strands (without removal), pars plana approach

♦§ **67031** Severing of vitreous strands, vitreous face adhesions, sheets, membranes or opacities, laser surgery (one or more stages)

♦§ **67036** Vitrectomy, mechanical, pars plana approach;

♦§ **67038** with epiretinal membrane stripping

♦§ **67039** with focal endolaser photocoagulation

♦§ **67040** with endolaser panretinal photocoagulation

(For use of ophthalmic endoscope with 67038, 67039, 67040, use 66990)

(For associated lensectomy, use 66850)

(For use of vitrectomy in retinal detachment surgery, use 67108)

(For associated removal of foreign body, see 65260, 65265)

(For unlisted procedures on vitreous, use 67299)

Retina or Choroid

Repair

(If diathermy, cryotherapy and/or photocoagulation are combined, report under principal modality used)

♦§ **67101** Repair of retinal detachment, one or more sessions; cryotherapy or diathermy, with or without drainage of subretinal fluid

♦§ **67105** photocoagulation, with or without drainage of subretinal fluid

♦§ **67107** Repair of retinal detachment; scleral buckling (such as lamellar scleral dissection, imbrication or encircling procedure), with or without implant, with or without cryotherapy, photocoagulation, and drainage of subretinal fluid

♦§ **67108** with vitrectomy, any method, with or without air or gas tamponade, focal endolaser photocoagulation, cryotherapy, drainage of subretinal fluid, scleral buckling, and/or removal of lens by same technique

♦§ **67110** by injection of air or other gas (eg, pneumatic retinopexy)

♦§ **67112** by scleral buckling or vitrectomy, on patient having previous ipsilateral retinal detachment repair(s) using scleral buckling or vitrectomy techniques

(For aspiration or drainage of subretinal or subchoroidal fluid, use 67015)

♦§ **67115** Release of encircling material (posterior segment)

♦§ **67120** Removal of implanted material, posterior segment; extraocular

♦§ **67121** intraocular

(For removal from anterior segment, use 65920)

(For removal of foreign body, see 65260, 65265)

Prophylaxis

Repetitive services. The services listed below are often performed in multiple sessions or groups of sessions. The methods of reporting vary.

The following descriptors are intended to include all sessions in a defined treatment period.

♦§ **67141** Prophylaxis of retinal detachment (eg, retinal break, lattice degeneration) without drainage, one or more sessions; cryotherapy, diathermy

♦§ **67145** photocoagulation (laser or xenon arc)

Destruction

♦§ **67208** Destruction of localized lesion of retina (eg, macular edema, tumors), one or more sessions; cryotherapy, diathermy

♦§ **67210** photocoagulation

♦§ **67218** radiation by implantation of source (includes removal of source)

♦§ **67220** Destruction of localized lesion of choroid (eg, choroidal neovascularization); photocoagulation (eg, laser), one or more sessions

(For destruction of macular drusen, photocoagulation, use Category III code 0017T)

(For destruction of localized lesion of choroid by transpupillary thermotherapy, use Category III code 0016T)

§ **67221** photodynamic therapy (includes intravenous infusion)
➔ *CPT Changes: An Insider's View* 2001

§+ **67225** photodynamic therapy, second eye, at single session (List separately in addition to code for primary eye treatment)
➔ *CPT Changes: An Insider's View* 2002

(Use 67225 in conjunction with 67221)

♦§ **67227** Destruction of extensive or progressive retinopathy (eg, diabetic retinopathy), one or more sessions; cryotherapy, diathermy

♦§ **67228** photocoagulation (laser or xenon arc)

(For unlisted procedures on retina, use 67299)

Sclera

Repair

(For excision lesion sclera, use 66130)

♦§ **67250** Scleral reinforcement (separate procedure); without graft

♦§ **67255** with graft

(For repair scleral staphyloma, see 66220, 66225)

Other Procedures

§ **67299** Unlisted procedure, posterior segment

Ocular Adnexa

Extraocular Muscles

♦§ **67311** Strabismus surgery, recession or resection procedure; one horizontal muscle

♦§ **67312** two horizontal muscles

♦§ **67314** one vertical muscle (excluding superior oblique)

♦§ **67316** two or more vertical muscles (excluding superior oblique)

(For adjustable sutures, use 67335 in addition to codes 67311-67334 for primary procedure reflecting number of muscles operated on)

♦§ **67318** Strabismus surgery, any procedure, superior oblique muscle

♦§+ **67320** Transposition procedure (eg, for paretic extraocular muscle), any extraocular muscle (specify) (List separately in addition to code for primary procedure)

(Use 67320 in conjunction with 67311-67318)

♦§+ **67331** Strabismus surgery on patient with previous eye surgery or injury that did not involve the extraocular muscles (List separately in addition to code for primary procedure)

(Use 67331 in conjunction with 67311-67318)

♦§+ **67332** Strabismus surgery on patient with scarring of extraocular muscles (eg, prior ocular injury, strabismus or retinal detachment surgery) or restrictive myopathy (eg, dysthyroid ophthalmopathy) (List separately in addition to code for primary procedure)

(Use 67332 in conjunction with 67311-67318)

♦§+ **67334** Strabismus surgery by posterior fixation suture technique, with or without muscle recession (List separately in addition to code for primary procedure)

(Use 67334 in conjunction with 67311-67318)

♦§+ **67335** Placement of adjustable suture(s) during strabismus surgery, including postoperative adjustment(s) of suture(s) (List separately in addition to code for specific strabismus surgery)

(Use 67335 in conjunction with 67311-67334)

♦§+ **67340** Strabismus surgery involving exploration and/or repair of detached extraocular muscle(s) (List separately in addition to code for primary procedure)

(Use 67340 in conjunction with 67311-67334)

♦§ **67343** Release of extensive scar tissue without detaching extraocular muscle (separate procedure)

(Use 67343 in conjunction with 67311-67340, when such procedures are performed other than on the affected muscle)

♦§ **67345** Chemodenervation of extraocular muscle

(For chemodenervation for blepharospasm and other neurological disorders, see 64612 and 64613)

Other Procedures

♦§ **67350** Biopsy of extraocular muscle

(For repair of wound, extraocular muscle, tendon or Tenon's capsule, use 65290)

♦§ **67399** Unlisted procedure, ocular muscle

Orbit

Exploration, Excision, Decompression

♦§ **67400** Orbitotomy without bone flap (frontal or transconjunctival approach); for exploration, with or without biopsy

♦§ **67405** with drainage only

♦§ **67412** with removal of lesion

♦§ **67413** with removal of foreign body

♦§ **67414** with removal of bone for decompression

♦§ **67415** Fine needle aspiration of orbital contents

(For exenteration, enucleation, and repair, see 65101 et seq; for optic nerve decompression, use 67570)

♦§ **67420** Orbitotomy with bone flap or window, lateral approach (eg, Kroenlein); with removal of lesion

♦§ **67430** with removal of foreign body

♦§ **67440** with drainage

♦§ **67445** with removal of bone for decompression

(For optic nerve sheath decompression, use 67570)

♦§ **67450** for exploration, with or without biopsy

(For orbitotomy, transcranial approach, see 61330-61334)

(For orbital implant, see 67550, 67560)

(For removal of eyeball or for repair after removal, see 65091-65175)

Other Procedures

♦❖ **67500** Retrobulbar injection; medication (separate procedure, does not include supply of medication)

♦§ **67505** alcohol

♦§ **67515** Injection of medication or other substance into Tenon's capsule

➲ *CPT Changes: An Insider's View* 2002

(For subconjunctival injection, use 68200)

♦§ **67550** Orbital implant (implant outside muscle cone); insertion

♦§ **67560** removal or revision

(For ocular implant (implant inside muscle cone), see 65093-65105, 65130-65175)

(For treatment of fractures of malar area, orbit, see 21355 et seq)

♦§ **67570** Optic nerve decompression (eg, incision or fenestration of optic nerve sheath)

§ **67599** Unlisted procedure, orbit

Eyelids

Incision

♦§ **67700** Blepharotomy, drainage of abscess, eyelid

♦§ **67710** Severing of tarsorrhaphy

♦§ **67715** Canthotomy (separate procedure)

(For canthoplasty, use 67950)

(For division of symblepharon, use 68340)

Excision

Codes for removal of lesion include more than skin (ie, involving lid margin, tarsus, and/or palpebral conjunctiva).

(For removal of lesion, involving mainly skin of eyelid, see 11310-11313; 11440-11446, 11640-11646; 17000-17004)

(For repair of wounds, blepharoplasty, grafts, reconstructive surgery, see 67930-67975)

§ **67800** Excision of chalazion; single

§ **67801** multiple, same lid

§ **67805** multiple, different lids

§ **67808** under general anesthesia and/or requiring hospitalization, single or multiple

§ **67810** Biopsy of eyelid

♦❖ **67820** Correction of trichiasis; epilation, by forceps only

§ **67825** epilation by other than forceps (eg, by electrosurgery, cryotherapy, laser surgery)

§ **67830** incision of lid margin

§ **67835** incision of lid margin, with free mucous membrane graft

§ **67840** Excision of lesion of eyelid (except chalazion) without closure or with simple direct closure

(For excision and repair of eyelid by reconstructive surgery, see 67961, 67966)

§ **67850** Destruction of lesion of lid margin (up to 1 cm)

(For Mohs micrographic surgery, see 17304-17310)

(For initiation or follow-up care of topical chemotherapy (eg, 5-FU or similar agents), see appropriate office visits)

Tarsorrhaphy

§ **67875** Temporary closure of eyelids by suture (eg, Frost suture)

§ **67880** Construction of intermarginal adhesions, median tarsorrhaphy, or canthorrhaphy;

§ **67882** with transposition of tarsal plate

(For severing of tarsorrhaphy, use 67710)

(For canthoplasty, reconstruction canthus, use 67950)

(For canthotomy, use 67715)

Repair (Brow Ptosis, Blepharoptosis, Lid Retraction, Ectropion, Entropion)

§ **67900** Repair of brow ptosis (supraciliary, mid-forehead or coronal approach)

(For forehead rhytidectomy, use 15824)

♦§ **67901** Repair of blepharoptosis; frontalis muscle technique with suture or other material

♦§ **67902** frontalis muscle technique with fascial sling (includes obtaining fascia)

♦§ **67903** (tarso) levator resection or advancement, internal approach

♦§ **67904** (tarso) levator resection or advancement, external approach

♦§ **67906** superior rectus technique with fascial sling (includes obtaining fascia)

♦§ **67908** conjunctivo-tarso-Muller's muscle-levator resection (eg, Fasanella-Servat type)

♦§ **67909** Reduction of overcorrection of ptosis

♦§ **67911** Correction of lid retraction

(For obtaining autogenous graft materials, see 20920, 20922 or 20926)

(For correction of trichiasis by mucous membrane graft, use 67835)

♦§ **67912** Correction of lagophthalmos, with implantation of upper eyelid lid load (eg, gold weight)

➔ *CPT Changes: An Insider's View* 2004

♦§ **67914** Repair of ectropion; suture

♦§ **67915** thermocauterization

♦§ **67916** excision tarsal wedge

➔ *CPT Changes: An Insider's View* 2004

♦§ **67917** extensive (eg, tarsal strip operations)

➔ *CPT Changes: An Insider's View* 2004

(For correction of everted punctum, use 68705)

♦§ **67921** Repair of entropion; suture

♦§ **67922** thermocauterization

♦§ **67923** excision tarsal wedge

➔ *CPT Changes: An Insider's View* 2004

♦§ **67924** extensive (eg, tarsal strip or capsulopalpebral fascia repairs operation)

➔ *CPT Changes: An Insider's View* 2004

(For repair of cicatricial ectropion or entropion requiring scar excision or skin graft, see also 67961 et seq)

Reconstruction

Codes for blepharoplasty involve more than skin (ie, involving lid margin, tarsus, and/or palpebral conjunctiva).

§ **67930** Suture of recent wound, eyelid, involving lid margin, tarsus, and/or palpebral conjunctiva direct closure; partial thickness

§ **67935** full thickness

❖ **67938** Removal of embedded foreign body, eyelid

(For repair of skin of eyelid, see 12011-12018; 12051-12057; 13150-13153)

(For tarsorrhaphy, canthorrhaphy, see 67880, 67882)

(For repair of blepharoptosis and lid retraction, see 67901-67911)

(For blepharoplasty for entropion, ectropion, see 67916, 67917, 67923, 67924)

(For correction of blepharochalasis (blepharorhytidectomy), see 15820-15823)

(For repair of skin of eyelid, adjacent tissue transfer, see 14060, 14061; preparation for graft, use 15000; free graft, see 15120, 15121, 15260, 15261)

(For excision of lesion of eyelid, use 67800 et seq)

(For repair of lacrimal canaliculi, use 68700)

§ **67950** Canthoplasty (reconstruction of canthus)

§ **67961** Excision and repair of eyelid, involving lid margin, tarsus, conjunctiva, canthus, or full thickness, may include preparation for skin graft or pedicle flap with adjacent tissue transfer or rearrangement; up to one-fourth of lid margin

§ **67966** over one-fourth of lid margin

(For canthoplasty, use 67950)

(For free skin grafts, see 15120, 15121, 15260, 15261)

(For tubed pedicle flap preparation, use 15576; for delay, use 15630; for attachment, use 15650)

§ **67971** Reconstruction of eyelid, full thickness by transfer of tarsoconjunctival flap from opposing eyelid; up to two-thirds of eyelid, one stage or first stage

§ **67973** total eyelid, lower, one stage or first stage

§ **67974** total eyelid, upper, one stage or first stage

§ **67975** second stage

Other Procedures

§ **67999** Unlisted procedure, eyelids

Conjunctiva

(For removal of foreign body, see 65205 et seq)

Incision and Drainage

§ **68020** Incision of conjunctiva, drainage of cyst

❖ **68040** Expression of conjunctival follicles (eg, for trachoma)

Excision and/or Destruction

§ **68100** Biopsy of conjunctiva

§ **68110** Excision of lesion, conjunctiva; up to 1 cm

§ **68115** over 1 cm

§ **68130** with adjacent sclera

§ **68135** Destruction of lesion, conjunctiva

Injection

(For injection into Tenon's capsule or retrobulbar injection, see 67500-67515)

♦❖ **68200** Subconjunctival injection

Conjunctivoplasty

(For wound repair, see 65270-65273)

§ **68320** Conjunctivoplasty; with conjunctival graft or extensive rearrangement

§ **68325** with buccal mucous membrane graft (includes obtaining graft)

§ **68326** Conjunctivoplasty, reconstruction cul-de-sac; with conjunctival graft or extensive rearrangement

§ **68328** with buccal mucous membrane graft (includes obtaining graft)

§ **68330** Repair of symblepharon; conjunctivoplasty, without graft

§ **68335** with free graft conjunctiva or buccal mucous membrane (includes obtaining graft)

§ **68340** division of symblepharon, with or without insertion of conformer or contact lens

Other Procedures

§ **68360** Conjunctival flap; bridge or partial (separate procedure)

§ **68362** total (such as Gunderson thin flap or purse string flap)

(For conjunctival flap for perforating injury, see 65280, 65285)

(For repair of operative wound, use 66250)

(For removal of conjunctival foreign body, see 65205, 65210)

§ **68371** Harvesting conjunctival allograft, living donor
➲ *CPT Changes: An Insider's View* 2004

§ **68399** Unlisted procedure, conjunctiva

Lacrimal System

Incision

§ **68400** Incision, drainage of lacrimal gland

§ **68420** Incision, drainage of lacrimal sac (dacryocystotomy or dacryocystostomy)

§ **68440** Snip incision of lacrimal punctum

Excision

§ **68500** Excision of lacrimal gland (dacryoadenectomy), except for tumor; total

§ **68505** partial

§ **68510** Biopsy of lacrimal gland

§ **68520** Excision of lacrimal sac (dacryocystectomy)

§ **68525** Biopsy of lacrimal sac

§ **68530** Removal of foreign body or dacryolith, lacrimal passages

§ **68540** Excision of lacrimal gland tumor; frontal approach

§ **68550** involving osteotomy

Repair

§ **68700** Plastic repair of canaliculi

§ **68705** Correction of everted punctum, cautery

§ **68720** Dacryocystorhinostomy (fistulization of lacrimal sac to nasal cavity)

§ **68745** Conjunctivorhinostomy (fistulization of conjunctiva to nasal cavity); without tube

§ **68750** with insertion of tube or stent

♦❖ **68760** Closure of the lacrimal punctum; by thermocauterization, ligation, or laser surgery

♦❖ **68761** by plug, each

§ **68770** Closure of lacrimal fistula (separate procedure)

Probing and/or Related Procedures

♦❖ **68801** Dilation of lacrimal punctum, with or without irrigation

(To report a bilateral procedure, use 68801 with modifier 50)

♦§ **68810** Probing of nasolacrimal duct, with or without irrigation;

(For bilateral procedure, report 68810 with modifier 50)

♦§ **68811** requiring general anesthesia

(For bilateral procedure, report 68811 with modifier 50)

♦§ **68815** with insertion of tube or stent

(See also 92018)

(For bilateral procedure, report 68815 with modifier 50)

Surgery: Ocular/Auditory System

❖ **68840** Probing of lacrimal canaliculi, with or without irrigation

☆ **68850** Injection of contrast medium for dacryocystography

(For radiological supervision and interpretation, see 70170, 78660)

Other Procedures

❖ **68899** Unlisted procedure, lacrimal system

Auditory System

(For diagnostic services (eg, audiometry, vestibular tests), see 92502 et seq)

External Ear

Incision

§ **69000** Drainage external ear, abscess or hematoma; simple

§ **69005** complicated

§ **69020** Drainage external auditory canal, abscess

☐ **69090** Ear piercing

Excision

§ **69100** Biopsy external ear

§ **69105** Biopsy external auditory canal

§ **69110** Excision external ear; partial, simple repair

§ **69120** complete amputation

(For reconstruction of ear, see 15120 et seq)

§ **69140** Excision exostosis(es), external auditory canal

§ **69145** Excision soft tissue lesion, external auditory canal

§ **69150** Radical excision external auditory canal lesion; without neck dissection
➔ *CPT Assistant* Jan 03:16

✿ **69155** with neck dissection

(For resection of temporal bone, use 69535)

(For skin grafting, see 15000-15261)

Removal of Foreign Body

♣ **69200** Removal foreign body from external auditory canal; without general anesthesia

§ **69205** with general anesthesia

✶♣ **69210** Removal impacted cerumen (separate procedure), one or both ears
➔ *CPT Assistant* Apr 03:9

♦§ **69220** Debridement, mastoidectomy cavity, simple (eg, routine cleaning)

(For bilateral procedure, report 69220 with modifier 50)

♦§ **69222** Debridement, mastoidectomy cavity, complex (eg, with anesthesia or more than routine cleaning)

(For bilateral procedure, report 69222 with modifier 50)

Repair

(For suture of wound or injury of external ear, see 12011-14300)

♦§ **69300** Otoplasty, protruding ear, with or without size reduction

(For bilateral procedure, report 69300 with modifier 50)

§ **69310** Reconstruction of external auditory canal (meatoplasty) (eg, for stenosis due to injury, infection) (separate procedure)
➔ *CPT Changes: An Insider's View* 2002

§ **69320** Reconstruction external auditory canal for congenital atresia, single stage

(For combination with middle ear reconstruction, see 69631, 69641)

(For other reconstructive procedures with grafts (eg, skin, cartilage, bone), see 13150-15760, 21230-21235)

Other Procedures

(For otoscopy under general anesthesia, use 92502)

§ **69399** Unlisted procedure, external ear

Middle Ear

Introduction

§ **69400** Eustachian tube inflation, transnasal; with catheterization

§ **69401** without catheterization

§ **69405** Eustachian tube catheterization, transtympanic

§ **69410** Focal application of phase control substance, middle ear (baffle technique)

Incision

♦§ **69420** Myringotomy including aspiration and/or eustachian tube inflation

♦§ **69421** Myringotomy including aspiration and/or eustachian tube inflation requiring general anesthesia

♦§ **69424** Ventilating tube removal requiring general anesthesia
➔ *CPT Changes: An Insider's View* 2003

(For bilateral procedure, report 69424 with modifier 50)

(Do not report code 69424 in conjunction with 69205, 69210, 69420, 69421, 69433-69676, 69710-69745, 69801-69930)

♦§ **69433** Tympanostomy (requiring insertion of ventilating tube), local or topical anesthesia

(For bilateral procedure, report 69433 with modifier 50)

♦§ **69436** Tympanostomy (requiring insertion of ventilating tube), general anesthesia

(For bilateral procedure, report 69436 with modifier 50)

♦§ **69440** Middle ear exploration through postauricular or ear canal incision

(For atticotomy, see 69601 et seq)

♦§ **69450** Tympanolysis, transcanal

Excision

♦§ **69501** Transmastoid antrotomy (simple mastoidectomy)

♦§ **69502** Mastoidectomy; complete

➲ *CPT Assistant* Jan 03:16

♦§ **69505** modified radical

♦§ **69511** radical

(For skin graft, see 15000 et seq)

(For mastoidectomy cavity debridement, see 69220, 69222)

♦§ **69530** Petrous apicectomy including radical mastoidectomy

♦✿ **69535** Resection temporal bone, external approach

(For middle fossa approach, see 69950-69970)

♦§ **69540** Excision aural polyp

♦§ **69550** Excision aural glomus tumor; transcanal

♦§ **69552** transmastoid

♦✿ **69554** extended (extratemporal)

Repair

♦§ **69601** Revision mastoidectomy; resulting in complete mastoidectomy

♦§ **69602** resulting in modified radical mastoidectomy

♦§ **69603** resulting in radical mastoidectomy

♦§ **69604** resulting in tympanoplasty

(For planned secondary tympanoplasty after mastoidectomy, see 69631, 69632)

♦§ **69605** with apicectomy

(For skin graft, see 15120, 15121, 15260, 15261)

♦§ **69610** Tympanic membrane repair, with or without site preparation of perforation for closure, with or without patch

♦§ **69620** Myringoplasty (surgery confined to drumhead and donor area)

♦§ **69631** Tympanoplasty without mastoidectomy (including canalplasty, atticotomy and/or middle ear surgery), initial or revision; without ossicular chain reconstruction

♦§ **69632** with ossicular chain reconstruction (eg, postfenestration)

♦§ **69633** with ossicular chain reconstruction and synthetic prosthesis (eg, partial ossicular replacement prosthesis (PORP), total ossicular replacement prosthesis (TORP))

♦§ **69635** Tympanoplasty with antrotomy or mastoidotomy (including canalplasty, atticotomy, middle ear surgery, and/or tympanic membrane repair); without ossicular chain reconstruction

♦§ **69636** with ossicular chain reconstruction

♦§ **69637** with ossicular chain reconstruction and synthetic prosthesis (eg, partial ossicular replacement prosthesis (PORP), total ossicular replacement prosthesis (TORP))

♦§ **69641** Tympanoplasty with mastoidectomy (including canalplasty, middle ear surgery, tympanic membrane repair); without ossicular chain reconstruction

♦§ **69642** with ossicular chain reconstruction

♦§ **69643** with intact or reconstructed wall, without ossicular chain reconstruction

♦§ **69644** with intact or reconstructed canal wall, with ossicular chain reconstruction

♦§ **69645** radical or complete, without ossicular chain reconstruction

♦§ **69646** radical or complete, with ossicular chain reconstruction

♦§ **69650** Stapes mobilization

♦§ **69660** Stapedectomy or stapedotomy with reestablishment of ossicular continuity, with or without use of foreign material;

♦§ **69661** with footplate drill out

♦§ **69662** Revision of stapedectomy or stapedotomy

♦§ **69666** Repair oval window fistula

♦§ **69667** Repair round window fistula

♦§ **69670** Mastoid obliteration (separate procedure)

♦§ **69676** Tympanic neurectomy

(For bilateral procedure, report 69676 with modifier 50)

Other Procedures

♦§ **69700** Closure postauricular fistula, mastoid (separate procedure)

☐ **69710** Implantation or replacement of electromagnetic bone conduction hearing device in temporal bone

(Replacement procedure includes removal of old device)

♦§ **69711** Removal or repair of electromagnetic bone conduction hearing device in temporal bone

♦§ **69714** Implantation, osseointegrated implant, temporal bone, with percutaneous attachment to external speech processor/cochlear stimulator; without mastoidectomy

➲ *CPT Changes: An Insider's View* 2001

♦§ **69715** with mastoidectomy

➲ *CPT Changes: An Insider's View* 2001

♦§ **69717** Replacement (including removal of existing device), osseointegrated implant, temporal bone, with percutaneous attachment to external speech processor/cochlear stimulator; without mastoidectomy

➲ *CPT Changes: An Insider's View* 2001

♦§ **69718** with mastoidectomy

➲ *CPT Changes: An Insider's View* 2001

♦§ **69720** Decompression facial nerve, intratemporal; lateral to geniculate ganglion

♦§ **69725** including medial to geniculate ganglion

♦§ **69740** Suture facial nerve, intratemporal, with or without graft or decompression; lateral to geniculate ganglion

♦§ **69745** including medial to geniculate ganglion

(For extracranial suture of facial nerve, use 64864)

♦§ **69799** Unlisted procedure, middle ear

Inner Ear

Incision and/or Destruction

♦§ **69801** Labyrinthotomy, with or without cryosurgery including other nonexcisional destructive procedures or perfusion of vestibuloactive drugs (single or multiple perfusions); transcanal

(69801 includes all required infusions performed on initial and subsequent days of treatment)

♦§ **69802** with mastoidectomy

♦§ **69805** Endolymphatic sac operation; without shunt

♦§ **69806** with shunt

♦§ **69820** Fenestration semicircular canal

♦§ **69840** Revision fenestration operation

Excision

♦§ **69905** Labyrinthectomy; transcanal

♦§ **69910** with mastoidectomy

♦§ **69915** Vestibular nerve section, translabyrinthine approach

(For transcranial approach, use 69950)

Introduction

♦§ **69930** Cochlear device implantation, with or without mastoidectomy

Other Procedures

♦§ **69949** Unlisted procedure, inner ear

Temporal Bone, Middle Fossa Approach

(For external approach, use 69535)

♦✿ **69950** Vestibular nerve section, transcranial approach

♦§ **69955** Total facial nerve decompression and/or repair (may include graft)

♦§ **69960** Decompression internal auditory canal

♦✿ **69970** Removal of tumor, temporal bone

Other Procedures

♦§ **69979** Unlisted procedure, temporal bone, middle fossa approach

Operating Microscope

The surgical microscope is employed when the surgical services are performed using the techniques of microsurgery. Code 69990 should be reported (without modifier 51 appended) in addition to the code for the primary procedure performed. Do not use 69990 for visualization with magnifying loupes or corrected vision. Do not report code 69990 in addition to procedures where use of the operating microscope is an inclusive component (15756-15758, 15842, 19364, 19368, 20955-20962, 20969-20973, 26551-26554, 26556, 31526, 31531, 31536, 31541, 31561, 31571, 43116, 43496, 49906, 61548, 63075-63078, 64727, 64820-64823, 65091-68850).

☆+ **69990** Microsurgical techniques, requiring use of operating microscope (List separately in addition to code for primary procedure)

➲ *CPT Assistant* Nov 98:20, Apr 99:11, Jun 99:11, Jul 99:11, Oct 99:10, May 00:1, Oct 02:8; *CPT Changes: An Insider's View* 2002

Surgery: Ocular/Auditory System

Notes

Radiology Guidelines (Including Nuclear Medicine and Diagnostic Ultrasound)

Items used by all physicians in reporting their services are presented in the **Introduction.** Some of the commonalities are repeated here for the convenience of those physicians referring to this section on **Radiology (Including Nuclear Medicine and Diagnostic Ultrasound).** Other definitions and items unique to Radiology are also listed.

Subject Listings

Subject listings apply when radiological services are performed by or under the responsible supervision of a physician.

Separate Procedures

Some of the procedures or services listed in *CPT* that are commonly carried out as an integral component of a total service or procedure have been identified by the inclusion of the term "separate procedure." The codes designated as "separate procedure" should not be reported in addition to the code for the total procedure or service of which it is considered an integral component.

However, when a procedure or service that is designated as a "separate procedure" is carried out independently or considered to be unrelated or distinct from other procedures/services provided at that time, it may be reported by itself, or in addition to other procedures/services by appending modifier 59 to the specific "separate procedure" code to indicate that the procedure is not considered to be a component of another procedure, but is a distinct, independent procedure. This may represent a different session or patient encounter, different procedure or surgery, different site or organ system, separate incision/excision, separate lesion, or separate injury (or area of injury in extensive injuries).

Subsection Information

Several of the subheadings or subsections have special needs or instructions unique to that section. Where these are indicated (eg, "Radiation Oncology") special **"Notes"** will be presented preceding those procedural terminology listings, referring to that subsection specifically. If there is an "Unlisted Procedure" code number (see section below) for the individual subsection, it will be shown. Those subsections with **"Notes"** are as follows:

Aorta and Arteries	75600-75790
►Veins and Lymphatics	75801-75893◄
►Transcatheter Procedures	75894-75989◄
Diagnostic Ultrasound	76506-76999
►Abdomen and Retroperitoneum	76700-76778◄
►Obstetrical	76801-76828◄
►Non-Obstetrical	76830-76857◄
Radiation Oncology	77261-77799
Clinical Treatment Planning	77261-77299
Radiation Treatment Management	77427-77499
Proton Beam Treatment Delivery	77520-77525
Hyperthermia	77600-77620
Clinical Brachytherapy	77750-77799
Nuclear Medicine	78000-78299
Musculoskeletal System	78300-78399
Cardiovascular System	78414-78499
►Therapeutic	79005-79999◄

Unlisted Service or Procedure

A service or procedure may be provided that is not listed in this edition of *CPT*. When reporting such a service, the appropriate "Unlisted Procedure" code may be used to indicate the service, identifying it by "Special Report" as discussed below. The "Unlisted Procedures" and accompanying codes for **Radiology (Including Nuclear Medicine and Diagnostic Ultrasound)** are as follows:

76496 Unlisted fluoroscopic procedure (eg, diagnostic, interventional)

76497 Unlisted computed tomography procedure (eg, diagnostic, interventional)

76498 Unlisted magnetic resonance procedure (eg, diagnostic, interventional)

76499 Unlisted diagnostic radiographic procedure

76999 Unlisted ultrasound procedure (eg, diagnostic, interventional)

77299 Unlisted procedure, therapeutic radiology clinical treatment planning

77399 Unlisted procedure, medical radiation physics, dosimetry and treatment devices, and special services

77499 Unlisted procedure, therapeutic radiology treatment management

77799 Unlisted procedure, clinical brachytherapy

78099 Unlisted endocrine procedure, diagnostic nuclear medicine

78199 Unlisted hematopoietic, reticuloendothelial and lymphatic procedure, diagnostic nuclear medicine

78299 Unlisted gastrointestinal procedure, diagnostic nuclear medicine

78399 Unlisted musculoskeletal procedure, diagnostic nuclear medicine

78499 Unlisted cardiovascular procedure, diagnostic nuclear medicine

78599 Unlisted respiratory procedure, diagnostic nuclear medicine

78699 Unlisted nervous system procedure, diagnostic nuclear medicine

78799 Unlisted genitourinary procedure, diagnostic nuclear medicine

78999 Unlisted miscellaneous procedure, diagnostic nuclear medicine

▲ **79999** Radiopharmaceutical therapy, unlisted procedure

Special Report

A service that is rarely provided, unusual, variable, or new may require a special report in determining medical appropriateness of the service. Pertinent information should include an adequate definition or description of the nature, extent, and need for the procedure; and the time, effort, and equipment necessary to provide the service. Additional items which may be included are:

- complexity of symptoms;
- final diagnosis;
- pertinent physical findings;
- diagnostic and therapeutic procedures;
- concurrent problems;
- follow-up care.

Supervision and Interpretation

When a procedure is performed by two physicians, the radiologic portion of the procedure is designated as "radiological supervision and interpretation." When a physician performs both the procedure and provides imaging supervision and interpretation, a combination of procedure codes outside the 70000 series and imaging supervision and interpretation codes are to be used.

(The Radiological Supervision and Interpretation codes are not applicable to the Radiation Oncology subsection.)

Administration of Contrast Material(s)

The phrase "with contrast" used in the codes for procedures performed using contrast for imaging enhancement represents contrast material administered intravascularly, intra-articularly or intrathecally.

For intra-articular injection, use the appropriate joint injection code. If radiographic arthrography is performed, also use the arthrography supervision and interpretation code for the appropriate joint (which includes fluoroscopy). If CT or MR arthrography are performed without radiographic arthrography, use the appropriate joint injection code, the appropriate CT or MR code ("with contrast" or "without followed by contrast"), and the appropriate imaging guidance code for needle placement for contrast injection.

For spine examinations using computed tomography, magnetic resonance imaging, magnetic resonance angiography, "with contrast" includes intrathecal or intravascular injection. For intrathecal injection, use also 61055 or 62284.

Injection of intravascular contrast material is part of the "with contrast" CT, CTA, MRI, MRA procedure.

Oral and/or rectal contrast administration alone does not qualify as a study "with contrast."

Written Report(s)

A written report, signed by the interpreting physician, should be considered an integral part of a radiologic procedure or interpretation.

Radiology

Diagnostic Radiology (Diagnostic Imaging)

Head and Neck

❖ **70010** Myelography, posterior fossa, radiological supervision and interpretation

❖ **70015** Cisternography, positive contrast, radiological supervision and interpretation

✢♣ **70030** Radiologic examination, eye, for detection of foreign body

♣ **70100** Radiologic examination, mandible; partial, less than four views

♣ **70110** complete, minimum of four views

✢♣ **70120** Radiologic examination, mastoids; less than three views per side

✢♣ **70130** complete, minimum of three views per side

♣ **70134** Radiologic examination, internal auditory meati, complete

♣ **70140** Radiologic examination, facial bones; less than three views

♣ **70150** complete, minimum of three views

♣ **70160** Radiologic examination, nasal bones, complete, minimum of three views

♣ **70170** Dacryocystography, nasolacrimal duct, radiological supervision and interpretation

♣ **70190** Radiologic examination; optic foramina

♣ **70200** orbits, complete, minimum of four views

♣ **70210** Radiologic examination, sinuses, paranasal, less than three views

♣ **70220** Radiologic examination, sinuses, paranasal, complete, minimum of three views

♣ **70240** Radiologic examination, sella turcica

♣ **70250** Radiologic examination, skull; less than four views
➲ *CPT Changes: An Insider's View* 2004

♣ **70260** complete, minimum of four views
➲ *CPT Changes: An Insider's View* 2004

♣ **70300** Radiologic examination, teeth; single view

♣ **70310** partial examination, less than full mouth

♣ **70320** complete, full mouth

⌘♣ **70328** Radiologic examination, temporomandibular joint, open and closed mouth; unilateral

✶♣ **70330** bilateral

✢❖ **70332** Temporomandibular joint arthrography, radiological supervision and interpretation

(Do not report 76003 in addition to 70332)

❖ **70336** Magnetic resonance (eg, proton) imaging, temporomandibular joint(s)
➲ *CPT Assistant* Jul 99:11, Jul 01:3; *CPT Changes: An Insider's View* 2001

♣ **70350** Cephalogram, orthodontic

♣ **70355** Orthopantogram

♣ **70360** Radiologic examination; neck, soft tissue

♣ **70370** pharynx or larynx, including fluoroscopy and/or magnification technique

♣ **70371** Complex dynamic pharyngeal and speech evaluation by cine or video recording

♣ **70373** Laryngography, contrast, radiological supervision and interpretation

♣ **70380** Radiologic examination, salivary gland for calculus

♣ **70390** Sialography, radiological supervision and interpretation

❖ **70450** Computed tomography, head or brain; without contrast material
➲ *CPT Assistant* Apr 96:11; *CPT Changes: An Insider's View* 2003

❖ **70460** with contrast material(s)
➲ *CPT Assistant* Apr 96:11

❖ **70470** without contrast material, followed by contrast material(s) and further sections
➲ *CPT Assistant* Apr 96:11

(For coronal, sagittal, and/or oblique sections, use 76375)

❖ **70480** Computed tomography, orbit, sella, or posterior fossa or outer, middle, or inner ear; without contrast material
➲ *CPT Changes: An Insider's View* 2003

❖ **70481** with contrast material(s)

❖ **70482** without contrast material, followed by contrast material(s) and further sections

(For coronal, sagittal, and/or oblique sections, use 76375)

❖ **70486** Computed tomography, maxillofacial area; without contrast material
➲ *CPT Assistant* Mar 02:11; *CPT Changes: An Insider's View* 2003

❖ **70487** with contrast material(s)

❖ **70488** without contrast material, followed by contrast material(s) and further sections

(For coronal, sagittal, and/or oblique sections, use 76375)

❖ **70490** Computed tomography, soft tissue neck; without contrast material
➔ *CPT Changes: An Insider's View* 2003

❖ **70491** with contrast material(s)

❖ **70492** without contrast material followed by contrast material(s) and further sections

(For coronal, sagittal, and/or oblique sections, use 76375)

(For cervical spine, see 72125, 72126)

❖ **70496** Computed tomographic angiography, head, without contrast material(s), followed by contrast material(s) and further sections, including image post-processing
➔ *CPT Assistant* Jul 01:3; *CPT Changes: An Insider's View* 2001

❖ **70498** Computed tomographic angiography, neck, without contrast material(s), followed by contrast material(s) and further sections, including image post-processing
➔ *CPT Assistant* Jul 01:3; *CPT Changes: An Insider's View* 2001

❖ **70540** Magnetic resonance (eg, proton) imaging, orbit, face, and neck; without contrast material(s)
➔ *CPT Assistant* Jul 01:3; *CPT Changes: An Insider's View* 2001

(For head or neck magnetic resonance angiography studies, see 70544-70546, 70547-70549)

❖ **70542** with contrast material(s)
➔ *CPT Assistant* Jul 01:3; *CPT Changes: An Insider's View* 2001

❖ **70543** without contrast material(s), followed by contrast material(s) and further sequences
➔ *CPT Assistant* Jul 01:3; *CPT Changes: An Insider's View* 2001

❖ **70544** Magnetic resonance angiography, head; without contrast material(s)
➔ *CPT Assistant* Sep 01:4; *CPT Changes: An Insider's View* 2001

❖ **70545** with contrast material(s)
➔ *CPT Assistant* Sep 01:4; *CPT Changes: An Insider's View* 2001

❖ **70546** without contrast material(s), followed by contrast material(s) and further sequences
➔ *CPT Assistant* Sep 01:4; *CPT Changes: An Insider's View* 2001

❖ **70547** Magnetic resonance angiography, neck; without contrast material(s)
➔ *CPT Assistant* Sep 01:4; *CPT Changes: An Insider's View* 2001

❖ **70548** with contrast material(s)
➔ *CPT Assistant* Sep 01:4; *CPT Changes: An Insider's View* 2001

❖ **70549** without contrast material(s), followed by contrast material(s) and further sequences
➔ *CPT Assistant* Sep 01:4; *CPT Changes: An Insider's View* 2001

❖ **70551** Magnetic resonance (eg, proton) imaging, brain (including brain stem); without contrast material
➔ *CPT Assistant* May 98:10

❖ **70552** with contrast material(s)
➔ *CPT Assistant* Jul 01:3

❖ **70553** without contrast material, followed by contrast material(s) and further sequences
➔ *CPT Assistant* Nov 97:24, Jul 01:3

(For magnetic spectroscopy, use 76390)

❖ **70557** Magnetic resonance (eg, proton) imaging, brain (including brain stem and skull base), during open intracranial procedure (eg, to assess for residual tumor or residual vascular malformation); without contrast material
➔ *CPT Changes: An Insider's View* 2004

❖ **70558** with contrast material(s)
➔ *CPT Changes: An Insider's View* 2004

❖ **70559** without contrast material(s), followed by contrast material(s) and further sequences
➔ *CPT Changes: An Insider's View* 2004

(For stereotactic biopsy of intracranial lesion with magnetic resonance guidance, use 61751. 70557, 70558 or 70559 may be reported only if a separate report is generated. Report only one of the above codes once per operative session. Do not use these codes in conjunction with 61751, 76393, 76394)

Chest

(For fluoroscopic or ultrasonic guidance for needle placement procedures (eg, biopsy, aspiration, injection, localization device) of the thorax, see 76003, 76942)

♣ **71010** Radiologic examination, chest; single view, frontal

♣ **71015** stereo, frontal

♣ **71020** Radiologic examination, chest, two views, frontal and lateral;
➔ *CPT Assistant* Sep 03:3

♣ **71021** with apical lordotic procedure

♣ **71022** with oblique projections

♣ **71023** with fluoroscopy
➔ *CPT Assistant* Aug 03:14

♣ **71030** Radiologic examination, chest, complete, minimum of four views;

♣ **71034** with fluoroscopy
➔ *CPT Assistant* Aug 03:14

(For separate chest fluoroscopy, use 76000)

♣ **71035** Radiologic examination, chest, special views (eg, lateral decubitus, Bucky studies)

⌘♣ **71040** Bronchography, unilateral, radiological supervision and interpretation

✶♣ **71060** Bronchography, bilateral, radiological supervision and interpretation

♣ **71090** Insertion pacemaker, fluoroscopy and radiography, radiological supervision and interpretation
➔ *CPT Assistant* Aug 02:11

(For procedure, see appropriate organ or site)

⌘♣ **71100** Radiologic examination, ribs, unilateral; two views

⌘♣ **71101** including posteroanterior chest, minimum of three views

✶♣ **71110** Radiologic examination, ribs, bilateral; three views

✶♣ **71111** including posteroanterior chest, minimum of four views

♣ **71120** Radiologic examination; sternum, minimum of two views

♣ **71130** sternoclavicular joint or joints, minimum of three views

❖ **71250** Computed tomography, thorax; without contrast material
➲ *CPT Changes: An Insider's View* 2003

❖ **71260** with contrast material(s)
➲ *CPT Assistant* Jul 01:3

❖ **71270** without contrast material, followed by contrast material(s) and further sections
➲ *CPT Assistant* Jun 01:10

(For coronal, sagittal, and/or oblique sections, use 76375)

❖ **71275** Computed tomographic angiography, chest, without contrast material(s), followed by contrast material(s) and further sections, including image post-processing
➲ *CPT Assistant* Jul 01:3; *CPT Changes: An Insider's View* 2001

❖ **71550** Magnetic resonance (eg, proton) imaging, chest (eg, for evaluation of hilar and mediastinal lymphadenopathy); without contrast material(s)
➲ *CPT Assistant* Jul 01:3; *CPT Changes: An Insider's View* 2001

❖ **71551** with contrast material(s)
➲ *CPT Assistant* Jul 01:3; *CPT Changes: An Insider's View* 2001

❖ **71552** without contrast material(s), followed by contrast material(s) and further sequences
➲ *CPT Assistant* Jul 01:3; *CPT Changes: An Insider's View* 2001

(For breast MRI, see 76093 and 76094)

✤ **71555** Magnetic resonance angiography, chest (excluding myocardium), with or without contrast material(s)

Spine and Pelvis

♣ **72010** Radiologic examination, spine, entire, survey study, anteroposterior and lateral
➲ *CPT Assistant* May 02:18

♣ **72020** Radiologic examination, spine, single view, specify level

♣ **72040** Radiologic examination, spine, cervical; two or three views
➲ *CPT Assistant* Sep 01:4; *CPT Changes: An Insider's View* 2001

♣ **72050** minimum of four views

♣ **72052** complete, including oblique and flexion and/or extension studies

♣ **72069** Radiologic examination, spine, thoracolumbar, standing (scoliosis)

♣ **72070** Radiologic examination, spine; thoracic, two views
➲ *CPT Assistant* Sep 01:4; *CPT Changes: An Insider's View* 2001

♣ **72072** thoracic, three views
➲ *CPT Assistant* Sep 01:4; *CPT Changes: An Insider's View* 2001

♣ **72074** thoracic, minimum of four views
➲ *CPT Assistant* Sep 01:4; *CPT Changes: An Insider's View* 2001

♣ **72080** thoracolumbar, two views
➲ *CPT Assistant* Sep 01:4; *CPT Changes: An Insider's View* 2001

♣ **72090** scoliosis study, including supine and erect studies

♣ **72100** Radiologic examination, spine, lumbosacral; two or three views
➲ *CPT Assistant* Sep 01:4; *CPT Changes: An Insider's View* 2001

♣ **72110** minimum of four views
➲ *CPT Assistant* Sep 01:4; *CPT Changes: An Insider's View* 2001

♣ **72114** complete, including bending views

♣ **72120** Radiologic examination, spine, lumbosacral, bending views only, minimum of four views

(Contrast material in CT of spine is either by intrathecal or intravenous injection. For intrathecal injection, use also 61055 or 62284. IV injection of contrast material is part of the CT procedure)

❖ **72125** Computed tomography, cervical spine; without contrast material
➲ *CPT Changes: An Insider's View* 2003

❖ **72126** with contrast material

❖ **72127** without contrast material, followed by contrast material(s) and further sections

(For intrathecal injection procedure, see 61055, 62284)

❖ **72128** Computed tomography, thoracic spine; without contrast material
➲ *CPT Changes: An Insider's View* 2003

❖ **72129** with contrast material

(For intrathecal injection procedure, see 61055, 62284)

❖ **72130** without contrast material, followed by contrast material(s) and further sections

(For intrathecal injection procedure, see 61055, 62284)

❖ **72131** Computed tomography, lumbar spine; without contrast material
➲ *CPT Changes: An Insider's View* 2003

❖ **72132** with contrast material
➲ *CPT Assistant* Fall 93:13

❖ **72133** without contrast material, followed by contrast material(s) and further sections

(For intrathecal injection procedure, see 61055, 62284)

(For coronal, sagittal, and/or oblique sections, use 76375)

❖ 72141 Magnetic resonance (eg, proton) imaging, spinal canal and contents, cervical; without contrast material

❖ 72142 with contrast material(s)

(For cervical spinal canal imaging without contrast material followed by contrast material, use 72156)

❖ 72146 Magnetic resonance (eg, proton) imaging, spinal canal and contents, thoracic; without contrast material
➲ *CPT Assistant* May 99:10

❖ 72147 with contrast material(s)
➲ *CPT Assistant* May 99:10

(For thoracic spinal canal imaging without contrast material followed by contrast material, use 72157)

❖ 72148 Magnetic resonance (eg, proton) imaging, spinal canal and contents, lumbar; without contrast material

❖ 72149 with contrast material(s)

(For lumbar spinal canal imaging without contrast material followed by contrast material, use 72158)

❖ 72156 Magnetic resonance (eg, proton) imaging, spinal canal and contents, without contrast material, followed by contrast material(s) and further sequences; cervical

❖ 72157 thoracic

❖ 72158 lumbar

□ 72159 Magnetic resonance angiography, spinal canal and contents, with or without contrast material(s)

♣ 72170 Radiologic examination, pelvis; one or two views
➲ *CPT Assistant* Sep 01:4; *CPT Changes: An Insider's View* 2001

♣ 72190 complete, minimum of three views

(For pelvimetry, use 74710)

❖ 72191 Computed tomographic angiography, pelvis, without contrast material(s), followed by contrast material(s) and further sections, including image post-processing
➲ *CPT Assistant* Jul 01:3; *CPT Changes: An Insider's View* 2001

(For CTA aorto-iliofemoral runoff, use 75635)

❖ 72192 Computed tomography, pelvis; without contrast material
➲ *CPT Changes: An Insider's View* 2003

❖ 72193 with contrast material(s)

❖ 72194 without contrast material, followed by contrast material(s) and further sections

(For coronal, sagittal, and/or oblique sections, use 76375)

►(For computed tomographic colonography, see Category III codes 0066T, 0067T. Do not report 72192-72194 in conjunction with 0066T, 0067T)◄

❖ 72195 Magnetic resonance (eg, proton) imaging, pelvis; without contrast material(s)
➲ *CPT Assistant* Jul 01:3; *CPT Changes: An Insider's View* 2001

❖ 72196 with contrast material(s)
➲ *CPT Assistant* Jul 01:3; *CPT Changes: An Insider's View* 2001

❖ 72197 without contrast material(s), followed by contrast material(s) and further sequences
➲ *CPT Assistant* Jul 01:3; *CPT Changes: An Insider's View* 2001

✤ 72198 Magnetic resonance angiography, pelvis, with or without contrast material(s)

♣ 72200 Radiologic examination, sacroiliac joints; less than three views

♣ 72202 three or more views

♣ 72220 Radiologic examination, sacrum and coccyx, minimum of two views

❖ 72240 Myelography, cervical, radiological supervision and interpretation
➲ *CPT Assistant* Fall 93:13

(For complete cervical myelography, see 61055, 62284, 72240)

❖ 72255 Myelography, thoracic, radiological supervision and interpretation

(For complete thoracic myelography, see 61055, 62284, 72255)

❖ 72265 Myelography, lumbosacral, radiological supervision and interpretation
➲ *CPT Assistant* Fall 93:13, Aug 00:7

(For complete lumbosacral myelography, see 61055, 62284, 72265)

❖ 72270 Myelography, two or more regions (eg, lumbar/thoracic, cervical/thoracic, lumbar/cervical, lumbar/thoracic/cervical), radiological supervision and interpretation
➲ *CPT Changes: An Insider's View* 2004

(For complete myelography of entire spinal canal, see 61055, 62284, 72270)

❖ 72275 Epidurography, radiological supervision and interpretation
➲ *CPT Assistant* Nov 99:40, Jan 00:1, Aug 00:7; *CPT Changes: An Insider's View* 2000

(72275 includes 76005)

(For injection procedure, see 62280-62282, 62310-62319, 64479-64484, 0027T)

(Use 72275 only when an epidurogram is performed, images documented, and a formal radiologic report is issued)

❖ 72285 Diskography, cervical or thoracic, radiological supervision and interpretation
➲ *CPT Assistant* Nov 99:35, 40; *CPT Changes: An Insider's View* 2000

❖ 72295 Diskography, lumbar, radiological supervision and interpretation
➲ *CPT Assistant* Apr 03:27

Upper Extremities

(For stress views, any joint, use 76006)

+♣ **73000** Radiologic examination; clavicle, complete

+♣ **73010** scapula, complete

+♣ **73020** Radiologic examination, shoulder; one view

+♣ **73030** complete, minimum of two views

+❖ **73040** Radiologic examination, shoulder, arthrography, radiological supervision and interpretation
➲ *CPT Assistant* Jul 01:3

(Do not report 76003 in addition to 73040)

✶♣ **73050** Radiologic examination; acromioclavicular joints, bilateral, with or without weighted distraction

+♣ **73060** humerus, minimum of two views

+♣ **73070** Radiologic examination, elbow; two views
➲ *CPT Assistant* Sep 01:4; *CPT Changes: An Insider's View* 2001

+♣ **73080** complete, minimum of three views

+❖ **73085** Radiologic examination, elbow, arthrography, radiological supervision and interpretation

(Do not report 76003 in addition to 73085)

+♣ **73090** Radiologic examination; forearm, two views
➲ *CPT Assistant* Sep 01:4, Apr 02:14; *CPT Changes: An Insider's View* 2001

+♣ **73092** upper extremity, infant, minimum of two views

+♣ **73100** Radiologic examination, wrist; two views
➲ *CPT Assistant* Sep 01:4, May 03:16; *CPT Changes: An Insider's View* 2001

+♣ **73110** complete, minimum of three views
➲ *CPT Assistant* Mar 97:10

+❖ **73115** Radiologic examination, wrist, arthrography, radiological supervision and interpretation

(Do not report 76003 in addition to 73115)

+♣ **73120** Radiologic examination, hand; two views

+♣ **73130** minimum of three views

+♣ **73140** Radiologic examination, finger(s), minimum of two views

+❖ **73200** Computed tomography, upper extremity; without contrast material
➲ *CPT Changes: An Insider's View* 2003

+❖ **73201** with contrast material(s)

+❖ **73202** without contrast material, followed by contrast material(s) and further sections

(For coronal, sagittal, and/or oblique sections, use 76375)

❖ **73206** Computed tomographic angiography, upper extremity, without contrast material(s), followed by contrast material(s) and further sections, including image post-processing
➲ *CPT Assistant* Jul 01:3; *CPT Changes: An Insider's View* 2001

+❖ **73218** Magnetic resonance (eg, proton) imaging, upper extremity, other than joint; without contrast material(s)
➲ *CPT Assistant* Jul 01:3; *CPT Changes: An Insider's View* 2001

+❖ **73219** with contrast material(s)
➲ *CPT Assistant* Jul 01:3; *CPT Changes: An Insider's View* 2001

+❖ **73220** without contrast material(s), followed by contrast material(s) and further sequences
➲ *CPT Assistant* Jul 01:3; *CPT Changes: An Insider's View* 2001

+❖ **73221** Magnetic resonance (eg, proton) imaging, any joint of upper extremity; without contrast material(s)
➲ *CPT Assistant* Jul 01:3; *CPT Changes: An Insider's View* 2001

+❖ **73222** with contrast material(s)
➲ *CPT Assistant* Jul 01:3; *CPT Changes: An Insider's View* 2001

+❖ **73223** without contrast material(s), followed by contrast material(s) and further sequences
➲ *CPT Assistant* Jul 01:3; *CPT Changes: An Insider's View* 2001

□ **73225** Magnetic resonance angiography, upper extremity, with or without contrast material(s)

Lower Extremities

(For stress views, any joint, use 76006)

⌘♣ **73500** Radiologic examination, hip, unilateral; one view

⌘♣ **73510** complete, minimum of two views
➲ *CPT Assistant* Spring 92:9, May 99:10, Apr 02:19, Mar 03:23

✶♣ **73520** Radiologic examination, hips, bilateral, minimum of two views of each hip, including anteroposterior view of pelvis
➲ *CPT Assistant* Apr 02:19, May 03:15

+❖ **73525** Radiologic examination, hip, arthrography, radiological supervision and interpretation

(Do not report 76003 in addition to 73525)

♣ **73530** Radiologic examination, hip, during operative procedure

♣ **73540** Radiologic examination, pelvis and hips, infant or child, minimum of two views

❖ **73542** Radiological examination, sacroiliac joint arthrography, radiological supervision and interpretation
➲ *CPT Assistant* Nov 99:40-41; *CPT Changes: An Insider's View* 2000

(Do not report 76003 in addition to 73542)

(For procedure, use 27096. If formal arthrography is not performed, recorded, and a formal radiologic report is not issued, use 76005 for fluoroscopic guidance for sacroiliac joint injections)

+♣ **73550** Radiologic examination, femur, two views
➲ *CPT Assistant* Sep 01:4; *CPT Changes: An Insider's View* 2001

+♣ **73560** Radiologic examination, knee; one or two views

+♣ **73562** three views
➲ *CPT Assistant* Apr 02:15

+♣ **73564** complete, four or more views
➲ *CPT Assistant* Jun 98:11, Nov 98:21

✶♣ **73565** both knees, standing, anteroposterior

+❖ 73580 Radiologic examination, knee, arthrography, radiological supervision and interpretation

(Do not report 76003 in addition to 73580)

+♣ 73590 Radiologic examination; tibia and fibula, two views

+♣ 73592 lower extremity, infant, minimum of two views

+♣ 73600 Radiologic examination, ankle; two views

➲ *CPT Assistant* Sep 01:4, Apr 02:15, Mar 03:17, 19, Mar 03:9; *CPT Changes: An Insider's View* 2001

+♣ 73610 complete, minimum of three views

➲ *CPT Assistant* Apr 02:15, Mar 03:9, 18, 19

+❖ 73615 Radiologic examination, ankle, arthrography, radiological supervision and interpretation

(Do not report 76003 in addition to 73615)

+♣ 73620 Radiologic examination, foot; two views

➲ *CPT Assistant* Sep 01:4, Apr 02:15, Mar 03:17, 19; *CPT Changes: An Insider's View* 2001

+♣ 73630 complete, minimum of three views

+♣ 73650 Radiologic examination; calcaneus, minimum of two views

+♣ 73660 toe(s), minimum of two views

❖ 73700 Computed tomography, lower extremity; without contrast material

➲ *CPT Changes: An Insider's View* 2003

❖ 73701 with contrast material(s)

❖ 73702 without contrast material, followed by contrast material(s) and further sections

(For coronal, sagittal, and/or oblique sections, use 76375)

❖ 73706 Computed tomographic angiography, lower extremity, without contrast material(s), followed by contrast material(s) and further sections, including image post-processing

➲ *CPT Assistant* Jul 01:3; *CPT Changes: An Insider's View* 2001

(For CTA aorto-iliofemoral runoff, use 75635)

❖ 73718 Magnetic resonance (eg, proton) imaging, lower extremity other than joint; without contrast material(s)

➲ *CPT Assistant* Jul 01:3; *CPT Changes: An Insider's View* 2001

❖ 73719 with contrast material(s)

➲ *CPT Assistant* Jul 01:3; *CPT Changes: An Insider's View* 2001

❖ 73720 without contrast material(s), followed by contrast material(s) and further sequences

➲ *CPT Assistant* Jul 01:3; *CPT Changes: An Insider's View* 2001

❖ 73721 Magnetic resonance (eg, proton) imaging, any joint of lower extremity; without contrast material

➲ *CPT Assistant* Jul 01:3; *CPT Changes: An Insider's View* 2001

❖ 73722 with contrast material(s)

➲ *CPT Assistant* Jul 01:3; *CPT Changes: An Insider's View* 2001

❖ 73723 without contrast material(s), followed by contrast material(s) and further sequences

➲ *CPT Assistant* Jul 01:3; *CPT Changes: An Insider's View* 2001

⚘ 73725 Magnetic resonance angiography, lower extremity, with or without contrast material(s)

Abdomen

♣ 74000 Radiologic examination, abdomen; single anteroposterior view

➲ *CPT Assistant* Nov 98:21

♣ 74010 anteroposterior and additional oblique and cone views

♣ 74020 complete, including decubitus and/or erect views

♣ 74022 complete acute abdomen series, including supine, erect, and/or decubitus views, single view chest

➲ *CPT Changes: An Insider's View* 2003

❖ 74150 Computed tomography, abdomen; without contrast material

➲ *CPT Assistant* Oct 02:12; *CPT Changes: An Insider's View* 2003

❖ 74160 with contrast material(s)

❖ 74170 without contrast material, followed by contrast material(s) and further sections

(For coronal, sagittal, and/or oblique sections, use 76375)

►(For computed tomographic colonography, see Category III codes 0066T, 0067T. Do not report 74150-74170 in conjunction with 0066T, 0067T)◄

❖ 74175 Computed tomographic angiography, abdomen, without contrast material(s), followed by contrast material(s) and further sections, including image post-processing

➲ *CPT Assistant* Jul 01:3; *CPT Changes: An Insider's View* 2001

(For CTA aorto-iliofemoral runoff, use 75635)

❖ 74181 Magnetic resonance (eg, proton) imaging, abdomen; without contrast material(s)

➲ *CPT Assistant* Jul 01:3; *CPT Changes: An Insider's View* 2001

❖ 74182 with contrast material(s)

➲ *CPT Assistant* Jul 01:3; *CPT Changes: An Insider's View* 2001

❖ 74183 without contrast material(s), followed by with contrast material(s) and further sequences

➲ *CPT Assistant* Jul 01:3; *CPT Changes: An Insider's View* 2001

⚘ 74185 Magnetic resonance angiography, abdomen, with or without contrast material(s)

♣ 74190 Peritoneogram (eg, after injection of air or contrast), radiological supervision and interpretation

(For procedure, use 49400)

(For computed tomography, see 72192 or 74150)

Gastrointestinal Tract

(For percutaneous placement of gastrostomy tube, use 43750)

❖ 74210 Radiologic examination; pharynx and/or cervical esophagus

❖ 74220 esophagus

Radiology

❖ **74230** Swallowing function, with cineradiography/videoradiography
➲ *CPT Changes: An Insider's View* 2002

❖ **74235** Removal of foreign body(s), esophageal, with use of balloon catheter, radiological supervision and interpretation

(For procedure, see 43215, 43247)

❖ **74240** Radiologic examination, gastrointestinal tract, upper; with or without delayed films, without KUB

❖ **74241** with or without delayed films, with KUB

❖ **74245** with small intestine, includes multiple serial films
➲ *CPT Changes: An Insider's View* 2002

❖ **74246** Radiological examination, gastrointestinal tract, upper, air contrast, with specific high density barium, effervescent agent, with or without glucagon; with or without delayed films, without KUB

❖ **74247** with or without delayed films, with KUB

❖ **74249** with small intestine follow-through
➲ *CPT Changes: An Insider's View* 2002

❖ **74250** Radiologic examination, small intestine, includes multiple serial films;
➲ *CPT Changes: An Insider's View* 2002

❖ **74251** via enteroclysis tube

❖ **74260** Duodenography, hypotonic

❖ **74270** Radiologic examination, colon; barium enema, with or without KUB

❖ **74280** air contrast with specific high density barium, with or without glucagon

❖ **74283** Therapeutic enema, contrast or air, for reduction of intussusception or other intraluminal obstruction (eg, meconium ileus)
➲ *CPT Assistant* Nov 97:24

❖ **74290** Cholecystography, oral contrast;

❖ **74291** additional or repeat examination or multiple day examination

♣ **74300** Cholangiography and/or pancreatography; intraoperative, radiological supervision and interpretation
➲ *CPT Assistant* Nov 99:41, Dec 00:14; *CPT Changes: An Insider's View* 2000

♣+ **74301** additional set intraoperative, radiological supervision and interpretation (List separately in addition to code for primary procedure)

(Use 74301 in conjunction with 74300)

♣ **74305** through existing catheter, radiological supervision and interpretation
➲ *CPT Assistant* Nov 99:41; *CPT Changes: An Insider's View* 2000, 2002

(For procedure, see 47505, 48400, 47560-47561, 47563)

(For biliary duct stone extraction, percutaneous, see 47630, 74327)

♣ **74320** Cholangiography, percutaneous, transhepatic, radiological supervision and interpretation

❖ **74327** Postoperative biliary duct calculus removal, percutaneous via T-tube tract, basket, or snare (eg, Burhenne technique), radiological supervision and interpretation
➲ *CPT Changes: An Insider's View* 2002

(For procedure, use 47630)

☆ **74328** Endoscopic catheterization of the biliary ductal system, radiological supervision and interpretation

(For procedure, see 43260-43272 as appropriate)

☆ **74329** Endoscopic catheterization of the pancreatic ductal system, radiological supervision and interpretation

(For procedure, see 43260-43272 as appropriate)

☆ **74330** Combined endoscopic catheterization of the biliary and pancreatic ductal systems, radiological supervision and interpretation

(For procedure, see 43260-43272 as appropriate)

♣ **74340** Introduction of long gastrointestinal tube (eg, Miller-Abbott), including multiple fluoroscopies and films, radiological supervision and interpretation

(For tube placement, use 44500)

♣ **74350** Percutaneous placement of gastrostomy tube, radiological supervision and interpretation

♣ **74355** Percutaneous placement of enteroclysis tube, radiological supervision and interpretation

❖ **74360** Intraluminal dilation of strictures and/or obstructions (eg, esophagus), radiological supervision and interpretation
➲ *CPT Assistant* Spring 94:3

❖ **74363** Percutaneous transhepatic dilation of biliary duct stricture with or without placement of stent, radiological supervision and interpretation
➲ *CPT Changes: An Insider's View* 2002

(For procedure, see 47510, 47511, 47555, 47556)

Urinary Tract

❖ **74400** Urography (pyelography), intravenous, with or without KUB, with or without tomography

❖ **74410** Urography, infusion, drip technique and/or bolus technique;

❖ **74415** with nephrotomography

❖ **74420** Urography, retrograde, with or without KUB
➲ *CPT Assistant* Sep 00:11

❖ **74425** Urography, antegrade, (pyelostogram, nephrostogram, loopogram), radiological supervision and interpretation
➲ *CPT Assistant* Fall 93:14, Dec 97:7

❖ **74430** Cystography, minimum of three views, radiological supervision and interpretation

❖ **74440** Vasography, vesiculography, or epididymography, radiological supervision and interpretation

❖ **74445** Corpora cavernosography, radiological supervision and interpretation

❖ **74450** Urethrocystography, retrograde, radiological supervision and interpretation

❖ **74455** Urethrocystography, voiding, radiological supervision and interpretation

♣ **74470** Radiologic examination, renal cyst study, translumbar, contrast visualization, radiological supervision and interpretation

❖ **74475** Introduction of intracatheter or catheter into renal pelvis for drainage and/or injection, percutaneous, radiological supervision and interpretation

❖ **74480** Introduction of ureteral catheter or stent into ureter through renal pelvis for drainage and/or injection, percutaneous, radiological supervision and interpretation

(For transurethral surgery (ureter and pelvis), see 52320-52355)

❖ **74485** Dilation of nephrostomy, ureters, or urethra, radiological supervision and interpretation

(For dilation of ureter without radiologic guidance, use 52341, 52344)

(For change of nephrostomy or pyelostomy tube, use 50398)

Gynecological and Obstetrical

(For abdomen and pelvis, see 72170-72190, 74000-74170)

♣ **74710** Pelvimetry, with or without placental localization

♣ **74740** Hysterosalpingography, radiological supervision and interpretation
➲ *CPT Assistant* Nov 97:24, Jul 99:8

(For introduction of saline or contrast for hysterosalpingography, see 58340)

♣ **74742** Transcervical catheterization of fallopian tube, radiological supervision and interpretation

(For procedure, use 58345)

❖ **74775** Perineogram (eg, vaginogram, for sex determination or extent of anomalies)

Heart

(For separate injection procedures for vascular radiology, see **Surgery** section, 36000-36299)

(For cardiac catheterization procedures, see 93501-93556)

❖ **75552** Cardiac magnetic resonance imaging for morphology; without contrast material
➲ *CPT Assistant* Fall 95:1

❖ **75553** with contrast material
➲ *CPT Assistant* Fall 95:1

❖ **75554** Cardiac magnetic resonance imaging for function, with or without morphology; complete study
➲ *CPT Assistant* Fall 95:2

❖ **75555** limited study
➲ *CPT Assistant* Fall 95:2

☐ **75556** Cardiac magnetic resonance imaging for velocity flow mapping
➲ *CPT Assistant* Fall 95:2

▸Vascular Procedures◂

Aorta and Arteries

Selective vascular catheterizations should be coded to include introduction and all lesser order selective catheterizations used in the approach (eg, the description for a selective right middle cerebral artery catheterization includes the introduction and placement catheterization of the right common and internal carotid arteries).

Additional second and/or third order arterial catheterizations within the same family of arteries supplied by a single first order artery should be expressed by 36218 or 36248. Additional first order or higher catheterizations in vascular families supplied by a first order vessel different from a previously selected and coded family should be separately coded using the conventions described above.

▸For angiography performed in conjunction with therapeutic transcatheter radiological supervision and interpretation services, see the Radiology Transcatheter Procedures guidelines.◂

▸Diagnostic angiography (radiological supervision and interpretation) codes should NOT be used with interventional procedures for:◂

▸ 1) Contrast injections, angiography, roadmapping, and/or fluoroscopic guidance for the intervention,◂

▸ 2) Vessel measurement, and◂

▸ 3) Post-angioplasty/stent angiography◂

▸as this work is captured in the interventional procedure code(s).◂

▸Diagnostic angiography performed at the time of an interventional procedure is separately reportable if:◂

▸ 1) No prior catheter-based angiographic study is available and a full diagnostic study is performed, and the decision to intervene is based on the diagnostic study, OR◂

▸ 2) A prior study is available, but as documented in the medical record:◂

▸ a) The patient's condition with respect to the clinical indication has changed since the prior study, OR◂

Radiology

► b) There is inadequate visualization of the anatomy and/or pathology, OR◄

► c) There is a clinical change during the procedure that requires new evaluation outside the target area of intervention◄

►Diagnostic angiography performed at a separate setting from an interventional procedure is separately reported.◄

►Diagnostic angiography performed at the time of an interventional procedure is NOT separately reportable if it is specifically included in the interventional code descriptor.◄

(For intravenous procedure, see 36000-36013, 36400-36425 and 36100-36248 for intra-arterial procedure)

(For radiological supervision and interpretation, see 75600-75978)

❖ **75600** Aortography, thoracic, without serialography, radiological supervision and interpretation

(For injection procedure, use 93544)

❖ **75605** Aortography, thoracic, by serialography, radiological supervision and interpretation

➲ *CPT Assistant* Spring 94:29, Dec 98:9

(For injection procedure, use 93544)

❖ **75625** Aortography, abdominal, by serialography, radiological supervision and interpretation

➲ *CPT Assistant* Fall 93:16, Jan 01:14

(For injection procedure, use 93544)

❖ **75630** Aortography, abdominal plus bilateral iliofemoral lower extremity, catheter, by serialography, radiological supervision and interpretation

➲ *CPT Assistant* Fall 93:16, Jan 01:14

❖ **75635** Computed tomographic angiography, abdominal aorta and bilateral iliofemoral lower extremity runoff, radiological supervision and interpretation, without contrast material(s), followed by contrast material(s) and further sections, including image post-processing

➲ *CPT Assistant* Jul 01:3; *CPT Changes: An Insider's View* 2001

❖ **75650** Angiography, cervicocerebral, catheter, including vessel origin, radiological supervision and interpretation

➲ *CPT Assistant* Spring 94:29, Apr 98:3, Oct 00:4

❖ **75658** Angiography, brachial, retrograde, radiological supervision and interpretation

⌘❖ **75660** Angiography, external carotid, unilateral, selective, radiological supervision and interpretation

✶❖ **75662** Angiography, external carotid, bilateral, selective, radiological supervision and interpretation

⌘❖ **75665** Angiography, carotid, cerebral, unilateral, radiological supervision and interpretation

✶❖ **75671** Angiography, carotid, cerebral, bilateral, radiological supervision and interpretation

➲ *CPT Assistant* Oct 00:4

⌘❖ **75676** Angiography, carotid, cervical, unilateral, radiological supervision and interpretation

➲ *CPT Assistant* Oct 00:4

✶❖ **75680** Angiography, carotid, cervical, bilateral, radiological supervision and interpretation

➲ *CPT Assistant* Oct 00:4

❖ **75685** Angiography, vertebral, cervical, and/or intracranial, radiological supervision and interpretation

➲ *CPT Assistant* Oct 00:4

❖ **75705** Angiography, spinal, selective, radiological supervision and interpretation

❖ **75710** Angiography, extremity, unilateral, radiological supervision and interpretation

➲ *CPT Assistant* Apr 99:11, Jan 01:14, Apr 03:12

✶❖ **75716** Angiography, extremity, bilateral, radiological supervision and interpretation

➲ *CPT Assistant* Fall 93:16, Jan 01:14, Apr 03:12

⌘❖ **75722** Angiography, renal, unilateral, selective (including flush aortogram), radiological supervision and interpretation

➲ *CPT Assistant* Apr 03:12

✶❖ **75724** Angiography, renal, bilateral, selective (including flush aortogram), radiological supervision and interpretation

➲ *CPT Assistant* Apr 03:12

❖ **75726** Angiography, visceral, selective or supraselective, (with or without flush aortogram), radiological supervision and interpretation

(For selective angiography, each additional visceral vessel studied after basic examination, use 75774)

⌘❖ **75731** Angiography, adrenal, unilateral, selective, radiological supervision and interpretation

✶❖ **75733** Angiography, adrenal, bilateral, selective, radiological supervision and interpretation

❖ **75736** Angiography, pelvic, selective or supraselective, radiological supervision and interpretation

⌘❖ **75741** Angiography, pulmonary, unilateral, selective, radiological supervision and interpretation

(For injection procedure, use 93541)

✶❖ **75743** Angiography, pulmonary, bilateral, selective, radiological supervision and interpretation

➲ *CPT Assistant* Spring 94:29, Apr 98:3

(For injection procedure, use 93541)

❖ **75746** Angiography, pulmonary, by nonselective catheter or venous injection, radiological supervision and interpretation

(For injection procedure, use 93541)

(For introduction of catheter, injection procedure, see 93501-93533, 93539, 93540, 93545, 93556)

(For introduction of catheter, injection procedure, see 93501-93533, 93545, 93556)

(For introduction of catheter, injection procedure, see 93501-93533, 93539, 93540, 93545, 93556)

❖ 75756 Angiography, internal mammary, radiological supervision and interpretation

(For introduction of catheter, injection procedure, see 93501-93533, 93545, 93556)

❖+ 75774 Angiography, selective, each additional vessel studied after basic examination, radiological supervision and interpretation (List separately in addition to code for primary procedure)

➲ *CPT Assistant* Fall 93:17, Spring 94:29

(Use 75774 in addition to code for specific initial vessel studied)

(For angiography, see codes 75600-75790)

(For catheterizations, see codes 36215-36248)

(For introduction of catheter, injection procedure, see 93501-93533, 93545, 93555, 93556)

❖ 75790 Angiography, arteriovenous shunt (eg, dialysis patient), radiological supervision and interpretation

➲ *CPT Assistant* May 01:1

(For introduction of catheter, use 36140, 36145, 36215-36217, 36245-36247)

Veins and Lymphatics

►For venography performed in conjunction with therapeutic transcatheter radiological supervision and interpretation services, see the Radiology Transcatheter Procedures guidelines.◄

►Diagnostic venography (radiological supervision and interpretation) codes should NOT be used with interventional procedures for:◄

► 1) Contrast injections, venography, roadmapping, and/or fluoroscopic guidance for the intervention,◄

► 2) Vessel measurement, and◄

► 3) Post-angioplasty/stent venography◄

►as this work is captured in the interventional procedure code(s).◄

►Diagnostic venography performed at the time of an interventional procedure is separately reportable if:◄

► 1) No prior catheter-based venographic study is available and a full diagnostic study is performed, and decision to intervene is based on the diagnostic study, OR◄

► 2) A prior study is available, but as documented in the medical record:◄

► a) The patient's condition with respect to the clinical indication has changed since the prior study, OR◄

► b) There is inadequate visualization of the anatomy and/or pathology, OR◄

► c) There is a clinical change during the procedure that requires new evaluation outside the target area of intervention◄

►Diagnostic venography performed at a separate setting from an interventional procedure is separately reported.◄

►Diagnostic venography performed at the time of an interventional procedure is NOT separately reportable if it is specifically included in the interventional code descriptor.◄

(For injection procedure for venous system, see 36000-36015, 36400-36510)

(For injection procedure for lymphatic system, use 38790)

⌘♣ 75801 Lymphangiography, extremity only, unilateral, radiological supervision and interpretation

✶♣ 75803 Lymphangiography, extremity only, bilateral, radiological supervision and interpretation

➲ *CPT Assistant* May 03:10

⌘♣ 75805 Lymphangiography, pelvic/abdominal, unilateral, radiological supervision and interpretation

✶♣ 75807 Lymphangiography, pelvic/abdominal, bilateral, radiological supervision and interpretation

♣ 75809 Shuntogram for investigation of previously placed indwelling nonvascular shunt (eg, LeVeen shunt, ventriculoperitoneal shunt, indwelling infusion pump), radiological supervision and interpretation

➲ *CPT Changes: An Insider's View* 2001

(For procedure, see 49427 or 61070)

❖ 75810 Splenoportography, radiological supervision and interpretation

⌘❖ 75820 Venography, extremity, unilateral, radiological supervision and interpretation

➲ *CPT Assistant* Oct 97:10

✶❖ 75822 Venography, extremity, bilateral, radiological supervision and interpretation

❖ 75825 Venography, caval, inferior, with serialography, radiological supervision and interpretation

❖ 75827 Venography, caval, superior, with serialography, radiological supervision and interpretation

➲ *CPT Assistant* Apr 98:3

⌘❖ 75831 Venography, renal, unilateral, selective, radiological supervision and interpretation

✶❖ 75833 Venography, renal, bilateral, selective, radiological supervision and interpretation

⌘❖ 75840 Venography, adrenal, unilateral, selective, radiological supervision and interpretation

✶❖ 75842 Venography, adrenal, bilateral, selective, radiological supervision and interpretation

Radiology

❖ **75860** Venography, venous sinus (eg, petrosal and inferior sagittal) or jugular, catheter, radiological supervision and interpretation

➲ *CPT Changes: An Insider's View* 2004

❖ **75870** Venography, superior sagittal sinus, radiological supervision and interpretation

❖ **75872** Venography, epidural, radiological supervision and interpretation

❖ **75880** Venography, orbital, radiological supervision and interpretation

❖ **75885** Percutaneous transhepatic portography with hemodynamic evaluation, radiological supervision and interpretation

➲ *CPT Assistant* Oct 96:4, Mar 02:10, Dec 03:1

❖ **75887** Percutaneous transhepatic portography without hemodynamic evaluation, radiological supervision and interpretation

➲ *CPT Assistant* Mar 02:10, Dec 03:1

❖ **75889** Hepatic venography, wedged or free, with hemodynamic evaluation, radiological supervision and interpretation

❖ **75891** Hepatic venography, wedged or free, without hemodynamic evaluation, radiological supervision and interpretation

☆ **75893** Venous sampling through catheter, with or without angiography (eg, for parathyroid hormone, renin), radiological supervision and interpretation

(For procedure, use 36500)

Transcatheter Procedures

►Therapeutic transcatheter radiological supervision and interpretation code(s) include the following services associated with that intervention:◄

► 1) Contrast injections, angiography/venography, roadmapping, and fluoroscopic guidance for the intervention,◄

► 2) Vessel measurement, and◄

► 3) Completion angiography/venography (except for those uses permitted by 75898).◄

►Unless specifically included in the code descriptor, diagnostic angiography/venography performed at the time of transcatheter therapeutic radiological and interpretation service(s) is separately reportable (eg, no prior catheter-based diagnostic angiography/venography study of the target vessel is available, prior diagnostic study is inadequate, patient's condition with respect to the clinical indication has changed since the prior study or during the intervention). See 75600-75893.◄

❖ **75894** Transcatheter therapy, embolization, any method, radiological supervision and interpretation

➲ *CPT Assistant* Sep 98:7

❖ **75896** Transcatheter therapy, infusion, any method (eg, thrombolysis other than coronary), radiological supervision and interpretation

(For infusion for coronary disease, see 92975, 92977)

♣ **75898** Angiography through existing catheter for follow-up study for transcatheter therapy, embolization or infusion

➲ *CPT Changes: An Insider's View* 2002

✿ **75900** Exchange of a previously placed arterial catheter during thrombolytic therapy with contrast monitoring, radiological supervision and interpretation

(For procedure, use 37209)

♣ **75901** Mechanical removal of pericatheter obstructive material (eg, fibrin sheath) from central venous device via separate venous access, radiologic supervision and interpretation

➲ *CPT Changes: An Insider's View* 2003

(For procedure, use 36595)

(For venous catheterization, see 36010-36012)

♣ **75902** Mechanical removal of intraluminal (intracatheter) obstructive material from central venous device through device lumen, radiologic supervision and interpretation

➲ *CPT Changes: An Insider's View* 2003

(For procedure, use 36596)

(For venous catheterization, see 36010-36012)

§ **75940** Percutaneous placement of IVC filter, radiological supervision and interpretation

➲ *CPT Assistant* Nov 00:11

❖ **75945** Intravascular ultrasound (non-coronary vessel), radiological supervision and interpretation; initial vessel

❖+ **75946** each additional non-coronary vessel (List separately in addition to code for primary procedure)

(Use 75946 in conjunction with 75945)

(For catheterizations, see codes 36215-36248)

(For transcatheter therapies, see codes 37200-37208, 61624, 61626)

(For procedure, see 37250, 37251)

✿ **75952** Endovascular repair of infrarenal abdominal aortic aneurysm or dissection, radiological supervision and interpretation

➲ *CPT Changes: An Insider's View* 2001

(For implantation of endovascular grafts, see 34800-34808)

►(For radiologic supervision and interpretation of endovascular repair of abdominal aortic aneurysm involving visceral vessels, see Category III codes 0078T-0081T)◄

Radiology

✿ **75953** Placement of proximal or distal extension prosthesis for endovascular repair of infrarenal aortic or iliac artery aneurysm, pseudoaneurysm, or dissection, radiological supervision and interpretation

➲ *CPT Assistant* Feb 03:1, ; *CPT Changes: An Insider's View* 2001, 2003

(For implantation of endovascular extension prostheses, see 34825, 34826)

✿ **75954** Endovascular repair of iliac artery aneurysm, pseudoaneurysm, arteriovenous malformation, or trauma, radiological supervision and interpretation

➲ *CPT Assistant* Feb 03:1; *CPT Changes: An Insider's View* 2003

(For implantation of endovascular graft, see 34900)

❖▲ **75960** Transcatheter introduction of intravascular stent(s), (except coronary, carotid, and vertebral vessel), percutaneous and/or open, radiological supervision and interpretation, each vessel

➲ *CPT Assistant* Fall 93:18, Oct 96:2, May 01:1, Dec 03:1; *CPT Changes: An Insider's View* 2005

(For procedure, see 37205-37208)

(For radiologic supervision and interpretation for transcatheter placement of extracranial ►vertebral or intrathoracic carotid◄ artery stent(s), ►see◄ Category III codes ►0075T, 0076T◄)

❖ **75961** Transcatheter retrieval, percutaneous, of intravascular foreign body (eg, fractured venous or arterial catheter), radiological supervision and interpretation

(For procedure, use 37203)

❖ **75962** Transluminal balloon angioplasty, peripheral artery, radiological supervision and interpretation

➲ *CPT Assistant* Fall 93:18, May 01:1

❖✚ **75964** Transluminal balloon angioplasty, each additional peripheral artery, radiological supervision and interpretation (List separately in addition to code for primary procedure)

(Use 75964 in conjunction with 75962)

❖ **75966** Transluminal balloon angioplasty, renal or other visceral artery, radiological supervision and interpretation

❖✚ **75968** Transluminal balloon angioplasty, each additional visceral artery, radiological supervision and interpretation (List separately in addition to code for primary procedure)

(Use 75968 in conjunction with 75966)

(For percutaneous transluminal coronary angioplasty, see 92982-92984)

❖ **75970** Transcatheter biopsy, radiological supervision and interpretation

(For injection procedure only for transcatheter therapy or biopsy, see 36100-36299)

(For transcatheter renal and ureteral biopsy, use 52007)

(For percutaneous needle biopsy of pancreas, use 48102; of retroperitoneal lymph node or mass, use 49180)

❖ **75978** Transluminal balloon angioplasty, venous (eg, subclavian stenosis), radiological supervision and interpretation

➲ *CPT Assistant* Oct 96:4, May 01:1

❖ **75980** Percutaneous transhepatic biliary drainage with contrast monitoring, radiological supervision and interpretation

❖ **75982** Percutaneous placement of drainage catheter for combined internal and external biliary drainage or of a drainage stent for internal biliary drainage in patients with an inoperable mechanical biliary obstruction, radiological supervision and interpretation

♣ **75984** Change of percutaneous tube or drainage catheter with contrast monitoring (eg, gastrointestinal system, genitourinary system, abscess), radiological supervision and interpretation

(For change of nephrostomy or pyelostomy tube only, use 50398)

(For introduction procedure only for percutaneous biliary drainage, see 47510, 47511)

(For percutaneous cholecystostomy, use 47490)

(For change of percutaneous biliary drainage catheter only, use 47525)

(For percutaneous nephrostolithotomy or pyelostolithotomy, see 50080, 50081)

☆ **75989** Radiological guidance (ie, fluoroscopy, ultrasound, or computed tomography), for percutaneous drainage (eg, abscess, specimen collection), with placement of catheter, radiological supervision and interpretation

➲ *CPT Assistant* Nov 97:24, Mar 98:8; *CPT Changes: An Insider's View* 2001, 2002

Transluminal Atherectomy

❖ **75992** Transluminal atherectomy, peripheral artery, radiological supervision and interpretation

(For procedure, see 35481-35485, 35491-35495)

❖✚ **75993** Transluminal atherectomy, each additional peripheral artery, radiological supervision and interpretation (List separately in addition to code for primary procedure)

(Use 75993 in conjunction with 75992)

(For procedure, see 35481-35485, 35491-35495)

❖ **75994** Transluminal atherectomy, renal, radiological supervision and interpretation

(For procedure, see 35480, 35490)

❖ **75995** Transluminal atherectomy, visceral, radiological supervision and interpretation

(For procedure, see 35480, 35490)

❖✚ **75996** Transluminal atherectomy, each additional visceral artery, radiological supervision and interpretation (List separately in addition to code for primary procedure)

(Use 75996 in conjunction with 75995)

(For procedure, see 35480, 35490)

Other Procedures

(For computed tomography cerebral perfusion analysis, see Category III code 0042T)

(For arthrography of shoulder, use 73040; elbow, use 73085; wrist, use 73115; hip, use 73525; knee, use 73580; ankle, use 73615)

☆✚ **75998** Fluoroscopic guidance for central venous access device placement, replacement (catheter only or complete), or removal (includes fluoroscopic guidance for vascular access and catheter manipulation, any necessary contrast injections through access site or catheter with related venography radiologic supervision and interpretation, and radiographic documentation of final catheter position) (List separately in addition to code for primary procedure)

➲ *CPT Changes: An Insider's View* 2004

(Do not use 76003 in conjunction with 75998)

(If formal extremity venography is performed from separate venous access and separately interpreted, use 36005 and 75820, 75822, 75825 or 75827)

♣ **76000** Fluoroscopy (separate procedure), up to one hour physician time, other than 71023 or 71034 (eg, cardiac fluoroscopy)

➲ *CPT Assistant* Apr 96:10, Nov 99:32, Dec 00:14, Apr 03:11, Jul 03:16, Aug 03:14; *CPT Changes: An Insider's View* 2000

☆ **76001** Fluoroscopy, physician time more than one hour, assisting a non-radiologic physician (eg, nephrostolithotomy, ERCP, bronchoscopy, transbronchial biopsy)

☆ **76003** Fluoroscopic guidance for needle placement (eg, biopsy, aspiration, injection, localization device)

➲ *CPT Assistant* Fall 93:14, Jul 01:3; *CPT Changes: An Insider's View* 2001

(See appropriate surgical code for procedure and anatomic location)

(Fluoroscopy 76003 is considered inclusive of all radiographic arthrography with the exception of supervision and interpretation for CT and MR arthrography)

(Do not report 76003 in addition to 70332, 73040, 73085, 73115, 73525, 73580, 73615)

(Fluoroscopy 76003 is considered inclusive of organ/anatomic specific radiological supervision and interpretation procedures 74320, 74350, 74355, 74445, 74470, 74475, 75809, 75810, 75885, 75887, 75980, 75982, 75989)

☆ **76005** Fluoroscopic guidance and localization of needle or catheter tip for spine or paraspinous diagnostic or therapeutic injection procedures (epidural, transforaminal epidural, subarachnoid, paravertebral facet joint, paravertebral facet joint nerve or sacroiliac joint), including neurolytic agent destruction

➲ *CPT Assistant* Nov 99:32, 34, 41, Jan 00:1, Feb 00:4, Aug 00:7, Sep 02:11; *CPT Changes: An Insider's View* 2000

(Injection of contrast during fluoroscopic guidance and localization is an inclusive component of codes 62263, 62264, 62270-62273, 62280-62282, 62310-62319, 0027T)

(Fluoroscopic guidance for subarachnoid puncture for diagnostic radiographic myelography is included in supervision and interpretation codes 72240, 72255, 72265, 72270)

(For epidural or subarachnoid needle or catheter placement and injection, see codes 62270-62273, 62280-62282, 62310-62319)

(For sacroiliac joint arthrography, see 27096, 73542. If formal arthrography is not performed, recorded, and a formal radiographic report is not issued, use 76005 for fluoroscopic guidance for sacroiliac joint injections)

(For paravertebral facet joint injection, see 64470-64476. For transforaminal epidural needle placement and injection, see 64479-64484)

(For destruction by neurolytic agent, see 64600-64680)

(For percutaneous or endoscopic lysis of epidural adhesions, codes 62263, 62264, 0027T include fluoroscopic guidance and localization)

✚♣ **76006** Manual application of stress performed by physician for joint radiography, including contralateral joint if indicated

➲ *CPT Assistant* Nov 98:21; *CPT Changes: An Insider's View* 2003

(For radiographic interpretation of stressed images, see appropriate anatomic site and number of views)

♣ **76010** Radiologic examination from nose to rectum for foreign body, single view, child

➲ *CPT Changes: An Insider's View* 2001

❖ **76012** Radiological supervision and interpretation, percutaneous vertebroplasty, per vertebral body; under fluoroscopic guidance

➲ *CPT Assistant* Mar 01:1 ; *CPT Changes: An Insider's View* 2001

❖ **76013** under CT guidance

➲ *CPT Assistant* Mar 01:1; *CPT Changes: An Insider's View* 2001

(For procedure, see 22520-22522)

♣ **76020** Bone age studies

♣ **76040** Bone length studies (orthoroentgenogram, scanogram)

♣ **76061** Radiologic examination, osseous survey; limited (eg, for metastases)

♣ **76062** complete (axial and appendicular skeleton)

♣ **76065** Radiologic examination, osseous survey, infant

♣ **76066** Joint survey, single view, two or more joints (specify)

➲ *CPT Changes: An Insider's View* 2002

❖ **76070** Computed tomography, bone mineral density study, one or more sites; axial skeleton (eg, hips, pelvis, spine)

❖ **76071** appendicular skeleton (peripheral) (eg, radius, wrist, heel)

➲ *CPT Changes: An Insider's View* 2003

❖▲ **76075** Dual energy x-ray absorptiometry (DXA), bone density study, one or more sites; axial skeleton (eg, hips, pelvis, spine)
➔ *CPT Assistant* Nov 97:24; *CPT Changes: An Insider's View* 2005

❖ **76076** appendicular skeleton (peripheral) (eg, radius, wrist, heel)
➔ *CPT Assistant* Nov 97:24; *CPT Changes: An Insider's View* 2005

♣● **76077** vertebral fracture assessment
➔ *CPT Changes: An Insider's View* 2005

(To report dual energy x-ray absorptiometry (►DXA◄) body composition study, one or more sites, use Category III code 0028T)

♣ **76078** Radiographic absorptiometry (eg, photodensitometry, radiogrammetry), one or more sites
➔ *CPT Assistant* Nov 97:24; *CPT Changes: An Insider's View* 2002

♣ **76080** Radiologic examination, abscess, fistula or sinus tract study, radiological supervision and interpretation
➔ *CPT Assistant* Nov 03:14

♠+ **76082** Computer aided detection (computer algorithm analysis of digital image data for lesion detection) with further physician review for interpretation, with or without digitization of film radiographic images; diagnostic mammography (List separately in addition to code for primary procedure)
➔ *CPT Changes: An Insider's View* 2004

(Use 76082 in conjunction with 76090 or 76091)

♠+ **76083** screening mammography (List separately in addition to code for primary procedure)
➔ *CPT Changes: An Insider's View* 2004

(Use 76083 in conjunction with 76092)

(76085 has been deleted. To report, see 76082, 76083)

♣ **76086** Mammary ductogram or galactogram, single duct, radiological supervision and interpretation

(For mammary ductogram or galactogram injection, use 19030)

♣ **76088** Mammary ductogram or galactogram, multiple ducts, radiological supervision and interpretation

⌘♠ **76090** Mammography; unilateral
➔ *CPT Assistant* Jul 96:6, Jun 99:10; *CPT Changes: An Insider's View* 2004

✶♠ **76091** bilateral
➔ *CPT Assistant* Jul 96:6; *CPT Changes: An Insider's View* 2004

(Use 76082 in conjunction with 76090 or 76091 for computer aided detection applied to a diagnostic mammogram)

✶♠ **76092** Screening mammography, bilateral (two view film study of each breast)
➔ *CPT Assistant* Jul 96:6, Jun 99:10; *CPT Changes: An Insider's View* 2004

(Use 76083 in conjunction with 76092 for computer aided detection applied to a screening mammogram)

(To report electrical impedance scan of the breast, bilateral, use Category III code 0060T)

⌘□ **76093** Magnetic resonance imaging, breast, without and/or with contrast material(s); unilateral

✶□ **76094** bilateral

§ **76095** Stereotactic localization guidance for breast biopsy or needle placement (eg, for wire localization or for injection), each lesion, radiological supervision and interpretation
➔ *CPT Assistant* Apr 96:9, Nov 97:24; *CPT Changes: An Insider's View* 2001

(For procedure, see 10022, 19000, 19001, 19102, 19103, 19290, 19291)

(For injection for sentinel node localization without lymphoscintigraphy, use 38792)

♣ **76096** Mammographic guidance for needle placement, breast (eg, for wire localization or for injection), each lesion, radiological supervision and interpretation
➔ *CPT Assistant* Jan 01:8; *CPT Changes: An Insider's View* 2001

(For procedure, see 10022, 19000, 19102, 19103, 19290, 19291)

(For injection for sentinel node localization without lymphoscintigraphy, use 38792)

♣ **76098** Radiological examination, surgical specimen

♣ **76100** Radiologic examination, single plane body section (eg, tomography), other than with urography

⌘♣ **76101** Radiologic examination, complex motion (ie, hypercycloidal) body section (eg, mastoid polytomography), other than with urography; unilateral

✶♣ **76102** bilateral

(For nephrotomography, use 74415)

♣ **76120** Cineradiography/videoradiography, except where specifically included
➔ *CPT Assistant* Sep 00:4, Apr 04:15; *CPT Changes: An Insider's View* 2002

♣+ **76125** Cineradiography/videoradiography to complement routine examination (List separately in addition to code for primary procedure)
➔ *CPT Assistant* Feb 03: 8

□ **76140** Consultation on x-ray examination made elsewhere, written report

♣ **76150** Xeroradiography

(76150 is to be used for non-mammographic studies only)

☆ **76350** Subtraction in conjunction with contrast studies

❖ **76355** Computed tomography guidance for stereotactic localization
➔ *CPT Changes: An Insider's View* 2002, 2003

❖ **76360** Computed tomography guidance for needle placement (eg, biopsy, aspiration, injection, localization device), radiological supervision and interpretation
➔ *CPT Assistant* Fall 93:12, Jan 01:8; *CPT Changes: An Insider's View* 2001, 2002, 2003

❖ **76362** Computed tomography guidance for, and monitoring of, visceral tissue ablation

➲ *CPT Changes: An Insider's View* 2002, 2004

(For percutaneous radiofrequency ablation, use 47382)

❖ **76370** Computed tomography guidance for placement of radiation therapy fields

➲ *CPT Assistant* Fall 91:12; *CPT Changes: An Insider's View* 2002, 2003

❖ **76375** Coronal, sagittal, multiplanar, oblique, 3-dimensional and/or holographic reconstruction of computed tomography, magnetic resonance imaging, or other tomographic modality

➲ *CPT Assistant* Apr 96:11, Nov 97:25, Jul 01:3, Sep 01:4, Mar 02:11, Oct 02:12; *CPT Changes: An Insider's View* 2002

(Use 76375 in addition to code for imaging procedure)

►(For computed tomographic colonography, see Category III codes 0066T, 0067T. Do not report 76375 in conjunction with 0066T, 0067T)◄

❖ **76380** Computed tomography, limited or localized follow-up study

➲ *CPT Changes: An Insider's View* 2002, 2003

☐ **76390** Magnetic resonance spectroscopy

(For magnetic resonance imaging, use appropriate MRI body site code)

❖ **76393** Magnetic resonance guidance for needle placement (eg, for biopsy, needle aspiration, injection, or placement of localization device) radiological supervision and interpretation

➲ *CPT Assistant* Jan 01:8; *CPT Changes: An Insider's View* 2001, 2002

(For procedure see appropriate organ or site)

❖ **76394** Magnetic resonance guidance for, and monitoring of, visceral tissue ablation

➲ *CPT Assistant* Oct 02:1; *CPT Changes: An Insider's View* 2002, 2004

(For percutaneous radiofrequency ablation, use 47382)

►(For focused ultrasound ablation treatment of uterine leiomyomata, see Category III codes 0071T, 0072T)◄

❖ **76400** Magnetic resonance (eg, proton) imaging, bone marrow blood supply

(76490 has been deleted. To report, use 76940)

♣ **76496** Unlisted fluoroscopic procedure (eg, diagnostic, interventional)

➲ *CPT Changes: An Insider's View* 2003

❖ **76497** Unlisted computed tomography procedure (eg, diagnostic, interventional)

➲ *CPT Changes: An Insider's View* 2003

❖ **76498** Unlisted magnetic resonance procedure (eg, diagnostic, interventional)

➲ *CPT Changes: An Insider's View* 2003

♣ **76499** Unlisted diagnostic radiographic procedure

➲ *CPT Assistant* Jul 99:10, Sep 00:4, Apr 04:15; *CPT Changes: An Insider's View* 2003

Diagnostic Ultrasound

►All diagnostic ultrasound examinations require permanently recorded images with measurements, when such measurements are clinically indicated. For those codes whose sole diagnostic goal is a biometric measure (ie, 76514, 76516, and 76519), permanently recorded images are not required. A final, written report should be issued for inclusion in the patient's medical record. The prescription form for the intraocular lens satisfies the written report requirement for 76519. For those anatomic regions that have "complete" and "limited" ultrasound codes, note the elements that comprise a "complete" exam. The report should contain a description of these elements or the reason that an element could not be visualized (eg, obscured by bowel gas, surgically absent etc.).◄

►If less than the required elements for a "complete" exam are reported (eg, limited number of organs or limited portion of region evaluated), the "limited" code for that anatomic region should be used once per patient exam session. A "limited" exam of an anatomic region should not be reported for the same exam session as a "complete" exam of that same region.◄

►Doppler evaluation of vascular structures (other than color flow used only for anatomic structure identification) is separately reportable. To report, see Non-Invasive Vascular Diagnostic Studies (93875-93990).◄

►Ultrasound guidance procedures also require permanently recorded images of the site to be localized, as well as a documented description of the localization process, either separately or within the report of the procedure for which the guidance is utilized.◄

►Use of ultrasound, without thorough evaluation of organ(s) or anatomic region, image documentation, and final, written report, is not separately reportable.◄

Definitions

A-mode implies a one-dimensional ultrasonic measurement procedure.

M-mode implies a one-dimensional ultrasonic measurement procedure with movement of the trace to record amplitude and velocity of moving echo-producing structures.

B-scan implies a two-dimensional ultrasonic scanning procedure with a two-dimensional display.

Real-time scan implies a two-dimensional ultrasonic scanning procedure with display of both two-dimensional structure and motion with time.

(To report diagnostic vascular ultrasound studies, see 93875-93990)

►(For focused ultrasound ablation treatment of uterine leiomyomata, see Category III codes 0071T, 0072T)◄

Head and Neck

❖ **76506** Echoencephalography, B-scan and/or real time with image documentation (gray scale) (for determination of ventricular size, delineation of cerebral contents and detection of fluid masses or other intracranial abnormalities), including A-mode encephalography as secondary component where indicated

+❖● **76510** Ophthalmic ultrasound, diagnostic; B-scan and quantitative A-scan performed during the same patient encounter

➲ *CPT Changes: An Insider's View* 2005

+❖▲ **76511** quantitative A-scan only

➲ *CPT Assistant* Oct 96:9, Nov 99:42; *CPT Changes: An Insider's View* 2005

+❖▲ **76512** B-scan (with or without superimposed non-quantitative A-scan)

➲ *CPT Assistant* Oct 96:9

+❖ **76513** anterior segment ultrasound, immersion (water bath) B-scan or high resolution biomicroscopy

➲ *CPT Assistant* Nov 99:42; *CPT Changes: An Insider's View* 2000

✶♣ **76514** corneal pachymetry, unilateral or bilateral (determination of corneal thickness)

➲ *CPT Changes: An Insider's View* 2004

✶❖ **76516** Ophthalmic biometry by ultrasound echography, A-scan;

✶❖ **76519** with intraocular lens power calculation

(For partial coherence interferometry, use 92136)

+❖ **76529** Ophthalmic ultrasonic foreign body localization

❖ **76536** Ultrasound, soft tissues of head and neck (eg, thyroid, parathyroid, parotid), B-scan and/or real time with image documentation

➲ *CPT Changes: An Insider's View* 2002

Chest

❖ **76604** Ultrasound, chest, B-scan (includes mediastinum) and/or real time with image documentation

➲ *CPT Changes: An Insider's View* 2002

✶❖ **76645** Ultrasound, breast(s) (unilateral or bilateral), B-scan and/or real time with image documentation

➲ *CPT Changes: An Insider's View* 2002

Abdomen and Retroperitoneum

►A complete ultrasound examination of the abdomen (76700) consists of B mode scans of: liver, gall bladder, common bile duct, pancreas, spleen, kidneys, and the upper abdominal aorta and inferior vena cava including any demonstrated abdominal abnormality.◄

►A complete ultrasound examination of the retroperitoneum (76770) consists of B mode scans of: kidneys, abdominal aorta, common iliac artery origins, and inferior vena cava, including any demonstrated retroperitoneal abnormality. Alternatively, if clinical history suggests urinary tract pathology, complete evaluation of the kidneys and urinary bladder also comprises a complete retroperitoneal ultrasound.◄

►Use of ultrasound, without thorough evaluation of organ(s) or anatomic region, image documentation and final, written report, is not separately reportable.◄

❖ **76700** Ultrasound, abdominal, B-scan and/or real time with image documentation; complete

➲ *CPT Assistant* Fall 93:13, Oct 01:1; *CPT Changes: An Insider's View* 2002

❖ **76705** limited (eg, single organ, quadrant, follow-up)

➲ *CPT Assistant* Fall 93:13, Oct 01:1, Apr 03:27

❖ **76770** Ultrasound, retroperitoneal (eg, renal, aorta, nodes), B-scan and/or real time with image documentation; complete

➲ *CPT Assistant* May 99:10, Jun 99:10; *CPT Changes: An Insider's View* 2002

❖ **76775** limited

➲ *CPT Assistant* May 99:10, Jun 99:10

❖ **76778** Ultrasound, transplanted kidney, B-scan and/or real time with image documentation, with or without duplex Doppler study

➲ *CPT Changes: An Insider's View* 2002

Spinal Canal

❖ **76800** Ultrasound, spinal canal and contents

➲ *CPT Assistant* Apr 98:15; *CPT Changes: An Insider's View* 2002

Pelvis

Obstetrical

Codes 76801 and 76802 include determination of the number of gestational sacs and fetuses, gestational sac/fetal measurements appropriate for gestation (<14 weeks 0 days), survey of visible fetal and placental anatomic structure, qualitative assessment of amniotic fluid volume/gestational sac shape and examination of the maternal uterus and adnexa.

Codes 76805 and 76810 include determination of number of fetuses and amniotic/chorionic sacs, measurements appropriate for gestational age (> or = 14 weeks 0 days), survey of intracranial/spinal/abdominal anatomy, 4 chambered heart, umbilical cord insertion site, placenta location and amniotic fluid assessment and, when visible, examination of maternal adnexa.

Codes 76811 and 76812 include all elements of codes 76805 and 76810 plus detailed anatomic evaluation of the fetal brain/ventricles, face, heart/outflow tracts and chest anatomy, abdominal organ specific anatomy, number/length/architecture of limbs and detailed evaluation of the umbilical cord and placenta and other fetal anatomy as clinically indicated.

Report should document the results of the evaluation of each element described above or the reason for non-visualization.

Code 76815 represents a focused "quick look" exam limited to the assessment of one or more of the elements listed in code 76815.

Code 76816 describes an examination designed to reassess fetal size and interval growth or reevaluate one or more anatomic abnormalities of a fetus previously demonstrated on ultrasound, and should be coded once for each fetus requiring reevaluation using modifier 59 for each fetus after the first.

Code 76817 describes a transvaginal obstetric ultrasound performed separately or in addition to one of the transabdominal examinations described above. For transvaginal examinations performed for non-obstetrical purposes, use code 76830.

❖ **76801** Ultrasound, pregnant uterus, real time with image documentation, fetal and maternal evaluation, first trimester (<14 weeks 0 days), transabdominal approach; single or first gestation

➔ *CPT Assistant* Mar 03:7; *CPT Changes: An Insider's View* 2003

❖+ **76802** each additional gestation (List separately in addition to code for primary procedure)

➔ *CPT Assistant* Mar 03:7; *CPT Changes: An Insider's View* 2003

(Use 76802 in conjunction with 76801)

❖ **76805** Ultrasound, pregnant uterus, real time with image documentation, fetal and maternal evaluation, after first trimester (> or = 14 weeks 0 days), transabdominal approach; single or first gestation

➔ *CPT Assistant* Apr 97:2, Nov 97:25, Oct 01:1, Mar 03:7; *CPT Changes: An Insider's View* 2002, 2003

❖+ **76810** each additional gestation (List separately in addition to code for primary procedure)

➔ *CPT Assistant* Apr 97:2, Oct 01:1, Mar 03:7; *CPT Changes: An Insider's View* 2003

(Use 76810 in conjunction with 76805)

❖ **76811** Ultrasound, pregnant uterus, real time with image documentation, fetal and maternal evaluation plus detailed fetal anatomic examination, transabdominal approach; single or first gestation

➔ *CPT Assistant* Mar 03:7; *CPT Changes: An Insider's View* 2003

❖+ **76812** each additional gestation (List separately in addition to code for primary procedure)

➔ *CPT Assistant* Mar 03:7; *CPT Changes: An Insider's View* 2003

(Use 76812 in conjunction with 76811)

❖ **76815** Ultrasound, pregnant uterus, real time with image documentation, limited (eg, fetal heart beat, placental location, fetal position and/or qualitative amniotic fluid volume), one or more fetuses

➔ *CPT Assistant* Apr 97:2, Nov 97:25, Oct 01:1, Dec 01:6, Mar 03:7, Nov 03:14; *CPT Changes: An Insider's View* 2003

(Use 76815 only once per exam and not per element)

❖ **76816** Ultrasound, pregnant uterus, real time with image documentation, follow-up (eg, re-evaluation of fetal size by measuring standard growth parameters and amniotic fluid volume, re-evaluation of organ system(s) suspected or confirmed to be abnormal on a previous scan), transabdominal approach, per fetus

➔ *CPT Assistant* Apr 97:2, Oct 01:1, Mar 03:7; *CPT Changes: An Insider's View* 2003

(Report 76816 with modifier 59 for each additional fetus examined in a multiple pregnancy)

❖ **76817** Ultrasound, pregnant uterus, real time with image documentation, transvaginal

➔ *CPT Assistant* Mar 03:7; *CPT Changes: An Insider's View* 2003

(For non-obstetrical transvaginal ultrasound, use 76830)

(If transvaginal examination is done in addition to transabdominal obstetrical ultrasound exam, use 76817 in addition to appropriate transabdominal exam code)

❖ **76818** Fetal biophysical profile; with non-stress testing

➔ *CPT Assistant* Apr 97:2, May 98:10, Sep 01:4, Dec 01:6, Mar 03:7; *CPT Changes: An Insider's View* 2001

❖ **76819** without non-stress testing

➔ *CPT Assistant* Sep 01:4, Dec 01:6; *CPT Changes: An Insider's View* 2001, 2002

(Fetal biophysical profile assessments for the second and any additional fetuses, should be reported separately by code 76818 or 76819 with the modifier 59 appended)

(For amniotic fluid index without non-stress test, use 76815)

❖● **76820** Doppler velocimetry, fetal; umbilical artery

➔ *CPT Changes: An Insider's View* 2005

❖● **76821** middle cerebral artery

➔ *CPT Changes: An Insider's View* 2005

❖ **76825** Echocardiography, fetal, cardiovascular system, real time with image documentation (2D), with or without M-mode recording;

➔ *CPT Assistant* Apr 97:2

❖ **76826** follow-up or repeat study

➔ *CPT Assistant* Apr 97:2

❖▲ **76827** Doppler echocardiography, fetal, pulsed wave and/or continuous wave with spectral display; complete

➔ *CPT Assistant* Apr 97:2

❖ **76828** follow-up or repeat study

➔ *CPT Assistant* Apr 97:2

(To report the use of color mapping, use 93325)

Non-Obstetrical

►Code 76856 includes the complete evaluation of the female pelvic anatomy. Elements of this examination include a description and measurements of the uterus and adnexal structures, measurement of the endometrium, measurement of the bladder (when applicable), and a description of any pelvic pathology (eg, ovarian cysts, uterine leiomyomata, free pelvic fluid).◄

►Code 76856 is also applicable to a complete evaluation of the male pelvis. Elements of the examination include evaluation and measurement (when applicable) of the urinary bladder, evaluation of the prostate and seminal vesicles to the extent that they are visualized transabdominally, and any pelvic pathology (eg, bladder tumor, enlarged prostate, free pelvic fluid, pelvic abscess).◄

►Code 76857 represents a focused examination limited to the assessment of one or more elements listed in code 76856 and/or the reevaluation of one or more pelvic abnormalities previously demonstrated on ultrasound. Code 76857, rather than 76770, should be utilized if the urinary bladder alone (ie, not including the kidneys) is imaged, whereas code 51798 should be utilized if a bladder volume or post-void residual measurement is obtained without imaging the bladder.◄

►Use of ultrasound, without thorough evaluation of organ(s) or anatomic region, image documentation, and final, written report, is not separately reportable.◄

❖ **76830** Ultrasound, transvaginal

➔ *CPT Assistant* Aug 96:10, Jul 99:8; *CPT Changes: An Insider's View* 2002

(For obstetrical transvaginal ultrasound, use 76817)

(If transvaginal examination is done in addition to transabdominal non-obstetrical ultrasound exam, use 76830 in addition to appropriate transabdominal exam code)

❖ **76831** Saline infusion sonohysterography (SIS), including color flow Doppler, when performed

➔ *CPT Assistant* Nov 97:25, Jul 99:8; *CPT Changes: An Insider's View* 2004

(For introduction of saline for saline infusion sonohysterography, use 58340)

❖ **76856** Ultrasound, pelvic (nonobstetric), B-scan and/or real time with image documentation; complete

➔ *CPT Assistant* Oct 01:1; *CPT Changes: An Insider's View* 2002

❖ **76857** limited or follow-up (eg, for follicles)

Genitalia

❖ **76870** Ultrasound, scrotum and contents

➔ *CPT Changes: An Insider's View* 2002

❖ **76872** Ultrasound, transrectal;

➔ *CPT Assistant* May 96:3, Nov 99:42; *CPT Changes: An Insider's View* 2000, 2004

❖ **76873** prostate volume study for brachytherapy treatment planning (separate procedure)

➔ *CPT Assistant* Nov 99:42; *CPT Changes: An Insider's View* 2000

Extremities

❖ **76880** Ultrasound, extremity, non-vascular, B-scan and/or real time with image documentation

➔ *CPT Changes: An Insider's View* 2002

❖ **76885** Ultrasound, infant hips, real time with imaging documentation; dynamic (requiring physician manipulation)

➔ *CPT Assistant* Nov 97:25; *CPT Changes: An Insider's View* 2002

❖ **76886** limited, static (not requiring physician manipulation)

➔ *CPT Assistant* Nov 97:25; *CPT Changes: An Insider's View* 2002

Ultrasonic Guidance Procedures

❖ **76930** Ultrasonic guidance for pericardiocentesis, imaging supervision and interpretation

➔ *CPT Changes: An Insider's View* 2001

❖ **76932** Ultrasonic guidance for endomyocardial biopsy, imaging supervision and interpretation

➔ *CPT Changes: An Insider's View* 2001

❖ **76936** Ultrasound guided compression repair of arterial pseudoaneurysm or arteriovenous fistulae (includes diagnostic ultrasound evaluation, compression of lesion and imaging)

☆✚ **76937** Ultrasound guidance for vascular access requiring ultrasound evaluation of potential access sites, documentation of selected vessel patency, concurrent realtime ultrasound visualization of vascular needle entry, with permanent recording and reporting (List separately in addition to code for primary procedure)

➔ *CPT Changes: An Insider's View* 2004

(Do not use 76937 in conjunction with 76942)

(If extremity venous non-invasive vascular diagnostic study is performed separate from venous access guidance, use 93965, 93970 or 93971)

❖ **76940** Ultrasound guidance for, and monitoring of, visceral tissue ablation

➔ *CPT Changes: An Insider's View* 2004

(Do not report 76940 in conjunction with 76986)

(For ablation, see 47370-47382)

❖ **76941** Ultrasonic guidance for intrauterine fetal transfusion or cordocentesis, imaging supervision and interpretation

➔ *CPT Changes: An Insider's View* 2001

(For procedure, see 36460, 59012)

❖ **76942** Ultrasonic guidance for needle placement (eg, biopsy, aspiration, injection, localization device), imaging supervision and interpretation

➔ *CPT Assistant* Fall 93:12, May 96:3, Jun 97:5, Oct 01:1; *CPT Changes: An Insider's View* 2001

(Do not report 76942 in conjunction with 43232, 43237, 43242, 45341, 45342, or 76975)

(For microwave thermotherapy of the breast, use Category III code 0061T)

❖ **76945** Ultrasonic guidance for chorionic villus sampling, imaging supervision and interpretation

➔ *CPT Changes: An Insider's View* 2001

(For procedure, use 59015)

❖ **76946** Ultrasonic guidance for amniocentesis, imaging supervision and interpretation

➔ *CPT Changes: An Insider's View* 2001

❖ **76948** Ultrasonic guidance for aspiration of ova, imaging supervision and interpretation

➔ *CPT Changes: An Insider's View* 2001

❖ **76950** Ultrasonic guidance for placement of radiation therapy fields

➔ *CPT Changes: An Insider's View* 2001

❖ **76965** Ultrasonic guidance for interstitial radioelement application

Other Procedures

❖ **76970** Ultrasound study follow-up (specify)

❖ **76975** Gastrointestinal endoscopic ultrasound, supervision and interpretation

➔ *CPT Assistant* Spring 94:5; *CPT Changes: An Insider's View* 2001

(Do not report 76975 in conjunction with 43231, 43232, 43237, 43238, 43242, 43259, 45341, 45342, or 76942)

♣ **76977** Ultrasound bone density measurement and interpretation, peripheral site(s), any method

➔ *CPT Assistant* Nov 98:21

❖ **76986** Ultrasonic guidance, intraoperative

➔ *CPT Changes: An Insider's View* 2001

(Do not report 76986 in addition to 47370-47382)

(For ultrasound guidance for open and laparoscopic radiofrequency tissue ablation, use 76940)

❖ **76999** Unlisted ultrasound procedure (eg, diagnostic, interventional)

➔ *CPT Changes: An Insider's View* 2003

Radiation Oncology

Listings for Radiation Oncology provide for teletherapy and brachytherapy to include initial consultation, clinical treatment planning, simulation, medical radiation physics, dosimetry, treatment devices, special services, and clinical treatment management procedures. They include normal follow-up care during course of treatment and for three months following its completion.

When a service or procedure is provided that is not listed in this edition of *CPT* it should be identified by a Special Report (see page 274) and one of the unlisted procedure codes listed below:

77299 Unlisted procedure, therapeutic radiology clinical treatment planning

77399 Unlisted procedure, medical radiation physics, dosimetry and treatment devices, and special services

77499 Unlisted procedure, therapeutic radiology treatment management

77799 Unlisted procedure, clinical brachytherapy

For treatment by injectable or ingestible isotopes, see subsection **Nuclear Medicine.**

Consultation: Clinical Management

Preliminary consultation, evaluation of patient prior to decision to treat, or full medical care (in addition to treatment management) when provided by the therapeutic radiologist may be identified by the appropriate procedure codes from **Evaluation and Management, Medicine,** or **Surgery** sections.

Clinical Treatment Planning (External and Internal Sources)

The clinical treatment planning process is a complex service including interpretation of special testing, tumor localization, treatment volume determination, treatment time/dosage determination, choice of treatment modality, determination of number and size of treatment ports, selection of appropriate treatment devices, and other procedures.

Definitions

Simple planning requires a single treatment area of interest encompassed in a single port or simple parallel opposed ports with simple or no blocking.

Intermediate planning requires three or more converging ports, two separate treatment areas, multiple blocks, or special time dose constraints.

Complex planning requires highly complex blocking, custom shielding blocks, tangential ports, special wedges or compensators, three or more separate treatment areas, rotational or special beam considerations, combination of therapeutic modalities.

☐ **77261** Therapeutic radiology treatment planning; simple

☐ **77262** intermediate

☐ **77263** complex

Definitions

Simple simulation of a single treatment area with either a single port or parallel opposed ports. Simple or no blocking.

Intermediate simulation of three or more converging ports, two separate treatment areas, multiple blocks.

Complex simulation of tangential portals, three or more treatment areas, rotation or arc therapy, complex blocking, custom shielding blocks, brachytherapy source verification, hyperthermia probe verification, any use of contrast materials.

Three-dimensional computer-generated three dimensional reconstruction of tumor volume and surrounding critical normal tissue structures from direct CT scans and/or MRI data in preparation for non-coplanar or coplanar therapy. The simulation utilizes documented three-dimensional beam's eye view volume-dose displays of multiple or moving beams. Documentation with three-dimensional volume reconstruction and dose distribution is required.

Simulation may be carried out on a dedicated simulator, a radiation therapy treatment unit, or diagnostic x-ray machine.

♣ **77280** Therapeutic radiology simulation-aided field setting; simple
➲ *CPT Assistant* Oct 97:1, Nov 97:26

♣ **77285** intermediate
➲ *CPT Assistant* Oct 97:1

♣ **77290** complex
➲ *CPT Assistant* Fall 91:12, Oct 97:1

♣ **77295** three-dimensional
➲ *CPT Assistant* Oct 97:1, Nov 97:26

☐ **77299** Unlisted procedure, therapeutic radiology clinical treatment planning

Medical Radiation Physics, Dosimetry, Treatment Devices, and Special Services

♣ **77300** Basic radiation dosimetry calculation, central axis depth dose calculation, TDF, NSD, gap calculation, off axis factor, tissue inhomogeneity factors, calculation of non-ionizing radiation surface and depth dose, as required during course of treatment, only when prescribed by the treating physician
➲ *CPT Assistant* Fall 91:13, Oct 97:1; *CPT Changes: An Insider's View* 2002

♣ **77301** Intensity modulated radiotherapy plan, including dose-volume histograms for target and critical structure partial tolerance specifications
➲ *CPT Changes: An Insider's View* 2002

(Dose plan is optimized using inverse or forward planning technique for modulated beam delivery (eg, binary, dynamic MLC) to create highly conformal dose distribution. Computer plan distribution must be verified for positional accuracy based on dosimetric verification of the intensity map with verification of treatment set-up and interpretation of verification methodology)

♣ **77305** Teletherapy, isodose plan (whether hand or computer calculated); simple (one or two parallel opposed unmodified ports directed to a single area of interest)
➲ *CPT Assistant* Oct 97:1

♣ **77310** intermediate (three or more treatment ports directed to a single area of interest)
➲ *CPT Assistant* Oct 97:1

♣ **77315** complex (mantle or inverted Y, tangential ports, the use of wedges, compensators, complex blocking, rotational beam, or special beam considerations)
➲ *CPT Assistant* Fall 91:13, Oct 97:1

(Only one teletherapy isodose plan may be reported for a given course of therapy to a specific treatment area)

♣ **77321** Special teletherapy port plan, particles, hemibody, total body

♣ **77326** Brachytherapy isodose plan; simple (calculation made from single plane, one to four sources/ribbon application, remote afterloading brachytherapy, 1 to 8 sources)
➲ *CPT Assistant* Winter 91:17; *CPT Changes: An Insider's View* 2003

(For definition of source/ribbon, see page 297)

♣ **77327** intermediate (multiplane dosage calculations, application involving 5 to 10 sources/ribbons, remote afterloading brachytherapy, 9 to 12 sources)
➲ *CPT Assistant* Winter 91:17

♣ **77328** complex (multiplane isodose plan, volume implant calculations, over 10 sources/ribbons used, special spatial reconstruction, remote afterloading brachytherapy, over 12 sources)
➲ *CPT Assistant* Winter 91:17

♣ **77331** Special dosimetry (eg, TLD, microdosimetry) (specify), only when prescribed by the treating physician
➲ *CPT Assistant* Fall 91:13, Oct 97:1

♣ **77332** Treatment devices, design and construction; simple (simple block, simple bolus)
➲ *CPT Assistant* Oct 97:1

♣ **77333** intermediate (multiple blocks, stents, bite blocks, special bolus)
➲ *CPT Assistant* Oct 97:1

♣ **77334** complex (irregular blocks, special shields, compensators, wedges, molds or casts)
➲ *CPT Assistant* Fall 91:13, Oct 97:1

♣ **77336** Continuing medical physics consultation, including assessment of treatment parameters, quality assurance of dose delivery, and review of patient treatment documentation in support of the radiation oncologist, reported per week of therapy
➲ *CPT Assistant* Fall 91:13, Oct 97:1, Nov 98:21

♣ **77370** Special medical radiation physics consultation
➲ *CPT Assistant* Fall 91:14, Oct 97:1

♣ **77399** Unlisted procedure, medical radiation physics, dosimetry and treatment devices, and special services
➲ *CPT Assistant* Nov 98:21

Radiation Treatment Delivery

(Radiation treatment delivery (77401-77416) recognizes the technical component and the various energy levels.)

►(For stereotactic body radiation therapy treatment delivery, use Category III code 0082T)◄

❖ **77401** Radiation treatment delivery, superficial and/or ortho voltage
➲ *CPT Assistant* Apr 03:13, 14, Aug 03:10

❖ **77402** Radiation treatment delivery, single treatment area, single port or parallel opposed ports, simple blocks or no blocks; up to 5 MeV
➲ *CPT Assistant* Apr 03:13, 14, Aug 03:10

❖ **77403** 6-10 MeV
➲ *CPT Assistant* Apr 03:13, 14, Aug 03:10

❖ **77404** 11-19 MeV
➲ *CPT Assistant* Apr 03:13, 14, Aug 03:10

❖ **77406** 20 MeV or greater
➲ *CPT Assistant* Apr 03:13, 14, Aug 03:10

❖ **77407** Radiation treatment delivery, two separate treatment areas, three or more ports on a single treatment area, use of multiple blocks; up to 5 MeV
➲ *CPT Assistant* Apr 03:13, 14, Aug 03:10

❖ **77408** 6-10 MeV
➲ *CPT Assistant* Apr 03:13, 14, Aug 03:10

❖ **77409** 11-19 MeV
➲ *CPT Assistant* Apr 03:13, 14, Aug 03:10

❖ **77411** 20 MeV or greater
➲ *CPT Assistant* Apr 03:13, 14, Aug 03:10

❖ **77412** Radiation treatment delivery, three or more separate treatment areas, custom blocking, tangential ports, wedges, rotational beam, compensators, special particle beam (eg, electron or neutrons); up to 5 MeV
➲ *CPT Assistant* Apr 03:13, 14, Aug 03:10

❖ **77413** 6-10 MeV
➲ *CPT Assistant* Fall 91:14, Apr 03:13, 14, Aug 03:10

❖ **77414** 11-19 MeV
➲ *CPT Assistant* Apr 03:13, 14, Aug 03:10

❖ **77416** 20 MeV or greater
➲ *CPT Assistant* Apr 03:13, 14, Aug 03:10

♣ **77417** Therapeutic radiology port film(s)
➲ *CPT Assistant* Fall 91:14, Dec 97:11

❖▲ **77418** Intensity modulated treatment delivery, single or multiple fields/arcs, via narrow spatially and temporally modulated beams, binary, dynamic MLC, per treatment session
➲ *CPT Changes: An Insider's View* 2002, 2005

(For intensity modulated treatment planning, use 77301)

►(For compensator-based beam modulation treatment delivery, use Category III code 0073T)◄

Radiation Treatment Management

Radiation treatment management is reported in units of five fractions or treatment sessions, regardless of the actual time period in which the services are furnished. The services need not be furnished on consecutive days. Multiple fractions representing two or more treatment sessions furnished on the same day may be counted separately as long as there has been a distinct break in therapy sessions, and the fractions are of the character usually furnished on different days. Code 77427 is also reported if there are three or four fractions beyond a multiple of five at the end of a course of treatment; one or two fractions beyond a multiple of five at the end of a course of treatment are not reported separately. The professional services furnished during treatment management typically consist of:

- Review of port films;
- Review of dosimetry, dose delivery, and treatment parameters;
- Review of patient treatment set-up;
- Examination of patient for medical evaluation and management (eg, assessment of the patient's response to treatment, coordination of care and treatment, review of imaging and/or lab test results).

□ **77427** Radiation treatment management, five treatments

□ **77431** Radiation therapy management with complete course of therapy consisting of one or two fractions only

(77431 is not to be used to fill in the last week of a long course of therapy)

□ **77432** Stereotactic radiation treatment management of cerebral lesion(s) (complete course of treatment consisting of one session)

►(For stereotactic body radiation therapy treatment management, use Category III code 0083T)◄

❖ **77470** Special treatment procedure (eg, total body irradiation, hemibody radiation, per oral, endocavitary or intraoperative cone irradiation)
➲ *CPT Assistant* Winter 91:22, Oct 97:1; *CPT Changes: An Insider's View* 2001

(77470 assumes that the procedure is performed one or more times during the course of therapy, in addition to daily or weekly patient management)

□ **77499** Unlisted procedure, therapeutic radiology treatment management

Proton Beam Treatment Delivery

Definitions

Simple proton treatment delivery to a single treatment area utilizing a single non-tangential/oblique port, custom block with compensation (77522) and without compensation (77520).

Intermediate proton treatment delivery to one or more treatment areas utilizing two or more ports or one or more tangential/oblique ports, with custom blocks and compensators.

Complex proton treatment delivery to one or more treatment areas utilizing two or more ports per treatment area with matching or patching fields and/or multiple isocenters, with custom blocks and compensators.

❖ **77520** Proton treatment delivery; simple, without compensation
➲ *CPT Assistant* Nov 99:43; *CPT Changes: An Insider's View* 2000, 2001

❖ **77522** simple, with compensation
➲ *CPT Changes: An Insider's View* 2001

❖ **77523** intermediate
➲ *CPT Assistant* Nov 99:43; *CPT Changes: An Insider's View* 2000, 2001

❖ **77525** complex
➲ *CPT Changes: An Insider's View* 2001

Hyperthermia

Hyperthermia treatments as listed in this section include external (superficial and deep), interstitial, and intracavitary.

Radiation therapy when given concurrently is listed separately.

Hyperthermia is used only as an adjunct to radiation therapy or chemotherapy. It may be induced by a variety of sources (eg, microwave, ultrasound, low energy radio-frequency conduction, or by probes).

The listed treatments include management during the course of therapy and follow-up care for three months after completion.

Preliminary consultation is not included (see **Medicine** 99241-99263).

Physics planning and interstitial insertion of temperature sensors, and use of external or interstitial heat generating sources are included.

The following descriptors are included in the treatment schedule:

❖⊙ **77600** Hyperthermia, externally generated; superficial (ie, heating to a depth of 4 cm or less)
➲ *CPT Assistant* Winter 91:22

❖⊙ **77605** deep (ie, heating to depths greater than 4 cm)
➲ *CPT Assistant* Winter 91:22

❖⊙ **77610** Hyperthermia generated by interstitial probe(s); 5 or fewer interstitial applicators
➲ *CPT Assistant* Winter 91:22

❖⊙ **77615** more than 5 interstitial applicators
➲ *CPT Assistant* Winter 91:22

Clinical Intracavitary Hyperthermia

❖ **77620** Hyperthermia generated by intracavitary probe(s)

Clinical Brachytherapy

Clinical brachytherapy requires the use of either natural or man-made radioelements applied into or around a treatment field of interest. The supervision of radioelements and dose interpretation are performed solely by the therapeutic radiologist.

Services 77750-77799 include admission to the hospital and daily visits.

For insertion of ovoids and tandems, use 57155.

For insertion of Heyman capsules, use 58346.

Definitions

(Sources refer to intracavitary placement or permanent interstitial placement; ribbons refer to temporary interstitial placement)

A ***simple*** application has one to four sources/ribbons.

An ***intermediate*** application has five to ten sources/ribbons.

A ***complex*** application has greater than ten sources/ribbons.

❖▲ **77750** Infusion or instillation of radioelement solution (includes three months follow-up care)
➲ *CPT Assistant* Apr 03:11; *CPT Changes: An Insider's View* 2005

(For administration of radiolabeled monoclonal antibodies, ►use◄ 79403)

►(For non-antibody radiopharmaceutical therapy by intravenous administration only, not including three month follow-up care, use 79101)◄

❖ **77761** Intracavitary radiation source application; simple
➲ *CPT Assistant* Winter 91:23, Jan 96:7, Mar 99:3; *CPT Changes: An Insider's View* 2001

❖ **77762** intermediate
➲ *CPT Assistant* Winter 91:23

❖ **77763** complex
➲ *CPT Assistant* Winter 91:23, Mar 99:3

❖ **77776** Interstitial radiation source application; simple
➲ *CPT Assistant* Winter 91:23, Apr 03: 7; *CPT Changes: An Insider's View* 2001

❖ **77777** intermediate
➲ *CPT Assistant* Winter 91:23, Apr 03:7

❖ **77778** complex
➲ *CPT Assistant* Winter 91:23, Apr 03:7; *CPT Changes: An Insider's View* 2005

❖ **77781** Remote afterloading high intensity brachytherapy; 1-4 source positions or catheters
➲ *CPT Assistant* Winter 91:23, Mar 99:3, Apr 03:8

❖ **77782** 5-8 source positions or catheters
➲ *CPT Assistant* Winter 91:23, Mar 99:3, Apr 03:8

❖ **77783** 9-12 source positions or catheters
➲ *CPT Assistant* Winter 91:23, Mar 99:3, Apr 03:8

❖ **77784** over 12 source positions or catheters
➲ *CPT Assistant* Winter 91:23, Mar 99:3, Apr 03:8

❖ **77789** Surface application of radiation source
➲ *CPT Changes: An Insider's View* 2001

☆ **77790** Supervision, handling, loading of radiation source
➔ *CPT Changes: An Insider's View* 2001

❖ **77799** Unlisted procedure, clinical brachytherapy

Nuclear Medicine

Listed procedures may be performed independently or in the course of overall medical care. If the physician providing these services is also responsible for diagnostic work-up and/or follow-up care of patient, see appropriate sections also.

Radioimmunoassay tests are found in the **Clinical Pathology** section (codes 82000-84999). These codes can be appropriately used by any specialist performing such tests in a laboratory licensed and/or certified for radioimmunoassays. The reporting of these tests is not confined to clinical pathology laboratories alone.

The services listed do not include the provision of radium or other radioelements. ►Diagnostic and therapeutic radiopharmaceuticals supplied by the physician should be reported separately.◄

Diagnostic

Endocrine System

❖ **78000** Thyroid uptake; single determination

❖ **78001** multiple determinations

❖ **78003** stimulation, suppression or discharge (not including initial uptake studies)

❖ **78006** Thyroid imaging, with uptake; single determination

❖ **78007** multiple determinations

❖ **78010** Thyroid imaging; only

❖ **78011** with vascular flow

❖ **78015** Thyroid carcinoma metastases imaging; limited area (eg, neck and chest only)
➔ *CPT Assistant* Nov 98:21

❖ **78016** with additional studies (eg, urinary recovery)

❖ **78018** whole body

❖+ **78020** Thyroid carcinoma metastases uptake (List separately in addition to code for primary procedure)
➔ *CPT Assistant* Nov 98:21, Apr 99:4

(Use 78020 in conjunction with 78018 only)

❖ **78070** Parathyroid imaging

❖ **78075** Adrenal imaging, cortex and/or medulla

❖ **78099** Unlisted endocrine procedure, diagnostic nuclear medicine

(For chemical analysis, see **Chemistry** section)

Hematopoietic, Reticuloendothelial and Lymphatic System

❖ **78102** Bone marrow imaging; limited area

❖ **78103** multiple areas

❖ **78104** whole body

❖ **78110** Plasma volume, radiopharmaceutical volume-dilution technique (separate procedure); single sampling

❖ **78111** multiple samplings

❖ **78120** Red cell volume determination (separate procedure); single sampling

❖ **78121** multiple samplings

❖ **78122** Whole blood volume determination, including separate measurement of plasma volume and red cell volume (radiopharmaceutical volume-dilution technique)

❖ **78130** Red cell survival study;

❖ **78135** differential organ/tissue kinetics, (eg, splenic and/or hepatic sequestration)

❖ **78140** Labeled red cell sequestration, differential organ/tissue, (eg, splenic and/or hepatic)

❖ **78160** Plasma radioiron disappearance (turnover) rate

❖ **78162** Radioiron oral absorption

❖ **78170** Radioiron red cell utilization

❖ **78172** Chelatable iron for estimation of total body iron

❖ **78185** Spleen imaging only, with or without vascular flow

(If combined with liver study, use procedures 78215 and 78216)

❖ **78190** Kinetics, study of platelet survival, with or without differential organ/tissue localization

❖ **78191** Platelet survival study

❖ **78195** Lymphatics and lymph nodes imaging
➔ *CPT Assistant* Nov 98:22, Nov 99:43, Dec 99:8; *CPT Changes: An Insider's View* 2000, 2002

(For sentinel node identification without scintigraphy imaging, use 38792)

(For sentinal node excision, see 38500-38542)

❖ **78199** Unlisted hematopoietic, reticuloendothelial and lymphatic procedure, diagnostic nuclear medicine

(For chemical analysis, see **Chemistry** section)

Gastrointestinal System

❖ **78201** Liver imaging; static only

❖ **78202** with vascular flow

(For spleen imaging only, use 78185)

❖ **78205** Liver imaging (SPECT);
➲ *CPT Assistant* Nov 98:22

❖ **78206** with vascular flow
➲ *CPT Assistant* Nov 98:22

❖ **78215** Liver and spleen imaging; static only

❖ **78216** with vascular flow

❖ **78220** Liver function study with hepatobiliary agents, with serial images

❖ **78223** Hepatobiliary ductal system imaging, including gallbladder, with or without pharmacologic intervention, with or without quantitative measurement of gallbladder function

❖ **78230** Salivary gland imaging;

❖ **78231** with serial images

❖ **78232** Salivary gland function study

❖ **78258** Esophageal motility

❖ **78261** Gastric mucosa imaging

❖ **78262** Gastroesophageal reflux study

❖ **78264** Gastric emptying study

♠ ▲ **78267** Urea breath test, C-14 (isotopic); acquisition for analysis
➲ *CPT Assistant* Nov 99:43; *CPT Changes: An Insider's View* 2000, 2005

♠ **78268** analysis
➲ *CPT Assistant* Nov 99:43; *CPT Changes: An Insider's View* 2000

❖ **78270** Vitamin B-12 absorption study (eg, Schilling test); without intrinsic factor

❖ **78271** with intrinsic factor

❖ **78272** Vitamin B-12 absorption studies combined, with and without intrinsic factor

❖ **78278** Acute gastrointestinal blood loss imaging

❖ **78282** Gastrointestinal protein loss

❖ **78290** Intestine imaging (eg, ectopic gastric mucosa, Meckel's localization, volvulus)
➲ *CPT Changes: An Insider's View* 2002

❖ **78291** Peritoneal-venous shunt patency test (eg, for LeVeen, Denver shunt)

(For injection procedure, use 49427)

❖ **78299** Unlisted gastrointestinal procedure, diagnostic nuclear medicine

Musculoskeletal System

Bone and joint imaging can be used in the diagnosis of a variety of inflammatory processes (eg, osteomyelitis), as well as for localization of primary and/or metastatic neoplasms.

❖ **78300** Bone and/or joint imaging; limited area
➲ *CPT Assistant* Mar 97:11

❖ **78305** multiple areas
➲ *CPT Assistant* Mar 97:11

❖ **78306** whole body
➲ *CPT Assistant* Mar 97:11, Jan 02:10

❖ **78315** three phase study
➲ *CPT Assistant* Jan 02:10

❖ **78320** tomographic (SPECT)
➲ *CPT Assistant* Mar 97:11

♣ **78350** Bone density (bone mineral content) study, one or more sites; single photon absorptiometry
➲ *CPT Assistant* Nov 97:26

□ **78351** dual photon absorptiometry, one or more sites

(For radiographic bone density (photodensitometry), use 76078)

❖ **78399** Unlisted musculoskeletal procedure, diagnostic nuclear medicine

Cardiovascular System

Myocardial perfusion and cardiac blood pool imaging studies may be performed at rest and/or during stress. When performed during exercise and/or pharmacologic stress, the appropriate stress testing code from the 93015-93018 series should be reported in addition to 78460-78465, 78472-78492.

❖ **78414** Determination of central c-v hemodynamics (non-imaging) (eg, ejection fraction with probe technique) with or without pharmacologic intervention or exercise, single or multiple determinations

❖ **78428** Cardiac shunt detection

❖ **78445** Non-cardiac vascular flow imaging (ie, angiography, venography)

❖ **78455** Venous thrombosis study (eg, radioactive fibrinogen)

❖ **78456** Acute venous thrombosis imaging, peptide
➲ *CPT Assistant* Nov 99:43; *CPT Changes: An Insider's View* 2000

⌘❖ **78457** Venous thrombosis imaging, venogram; unilateral
➲ *CPT Assistant* Nov 99:43; *CPT Changes: An Insider's View* 2000

✶❖ **78458** bilateral
➲ *CPT Assistant* Nov 99:43, May 03:15; *CPT Changes: An Insider's View* 2000

✤ **78459** Myocardial imaging, positron emission tomography (PET), metabolic evaluation

(For myocardial perfusion study, see 78491-78492)

Radiology

❖ **78460** Myocardial perfusion imaging; (planar) single study, at rest or stress (exercise and/or pharmacologic), with or without quantification

➲ *CPT Assistant* Mar 99:10, Apr 00:1

❖ **78461** multiple studies, (planar) at rest and/or stress (exercise and/or pharmacologic), and redistribution and/or rest injection, with or without quantification

➲ *CPT Assistant* Mar 99:10

❖▲ **78464** tomographic (SPECT), single study (including attenuation correction when performed), at rest or stress (exercise and/or pharmacologic), with or without quantification

➲ *CPT Assistant* Mar 99:10; *CPT Changes: An Insider's View* 2005

❖▲ **78465** tomographic (SPECT), multiple studies (including attenuation correction when performed), at rest and/or stress (exercise and/or pharmacologic) and redistribution and/or rest injection, with or without quantification

➲ *CPT Assistant* Aug 98:11, Mar 99:10; *CPT Changes: An Insider's View* 2005

❖ **78466** Myocardial imaging, infarct avid, planar; qualitative or quantitative

❖ **78468** with ejection fraction by first pass technique

❖ **78469** tomographic SPECT with or without quantification

❖ **78472** Cardiac blood pool imaging, gated equilibrium; planar, single study at rest or stress (exercise and/or pharmacologic), wall motion study plus ejection fraction, with or without additional quantitative processing

➲ *CPT Assistant* Nov 98:22, Jun 99:8, Nov 99:44; *CPT Changes: An Insider's View* 2000

(For assessment of cardiac function by first pass technique, use 78496)

❖ **78473** multiple studies, wall motion study plus ejection fraction, at rest and stress (exercise and/or pharmacologic), with or without additional quantification

❖+ **78478** Myocardial perfusion study with wall motion, qualitative or quantitative study (List separately in addition to code for primary procedure)

➲ *CPT Assistant* Mar 99:10

(Use 78478 in conjunction with 78460, 78461, 78464, 78465)

❖+ **78480** Myocardial perfusion study with ejection fraction (List separately in addition to code for primary procedure)

➲ *CPT Assistant* Mar 97:10

(Use 78480 in conjunction with 78460, 78461, 78464, 78465)

❖ **78481** Cardiac blood pool imaging, (planar), first pass technique; single study, at rest or with stress (exercise and/or pharmacologic), wall motion study plus ejection fraction, with or without quantification

❖ **78483** multiple studies, at rest and with stress (exercise and/ or pharmacologic), wall motion study plus ejection fraction, with or without quantification

(For cerebral blood flow study, use 78615)

☐ **78491** Myocardial imaging, positron emission tomography (PET), perfusion; single study at rest or stress

☐ **78492** multiple studies at rest and/or stress

❖ **78494** Cardiac blood pool imaging, gated equilibrium, SPECT, at rest, wall motion study plus ejection fraction, with or without quantitative processing

❖+ **78496** Cardiac blood pool imaging, gated equilibrium, single study, at rest, with right ventricular ejection fraction by first pass technique (List separately in addition to code for primary procedure)

➲ *CPT Assistant* Nov 98:22, Jun 99:3, 11

(Use 78496 in conjunction with 78472)

❖ **78499** Unlisted cardiovascular procedure, diagnostic nuclear medicine

Respiratory System

❖ **78580** Pulmonary perfusion imaging, particulate

➲ *CPT Assistant* Mar 99:4

❖ **78584** Pulmonary perfusion imaging, particulate, with ventilation; single breath

➲ *CPT Assistant* Mar 99:4

❖ **78585** rebreathing and washout, with or without single breath

➲ *CPT Assistant* Mar 99:4

❖ **78586** Pulmonary ventilation imaging, aerosol; single projection

➲ *CPT Assistant* Mar 99:4

❖ **78587** multiple projections (eg, anterior, posterior, lateral views)

➲ *CPT Assistant* Mar 99:4

❖ **78588** Pulmonary perfusion imaging, particulate, with ventilation imaging, aerosol, one or multiple projections

➲ *CPT Assistant* Nov 98:22, Mar 99:4

❖ **78591** Pulmonary ventilation imaging, gaseous, single breath, single projection

➲ *CPT Assistant* Mar 99:4

❖ **78593** Pulmonary ventilation imaging, gaseous, with rebreathing and washout with or without single breath; single projection

➲ *CPT Assistant* Mar 99:4

❖ **78594** multiple projections (eg, anterior, posterior, lateral views)

❖ **78596** Pulmonary quantitative differential function (ventilation/perfusion) study

❖ **78599** Unlisted respiratory procedure, diagnostic nuclear medicine

Nervous System

❖ **78600** Brain imaging, limited procedure; static

❖ **78601** with vascular flow

❖ **78605** Brain imaging, complete study; static

❖ **78606** with vascular flow

❖ **78607** tomographic (SPECT)

☐ **78608** Brain imaging, positron emission tomography (PET); metabolic evaluation

☐ **78609** perfusion evaluation

❖ **78610** Brain imaging, vascular flow only

❖ **78615** Cerebral vascular flow
➲ *CPT Changes: An Insider's View* 2002

❖ **78630** Cerebrospinal fluid flow, imaging (not including introduction of material); cisternography

(For injection procedure, see 61000-61070, 62270-62319)

❖ **78635** ventriculography

(For injection procedure, see 61000-61070, 62270-62294)

❖ **78645** shunt evaluation

(For injection procedure, see 61000-61070, 62270-62294)

❖ **78647** tomographic (SPECT)

❖ **78650** Cerebrospinal fluid leakage detection and localization
➲ *CPT Changes: An Insider's View* 2002

(For injection procedure, see 61000-61070, 62270-62294)

❖ **78660** Radiopharmaceutical dacryocystography

❖ **78699** Unlisted nervous system procedure, diagnostic nuclear medicine

Genitourinary System

❖ **78700** Kidney imaging; static only

❖ **78701** with vascular flow

❖ **78704** with function study (ie, imaging renogram)

❖ **78707** Kidney imaging with vascular flow and function; single study without pharmacological intervention
➲ *CPT Assistant* Nov 97:27

❖ **78708** single study, with pharmacological intervention (eg, angiotensin converting enzyme inhibitor and/or diuretic)
➲ *CPT Assistant* Nov 97:27

❖ **78709** multiple studies, with and without pharmacological intervention (eg, angiotensin converting enzyme inhibitor and/or diuretic)
➲ *CPT Assistant* Nov 97:27

❖ **78710** Kidney imaging, tomographic (SPECT)
➲ *CPT Assistant* Nov 97:27

❖ **78715** Kidney vascular flow only

❖ **78725** Kidney function study, non-imaging radioisotopic study
➲ *CPT Assistant* Nov 98:22

♣ **78730** Urinary bladder residual study

(For introduction of radioactive substance in association with cystotomy or cystostomy, use 51020; in association with cystourethroscopy, use 52250)

❖ **78740** Ureteral reflux study (radiopharmaceutical voiding cystogram)

(For catheterization, see 51701, 51702, 51703)

❖ **78760** Testicular imaging;

❖ **78761** with vascular flow

❖ **78799** Unlisted genitourinary procedure, diagnostic nuclear medicine

(For chemical analysis, see **Chemistry** section)

Other Procedures

(For specific organ, see appropriate heading)

(For radiophosphorus tumor identification, ocular, see 78800)

❖ **78800** Radiopharmaceutical localization of tumor or distribution of radiopharmaceutical agent(s); limited area
➲ *CPT Assistant* Apr 03:11; *CPT Changes: An Insider's View* 2004

(For specific organ, see appropriate heading)

❖ **78801** multiple areas
➲ *CPT Assistant* Apr 03:11

❖ **78802** whole body, single day imaging
➲ *CPT Assistant* Apr 03:11; *CPT Changes: An Insider's View* 2004

❖ **78803** tomographic (SPECT)
➲ *CPT Assistant* Apr 03:11

❖ **78804** whole body, requiring two or more days imaging
➲ *CPT Changes: An Insider's View* 2004

❖ **78805** Radiopharmaceutical localization of inflammatory process; limited area
➲ *CPT Assistant* Nov 99:44; *CPT Changes: An Insider's View* 2001

❖ **78806** whole body
➲ *CPT Assistant* Nov 99:44; *CPT Changes: An Insider's View* 2000

❖ **78807** tomographic (SPECT)

(For imaging bone infectious or inflammatory disease with a bone imaging radiopharmaceutical, see 78300, 78305, 78306)

►(78810 has been deleted. To report, see 78811-78813)◄

►(For PET of brain, see 78608, 78609)◄

►(For PET myocardial imaging, see 78491, 78492)◄

Radiology

□● **78811** Tumor imaging, positron emission tomography (PET); limited area (eg, chest, head/neck)
➔ *CPT Changes: An Insider's View* 2005

□● **78812** skull base to mid-thigh
➔ *CPT Changes: An Insider's View* 2005

□● **78813** whole body

□● **78814** Tumor imaging, positron emission tomography (PET) with concurrently acquired computed tomography (CT) for attenuation correction and anatomical localization; limited area (eg, chest, head/neck)
➔ *CPT Changes: An Insider's View* 2005

□● **78815** skull base to mid-thigh
➔ *CPT Changes: An Insider's View* 2005

□● **78816** whole body
➔ *CPT Changes: An Insider's View* 2005

►(Report 78811-78816 only once per imaging session)◄

►(Computed tomography (CT) performed for other than attenuation correction and anatomical localization is reported using the appropriate site specific CT code with modifier 59)◄

☆ **78890** Generation of automated data: interactive process involving nuclear physician and/or allied health professional personnel; simple manipulations and interpretation, not to exceed 30 minutes

☆ **78891** complex manipulations and interpretation, exceeding 30 minutes

(Use 78890 or 78891 in addition to primary procedure)

►(78990 has been deleted)◄

❖ **78999** Unlisted miscellaneous procedure, diagnostic nuclear medicine

Therapeutic

►The oral and intravenous administration codes in this section are inclusive of the mode of administration. For intra-arterial, intra-cavitary, and intra-articular administration, also use the appropriate injection and/or procedure codes, as well as imaging guidance and radiological supervision and interpretation codes, when appropriate.◄

►(79000, 79001 have been deleted. To report, use 79005)◄

❖● **79005** Radiopharmaceutical therapy, by oral administration
➔ *CPT Changes: An Insider's View* 2005

►(79020, 79030, 79035 have been deleted. To report, use 79005)◄

► (79100 has been deleted. To report, use 79101)◄

(For monoclonal antibody therapy, use 79403)

❖● **79101** Radiopharmaceutical therapy, by intravenous administration
➔ *CPT Changes: An Insider's View* 2005

►(Do not report 79101 in conjunction with 36400, 36410, 79403, 90780, 90784, 96408)◄

►(For radiolabeled monoclonal antibody by intravenous infusion, use 79403)◄

►(For infusion or instillation of non-antibody radioelement solution that includes three months follow-up care, use 77750)◄

❖▲ **79200** Radiopharmaceutical therapy, by intracavitary administration
➔ *CPT Changes: An Insider's View* 2005

❖▲ **79300** Radiopharmaceutical therapy, by interstitial radioactive colloid administration
➔ *CPT Changes: An Insider's View* 2005

►(79400 has been deleted. To report, use 79101)◄

❖ **79403** Radiopharmaceutical therapy, radiolabeled monoclonal antibody by intravenous infusion
➔ *CPT Changes: An Insider's View* 2004

(For pre-treatment imaging, see 78802, 78804)

(Do not report 79403 in conjunction with ►79101◄)

►(79420 has been deleted. To report use 79445)◄

❖▲ **79440** Radiopharmaceutical therapy, by intra-articular administration
➔ *CPT Changes: An Insider's View* 2005

❖● **79445** Radiopharmaceutical therapy, by intra-arterial particulate administration
➔ *CPT Changes: An Insider's View* 2005

►(Do not report 79445 in conjunction with 90783, 96420)◄

►(Use appropriate procedural and radiological supervision and interpretation codes for the angiographic and interventional procedures provided pre-requisite to intra-arterial radiopharmaceutical therapy)◄

►(79900 has been deleted)◄

❖▲ **79999** Radiopharmaceutical therapy, unlisted procedure
➔ *CPT Changes: An Insider's View* 2005

Notes

Pathology and Laboratory Guidelines

Items used by all physicians in reporting their services are presented in the **Introduction.** Some of the commonalities are repeated here for the convenience of those physicians referring to this section on **Pathology and Laboratory.** Other definitions and items unique to Pathology and Laboratory are also listed.

Services in Pathology and Laboratory

Services in Pathology and Laboratory are provided by a physician or by technologists under responsible supervision of a physician.

Separate or Multiple Procedures

It is appropriate to designate multiple procedures that are rendered on the same date by separate entries.

Subsection Information

Several of the subheadings or subsections have special needs or instructions unique to that section. Where these are indicated, (eg, "Panel Tests"), special **"Notes"** will be presented preceding those procedural terminology listings referring to that subsection specifically. If there is an "Unlisted Procedure" code number (see section below) for the individual subsection, it will be shown. Those subsections with **"Notes"** are as follows:

Organ or Disease Panels	80048-80076
Drug Testing	80100-80103
Therapeutic Drug Assays	80150-80299
Evocative/Suppression Testing	80400-80440
Consultations (Clinical Pathology)	80500-80502
Urinalysis	81000-81099
Chemistry	82000-84999
Molecular Diagnostics	83890-83912
Infectious Agent: Detection of Antibodies	86602-86804
Microbiology	87001-87255
Infectious Agent Detection	87260-87999
Anatomic Pathology	88000-88099
Cytopathology	88104-88199
►**Cytogenetic Studies**	88230-88299◄
Surgical Pathology	88300-88399

Unlisted Service or Procedure

A service or procedure may be provided that is not listed in this edition of *CPT.* When reporting such a service, the appropriate "Unlisted Procedure" code may be used to indicate the service, identifying it by "Special Report" as discussed below. The "Unlisted Procedures" and accompanying codes for **Pathology and Laboratory** are as follows:

81099 Unlisted urinalysis procedure

84999 Unlisted chemistry procedure

85999 Unlisted hematology and coagulation procedure

86586 Unlisted antigen, each

86849 Unlisted immunology procedure

86999 Unlisted transfusion medicine procedure

87999 Unlisted microbiology procedure

88099 Unlisted necropsy (autopsy) procedure

88199 Unlisted cytopathology procedure

88299 Unlisted cytogenetic study

88399 Unlisted surgical pathology procedure

89240 Unlisted miscellaneous pathology test

Special Report

A service that is rarely provided, unusual, variable, or new may require a special report in determining medical appropriateness of the service. Pertinent information should include an adequate definition or description of the nature, extent, and need for the procedure; and the time, effort, and equipment necessary to provide the service. Additional items which may be included are:

- complexity of symptoms;
- final diagnosis;
- pertinent physical findings;
- diagnostic and therapeutic procedures;
- concurrent problems;
- follow-up care.

Notes

Pathology and Laboratory

Organ or Disease Oriented Panels

These panels were developed for coding purposes only and should not be interpreted as clinical parameters. The tests listed with each panel identify the defined components of that panel.

These panel components are not intended to limit the performance of other tests. If one performs tests in addition to those specifically indicated for a particular panel, those tests should be reported separately in addition to the panel code.

♠ **80048** Basic metabolic panel

This panel must include the following:

Calcium (82310)

Carbon dioxide (82374)

Chloride (82435)

Creatinine (82565)

Glucose (82947)

Potassium (84132)

Sodium (84295)

Urea nitrogen (BUN) (84520)

➔ *CPT Assistant* Jan 98:6, Nov 99:44, Jan 00:7; *CPT Changes: An Insider's View* 2000

(Do not use 80048 in addition to 80053)

☐ **80050** General health panel

This panel must include the following:

Comprehensive metabolic panel (80053)

Blood count, complete (CBC), automated and automated differential WBC count (85025 or 85027 and 85004)

OR

Blood count, complete (CBC), automated (85027) and appropriate manual differential WBC count (85007 or 85009)

Thyroid stimulating hormone (TSH) (84443)

➔ *CPT Assistant* Winter 92:14, Summer 93:14, Jun 97:10, Nov 97:28, Jan 00:6; *CPT Changes: An Insider's View* 2001, 2004

♠ **80051** Electrolyte panel

This panel must include the following:

Carbon dioxide (82374)

Chloride (82435)

Potassium (84132)

Sodium (84295)

➔ *CPT Assistant* Nov 97:28, Jan 98:6

♠ **80053** Comprehensive metabolic panel

This panel must include the following:

Albumin (82040)

Bilirubin, total (82247)

Calcium (82310)

Carbon dioxide (bicarbonate) (82374)

Chloride (82435)

Creatinine (82565)

Glucose (82947)

Phosphatase, alkaline (84075)

Potassium (84132)

Protein, total (84155)

Sodium (84295)

Transferase, alanine amino (ALT) (SGPT) (84460)

Transferase, aspartate amino (AST) (SGOT) (84450)

Urea nitrogen (BUN) (84520)

➔ *CPT Assistant* Jan 98:6, Nov 98:23, Nov 99:44, Dec 99:1, Jan 00:7, May 00:11; *CPT Changes: An Insider's View* 2000

(Do not use 80053 in addition to 80048, 80076)

☐ **80055** Obstetric panel

This panel must include the following:

Blood count, complete (CBC), automated and automated differential WBC count (85025 or 85027 and 85004)

OR

Blood count, complete (CBC), automated (85027) and appropriate manual differential WBC count (85007 or 85009)

Hepatitis B surface antigen (HBsAg) (87340)

Antibody, rubella (86762)

Syphilis test, qualitative (eg, VDRL, RPR, ART) (86592)

Antibody screen, RBC, each serum technique (86850)

Blood typing, ABO (86900) AND

Blood typing, Rh (D) (86901)

➔ *CPT Assistant* Winter 92:14, Summer 93:14, Jun 97:10; *CPT Changes: An Insider's View* 2004

♠ **80061** Lipid panel

This panel must include the following:

Cholesterol, serum, total (82465)

Lipoprotein, direct measurement, high density cholesterol (HDL cholesterol) (83718)

Triglycerides (84478)

➲ *CPT Assistant* Winter 92:14, Summer 93:14, Jun 97:10, Mar 00:11

♠ **80069** Renal function panel

This panel must include the following:

Albumin (82040)

Calcium (82310)

Carbon dioxide (bicarbonate) (82374)

Chloride (82435)

Creatinine (82565)

Glucose (82947)

Phosphorus inorganic (phosphate) (84100)

Potassium (84132)

Sodium (84295)

Urea nitrogen (BUN) (84520)

➲ *CPT Assistant* Nov 99:44, Jan 00:7; *CPT Changes: An Insider's View* 2000

♠ **80074** Acute hepatitis panel

This panel must include the following:

Hepatitis A antibody (HAAb), IgM antibody (86709)

Hepatitis B core antibody (HBcAb), IgM antibody (86705)

Hepatitis B surface antigen (HBsAg) (87340)

Hepatitis C antibody (86803)

➲ *CPT Assistant* Nov 99:45, Jan 00:7; *CPT Changes: An Insider's View* 2000

♠ **80076** Hepatic function panel

This panel must include the following:

Albumin (82040)

Bilirubin, total (82247)

Bilirubin, direct (82248)

Phosphatase, alkaline (84075)

Protein, total (84155)

Transferase, alanine amino (ALT) (SGPT) (84460)

Transferase, aspartate amino (AST) (SGOT) (84450)

➲ *CPT Assistant* Winter 92:14, Summer 93:14, Jun 97:10, Jan 98:6, Apr 99:6, Nov 99:45, Jan 00:7; *CPT Changes: An Insider's View* 2000

(Do not use 80076 in addition to 80053)

(80090 has been deleted. To report, see codes for specific tests)

Drug Testing

The following list contains examples of drugs or classes of drugs that are commonly assayed by qualitative screen, followed by confirmation with a second method.

Alcohols

Amphetamines

Barbiturates

Benzodiazepines

Cocaine and Metabolites

Methadones

Methaqualones

Opiates

Phencyclidines

Phenothiazines

Propoxyphenes

Tetrahydrocannabinoids

Tricyclic Antidepressants

Confirmed drugs may also be quantitated.

Use 80100 for each multiple drug class chromatographic procedure. Use 80102 for each procedure necessary for confirmation. For chromatography, each combination of stationary and mobile phase is to be counted as one procedure. For example, if detection of three drugs by chromatography requires one stationary phase with three mobile phases, use 80100 three (3) times. However, if multiple drugs can be detected using a single analysis (eg, one stationary phase with one mobile phase), use 80100 only once.

For quantitation of drugs screened, use appropriate code in **Chemistry** section (82000-84999) or **Therapeutic Drug Assay** section (80150-80299).

♠ **80100** Drug screen, qualitative; multiple drug classes chromatographic method, each procedure

➲ *CPT Assistant* Fall 93:26, Mar 00:1; *CPT Changes: An Insider's View* 2001

♠ **80101** single drug class method (eg, immunoassay, enzyme assay), each drug class

➲ *CPT Assistant* Fall 93:26, Mar 00:1; *CPT Changes: An Insider's View* 2001

♠ **80102** Drug confirmation, each procedure

➲ *CPT Assistant* Fall 93:26, Mar 00:1; *CPT Changes: An Insider's View* 2001

☆ **80103** Tissue preparation for drug analysis

➲ *CPT Assistant* Mar 00:1

Pathology and Laboratory

Therapeutic Drug Assays

The material for examination may be from any source. Examination is quantitative. For nonquantitative testing, see Drug Testing (80100-80103).

♠ **80150** Amikacin

♠ **80152** Amitriptyline

♠ **80154** Benzodiazepines

♠ **80156** Carbamazepine; total
➲ *CPT Changes: An Insider's View* 2001

♠ **80157** free
➲ *CPT Changes: An Insider's View* 2001

♠ **80158** Cyclosporine

♠ **80160** Desipramine

♠ **80162** Digoxin

♠ **80164** Dipropylacetic acid (valproic acid)

♠ **80166** Doxepin

♠ **80168** Ethosuximide

♠ **80170** Gentamicin

♠ **80172** Gold

♠ **80173** Haloperidol
➲ *CPT Changes: An Insider's View* 2001

♠ **80174** Imipramine

♠ **80176** Lidocaine

♠ **80178** Lithium

♠ **80182** Nortriptyline

♠ **80184** Phenobarbital

♠ **80185** Phenytoin; total

♠ **80186** free

♠ **80188** Primidone

♠ **80190** Procainamide;

♠ **80192** with metabolites (eg, n-acetyl procainamide)

♠ **80194** Quinidine

♠ **80196** Salicylate

♠ **80197** Tacrolimus

♠ **80198** Theophylline

♠ **80200** Tobramycin

♠ **80201** Topiramate

♠ **80202** Vancomycin

♠ **80299** Quantitation of drug, not elsewhere specified
➲ *CPT Assistant* Mar 00:3

Evocative/Suppression Testing

The following test panels involve the administration of evocative or suppressive agents, and the baseline and subsequent measurement of their effects on chemical constituents. These codes are to be used for the reporting of the laboratory component of the overall testing protocol. For the physician's administration of the evocative or suppressive agents, see 90780-90784; for the supplies and drugs, see 99070. To report physician attendance and monitoring during the testing, use the appropriate evaluation and management code, including the prolonged physician care codes if required. Prolonged physician care codes are not separately reported when evocative/suppression testing involves prolonged infusions reported with 90780 and 90781. In the code descriptors where reference is made to a particular analyte (eg, Cortisol (82533 x 2)) the "x 2" refers to the number of times the test for that particular analyte is performed.

♠ **80400** ACTH stimulation panel; for adrenal insufficiency

This panel must include the following:

Cortisol (82533 x 2)
➲ *CPT Assistant* Summer 94:1

♠ **80402** for 21 hydroxylase deficiency

This panel must include the following:

Cortisol (82533 x 2)

17 hydroxyprogesterone (83498 x 2)
➲ *CPT Assistant* Summer 94:1

♠ **80406** for 3 beta-hydroxydehydrogenase deficiency

This panel must include the following:

Cortisol (82533 x 2)

17 hydroxypregnenolone (84143 x 2)
➲ *CPT Assistant* Summer 94:1

♠ **80408** Aldosterone suppression evaluation panel (eg, saline infusion)

This panel must include the following:

Aldosterone (82088 x 2)

Renin (84244 x 2)
➲ *CPT Assistant* Summer 94:1

♠ **80410** Calcitonin stimulation panel (eg, calcium, pentagastrin)

This panel must include the following:

Calcitonin (82308 x 3)
➲ *CPT Assistant* Summer 94:1

♠ **80412** Corticotropic releasing hormone (CRH) stimulation panel

This panel must include the following:

Cortisol (82533 x 6)

Adrenocorticotropic hormone (ACTH) (82024 x 6)

➲ *CPT Assistant* Summer 94:1

♠ **80414** Chorionic gonadotropin stimulation panel; testosterone response

This panel must include the following:

Testosterone (84403 x 2 on three pooled blood samples)

➲ *CPT Assistant* Summer 94:1

♠ **80415** estradiol response

This panel must include the following:

Estradiol (82670 x 2 on three pooled blood samples)

➲ *CPT Assistant* Summer 94:1

♠ **80416** Renal vein renin stimulation panel (eg, captopril)

This panel must include the following:

Renin (84244 x 6)

➲ *CPT Assistant* Summer 94:1

♠ **80417** Peripheral vein renin stimulation panel (eg, captopril)

This panel must include the following:

Renin (84244 x 2)

♠ **80418** Combined rapid anterior pituitary evaluation panel

This panel must include the following:

Adrenocorticotropic hormone (ACTH) (82024 x 4)

Luteinizing hormone (LH) (83002 x 4)

Follicle stimulating hormone (FSH) (83001 x 4)

Prolactin (84146 x 4)

Human growth hormone (HGH) (83003 x 4)

Cortisol (82533 x 4)

Thyroid stimulating hormone (TSH) (84443 x 4)

➲ *CPT Assistant* Summer 94:1

♠ **80420** Dexamethasone suppression panel, 48 hour

This panel must include the following:

Free cortisol, urine (82530 x 2)

Cortisol (82533 x 2)

Volume measurement for timed collection (81050 x 2)

➲ *CPT Assistant* Summer 94:1

(For single dose dexamethasone, use 82533)

♠ **80422** Glucagon tolerance panel; for insulinoma

This panel must include the following:

Glucose (82947 x 3)

Insulin (83525 x 3)

➲ *CPT Assistant* Summer 94:1

♠ **80424** for pheochromocytoma

This panel must include the following:

Catecholamines, fractionated (82384 x 2)

➲ *CPT Assistant* Summer 94:1

♠ **80426** Gonadotropin releasing hormone stimulation panel

This panel must include the following:

Follicle stimulating hormone (FSH) (83001 x 4)

Luteinizing hormone (LH) (83002 x 4)

➲ *CPT Assistant* Summer 94:1

♠ **80428** Growth hormone stimulation panel (eg, arginine infusion, l-dopa administration)

This panel must include the following:

Human growth hormone (HGH) (83003 x 4)

➲ *CPT Assistant* Summer 94:1

♠ **80430** Growth hormone suppression panel (glucose administration)

This panel must include the following:

Glucose (82947 x 3)

Human growth hormone (HGH) (83003 x 4)

➲ *CPT Assistant* Summer 94:1

♠ **80432** Insulin-induced C-peptide suppression panel

This panel must include the following:

Insulin (83525)

C-peptide (84681 x 5)

Glucose (82947 x 5)

➲ *CPT Assistant* Summer 94:1

♠ **80434** Insulin tolerance panel; for ACTH insufficiency

This panel must include the following:

Cortisol (82533 x 5)

Glucose (82947 x 5)

➲ *CPT Assistant* Summer 94:1

♠ **80435** for growth hormone deficiency

This panel must include the following:

Glucose (82947 x 5)

Human growth hormone (HGH) (83003 x 5)

➲ *CPT Assistant* Summer 94:1

♠ **80436** Metyrapone panel

This panel must include the following:

Cortisol (82533 x 2)

11 deoxycortisol (82634 x 2)

➲ *CPT Assistant* Summer 94:1

♠ **80438** Thyrotropin releasing hormone (TRH) stimulation panel; one hour

This panel must include the following:

Thyroid stimulating hormone (TSH) (84443 x 3)

➲ *CPT Assistant* Summer 94:1

♠ **80439** two hour

This panel must include the following:

Thyroid stimulating hormone (TSH) (84443 x 4)

➲ *CPT Assistant* Summer 94:1

♠ **80440** for hyperprolactinemia

This panel must include the following:

Prolactin (84146 x 3)

➲ *CPT Assistant* Summer 94:1

Consultations (Clinical Pathology)

A clinical pathology consultation is a service, including a written report, rendered by the pathologist in response to a request from an attending physician in relation to a test result(s) requiring additional medical interpretive judgment.

Reporting of a test result(s) without medical interpretive judgment is not considered a clinical pathology consultation.

♣ **80500** Clinical pathology consultation; limited, without review of patient's history and medical records

➲ *CPT Assistant* Apr 97:9, Nov 02:9

♣ **80502** comprehensive, for a complex diagnostic problem, with review of patient's history and medical records

➲ *CPT Assistant* Apr 97:9, Nov 02:9

(These codes may also be used for pharmacokinetic consultations)

(For consultations involving the examination and evaluation of the patient, see 99241-99275)

Urinalysis

For specific analyses, see appropriate section.

(For urinalysis, infectious agent detection, semi-quantitative analysis of volatile compounds, use Category III code 0041T)

♠ **81000** Urinalysis, by dip stick or tablet reagent for bilirubin, glucose, hemoglobin, ketones, leukocytes, nitrite, pH, protein, specific gravity, urobilinogen, any number of these constituents; non-automated, with microscopy

➲ *CPT Assistant* Winter 90-91:10, Fall 93:25

♠ **81001** automated, with microscopy

♠ **81002** non-automated, without microscopy

➲ *CPT Assistant* Mar 98:3

♠ **81003** automated, without microscopy

♠ **81005** Urinalysis; qualitative or semiquantitative, except immunoassays

➲ *CPT Assistant* Winter 90-91:10, Fall 93:25

(For non-immunoassay reagent strip urinalysis, see 81000, 81002)

(For immunoassay, qualitative or semiquantitative, use 83518)

(For microalbumin, see 82043, 82044)

♠ **81007** bacteriuria screen, except by culture or dipstick

➲ *CPT Changes: An Insider's View* 2001

(For culture, see 87086-87088)

(For dipstick, use 81000 or 81002)

♠ **81015** microscopic only

♠ **81020** two or three glass test

➲ *CPT Assistant* Winter 90-91:10

♠ **81025** Urine pregnancy test, by visual color comparison methods

➲ *CPT Assistant* Mar 98:3

♠ **81050** Volume measurement for timed collection, each

♠ **81099** Unlisted urinalysis procedure

Chemistry

The material for examination may be from any source unless otherwise specified in the code descriptor. When an analyte is measured in multiple specimens from different sources, or in specimens that are obtained at different times, the analyte is reported separately for each source and for each specimen. The examination is quantitative unless specified. To report an organ or disease oriented panel, see codes 80048-80076.

When a code describes a method where measurement of multiple analytes may require one or several procedures, each procedure is coded separately (eg, 82491-82492, 82541-82544). For example, if two (2) analytes are measured using column chromatography using a single stationary or mobile phase, use 82492. If the same two analytes are measured using different stationary or mobile phase conditions, 82491 would be used twice. If a total of four (4) analytes are measured where two (2) analytes are measured with a single stationary and mobile phase, and the other two (2) analytes are measured using a different stationary and mobile phase, use 82492 twice. If a total of three (3) analytes are measured where two (2) analytes are measured using a single stationary or mobile phase condition, and the third analyte is measured separately using a different stationary or mobile phase procedure, use 82492 once for the (2) analytes measured under the same condition, and use 82491 once for the third analyte measured separately.

Clinical information derived from the results of laboratory data that is mathematically calculated (eg, free thyroxine index (T7)) is considered part of the test procedure and therefore is not a separately reportable service.

♠ **82000** Acetaldehyde, blood
➲ *CPT Assistant* Mar 00:1

♠ **82003** Acetaminophen

♠ **82009** Acetone or other ketone bodies, serum; qualitative

♠ **82010** quantitative

♠ **82013** Acetylcholinesterase

(Acid, gastric, see gastric acid, 82926, 82928)

(Acid phosphatase, see 84060-84066)

♠ **82016** Acylcarnitines; qualitative, each specimen
➲ *CPT Assistant* Nov 98:23

♠ **82017** quantitative, each specimen
➲ *CPT Assistant* Nov 98:23; *CPT Changes: An Insider's View* 2000

(For carnitine, use 82379)

♠ **82024** Adrenocorticotropic hormone (ACTH)

♠ **82030** Adenosine, 5-monophosphate, cyclic (cyclic AMP)

♠ **82040** Albumin; serum
➲ *CPT Assistant* Dec 99:2

♠ **82042** urine or other source, quantitative, each specimen
➲ *CPT Changes: An Insider's View* 2001

♠ **82043** urine, microalbumin, quantitative
➲ *CPT Assistant* Summer 94:2

♠ **82044** urine, microalbumin, semiquantitative (eg, reagent strip assay)
➲ *CPT Assistant* Summer 94:2, Mar 98:3, Sep 02:10

(For prealbumin, use 84134)

♠● **82045** ischemia modified
➲ *CPT Changes: An Insider's View* 2005

♠ **82055** Alcohol (ethanol); any specimen except breath

(For other volatiles, alcohol, use 84600)

♠ **82075** breath

♠ **82085** Aldolase

♠ **82088** Aldosterone

(Alkaline phosphatase, see 84075, 84080)

♠ **82101** Alkaloids, urine, quantitative

(Alphaketoglutarate, see 82009, 82010)

(Alpha tocopherol (Vitamin E), use 84446)

♠ **82103** Alpha-1-antitrypsin; total

♠ **82104** phenotype

♠ **82105** Alpha-fetoprotein; serum

♠ **82106** amniotic fluid

♠ **82108** Aluminum

♠ **82120** Amines, vaginal fluid, qualitative
➲ *CPT Assistant* Nov 99:45; *CPT Changes: An Insider's View* 2000

(For combined pH and amines test for vaginitis, use 82120 and 83986)

♠ **82127** Amino acids; single, qualitative, each specimen
➲ *CPT Assistant* Nov 98:24

♠ **82128** multiple, qualitative, each specimen
➲ *CPT Assistant* Nov 98:24

♠ **82131** single, quantitative, each specimen
➲ *CPT Assistant* May 98:11, Nov 98:24

♠ **82135** Aminolevulinic acid, delta (ALA)

♠ **82136** Amino acids, 2 to 5 amino acids, quantitative, each specimen
➲ *CPT Assistant* Nov 98:24

♠ **82139** Amino acids, 6 or more amino acids, quantitative, each specimen
➲ *CPT Assistant* Nov 98:24

♠ **82140** Ammonia

♠ **82143** Amniotic fluid scan (spectrophotometric)

(For L/S ratio, use 83661)

(Amobarbital, see 80100-80103 for qualitative analysis, 82205 for quantitative analysis)

♠ **82145** Amphetamine or methamphetamine

(For qualitative analysis, see 80100-80103)

♠ **82150** Amylase

♠ **82154** Androstanediol glucuronide
➲ *CPT Assistant* Summer 94:5

♠ **82157** Androstenedione

♠ **82160** Androsterone

♠ **82163** Angiotensin II

♠ **82164** Angiotensin I - converting enzyme (ACE)

(Antidiuretic hormone (ADH), use 84588)

(Antimony, use 83015)

(Antitrypsin, alpha-1-, see 82103, 82104)

♠ **82172** Apolipoprotein, each

♠ **82175** Arsenic

(For heavy metal screening, use 83015)

♠ **82180** Ascorbic acid (Vitamin C), blood

(Aspirin, see acetylsalicylic acid, 80196)

(Atherogenic index, blood, ultracentrifugation, quantitative, use 83716)

♠ **82190** Atomic absorption spectroscopy, each analyte

♠ **82205** Barbiturates, not elsewhere specified

(For qualitative analysis, see 80100-80103)

(For B-Natriuretic peptide, use 83880)

♠ **82232** Beta-2 microglobulin

(Bicarbonate, use 82374)

♠ **82239** Bile acids; total

♠ **82240** cholylglycine

(For bile pigments, urine, see 81000-81005)

♠ **82247** Bilirubin; total
➔ *CPT Assistant* Nov 98:24, Apr 99:6, Dec 99:1, Jan 00:7

♠ **82248** direct
➔ *CPT Assistant* Nov 98:24, Apr 99:6, Dec 99:1

♠ **82252** feces, qualitative

♠ **82261** Biotinidase, each specimen
➔ *CPT Assistant* Nov 98:24

♠ **82270** Blood, occult, by peroxidase activity (eg, guaiac), qualitative; feces, 1-3 simultaneous determinations
➔ *CPT Assistant* Sep 03:15; *CPT Changes: An Insider's View* 2002

♠ **82273** other sources
➔ *CPT Changes: An Insider's View* 2002

(Blood urea nitrogen (BUN), see 84520, 84525)

♠ **82274** Blood, occult, by fecal hemoglobin determination by immunoassay, qualitative, feces, 1-3 simultaneous determinations
➔ *CPT Changes: An Insider's View* 2002

♠ **82286** Bradykinin

♠ **82300** Cadmium

♠ **82306** Calcifediol (25-OH Vitamin D-3)

♠ **82307** Calciferol (Vitamin D)

(For 1,25-Dihydroxyvitamin D, use 82652)

♠ **82308** Calcitonin

♠ **82310** Calcium; total
➔ *CPT Assistant* Dec 99:1

♠ **82330** ionized

♠ **82331** after calcium infusion test

♠ **82340** urine quantitative, timed specimen

♠ **82355** Calculus; qualitative analysis
➔ *CPT Changes: An Insider's View* 2002

♠ **82360** quantitative analysis, chemical

♠ **82365** infrared spectroscopy

♠ **82370** x-ray diffraction
➔ *CPT Changes: An Insider's View* 2001

(Carbamates, see individual listings)

♠ **82373** Carbohydrate deficient transferrin
➔ *CPT Changes: An Insider's View* 2001

♠ **82374** Carbon dioxide (bicarbonate)
➔ *CPT Assistant* Dec 99:1

(See also 82803)

♠ **82375** Carbon monoxide, (carboxyhemoglobin); quantitative

♠ **82376** qualitative

(To report end-tidal carbon monoxide, use Category III code 0043T)

♠ **82378** Carcinoembryonic antigen (CEA)
➔ *CPT Assistant* Fall 93:25, Aug 96:11

♠ **82379** Carnitine (total and free), quantitative, each specimen
➔ *CPT Assistant* Nov 98:24

(For acylcarnitine, see 82016, 82017)

♠ **82380** Carotene

♠ **82382** Catecholamines; total urine

♠ **82383** blood

♠ **82384** fractionated

(For urine metabolites, see 83835, 84585)

♠ **82387** Cathepsin-D

♠ **82390** Ceruloplasmin

♠ **82397** Chemiluminescent assay
➔ *CPT Assistant* Fall 93:25

♠ **82415** Chloramphenicol

♠ **82435** Chloride; blood
➔ *CPT Assistant* Dec 99:1

♠ **82436** urine

♠ **82438** other source
➔ *CPT Assistant* Jul 03:7

(For sweat collection by iontophoresis, use 89230)

♠ **82441** Chlorinated hydrocarbons, screen

(Chlorpromazine, use 84022)

(Cholecalciferol (Vitamin D), use 82307)

♠ **82465** Cholesterol, serum or whole blood, total
➔ *CPT Assistant* Dec 99:1, Mar 00:11; *CPT Changes: An Insider's View* 2001

(For high density lipoprotein (HDL), use 83718)

♠ **82480** Cholinesterase; serum

♠ **82482** RBC

♠ **82485** Chondroitin B sulfate, quantitative

(Chorionic gonadotropin, see gonadotropin, 84702, 84703)

♠ **82486** Chromatography, qualitative; column (eg, gas liquid or HPLC), analyte not elsewhere specified
➔ *CPT Assistant* Nov 98:24-25

♠ **82487** paper, 1-dimensional, analyte not elsewhere specified

♠ **82488** paper, 2-dimensional, analyte not elsewhere specified

♠ **82489** thin layer, analyte not elsewhere specified

♠ **82491** Chromatography, quantitative, column (eg, gas liquid or HPLC); single analyte not elsewhere specified, single stationary and mobile phase
➲ *CPT Assistant* Fall 93:25, Nov 98:24-25, Mar 00:1

♠ **82492** multiple analytes, single stationary and mobile phase
➲ *CPT Assistant* Nov 98:24-25, Mar 00:1

♠ **82495** Chromium

♠ **82507** Citrate

♠ **82520** Cocaine or metabolite

(Cocaine, qualitative analysis, see 80100-80103)

(Codeine, qualitative analysis, see 80100-80103)

(Codeine, quantitative analysis, see 82101)

(Complement, see 86160-86162)

♠ **82523** Collagen cross links, any method

♠ **82525** Copper

(Coproporphyrin, see 84119, 84120)

(Corticosteroids, use 83491)

♠ **82528** Corticosterone

♠ **82530** Cortisol; free
➲ *CPT Assistant* Summer 94:3

♠ **82533** total
➲ *CPT Assistant* Summer 94:3

(C-peptide, use 84681)

♠ **82540** Creatine

♠ **82541** Column chromatography/mass spectrometry (eg, GC/MS, or HPLC/MS), analyte not elsewhere specified; qualitative, single stationary and mobile phase
➲ *CPT Assistant* Nov 98:24-25

♠ **82542** quantitative, single stationary and mobile phase
➲ *CPT Assistant* Nov 98:24-25

♠ **82543** stable isotope dilution, single analyte, quantitative, single stationary and mobile phase
➲ *CPT Assistant* Nov 98:24-25

♠ **82544** stable isotope dilution, multiple analytes, quantitative, single stationary and mobile phase
➲ *CPT Assistant* Nov 98:24-25, Dec 99:7

♠ **82550** Creatine kinase (CK), (CPK); total
➲ *CPT Assistant* Feb 98:1, Dec 99:1

♠ **82552** isoenzymes
➲ *CPT Assistant* Feb 98:1

♠ **82553** MB fraction only
➲ *CPT Assistant* Feb 98:1

♠ **82554** isoforms
➲ *CPT Assistant* Feb 98:1

♠ **82565** Creatinine; blood
➲ *CPT Assistant* Dec 99:1

♠ **82570** other source

♠ **82575** clearance

♠ **82585** Cryofibrinogen

♠ **82595** Cryoglobulin, qualitative or semi-quantitative (eg, cryocrit)
➲ *CPT Changes: An Insider's View* 2001

(For quantitative, cryoglobulin, see 82784, 82785)

(Crystals, pyrophosphate vs. urate, use 89060)

♠ **82600** Cyanide

♠ **82607** Cyanocobalamin (Vitamin B-12);

♠ **82608** unsaturated binding capacity

(Cyclic AMP, use 82030)

(Cyclic GMP, use 83008)

(Cyclosporine, use 80158)

♠ **82615** Cystine and homocystine, urine, qualitative

♠ **82626** Dehydroepiandrosterone (DHEA)
➲ *CPT Assistant* Summer 94:4

♠ **82627** Dehydroepiandrosterone-sulfate (DHEA-S)
➲ *CPT Assistant* Summer 94:4

(Delta-aminolevulinic acid (ALA), use 82135)

♠ **82633** Desoxycorticosterone, 11-

♠ **82634** Deoxycortisol, 11-

(Dexamethasone suppression test, use 80420)

(Diastase, urine, use 82150)

♠ **82638** Dibucaine number

(Dichloroethane, use 84600)

(Dichloromethane, use 84600)

(Diethylether, use 84600)

♠ **82646** Dihydrocodeinone

(For qualitative analysis, see 80100-80103)

♠ **82649** Dihydromorphinone

(For qualitative analysis, see 80100-80103)

♠ **82651** Dihydrotestosterone (DHT)

♠ **82652** Dihydroxyvitamin D, 1,25-

♠ **82654** Dimethadione

(For qualitative analysis, see 80100-80103)

(Diphenylhydantoin, use 80185)

(Dipropylacetic acid, use 80164)

(Dopamine, see 82382-82384)

(Duodenal contents, see individual enzymes; for intubation and collection, use 89100)

♠● **82656** Elastase, pancreatic (EL-1), fecal, qualitative or semi-quantitative
➲ *CPT Changes: An Insider's View* 2005

♠ **82657** Enzyme activity in blood cells, cultured cells, or tissue, not elsewhere specified; nonradioactive substrate, each specimen
➲ *CPT Assistant* Nov 98:25

♠ **82658** radioactive substrate, each specimen
➲ *CPT Assistant* Nov 98:25

♠ **82664** Electrophoretic technique, not elsewhere specified

(Endocrine receptor assays, see 84233-84235)

♠ **82666** Epiandrosterone

(Epinephrine, see 82382-82384)

♠ **82668** Erythropoietin

♠ **82670** Estradiol

♠ **82671** Estrogens; fractionated

♠ **82672** total

(Estrogen receptor assay, use 84233)

♠ **82677** Estriol

♠ **82679** Estrone

(Ethanol, see 82055 and 82075)

♠ **82690** Ethchlorvynol

(Ethyl alcohol, see 82055 and 82075)

♠ **82693** Ethylene glycol

♠ **82696** Etiocholanolone

(For fractionation of ketosteroids, use 83593)

♠ **82705** Fat or lipids, feces; qualitative

♠ **82710** quantitative

♠ **82715** Fat differential, feces, quantitative

♠ **82725** Fatty acids, nonesterified

♠ **82726** Very long chain fatty acids
➲ *CPT Assistant* Nov 98:25

♠ **82728** Ferritin

(Fetal hemoglobin, see hemoglobin 83030, 83033, and 85460)

(Fetoprotein, alpha-1, see 82105, 82106)

♠ **82731** Fetal fibronectin, cervicovaginal secretions, semi-quantitative
➲ *CPT Assistant* Nov 98:25

♠ **82735** Fluoride

♠ **82742** Flurazepam

(For qualitative analysis, see 80100-80103)

(Foam stability test, use 83662)

♠ **82746** Folic acid; serum

♠ **82747** RBC

(Follicle stimulating hormone (FSH), use 83001)

♠ **82757** Fructose, semen

(Fructosamine, use 82985)

(Fructose, TLC screen, use 84375)

♠ **82759** Galactokinase, RBC

♠ **82760** Galactose

♠ **82775** Galactose-1-phosphate uridyl transferase; quantitative

♠ **82776** screen

♠ **82784** Gammaglobulin; IgA, IgD, IgG, IgM, each
➲ *CPT Assistant* Spring 94:31, Aug 00:11

♠ **82785** IgE
➲ *CPT Assistant* Spring 94:31

(For allergen specific IgE, see 86003, 86005)

♠ **82787** immunoglobulin subclasses, (IgG1, 2, 3, or 4), each
➲ *CPT Changes: An Insider's View* 2001

(Gamma-glutamyltransferase (GGT), use 82977)

♠ **82800** Gases, blood, pH only

♠ **82803** Gases, blood, any combination of pH, pCO_2, pO_2, CO_2, HCO_3 (including calculated O_2 saturation);

(Use 82803 for two or more of the above listed analytes)

♠ **82805** with O_2 saturation, by direct measurement, except pulse oximetry

♠ **82810** Gases, blood, O_2 saturation only, by direct measurement, except pulse oximetry

(For pulse oximetry, use 94760)

♠ **82820** Hemoglobin-oxygen affinity (pO_2 for 50% hemoglobin saturation with oxygen)

♠ **82926** Gastric acid, free and total, each specimen

♠ **82928** Gastric acid, free or total, each specimen

♠ **82938** Gastrin after secretin stimulation

♠ **82941** Gastrin

(Gentamicin, use 80170)

(GGT, use 82977)

(GLC, gas liquid chromatography, use 82486)

♠ **82943** Glucagon

♠ **82945** Glucose, body fluid, other than blood
➲ *CPT Changes: An Insider's View* 2001

♠ **82946** Glucagon tolerance test

♠ **82947** Glucose; quantitative, blood (except reagent strip)
➲ *CPT Assistant* Summer 93:14, Summer 94:5, Sep 99:10, Dec 99:1, Jun 02:1, Jun 02:1-3; *CPT Changes: An Insider's View* 2001

♠ **82948** blood, reagent strip
➲ *CPT Assistant* Summer 94:5, Jan 99:10

♠ **82950** post glucose dose (includes glucose)
➲ *CPT Assistant* Sep 99:10, Jun 02:1-3

♠ **82951** tolerance test (GTT), three specimens (includes glucose)
➔ *CPT Assistant* Feb 01:10

♠ **82952** tolerance test, each additional beyond three specimens
➔ *CPT Assistant* Feb 01:10

♠ **82953** tolbutamide tolerance test

(For insulin tolerance test, see 80434, 80435)

(For leucine tolerance test, use 80428)

(For semiquantitative urine glucose, see 81000, 81002, 81005, 81099)

♠ **82955** Glucose-6-phosphate dehydrogenase (G6PD); quantitative

♠ **82960** screen

(For glucose tolerance test with medication, use 90784 in addition)

♠ **82962** Glucose, blood by glucose monitoring device(s) cleared by the FDA specifically for home use
➔ *CPT Assistant* Summer 94:4, Jan 99:10

♠ **82963** Glucosidase, beta

♠ **82965** Glutamate dehydrogenase

♠ **82975** Glutamine (glutamic acid amide)

♠ **82977** Glutamyltransferase, gamma (GGT)
➔ *CPT Assistant* Dec 99:1

♠ **82978** Glutathione

♠ **82979** Glutathione reductase, RBC

♠ **82980** Glutethimide

(Glycohemoglobin, use 83036)

♠ **82985** Glycated protein
➔ *CPT Assistant* Summer 94:2

(Gonadotropin, chorionic, see 84702, 84703)

♠ **83001** Gonadotropin; follicle stimulating hormone (FSH)

♠ **83002** luteinizing hormone (LH)

(For luteinizing releasing factor (LRH), use 83727)

♠ **83003** Growth hormone, human (HGH) (somatotropin)

(For antibody to human growth hormone, use 86277)

♠ **83008** Guanosine monophosphate (GMP), cyclic

♠● **83009** Helicobacter pylori, blood test analysis for urease activity, non-radioactive isotope (eg, C-13)
➔ *CPT Changes: An Insider's View* 2005

►(For H. pylori, breath test analysis for urease activity, see 83013, 83014)◄

♠ **83010** Haptoglobin; quantitative

♠ **83012** phenotypes

♠▲ **83013** Helicobacter pylori; breath test analysis for urease activity, non-radioactive isotope (eg, C-13)
➔ *CPT Assistant* Nov 98:25, Feb 99:8, Nov 99:45; *CPT Changes: An Insider's View* 2001, 2002, 2005

♠▲ **83014** drug administration
➔ *CPT Assistant* Nov 98:25, Feb 99:8, Nov 99:45; *CPT Changes: An Insider's View* 2005

(For H. pylori, stool, use 87338. For H. pylori, liquid scintillation counter, see 78267, 78268. For H. pylori, enzyme immunoassay, use 87339)

►(For H. pylori, blood test analysis for urease activity, use 83009)◄

♠ **83015** Heavy metal (eg, arsenic, barium, beryllium, bismuth, antimony, mercury); screen

♠ **83018** quantitative, each

♠ **83020** Hemoglobin fractionation and quantitation; electrophoresis (eg, A2, S, C, and/or F)
➔ *CPT Assistant* Nov 98:25

♠ **83021** chromatography (eg, A2, S, C, and/or F)
➔ *CPT Assistant* Nov 98:25, Dec 99:7

♠ **83026** Hemoglobin; by copper sulfate method, non-automated

♠ **83030** F (fetal), chemical

♠ **83033** F (fetal), qualitative
➔ *CPT Changes: An Insider's View* 2001

♠ **83036** glycated

(For fecal hemoglobin detection by immunoassay, use 82274)

♠ **83045** methemoglobin, qualitative

♠ **83050** methemoglobin, quantitative

♠ **83051** plasma

♠ **83055** sulfhemoglobin, qualitative

♠ **83060** sulfhemoglobin, quantitative

♠ **83065** thermolabile

♠ **83068** unstable, screen

♠ **83069** urine

♠ **83070** Hemosiderin; qualitative

♠ **83071** quantitative

(Heroin, see 80100-80103)

(HIAA, use 83497)

(High performance liquid chromatography (HPLC), use 82486)

♠ **83080** b-Hexosaminidase, each assay
➔ *CPT Assistant* Nov 98:25

♠ **83088** Histamine

(Hollander test, use 91052)

♠ **83090** Homocystine
➲ *CPT Assistant* Jan 01:13; *CPT Changes: An Insider's View* 2001

♠ **83150** Homovanillic acid (HVA)

(Hormones, see individual alphabetic listings in **Chemistry** section)

(Hydrogen breath test, use 91065)

♠ **83491** Hydroxycorticosteroids, 17- (17-OHCS)

(For cortisol, see 82530, 82533. For deoxycortisol, use 82634)

♠ **83497** Hydroxyindolacetic acid, 5-(HIAA)

(For urine qualitative test, use 81005)

(5-Hydroxytryptamine, use 84260)

♠ **83498** Hydroxyprogesterone, 17-d

♠ **83499** Hydroxyprogesterone, 20-

♠ **83500** Hydroxyproline; free

♠ **83505** total

♠ **83516** Immunoassay for analyte other than infectious agent antibody or infectious agent antigen, qualitative or semiquantitative; multiple step method
➲ *CPT Assistant* Nov 98:25

♠ **83518** single step method (eg, reagent strip)
➲ *CPT Assistant* Fall 93:26

♠ **83519** Immunoassay, analyte, quantitative; by radiopharmaceutical technique (eg, RIA)
➲ *CPT Assistant* Fall 93:26, Summer 94:2

♠ **83520** not otherwise specified
➲ *CPT Assistant* Fall 93:26

(For immunoassays for antibodies to infectious agent antigens, see analyte and method specific codes in the **Immunology** section)

(For immunoassay of tumor antigen not elsewhere specified, use 86316)

(Immunoglobulins, see 82784, 82785)

♠ **83525** Insulin; total

(For proinsulin, use 84206)

♠ **83527** free
➲ *CPT Assistant* Summer 94:5

♠ **83528** Intrinsic factor

(For intrinsic factor antibodies, use 86340)

♠ **83540** Iron
➲ *CPT Assistant* Fall 93:25

♠ **83550** Iron binding capacity

♠ **83570** Isocitric dehydrogenase (IDH)

(Isonicotinic acid hydrazide, INH, see code for specific method)

(Isopropyl alcohol, use 84600)

♠ **83582** Ketogenic steroids, fractionation

(Ketone bodies, for serum, see 82009, 82010; for urine, see 81000-81003)

♠ **83586** Ketosteroids, 17- (17-KS); total

♠ **83593** fractionation

♠ **83605** Lactate (lactic acid)

♠ **83615** Lactate dehydrogenase (LD), (LDH);
➲ *CPT Assistant* Fall 93:25, Feb 98:1, Dec 99:1

♠ **83625** isoenzymes, separation and quantitation
➲ *CPT Assistant* Fall 93:25, Feb 98:1

♠● **83630** Lactoferrin, fecal, qualitative
➲ *CPT Changes: An Insider's View* 2005

♠ **83632** Lactogen, human placental (HPL) human chorionic somatomammotropin

♠ **83633** Lactose, urine; qualitative

♠ **83634** quantitative

(For tolerance, see 82951, 82952)

(For breath hydrogen test for lactase deficiency, use 91065)

♠ **83655** Lead

♠ **83661** Fetal lung maturity assessment; lecithin sphingomyelin (L/S) ratio
➲ *CPT Changes: An Insider's View* 2001

♠ **83662** foam stability test

♠ **83663** fluorescence polarization
➲ *CPT Changes: An Insider's View* 2001

♠ **83664** lamellar body density
➲ *CPT Changes: An Insider's View* 2001

(For phosphatidylglycerol, use 84081)

♠ **83670** Leucine aminopeptidase (LAP)

♠ **83690** Lipase

♠ **83715** Lipoprotein, blood; electrophoretic separation and quantitation
➲ *CPT Assistant* Nov 98:25, Oct 99:11

♠ **83716** high resolution fractionation and quantitation of lipoproteins including lipoprotein subclasses when performed (eg, electrophoresis, nuclear magnetic resonance, ultracentrifugation)
➲ *CPT Assistant* Nov 98:25, Oct 99:11, Mar 00:11; *CPT Changes: An Insider's View* 2004

♠ **83718** Lipoprotein, direct measurement; high density cholesterol (HDL cholesterol)
➲ *CPT Assistant* Oct 99:11

♠ **83719** direct measurement, VLDL cholesterol
➲ *CPT Assistant* Oct 99:11

♠ **83721** direct measurement, LDL cholesterol
➲ *CPT Assistant* Nov 98:25, Oct 99:11

(For fractionation by nuclear magnetic resonance or high resolution electrophoresis, use 83716)

(To report direct measurement, intermediate density lipoproteins (remnant lipoproteins), use Category III code 0026T)

(Luteinizing hormone (LH), use 83002)

♠ **83727** Luteinizing releasing factor (LRH)

(For qualitative analysis, see 80100-80103)

(Macroglobulins, alpha-2, use 86329)

♠ **83735** Magnesium

♠ **83775** Malate dehydrogenase

(Maltose tolerance, see 82951, 82952)

(Mammotropin, use 84146)

♠ **83785** Manganese

(Marijuana, see 80100-80103)

♠ **83788** Mass spectrometry and tandem mass spectrometry (MS, MS/MS), analyte not elsewhere specified; qualitative, each specimen
➲ *CPT Assistant* Nov 98:26

♠ **83789** quantitative, each specimen
➲ *CPT Assistant* Nov 98:26

♠ **83805** Meprobamate

(For qualitative analysis, see 80100-80103)

♠ **83825** Mercury, quantitative

(Mercury screen, use 83015)

♠ **83835** Metanephrines

(For catecholamines, see 82382-82384)

♠ **83840** Methadone

(For methadone qualitative analysis, see 80100-80103)

(Methamphetamine, see 80100-80103, 82145)

(Methanol, use 84600)

♠ **83857** Methemalbumin

(Methemoglobin, see hemoglobin 83045, 83050)

♠ **83858** Methsuximide

(Methyl alcohol, use 84600)

(Microalbumin, see 82043 for quantitative, see 82044 for semiquantitative)

(Microglobulin, beta-2, use 82232)

♠ **83864** Mucopolysaccharides, acid; quantitative

♠ **83866** screen

♠ **83872** Mucin, synovial fluid (Ropes test)

♠ **83873** Myelin basic protein, cerebrospinal fluid
➲ *CPT Changes: An Insider's View* 2002

(For oligoclonal bands, use 83916)

♠ **83874** Myoglobin
➲ *CPT Assistant* Feb 98:1

(Nalorphine, use 83925)

♠ **83880** Natriuretic peptide
➲ *CPT Assistant* Jul 03:7; *CPT Changes: An Insider's View* 2003

♠ **83883** Nephelometry, each analyte not elsewhere specified

♠ **83885** Nickel

♠ **83887** Nicotine

Codes 83890-83912 are intended for use with molecular diagnostic techniques for analysis of nucleic acids.

Codes 83890-83912 are coded by procedure rather than analyte.

Code separately for each procedure used in an analysis. For example, a procedure requiring isolation of DNA, restriction endonuclease digestion, electrophoresis, and nucleic acid probe amplification would be coded 83890, 83892, 83894, and 83898.

►When molecular diagnostic procedures are performed to test for infectious disease, oncology, hematology, neurology or inherited disorder, use the appropriate modifier to specify probe type or condition tested. (See **Appendix I**).◄

(For microbial identification, see 87797, 87798)

♠ **83890** Molecular diagnostics; molecular isolation or extraction
➲ *CPT Assistant* Fall 93:26, Nov 98:26

♠ **83891** isolation or extraction of highly purified nucleic acid
➲ *CPT Assistant* Nov 98:26

♠ **83892** enzymatic digestion
➲ *CPT Assistant* Fall 93:26

♠ **83893** dot/slot blot production
➲ *CPT Assistant* Nov 98:26

♠ **83894** separation by gel electrophoresis (eg, agarose, polyacrylamide)
➲ *CPT Assistant* Fall 93:25, Nov 98:26

♠ **83896** nucleic acid probe, each
➲ *CPT Assistant* Fall 93:26, Aug 02:10

♠ **83897** nucleic acid transfer (eg, Southern, Northern)
➲ *CPT Assistant* Nov 98:26

♠ **83898** amplification of patient nucleic acid (eg, PCR, LCR), single primer pair, each primer pair
➲ *CPT Assistant* Fall 93:26, Nov 98:26; *CPT Changes: An Insider's View* 2001

♠ **83901** amplification of patient nucleic acid, multiplex, each multiplex reaction
➲ *CPT Assistant* Nov 98:26

♠ **83902** reverse transcription
➲ *CPT Changes: An Insider's View* 2001

♠ **83903** mutation scanning, by physical properties (eg, single strand conformational polymorphisms (SSCP), heteroduplex, denaturing gradient gel electrophoresis (DGGE), RNA'ase A), single segment, each
➲ *CPT Assistant* Nov 98:26

♠ **83904** mutation identification by sequencing, single segment, each segment
➲ *CPT Assistant* Nov 98:26

♠ **83905** mutation identification by allele specific transcription, single segment, each segment
➲ *CPT Assistant* Nov 98:26

♠ **83906** mutation identification by allele specific translation, single segment, each segment
➲ *CPT Assistant* Nov 98:26

♠ **83912** interpretation and report

♠ **83915** Nucleotidase 5-

♠ **83916** Oligoclonal immune (oligoclonal bands)
➲ *CPT Changes: An Insider's View* 2002

♠ **83918** Organic acids; total, quantitative, each specimen
➲ *CPT Assistant* Mar 96:11, Nov 98:26; *CPT Changes: An Insider's View* 2001

♠ **83919** qualitative, each specimen
➲ *CPT Assistant* Nov 98:26

♠ **83921** Organic acid, single, quantitative
➲ *CPT Changes: An Insider's View* 2001

♠ **83925** Opiates, (eg, morphine, meperidine)

♠ **83930** Osmolality; blood

♠ **83935** urine

♠ **83937** Osteocalcin (bone g1a protein)
➲ *CPT Assistant* Summer 94:5

♠ **83945** Oxalate

♠ **83950** Oncoprotein, HER-2/neu
➲ *CPT Changes: An Insider's View* 2002

(For tissue, see 88342, 88365)

♠ **83970** Parathormone (parathyroid hormone)

(Pesticide, quantitative, see code for specific method. For screen for chlorinated hydrocarbons, use 82441)

♠ **83986** pH, body fluid, except blood

(For blood pH, see 82800, 82803)

♠ **83992** Phencyclidine (PCP)

(For qualitative analysis, see 80100-80103)

(Phenobarbital, use 80184)

♠ **84022** Phenothiazine

(For qualitative analysis, see 80100, 80101)

♠ **84030** Phenylalanine (PKU), blood

(Phenylalanine-tyrosine ratio, see 84030, 84510)

♠ **84035** Phenylketones, qualitative

♠ **84060** Phosphatase, acid; total

♠ **84061** forensic examination

♠ **84066** prostatic

♠ **84075** Phosphatase, alkaline;
➲ *CPT Assistant* Dec 99:1

♠ **84078** heat stable (total not included)

♠ **84080** isoenzymes

♠ **84081** Phosphatidylglycerol

(Phosphates inorganic, use 84100)

(Phosphates, organic, see code for specific method. For cholinesterase, see 82480, 82482)

♠ **84085** Phosphogluconate, 6-, dehydrogenase, RBC

♠ **84087** Phosphohexose isomerase

♠ **84100** Phosphorus inorganic (phosphate);
➲ *CPT Assistant* Dec 99:1

♠ **84105** urine

(Pituitary gonadotropins, see 83001-83002)

(PKU, see 84030, 84035)

♠ **84106** Porphobilinogen, urine; qualitative

♠ **84110** quantitative

♠ **84119** Porphyrins, urine; qualitative

♠ **84120** quantitation and fractionation

♠ **84126** Porphyrins, feces; quantitative

♠ **84127** qualitative

(Porphyrin precursors, see 82135, 84106, 84110)

(For protoporphyrin, RBC, see 84202, 84203)

♠ **84132** Potassium; serum
➲ *CPT Assistant* Dec 99:1, Jun 02:1-3, Sep 03:7

♠ **84133** urine

♠ **84134** Prealbumin

(For microalbumin, see 82043, 82044)

♠ **84135** Pregnanediol

♠ **84138** Pregnanetriol

♠ **84140** Pregnenolone
➲ *CPT Assistant* Summer 94:6

♠ **84143** 17-hydroxypregnenolone
➲ *CPT Assistant* Summer 94:6

♠ **84144** Progesterone

(Progesterone receptor assay, use 84234)

(For proinsulin, use 84206)

♠ **84146** Prolactin

♠ **84150** Prostaglandin, each

♠ **84152** Prostate specific antigen (PSA); complexed (direct measurement)
➲ *CPT Changes: An Insider's View* 2001

♠ **84153** total
➲ *CPT Assistant* Fall 93:26, May 96:10, Aug 96:10, Jan 97:10, Nov 98:26, Aug 99:5, Dec 99:10

♠ **84154** free
➲ *CPT Assistant* Nov 98:26, Aug 99:5, Dec 99:10

♠ **84155** Protein, total, except by refractometry; serum
➲ *CPT Assistant* Dec 99:1, Jan 00:7; *CPT Changes: An Insider's View* 2004

♠ **84156** urine
➲ *CPT Changes: An Insider's View* 2004

♠ **84157** other source (eg, synovial fluid, cerebrospinal fluid)
➲ *CPT Changes: An Insider's View* 2004

♠ **84160** Protein, total, by refractometry, any source
➲ *CPT Changes: An Insider's View* 2004

(For urine total protein by dipstick method, use 81000-81003)

♠● **84163** Pregnancy-associated plasma protein-A (PAPP-A)
➲ *CPT Changes: An Insider's View* 2005

♠▲ **84165** Protein; electrophoretic fractionation and quantitation, serum
➲ *CPT Changes: An Insider's View* 2004, 2005

♠● **84166** electrophoretic fractionation and quantitation, other fluids with concentration (eg, urine, CSF)
➲ *CPT Changes: An Insider's View* 2005

♠ **84181** Western Blot, with interpretation and report, blood or other body fluid

♠ **84182** Western Blot, with interpretation and report, blood or other body fluid, immunological probe for band identification, each

(For Western Blot tissue analysis, use 88371)

♠ **84202** Protoporphyrin, RBC; quantitative

♠ **84203** screen

♠ **84206** Proinsulin

(Pseudocholinesterase, use 82480)

♠ **84207** Pyridoxal phosphate (Vitamin B-6)

♠ **84210** Pyruvate

♠ **84220** Pyruvate kinase

♠ **84228** Quinine

♠ **84233** Receptor assay; estrogen

♠ **84234** progesterone

♠ **84235** endocrine, other than estrogen or progesterone (specify hormone)

♠ **84238** non-endocrine (eg, acetylcholine) (specify receptor)

♠ **84244** Renin

♠ **84252** Riboflavin (Vitamin B-2)

(Salicylates, use 80196)

(Secretin test, see 99070, 89100 and appropriate analyses)

♠ **84255** Selenium

♠ **84260** Serotonin

(For urine metabolites (HIAA), use 83497)

♠ **84270** Sex hormone binding globulin (SHBG)
➲ *CPT Assistant* Summer 94:4

♠ **84275** Sialic acid

(Sickle hemoglobin, use 85660)

♠ **84285** Silica

♠ **84295** Sodium; serum
➲ *CPT Assistant* Dec 99:1

♠ **84300** urine

♠ **84302** other source
➲ *CPT Assistant* Jul 03:7; *CPT Changes: An Insider's View* 2003

(Somatomammotropin, use 83632)

(Somatotropin, use 83003)

♠ **84305** Somatomedin
➲ *CPT Assistant* Summer 94:4

♠ **84307** Somatostatin
➲ *CPT Assistant* Summer 94:4

♠ **84311** Spectrophotometry, analyte not elsewhere specified

♠ **84315** Specific gravity (except urine)

(For specific gravity, urine, see 81000-81003)

(Stone analysis, see 82355-82370)

♠ **84375** Sugars, chromatographic, TLC or paper chromatography

♠ **84376** Sugars (mono-, di-, and oligosaccharides); single qualitative, each specimen
➲ *CPT Assistant* Nov 98:26-27, Dec 99:7

♠ **84377** multiple qualitative, each specimen
➲ *CPT Assistant* Nov 98:26-27, Jul 03:7

♠ **84378** single quantitative, each specimen
➲ *CPT Assistant* Nov 98:26-27

♠ **84379** multiple quantitative, each specimen
➲ *CPT Assistant* Nov 98:26-27, Dec 99:7, Jul 03:7

♠ **84392** Sulfate, urine

(Sulfhemoglobin, see hemoglobin, 83055, 83060)

(T-3, see 84479-84481)

(T-4, see 84436-84439)

♠ **84402** Testosterone; free

♠ **84403** total

♠ **84425** Thiamine (Vitamin B-1)

♠ **84430** Thiocyanate

♠ **84432** Thyroglobulin
➲ *CPT Assistant* Summer 94:2

(Thyroglobulin, antibody, use 86800)

(Thyrotropin releasing hormone (TRH) test, see 80438, 80439)

♠ **84436** Thyroxine; total
➲ *CPT Assistant* Fall 93:25, Summer 94:3

♠ **84437** requiring elution (eg, neonatal)

♠ **84439** free

♠ **84442** Thyroxine binding globulin (TBG)

♠ **84443** Thyroid stimulating hormone (TSH)
➲ *CPT Assistant* Summer 94:3

♠ **84445** Thyroid stimulating immune globulins (TSI)
➲ *CPT Assistant* Summer 94:3; *CPT Changes: An Insider's View* 2002

(Tobramycin, use 80200)

♠ **84446** Tocopherol alpha (Vitamin E)

(Tolbutamide tolerance, use 82953)

♠ **84449** Transcortin (cortisol binding globulin)
➲ *CPT Assistant* Summer 94:6

♠ **84450** Transferase; aspartate amino (AST) (SGOT)
➲ *CPT Assistant* Dec 99:1

♠ **84460** alanine amino (ALT) (SGPT)
➲ *CPT Assistant* Dec 99:1

♠ **84466** Transferrin
➲ *CPT Assistant* Summer 94:4

(Iron binding capacity, use 83550)

♠ **84478** Triglycerides
➲ *CPT Assistant* Dec 99:1, Mar 00:11

♠ **84479** Thyroid hormone (T3 or T4) uptake or thyroid hormone binding ratio (THBR)
➲ *CPT Assistant* Fall 93:25, Summer 94:3

♠ **84480** Triiodothyronine T3; total (TT-3)

♠ **84481** free

♠ **84482** reverse
➲ *CPT Assistant* Summer 94:2

♠ **84484** Troponin, quantitative
➲ *CPT Assistant* Nov 97:29, Jan 98:6, Feb 98:1

(For troponin, qualitative assay, use 84512)

♠ **84485** Trypsin; duodenal fluid

♠ **84488** feces, qualitative

♠ **84490** feces, quantitative, 24-hour collection

♠ **84510** Tyrosine

(Urate crystal identification, use 89060)

♠ **84512** Troponin, qualitative
➲ *CPT Assistant* Nov 97:29, Jan 98:6, Feb 98:1

(For troponin, quantitative assay, use 84484)

♠ **84520** Urea nitrogen; quantitative
➲ *CPT Assistant* Dec 99:1

♠ **84525** semiquantitative (eg, reagent strip test)
➲ *CPT Assistant* Mar 98:3

♠ **84540** Urea nitrogen, urine

♠ **84545** Urea nitrogen, clearance

♠ **84550** Uric acid; blood
➲ *CPT Assistant* Dec 99:1

♠ **84560** other source

♠ **84577** Urobilinogen, feces, quantitative

♠ **84578** Urobilinogen, urine; qualitative

♠ **84580** quantitative, timed specimen

♠ **84583** semiquantitative

(Uroporphyrins, use 84120)

(Valproic acid (dipropylacetic acid), use 80164)

♠ **84585** Vanillylmandelic acid (VMA), urine

♠ **84586** Vasoactive intestinal peptide (VIP)
➲ *CPT Assistant* Summer 94:6

♠ **84588** Vasopressin (antidiuretic hormone, ADH)

♠ **84590** Vitamin A

(Vitamin B-1, use 84425)

(Vitamin B-2, use 84252)

(Vitamin B-6, use 84207)

(Vitamin B-12, use 82607)

(Vitamin B-12, absorption (Schilling), see 78270, 78271)

(Vitamin C, use 82180)

(Vitamin D, see 82306, 82307, 82652)

(Vitamin E, use 84446)

♠ **84591** Vitamin, not otherwise specified
➲ *CPT Changes: An Insider's View* 2001

♠ **84597** Vitamin K

(VMA, use 84585)

♠ **84600** Volatiles (eg, acetic anhydride, carbon tetrachloride, dichloroethane, dichloromethane, diethylether, isopropyl alcohol, methanol)

(For acetaldehyde, use 82000)

(Volume, blood, RISA or Cr-51, see 78110, 78111)

♠ **84620** Xylose absorption test, blood and/or urine

(For administration, use 99070)

♠ **84630** Zinc

♠ **84681** C-peptide

♠ **84702** Gonadotropin, chorionic (hCG); quantitative

♠ **84703** qualitative

(For urine pregnancy test by visual color comparison, use 81025)

♠ **84830** Ovulation tests, by visual color comparison methods for human luteinizing hormone

♠ **84999** Unlisted chemistry procedure
➲ *CPT Assistant* Oct 00:7

Hematology and Coagulation

(For blood banking procedures, see **Transfusion Medicine**)

(Agglutinins, see **Immunology**)

(Antiplasmin, use 85410)

(Antithrombin III, see 85300, 85301)

♠ **85002** Bleeding time

♠ **85004** Blood count; automated differential WBC count
➲ *CPT Assistant* Jan 04:26; *CPT Changes: An Insider's View* 2003

♠ **85007** blood smear, microscopic examination with manual differential WBC count
➲ *CPT Assistant* Jul 03:7, Jan 04:26; *CPT Changes: An Insider's View* 2003

♠ **85008** blood smear, microscopic examination without manual differential WBC count
➲ *CPT Assistant* Jul 03:7, Jan 04:26; *CPT Changes: An Insider's View* 2003

(For other fluids (eg, CSF), see 89050, 89051)

♠ **85009** manual differential WBC count, buffy coat
➲ *CPT Assistant* Jul 03:7, Jan 04:26; *CPT Changes: An Insider's View* 2003

(Eosinophils, nasal smear, use 89190)

♠ **85013** spun microhematocrit

♠ **85014** hematocrit (Hct)
➲ *CPT Assistant* Jan 04:26; *CPT Changes: An Insider's View* 2003

♠ **85018** hemoglobin (Hgb)
➲ *CPT Assistant* Jul 03:7; *CPT Changes: An Insider's View* 2003

(For other hemoglobin determination, see 83020-83069)

(For immunoassay, hemoglobin, fecal, use 82274)

(85021 has been deleted)

(85022 has been deleted)

(85023 has been deleted. To report, use 85007 and 85027)

(85024 has been deleted. To report, use 85025)

♠ **85025** complete (CBC), automated (Hgb, Hct, RBC, WBC and platelet count) and automated differential WBC count
➲ *CPT Assistant* Jul 00:11, Jul 03:7; *CPT Changes: An Insider's View* 2003

♠ **85027** complete (CBC), automated (Hgb, Hct, RBC, WBC and platelet count)
➲ *CPT Assistant* Jul 03:7; *CPT Changes: An Insider's View* 2003

(85031 has been deleted. To report, use 85014, 85018 and 85032)

♠ **85032** manual cell count (erythrocyte, leukocyte, or platelet) each
➲ *CPT Assistant* Jul 03:7, Nov 03:15; *CPT Changes: An Insider's View* 2003

♠ **85041** red blood cell (RBC), automated
➲ *CPT Assistant* Jul 03:7; *CPT Changes: An Insider's View* 2003

(Do not report code 85041 in conjunction with 85025 or 85027)

♠ **85044** reticulocyte, manual
➲ *CPT Assistant* Jul 03:7; *CPT Changes: An Insider's View* 2003

♠ **85045** reticulocyte, automated
➲ *CPT Assistant* Jul 03:7; *CPT Changes: An Insider's View* 2003

♠ ▲ **85046** reticulocytes, automated, including one or more cellular parameters (eg, reticulocyte hemoglobin content (CHr), immature reticulocyte fraction (IRF), reticulocyte volume (MRV), RNA content), direct measurement
➲ *CPT Assistant* Nov 98:27; *CPT Changes: An Insider's View* 2005

♠ **85048** leukocyte (WBC), automated
➲ *CPT Assistant* Jul 03:7; *CPT Changes: An Insider's View* 2003

♠ **85049** platelet, automated
➲ *CPT Changes: An Insider's View* 2003

♠ **85055** Reticulated platelet assay
➲ *CPT Changes: An Insider's View* 2004

♣ **85060** Blood smear, peripheral, interpretation by physician with written report

♣ **85097** Bone marrow, smear interpretation
➲ *CPT Assistant* Winter 92:17, Jul 98:4, Mar 03:22; *CPT Changes: An Insider's View* 2002

(For special stains, see 85540, 88312, 88313)

(For bone biopsy, see 20220, 20225, 20240, 20245, 20250, 20251)

♠ **85130** Chromogenic substrate assay

(Circulating anti-coagulant screen (mixing studies), see 85611, 85732)

♠ **85170** Clot retraction

♠ **85175** Clot lysis time, whole blood dilution

(Clotting factor I (fibrinogen), see 85384, 85385)

Pathology and Laboratory

♠ **85210** Clotting; factor II, prothrombin, specific

(See also 85610-85613)

♠ **85220** factor V (AcG or proaccelerin), labile factor

♠ **85230** factor VII (proconvertin, stable factor)

♠ **85240** factor VIII (AHG), one stage

♠ **85244** factor VIII related antigen

♠ **85245** factor VIII, VW factor, ristocetin cofactor

♠ **85246** factor VIII, VW factor antigen

♠ **85247** factor VIII, von Willebrand factor, multimetric analysis

♠ **85250** factor IX (PTC or Christmas)

♠ **85260** factor X (Stuart-Prower)

♠ **85270** factor XI (PTA)

♠ **85280** factor XII (Hageman)

♠ **85290** factor XIII (fibrin stabilizing)

♠ **85291** factor XIII (fibrin stabilizing), screen solubility

♠ **85292** prekallikrein assay (Fletcher factor assay)

♠ **85293** high molecular weight kininogen assay (Fitzgerald factor assay)

♠ **85300** Clotting inhibitors or anticoagulants; antithrombin III, activity

♠ **85301** antithrombin III, antigen assay

♠ **85302** protein C, antigen

♠ **85303** protein C, activity

♠ **85305** protein S, total

♠ **85306** protein S, free

♠ **85307** Activated Protein C (APC) resistance assay
➔ *CPT Changes: An Insider's View* 2001

♠ **85335** Factor inhibitor test

♠ **85337** Thrombomodulin

(For mixing studies for inhibitors, use 85732)

♠ **85345** Coagulation time; Lee and White

♠ **85347** activated

♠ **85348** other methods

(Differential count, see 85007 et seq)

(Duke bleeding time, use 85002)

(Eosinophils, nasal smear, use 89190)

♠ **85360** Euglobulin lysis

(Fetal hemoglobin, see 83030, 83033, 85460)

♠ **85362** Fibrin(ogen) degradation (split) products (FDP)(FSP); agglutination slide, semiquantitative

(Immunoelectrophoresis, use 86320)

♠ **85366** paracoagulation

♠ **85370** quantitative

♠ **85378** Fibrin degradation products, D-dimer; qualitative or semiquantitative
➔ *CPT Assistant* Jul 03:7; *CPT Changes: An Insider's View* 2003

♠ **85379** quantitative

(For ultrasensitive and standard sensitivity quantitative D-dimer, use 85379)

♠ **85380** ultrasensitive (eg, for evaluation for venous thromboembolism), qualitative or semiquantitative
➔ *CPT Assistant* Jul 03:7; *CPT Changes: An Insider's View* 2003

♠ **85384** Fibrinogen; activity

♠ **85385** antigen

♠ **85390** Fibrinolysins or coagulopathy screen, interpretation and report

☆ **85396** Coagulation/fibrinolysis assay, whole blood (eg, viscoelastic clot assessment), including use of any pharmacologic additive(s), as indicated, including interpretation and written report, per day
➔ *CPT Changes: An Insider's View* 2004

♠ **85400** Fibrinolytic factors and inhibitors; plasmin

♠ **85410** alpha-2 antiplasmin

♠ **85415** plasminogen activator

♠ **85420** plasminogen, except antigenic assay

♠ **85421** plasminogen, antigenic assay

(Fragility, red blood cell, see 85547, 85555-85557)

♠ **85441** Heinz bodies; direct

♠ **85445** induced, acetyl phenylhydrazine

(Hematocrit (PCV), see 85014, 85025, 85027)

(Hemoglobin, see 83020-83068, 85018, 85025, 85027)

♠ **85460** Hemoglobin or RBCs, fetal, for fetomaternal hemorrhage; differential lysis (Kleihauer-Betke)
➔ *CPT Assistant* Fall 93:25

(See also 83030, 83033)

(Hemolysins, see 86940, 86941)

♠ **85461** rosette

♠ **85475** Hemolysin, acid

(See also 86940, 86941)

♠ **85520** Heparin assay

♠ **85525** Heparin neutralization

♠ **85530** Heparin-protamine tolerance test

♠ **85536** Iron stain, peripheral blood
➔ *CPT Changes: An Insider's View* 2001

(For iron stains on bone marrow or other tissues with physician evaluation, use 88313)

♠ **85540** Leukocyte alkaline phosphatase with count

♠ **85547** Mechanical fragility, RBC

♠ **85549** Muramidase

(Nitroblue tetrazolium dye test, use 86384)

♠ **85555** Osmotic fragility, RBC; unincubated

♠ **85557** incubated

(Packed cell volume, use 85013)

(Partial thromboplastin time, see 85730, 85732)

(Parasites, blood (eg, malaria smears), use 87207)

(Plasmin, use 85400)

(Plasminogen, use 85420)

(Plasminogen activator, use 85415)

♠ **85576** Platelet, aggregation (in vitro), each agent
➲ *CPT Assistant* Jul 96:10; *CPT Changes: An Insider's View* 2003

(85585 has been deleted. To report, use 85008)

(85590 has been deleted. To report, use 85032)

(85595 has been deleted. To report, use 85049)

♠ **85597** Platelet neutralization

♠ **85610** Prothrombin time;

♠ **85611** substitution, plasma fractions, each

♠ **85612** Russell viper venom time (includes venom); undiluted

♠ **85613** diluted

(Red blood cell count, see 85025, 85027, 85041)

♠ **85635** Reptilase test

(Reticulocyte count, see 85044, 85045)

♠ **85651** Sedimentation rate, erythrocyte; non-automated

♠ **85652** automated

♠ **85660** Sickling of RBC, reduction

(Hemoglobin electrophoresis, use 83020)

(Smears (eg, for parasites, malaria), use 87207)

♠ **85670** Thrombin time; plasma

♠ **85675** titer

♠ **85705** Thromboplastin inhibition, tissue

(For individual clotting factors, see 85245-85247)

♠ **85730** Thromboplastin time, partial (PTT); plasma or whole blood

♠ **85732** substitution, plasma fractions, each

♠ **85810** Viscosity

(von Willebrand factor assay, see 85245-85247)

(WBC count, see 85025, 85027, 85048, 89050)

♠ **85999** Unlisted hematology and coagulation procedure

Immunology

(Acetylcholine receptor antibody, see 86255, 86256)

(Actinomyces, antibodies to, use 86602)

(Adrenal cortex antibodies, see 86255, 86256)

(For tuberculosis test, cell mediated immunity measurement of gamma interferon antigen response, use Category III code 0010T)

♠ **86000** Agglutinins, febrile (eg, Brucella, Francisella, Murine typhus, Q fever, Rocky Mountain spotted fever, scrub typhus), each antigen

(For antibodies to infectious agents, see 86602-86804)

♠ **86001** Allergen specific IgG quantitative or semiquantitative, each allergen
➲ *CPT Changes: An Insider's View* 2001

(Agglutinins and autohemolysins, see 86940, 86941)

♠ **86003** Allergen specific IgE; quantitative or semiquantitative, each allergen
➲ *CPT Assistant* Spring 94:31

(For total quantitative IgE, use 82785)

♠ **86005** qualitative, multiallergen screen (dipstick, paddle or disk)
➲ *CPT Assistant* Spring 94:31

(For total qualitative IgE, use 83518)

(Alpha-1 antitrypsin, see 82103, 82104)

(Alpha-1 feto-protein, see 82105, 82106)

(Anti-AChR (acetylcholine receptor) antibody titer, see 86255, 86256)

(Anticardiolipin antibody, use 86147)

(Anti-DNA, use 86225)

(Anti-deoxyribonuclease titer, use 86215)

♠ **86021** Antibody identification; leukocyte antibodies

♠ **86022** platelet antibodies

♠ **86023** platelet associated immunoglobulin assay

♠ **86038** Antinuclear antibodies (ANA);

♠ **86039** titer

(Antistreptococcal antibody, ie, anti-DNAse, use 86215)

(Antistreptokinase titer, use 86590)

♠ **86060** Antistreptolysin O; titer

(For antibodies to infectious agents, see 86602-86804)

♠ **86063** screen

(For antibodies to infectious agents, see 86602-86804)

(Blastomyces, antibodies to, use 86612)

♠● **86064** B cells, total count
➔ *CPT Changes: An Insider's View* 2005

►(For flow cytometric immunophenotyping for the assessment of potential hematolymphoid neoplasia, see 88182, 88184-88189)◄

♣ **86077** Blood bank physician services; difficult cross match and/or evaluation of irregular antibody(s), interpretation and written report

♣ **86078** investigation of transfusion reaction including suspicion of transmissible disease, interpretation and written report

♣ **86079** authorization for deviation from standard blood banking procedures (eg, use of outdated blood, transfusion of Rh incompatible units), with written report

(Brucella, antibodies to, use 86622)

(Candida, antibodies to, use 86628. For skin testing, use 86485)

♠ **86140** C-reactive protein;
➔ *CPT Changes: An Insider's View* 2002

(Candidiasis, use 86628)

♠ **86141** high sensitivity (hsCRP)
➔ *CPT Changes: An Insider's View* 2002

♠ **86146** Beta 2 Glycoprotein I antibody, each
➔ *CPT Changes: An Insider's View* 2001

♠ **86147** Cardiolipin (phospholipid) antibody, each Ig class
➔ *CPT Changes: An Insider's View* 2001

♠ **86148** Anti-phosphatidylserine (phospholipid) antibody
➔ *CPT Assistant* Nov 97:30, Jul 03:7, Nov 03:5

(To report antiprothrombin (phospholipid cofactor) antibody, use Category III code 0030T)

♠ **86155** Chemotaxis assay, specify method

(Clostridium difficile toxin, use 87230)

(Coccidioides, antibodies to, see 86635. For skin testing, use 86490)

♠ **86156** Cold agglutinin; screen

♠ **86157** titer

♠ **86160** Complement; antigen, each component

♠ **86161** functional activity, each component

♠ **86162** total hemolytic (CH50)

♠ **86171** Complement fixation tests, each antigen

(Coombs test, see 86880-86886)

♠ **86185** Counterimmunoelectrophoresis, each antigen

(Cryptococcus, antibodies to, use 86641)

♠ **86215** Deoxyribonuclease, antibody

♠ **86225** Deoxyribonucleic acid (DNA) antibody; native or double stranded

(Echinococcus, antibodies to, see code for specific method)

(For HIV antibody tests, see 86701-86703)

♠ **86226** single stranded

(Anti D.S., DNA, IFA, eg, using C.Lucilae, see 86255 and 86256)

♠ **86235** Extractable nuclear antigen, antibody to, any method (eg, nRNP, SS-A, SS-B, Sm, RNP, Sc170, J01), each antibody

♠ **86243** Fc receptor

(Filaria, antibodies to, see code for specific method)

♠ **86255** Fluorescent noninfectious agent antibody; screen, each antibody
➔ *CPT Assistant* Nov 98:27

♠ **86256** titer, each antibody

(Fluorescent technique for antigen identification in tissue, use 88346; for indirect fluorescence, use 88347)

(FTA, see 86781)

(Gel (agar) diffusion tests, use 86331)

♠ **86277** Growth hormone, human (HGH), antibody

♠ **86280** Hemagglutination inhibition test (HAI)

(For rubella, use 86762)

(For antibodies to infectious agents, see 86602-86804)

♠ **86294** Immunoassay for tumor antigen, qualitative or semiquantitative (eg, bladder tumor antigen)
➔ *CPT Changes: An Insider's View* 2001

♠ **86300** Immunoassay for tumor antigen, quantitative; CA 15-3 (27.29)
➔ *CPT Changes: An Insider's View* 2001

♠ **86301** CA 19-9
➔ *CPT Changes: An Insider's View* 2001

♠ **86304** CA 125
➔ *CPT Changes: An Insider's View* 2001

(For measurement of serum HER-2/neu oncoprotein, see 83950)

(For hepatitis delta agent, antibody, use 86692)

♠ **86308** Heterophile antibodies; screening

(For antibodies to infectious agents, see 86602-86804)

♠ **86309** titer

(For antibodies to infectious agents, see 86602-86804)

♠ **86310** titers after absorption with beef cells and guinea pig kidney

(Histoplasma, antibodies to, use 86698. For skin testing, use 86510)

(For antibodies to infectious agents, see 86602-86804)

(Human growth hormone antibody, use 86277)

♠ 86316 Immunoassay for tumor antigen, other antigen, quantitative (eg, CA 50, 72-4, 549), each
➲ *CPT Assistant* May 96:11, Aug 96:11, Apr 98:15, Aug 99:5, Dec 99:10; *CPT Changes: An Insider's View* 2001

♠ 86317 Immunoassay for infectious agent antibody, quantitative, not otherwise specified
➲ *CPT Assistant* Nov 97:30-31

(For immunoassay techniques for antigens, see 83516, 83518, 83519, 83520, 87301-87450, 87810-87899)

(For particle agglutination procedures, use 86403)

♠ 86318 Immunoassay for infectious agent antibody, qualitative or semiquantitative, single step method (eg, reagent strip)

♠ 86320 Immunoelectrophoresis; serum

♠ 86325 other fluids (eg, urine, cerebrospinal fluid) with concentration
➲ *CPT Changes: An Insider's View* 2002

♠ 86327 crossed (2-dimensional assay)

♠ 86329 Immunodiffusion; not elsewhere specified
➲ *CPT Assistant* Aug 00:11

♠ 86331 gel diffusion, qualitative (Ouchterlony), each antigen or antibody

♠ 86332 Immune complex assay

♠▲ 86334 Immunofixation electrophoresis; serum
➲ *CPT Changes: An Insider's View* 2005

♠● 86335 other fluids with concentration (eg, urine, CSF)
➲ *CPT Changes: An Insider's View* 2005

♠ 86336 Inhibin A
➲ *CPT Changes: An Insider's View* 2002

♠ 86337 Insulin antibodies

♠ 86340 Intrinsic factor antibodies

(Leptospira, antibodies to, use 86720)

(Leukoagglutinins, use 86021)

♠ 86341 Islet cell antibody
➲ *CPT Assistant* Summer 94:6

♠ 86343 Leukocyte histamine release test (LHR)

♠ 86344 Leukocyte phagocytosis

♠ 86353 Lymphocyte transformation, mitogen (phytomitogen) or antigen induced blastogenesis

(Lymphocytes immunophenotyping, ►see 88182, 88189◄ for cytometry; see 88342, 88346 for microscopic techniques)

(Malaria antibodies, use 86750)

♠ 86359 T cells; total count
➲ *CPT Assistant* Nov 97:30

♠ 86360 absolute CD4 and CD8 count, including ratio
➲ *CPT Assistant* Nov 97:30

♠ 86361 absolute CD4 count
➲ *CPT Assistant* Nov 97:30

♠ 86376 Microsomal antibodies (eg, thyroid or liver-kidney), each

♠ 86378 Migration inhibitory factor test (MIF)

(Mitochondrial antibody, liver, see 86255, 86256)

(Mononucleosis, see 86308-86310)

♠● 86379 Natural killer (NK) cells, total count
➲ *CPT Changes: An Insider's View* 2005

►(For flow cytometric immunophenotyping for the assessment of potential hematolymphoid neoplasia, see 88182, 88184-88189)◄

♠ 86382 Neutralization test, viral

♠ 86384 Nitroblue tetrazolium dye test (NTD)

(Ouchterlony diffusion, use 86331)

(Platelet antibodies, see 86022, 86023)

♠ 86403 Particle agglutination; screen, each antibody

♠ 86406 titer, each antibody

(Pregnancy test, see 84702, 84703)

(Rapid plasma reagin test (RPR), see 86592, 86593)

♠ 86430 Rheumatoid factor; qualitative

♠ 86431 quantitative

(Serologic test for syphilis, see 86592, 86593)

♣ 86485 Skin test; candida

(For antibody, candida, use 86628)

♣ 86490 coccidioidomycosis

♣ 86510 histoplasmosis

(For histoplasma, antibody, use 86698)

♣ 86580 tuberculosis, intradermal

♣ 86585 tuberculosis, tine test

(For tuberculosis test, cell mediated immunity measurement of gamma interferon antigen response, use Category III code 0010T)

(For skin tests for allergy, see 95010-95199)

(Smooth muscle antibody, see 86255, 86256)

(Sporothrix, antibodies to, see code for specific method)

♣ 86586 Unlisted antigen, each
➲ *CPT Assistant* Jul 98:11; *CPT Changes: An Insider's View* 2000

♠● 86587 Stem cells (ie, CD34), total count
➲ *CPT Changes: An Insider's View* 2005

►(For flow cytometric immunophenotyping for the assessment of potential hematolymphoid neoplasia, see 88182, 88189)◄

♠ 86590 Streptokinase, antibody

(For antibodies to infectious agents, see 86602-86804)

(Streptolysin O antibody, see antistreptolysin O, 86060, 86063)

♠ **86592** Syphilis test; qualitative (eg, VDRL, RPR, ART)

(For antibodies to infectious agents, see 86602-86804)

♠ **86593** quantitative

(For antibodies to infectious agents, see 86602-86804)

(Tetanus antibody, use 86774)

(Thyroglobulin antibody, use 86800)

(Thyroglobulin, use 84432)

(Thyroid microsomal antibody, use 86376)

(For toxoplasma antibody, see 86777-86778)

The following codes (86602-86804) are qualitative or semiquantitative immunoassays performed by multiple step methods for the detection of antibodies to infectious agents. For immunoassays by single step method (eg, reagent strips), use code 86318. Procedures for the identification of antibodies should be coded as precisely as possible. For example, an antibody to a virus could be coded with increasing specificity for virus, family, genus, species, or type. In some cases, further precision may be added to codes by specifying the class of immunoglobulin being detected. When multiple tests are done to detect antibodies to organisms classified more precisely than the specificity allowed by available codes, it is appropriate to code each as a separate service. For example, a test for antibody to an enterovirus is coded as 86658. Coxsackie viruses are enteroviruses, but there are no codes for the individual species of enterovirus. If assays are performed for antibodies to coxsackie A and B species, each assay should be separately coded. Similarly, if multiple assays are performed for antibodies of different immunoglobulin classes, each assay should be coded separately.

(For the detection of antibodies other than those to infectious agents, see specific antibody (eg, 86021, 86022, 86023, 86376, 86800, 86850-86870) or specific method (eg, 83516, 86255, 86256)).

(For infectious agent/antigen detection, see 87260-87899)

♠ **86602** Antibody; actinomyces

♠ **86603** adenovirus

♠ **86606** Aspergillus

♠ **86609** bacterium, not elsewhere specified

♠ **86611** Bartonella
➲ *CPT Changes: An Insider's View* 2001

♠ **86612** Blastomyces

♠ **86615** Bordetella

♠ **86617** Borrelia burgdorferi (Lyme disease) confirmatory test (eg, Western Blot or immunoblot)

♠ **86618** Borrelia burgdorferi (Lyme disease)

♠ **86619** Borrelia (relapsing fever)

♠ **86622** Brucella

♠ **86625** Campylobacter

♠ **86628** Candida

(For skin test, candida, use 86485)

♠ **86631** Chlamydia

♠ **86632** Chlamydia, IgM
➲ *CPT Assistant* Nov 97:31

(For chlamydia antigen, see 87270, 87320. For fluorescent antibody technique, see 86255, 86256)

♠ **86635** Coccidioides

♠ **86638** Coxiella burnetii (Q fever)

♠ **86641** Cryptococcus

♠ **86644** cytomegalovirus (CMV)

♠ **86645** cytomegalovirus (CMV), IgM
➲ *CPT Assistant* Jul 03:7

♠ **86648** Diphtheria

♠ **86651** encephalitis, California (La Crosse)

♠ **86652** encephalitis, Eastern equine

♠ **86653** encephalitis, St. Louis

♠ **86654** encephalitis, Western equine

♠ **86658** enterovirus (eg, coxsackie, echo, polio)

(Trichinella, antibodies to, use 86784)

(Trypanosoma, antibodies to, see code for specific method)

(Tuberculosis, use 86580 for skin testing)

(Viral antibodies, see code for specific method)

♠ **86663** Epstein-Barr (EB) virus, early antigen (EA)

♠ **86664** Epstein-Barr (EB) virus, nuclear antigen (EBNA)

♠ **86665** Epstein-Barr (EB) virus, viral capsid (VCA)

♠ **86666** Ehrlichia
➲ *CPT Changes: An Insider's View* 2001

♠ **86668** Francisella tularensis

♠ **86671** fungus, not elsewhere specified

♠ **86674** Giardia lamblia

♠ **86677** Helicobacter pylori

♠ **86682** helminth, not elsewhere specified

♠ **86684** Haemophilus influenza

♠ **86687** HTLV-I

♠ **86688** HTLV-II

♠ **86689** HTLV or HIV antibody, confirmatory test (eg, Western Blot)

♠ **86692** hepatitis, delta agent
➲ *CPT Assistant* Nov 97:31

(For hepatitis delta agent, antigen, use 87380)

♠ **86694** herpes simplex, non-specific type test

♠ **86695** herpes simplex, type 1

♠ **86696** herpes simplex, type 2
➲ *CPT Changes: An Insider's View* 2001

♠ **86698** histoplasma

♠ **86701** HIV-1

♠ **86702** HIV-2

♠ **86703** HIV-1 and HIV-2, single assay
➲ *CPT Assistant* Nov 97:31

(For HIV-1 antigen, use 87390)

(For HIV-2 antigen, use 87391)

(For confirmatory test for HIV antibody (eg, Western Blot), use 86689)

♠ **86704** Hepatitis B core antibody (HBcAb); total
➲ *CPT Assistant* Nov 97:31-32; *CPT Changes: An Insider's View* 2001

♠ **86705** IgM antibody
➲ *CPT Assistant* Nov 97:31-32

♠ **86706** Hepatitis B surface antibody (HBsAb)
➲ *CPT Assistant* Nov 97:31-32

♠ **86707** Hepatitis Be antibody (HBeAb)
➲ *CPT Assistant* Nov 97:31-32

♠ **86708** Hepatitis A antibody (HAAb); total
➲ *CPT Assistant* Nov 97:31-32, Jun 00:11; *CPT Changes: An Insider's View* 2001

♠ **86709** IgM antibody
➲ *CPT Assistant* Nov 97:31-32, Jun 00:11

♠ **86710** Antibody; influenza virus

♠ **86713** Legionella

♠ **86717** Leishmania

♠ **86720** Leptospira

♠ **86723** Listeria monocytogenes

♠ **86727** lymphocytic choriomeningitis

♠ **86729** lymphogranuloma venereum

♠ **86732** mucormycosis

♠ **86735** mumps

♠ **86738** mycoplasma

♠ **86741** Neisseria meningitidis

♠ **86744** Nocardia

♠ **86747** parvovirus

♠ **86750** Plasmodium (malaria)

♠ **86753** protozoa, not elsewhere specified

♠ **86756** respiratory syncytial virus

♠ **86757** Rickettsia
➲ *CPT Changes: An Insider's View* 2001

♠ **86759** rotavirus

♠ **86762** rubella

♠ **86765** rubeola

♠ **86768** Salmonella

♠ **86771** Shigella

♠ **86774** tetanus

♠ **86777** Toxoplasma

♠ **86778** Toxoplasma, IgM

♠ **86781** Treponema pallidum, confirmatory test (eg, FTA-abs)

♠ **86784** Trichinella

♠ **86787** varicella-zoster

♠ **86790** virus, not elsewhere specified

♠ **86793** Yersinia

♠ **86800** Thyroglobulin antibody

(For thyroglobulin, use 84432)

♠ **86803** Hepatitis C antibody;
➲ *CPT Assistant* Nov 97:31-32

♠ **86804** confirmatory test (eg, immunoblot)
➲ *CPT Assistant* Nov 97:31-32

Tissue Typing

(For pretransplant cross-match, see appropriate code or codes)

♠ **86805** Lymphocytotoxicity assay, visual crossmatch; with titration

♠ **86806** without titration

♠ **86807** Serum screening for cytotoxic percent reactive antibody (PRA); standard method
➲ *CPT Assistant* Jun 01:11

♠ **86808** quick method
➲ *CPT Assistant* Jun 01:11

♠ **86812** HLA typing; A, B, or C (eg, A10, B7, B27), single antigen
➲ *CPT Assistant* Mar 03:23

♠ **86813** A, B, or C, multiple antigens
➲ *CPT Assistant* Mar 03:23

♠ **86816** DR/DQ, single antigen
➲ *CPT Assistant* Mar 03:23

♠ **86817** DR/DQ, multiple antigens
➲ *CPT Assistant* Mar 03:23

♠ **86821** lymphocyte culture, mixed (MLC)
➲ *CPT Assistant* Mar 03:23

♠ **86822** lymphocyte culture, primed (PLC)
➲ *CPT Assistant* Mar 03:23

♠ **86849** Unlisted immunology procedure
➲ *CPT Assistant* Mar 98:10

Pathology and Laboratory

Transfusion Medicine

(For apheresis, use 36511, 36512)

(For therapeutic phlebotomy, use 99195)

♣ **86850** Antibody screen, RBC, each serum technique
➲ *CPT Assistant* Fall 93:25

♣ **86860** Antibody elution (RBC), each elution

♣ **86870** Antibody identification, RBC antibodies, each panel for each serum technique
➲ *CPT Assistant* Fall 93:25, Mar 01:10

♣ **86880** Antihuman globulin test (Coombs test); direct, each antiserum

♣ **86885** indirect, qualitative, each antiserum

♣ **86886** indirect, titer, each antiserum

♣ **86890** Autologous blood or component, collection processing and storage; predeposited
➲ *CPT Assistant* Apr 96:2

♣ **86891** intra- or postoperative salvage

(For physician services to autologous donors, see 99201-99204)

♣ **86900** Blood typing; ABO

♣ **86901** Rh (D)
➲ *CPT Assistant* Fall 93:25

♣ **86903** antigen screening for compatible blood unit using reagent serum, per unit screened

♣ **86904** antigen screening for compatible unit using patient serum, per unit screened

♣ **86905** RBC antigens, other than ABO or Rh (D), each

♣ **86906** Rh phenotyping, complete

☐ **86910** Blood typing, for paternity testing, per individual; ABO, Rh and MN

☐ **86911** each additional antigen system

(86915 has been deleted. To report, see 38210-38213)

♣ **86920** Compatibility test each unit; immediate spin technique

♣ **86921** incubation technique

♣ **86922** antiglobulin technique

♣ **86927** Fresh frozen plasma, thawing, each unit

♣ **86930** Frozen blood, each unit; freezing (includes preparation)
➲ *CPT Assistant* Apr 96:2, Jul 03:7; *CPT Changes: An Insider's View* 2002

♣ **86931** thawing
➲ *CPT Assistant* Jul 03:7; *CPT Changes: An Insider's View* 2003

♣ **86932** freezing (includes preparation) and thawing
➲ *CPT Assistant* Jul 03:7; *CPT Changes: An Insider's View* 2003

♠ **86940** Hemolysins and agglutinins; auto, screen, each

♠ **86941** incubated

♣ **86945** Irradiation of blood product, each unit

♣ **86950** Leukocyte transfusion

(For leukapheresis, use 36511)

♣ **86965** Pooling of platelets or other blood products

♣ **86970** Pretreatment of RBCs for use in RBC antibody detection, identification, and/or compatibility testing; incubation with chemical agents or drugs, each

♣ **86971** incubation with enzymes, each

♣ **86972** by density gradient separation

♣ **86975** Pretreatment of serum for use in RBC antibody identification; incubation with drugs, each

♣ **86976** by dilution

♣ **86977** incubation with inhibitors, each

♣ **86978** by differential red cell absorption using patient RBCs or RBCs of known phenotype, each absorption

♣ **86985** Splitting of blood or blood products, each unit
➲ *CPT Assistant* Apr 96:2

♣ **86999** Unlisted transfusion medicine procedure

Microbiology

Includes bacteriology, mycology, parasitology, and virology.

Presumptive identification of microorganisms is defined as identification by colony morphology, growth on selective media, Gram stains, or up to three tests (eg, catalase, oxidase, indole, urease). Definitive identification of microorganisms is defined as an identification to the genus or species level that requires additional tests (eg, biochemical panels, slide cultures). If additional studies involve molecular probes, chromatography, or immunologic techniques, these should be separately coded in addition to definitive identification codes (87140-87158). For multiple specimens/sites use modifier 59. For repeat laboratory tests performed on the same day, use modifier 91.

♠ **87001** Animal inoculation, small animal; with observation

♠ **87003** with observation and dissection

♠ **87015** Concentration (any type), for infectious agents
➲ *CPT Changes: An Insider's View* 2001

(Do not report 87015 in conjunction with 87177)

♠ **87040** Culture, bacterial; blood, aerobic, with isolation and presumptive identification of isolates (includes anaerobic culture, if appropriate)
➲ *CPT Assistant* Jun 02:1-3; *CPT Changes: An Insider's View* 2004

♠ **87045** stool, aerobic, with isolation and preliminary examination (eg, KIA, LIA), Salmonella and Shigella species
➲ *CPT Changes: An Insider's View* 2001, 2002, 2004

♠▲ 87046 stool, aerobic, additional pathogens, isolation and presumptive identification of isolates, each plate
➲ CPT Changes: An Insider's View 2001, 2002, 2004, 2005

♠ 87070 any other source except urine, blood or stool, aerobic, with isolation and presumptive identification of isolates
➲ CPT Assistant Aug 97:18, Nov 01:10, Oct 03:10; CPT Changes: An Insider's View 2004

(For urine, use 87088)

♠ 87071 quantitative, aerobic with isolation and presumptive identification of isolates, any source except urine, blood or stool
➲ CPT Assistant Jun 02:1-3, Sep 03:3; CPT Changes: An Insider's View 2001

(For urine, use 87088)

♠ 87073 quantitative, anaerobic with isolation and presumptive identification of isolates, any source except urine, blood or stool
➲ CPT Assistant Jun 02:1-3, Sep 03:3; CPT Changes: An Insider's View 2001

(For definitive identification of isolates, use 87076 or 87077. For typing of isolates see 87140-87158)

♠ 87075 any source, except blood, anaerobic with isolation and presumptive identification of isolates
➲ CPT Changes: An Insider's View 2001, 2004

♠ 87076 anaerobic isolate, additional methods required for definitive identification, each isolate

(For gas liquid chromatography (GLC) or high pressure liquid chromatography (HPLC), use 87143)

♠ 87077 aerobic isolate, additional methods required for definitive identification, each isolate
➲ CPT Assistant Nov 01:10; CPT Changes: An Insider's View 2001

(For gas liquid chromatography (GLC) or high pressure liquid chromatography (HPLC), use 87143)

♠ 87081 Culture, presumptive, pathogenic organisms, screening only;
➲ CPT Assistant Nov 01:10; CPT Changes: An Insider's View 2001

♠ 87084 with colony estimation from density chart

♠ 87086 Culture, bacterial; quantitative colony count, urine
➲ CPT Changes: An Insider's View 2001

♠ 87088 with isolation and presumptive identification of isolates, urine
➲ CPT Changes: An Insider's View 2001

♠ 87101 Culture, fungi (mold or yeast) isolation, with presumptive identification of isolates; skin, hair, or nail
➲ CPT Assistant Sep 99:10; CPT Changes: An Insider's View 2001

♠ 87102 other source (except blood)

♠ 87103 blood

♠ 87106 Culture, fungi, definitive identification, each organism; yeast
➲ CPT Changes: An Insider's View 2001

(Use 87106 in addition to codes 87101, 87102, or 87103 when appropriate)

♠ 87107 mold
➲ CPT Changes: An Insider's View 2001

♠ 87109 Culture, mycoplasma, any source

♠ 87110 Culture, chlamydia, any source
➲ CPT Changes: An Insider's View 2001

(For immunofluorescence staining of shell vials, use 87140)

♠ 87116 Culture, tubercle or other acid-fast bacilli (eg, TB, AFB, mycobacteria) any source, with isolation and presumptive identification of isolates
➲ CPT Changes: An Insider's View 2001

(For concentration, use 87015)

♠ 87118 Culture, mycobacterial, definitive identification, each isolate
➲ CPT Changes: An Insider's View 2001

(For nucleic acid probe identification, use 87149)

(For GLC or HPLC identification, use 87143)

♠ 87140 Culture, typing; immunofluorescent method, each antiserum
➲ CPT Assistant Nov 01:10, Sep 03:3

♠ 87143 gas liquid chromatography (GLC) or high pressure liquid chromatography (HPLC) method
➲ CPT Assistant Sep 03:3

♠ 87147 immunologic method, other than immunofluoresence (eg, agglutination grouping), per antiserum
➲ CPT Assistant Apr 02:18, Sep 03:3

♠ 87149 identification by nucleic acid probe
➲ CPT Assistant Nov 01:10, Sep 03:3

♠ 87152 identification by pulse field gel typing
➲ CPT Assistant Sep 03:3

♠ 87158 other methods
➲ CPT Assistant Nov 01:10, Sep 03:3

♠ 87164 Dark field examination, any source (eg, penile, vaginal, oral, skin); includes specimen collection

♠ 87166 without collection

♠ 87168 Macroscopic examination; arthropod
➲ CPT Changes: An Insider's View 2001

♠ 87169 parasite
➲ CPT Changes: An Insider's View 2001

♠ 87172 Pinworm exam (eg, cellophane tape prep)
➲ CPT Changes: An Insider's View 2001

♠ 87176 Homogenization, tissue, for culture
➲ CPT Changes: An Insider's View 2001

♠ **87177** Ova and parasites, direct smears, concentration and identification
➲ *CPT Assistant* Jul 03:7, Nov 03:15

(Do not report 87177 in conjunction with 87015)

(For direct smears from a primary source, use 87207)

(For coccidia or microsporidia exam, use 87207)

(For trichrome, iron hemotoxylin and other special stains, use 88313)

(For nucleic acid probes in cytologic material, use 88365)

(For molecular diagnostics, see 83890-83898, 87470-87799)

♠ **87181** Susceptibility studies, antimicrobial agent; agar dilution method, per agent (eg, antibiotic gradient strip)
➲ *CPT Assistant* Nov 01:10; *CPT Changes: An Insider's View* 2001

♠ **87184** disk method, per plate (12 or fewer agents)
➲ *CPT Assistant* Nov 01:10; *CPT Changes: An Insider's View* 2001

♠ **87185** enzyme detection (eg, beta lactamase), per enzyme

♠ **87186** microdilution or agar dilution (minimum inhibitory concentration (MIC) or breakpoint), each multi-antimicrobial, per plate
➲ *CPT Assistant* Nov 01:10; *CPT Changes: An Insider's View* 2001

♠+ **87187** microdilution or agar dilution, minimum lethal concentration (MLC), each plate (List separately in addition to code for primary procedure)
➲ *CPT Assistant* Nov 01:10; *CPT Changes: An Insider's View* 2001

(Use 87187 in conjunction with 87186 or 87188)

♠ **87188** macrobroth dilution method, each agent
➲ *CPT Assistant* Nov 01:10; *CPT Changes: An Insider's View* 2001

♠ **87190** mycobacteria, proportion method, each agent
➲ *CPT Changes: An Insider's View* 2001

(For other mycobacterial susceptibility studies, see 87181, 87184, 87186, or 87188)

♠ **87197** Serum bactericidal titer (Schlicter test)

♠ **87205** Smear, primary source with interpretation; Gram or Giemsa stain for bacteria, fungi, or cell types
➲ *CPT Changes: An Insider's View* 2001

♠ **87206** fluorescent and/or acid fast stain for bacteria, fungi, parasites, viruses or cell types
➲ *CPT Changes: An Insider's View* 2001

♠ **87207** special stain for inclusion bodies or parasites (eg, malaria, coccidia, microsporidia, trypanosomes, herpes viruses
➲ *CPT Assistant* Jul 03:7; *CPT Changes: An Insider's View* 2001, 2003

(For direct smears with concentration and identification, use 87177)

(For thick smear preparation, use 87015)

(For complex special stains, see 88312, 88313)

(For fat, meat, fibers, nasal eosinophils, and starch, see miscellaneous section)

♠ **87210** wet mount for infectious agents (eg, saline, India ink, KOH preps)
➲ *CPT Changes: An Insider's View* 2001

(For KOH examination of skin, hair or nails, see 87220)

♠ **87220** Tissue examination by KOH slide of samples from skin, hair, or nails for fungi or ectoparasite ova or mites (eg, scabies)
➲ *CPT Changes: An Insider's View* 2001

♠ **87230** Toxin or antitoxin assay, tissue culture (eg, Clostridium difficile toxin)

♠ **87250** Virus isolation; inoculation of embryonated eggs, or small animal, includes observation and dissection
➲ *CPT Changes: An Insider's View* 2001

♠ **87252** tissue culture inoculation, observation, and presumptive identification by cytopathic effect
➲ *CPT Changes: An Insider's View* 2001

♠ **87253** tissue culture, additional studies or definitive identification (eg, hemabsorption, neutralization, immunofluoresence stain), each isolate
➲ *CPT Changes: An Insider's View* 2001

(Electron microscopy, use 88348)

(Inclusion bodies in tissue sections, see 88304-88309; in smears, see 87207-87210; in fluids, use 88106)

♠ **87254** centrifuge enhanced (shell vial) technique, includes identification with immunofluorescence stain, each virus
➲ *CPT Assistant* Jul 03:7; *CPT Changes: An Insider's View* 2001, 2003

(Report 87254 in addition to 87252 as appropriate)

♠ **87255** including identification by non-immunologic method, other than by cytopathic effect (eg, virus specific enzymatic activity)
➲ *CPT Assistant* Jul 03:7; *CPT Changes: An Insider's View* 2003

These codes are intended for primary source only. For similar studies on culture material, refer to codes 87140-87158. Infectious agents by antigen detection, immunofluorescence microscopy, or nucleic acid probe techniques should be reported as precisely as possible. The most specific code possible should be reported. If there is no specific agent code, the general methodology code (eg, 87299, 87449, 87450, 87797, 87798, 87799, 87899) should be used. For identification of antibodies to many of the listed infectious agents, see 86602-86804. When separate assays are performed for different species or strain(s) of organisms, each assay should be reported separately.

♠ **87260** Infectious agent antigen detection by immunofluorescent technique; adenovirus
➲ *CPT Changes: An Insider's View* 2001

♠ **87265** Bordetella pertussis/parapertussis
➲ *CPT Assistant* Nov 97:32

♠ 87267 Enterovirus, direct fluorescent antibody (DFA)
➲ *CPT Assistant* Jul 03:7

♠ 87269 giardia
➲ *CPT Changes: An Insider's View* 2004

♠ 87270 Chlamydia trachomatis
➲ *CPT Assistant* Nov 97:32

♠ 87271 Cytomegalovirus, direct fluorescent antibody (DFA)
➲ *CPT Assistant* Jul 03:7

♠ 87272 cryptosporidium
➲ *CPT Assistant* Nov 97:32; *CPT Changes: An Insider's View* 2004

♠ 87273 Herpes simplex virus type 2
➲ *CPT Changes: An Insider's View* 2001

♠ 87274 Herpes simplex virus type 1
➲ *CPT Assistant* Nov 97:32; *CPT Changes: An Insider's View* 2001

♠ 87275 influenza B virus
➲ *CPT Changes: An Insider's View* 2001

♠ 87276 influenza A virus
➲ *CPT Assistant* Nov 97:32

♠ 87277 Legionella micdadei
➲ *CPT Changes: An Insider's View* 2001

♠ 87278 Legionella pneumophila
➲ *CPT Assistant* Nov 97:32

♠ 87279 Parainfluenza virus, each type
➲ *CPT Changes: An Insider's View* 2001

♠ 87280 respiratory syncytial virus
➲ *CPT Assistant* Nov 97:32

♠ 87281 Pneumocystis carinii
➲ *CPT Changes: An Insider's View* 2001

♠ 87283 Rubeola
➲ *CPT Changes: An Insider's View* 2001

♠ 87285 Treponema pallidum
➲ *CPT Assistant* Nov 97:32

♠ 87290 Varicella zoster virus
➲ *CPT Assistant* Nov 97:32

♠ 87299 not otherwise specified, each organism
➲ *CPT Assistant* Nov 97:32, Nov 01:10; *CPT Changes: An Insider's View* 2001

♠ 87300 Infectious agent antigen detection by immunofluorescent technique, polyvalent for multiple organisms, each polyvalent antiserum
➲ *CPT Changes: An Insider's View* 2001

(For physician evaluation of infectious disease agents by immunofluorescence, use 88346)

♠ 87301 Infectious agent antigen detection by enzyme immunoassay technique, qualitative or semiquantitative, multiple step method; adenovirus enteric types 40/41
➲ *CPT Assistant* Nov 97:32, Nov 99:46

♠ 87320 Chlamydia trachomatis
➲ *CPT Assistant* Nov 97:32

♠ 87324 Clostridium difficile toxin(s)
➲ *CPT Assistant* Nov 97:32; *CPT Changes: An Insider's View* 2001

♠ 87327 Cryptococcus neoformans
➲ *CPT Changes: An Insider's View* 2001

(For Cryptococcus latex agglutination, use 86403)

♠ 87328 cryptosporidium
➲ *CPT Assistant* Nov 97:32; *CPT Changes: An Insider's View* 2004

♠ 87329 giardia
➲ *CPT Changes: An Insider's View* 2004

♠ 87332 cytomegalovirus
➲ *CPT Assistant* Nov 97:32

♠ 87335 Escherichia coli 0157
➲ *CPT Assistant* Nov 97:32

(For giardia antigen, use ►87329◄)

♠ 87336 Entamoeba histolytica dispar group
➲ *CPT Changes: An Insider's View* 2001

♠ 87337 Entamoeba histolytica group
➲ *CPT Changes: An Insider's View* 2001

♠ 87338 Helicobacter pylori, stool
➲ *CPT Assistant* Nov 99:46; *CPT Changes: An Insider's View* 2000

♠ 87339 Helicobacter pylori
➲ *CPT Changes: An Insider's View* 2001

(For H. pylori, stool, use 87338. For H. pylori, breath and blood by mass spectrometry, see 83013, 83014. For H. pylori, liquid scintillation counter, see 78267, 78268)

♠ 87340 hepatitis B surface antigen (HBsAg)

♠ 87341 hepatitis B surface antigen (HBsAg) neutralization
➲ *CPT Changes: An Insider's View* 2001

♠ 87350 hepatitis Be antigen (HBeAg)
➲ *CPT Assistant* Nov 97:32

♠ 87380 hepatitis, delta agent
➲ *CPT Assistant* Nov 97:32

♠ 87385 Histoplasma capsulatum
➲ *CPT Assistant* Nov 97:32

♠ 87390 HIV-1
➲ *CPT Assistant* Nov 97:32

♠ 87391 HIV-2
➲ *CPT Assistant* Nov 97:32

♠ 87400 Influenza, A or B, each
➲ *CPT Assistant* Jun 01:11, Dec 01:6; *CPT Changes: An Insider's View* 2001

♠ 87420 respiratory syncytial virus
➲ *CPT Assistant* Nov 97:32

♠ 87425 rotavirus
➲ *CPT Assistant* Nov 97:32

♠ **87427** Shiga-like toxin

➲ *CPT Changes: An Insider's View* 2001

♠ **87430** Streptococcus, group A

♠ **87449** Infectious agent antigen detection by enzyme immunoassay technique qualitative or semiquantitative; multiple step method, not otherwise specified, each organism

➲ *CPT Assistant* Nov 97:32, Jan 00:11, Nov 01:10; *CPT Changes: An Insider's View* 2001

♠ **87450** single step method, not otherwise specified, each organism

➲ *CPT Assistant* Nov 97:33; *CPT Changes: An Insider's View* 2001

♠ **87451** multiple step method, polyvalent for multiple organisms, each polyvalent antiserum

➲ *CPT Changes: An Insider's View* 2001

♠ **87470** Infectious agent detection by nucleic acid (DNA or RNA); Bartonella henselae and Bartonella quintana, direct probe technique

➲ *CPT Assistant* Nov 97:33-34

♠ **87471** Bartonella henselae and Bartonella quintana, amplified probe technique

♠ **87472** Bartonella henselae and Bartonella quintana, quantification

♠ **87475** Borrelia burgdorferi, direct probe technique

♠ **87476** Borrelia burgdorferi, amplified probe technique

♠ **87477** Borrelia burgdorferi, quantification

♠ **87480** Candida species, direct probe technique

♠ **87481** Candida species, amplified probe technique

♠ **87482** Candida species, quantification

♠ **87485** Chlamydia pneumoniae, direct probe technique

♠ **87486** Chlamydia pneumoniae, amplified probe technique

♠ **87487** Chlamydia pneumoniae, quantification

♠ **87490** Chlamydia trachomatis, direct probe technique

♠ **87491** Chlamydia trachomatis, amplified probe technique

♠ **87492** Chlamydia trachomatis, quantification

♠ **87495** cytomegalovirus, direct probe technique

♠ **87496** cytomegalovirus, amplified probe technique

♠ **87497** cytomegalovirus, quantification

♠ **87510** Gardnerella vaginalis, direct probe technique

♠ **87511** Gardnerella vaginalis, amplified probe technique

♠ **87512** Gardnerella vaginalis, quantification

♠ **87515** hepatitis B virus, direct probe technique

♠ **87516** hepatitis B virus, amplified probe technique

♠ **87517** hepatitis B virus, quantification

♠ **87520** hepatitis C, direct probe technique

♠ **87521** hepatitis C, amplified probe technique

♠ **87522** hepatitis C, quantification

♠ **87525** hepatitis G, direct probe technique

♠ **87526** hepatitis G, amplified probe technique

♠ **87527** hepatitis G, quantification

♠ **87528** Herpes simplex virus, direct probe technique

♠ **87529** Herpes simplex virus, amplified probe technique

♠ **87530** Herpes simplex virus, quantification

♠ **87531** Herpes virus-6, direct probe technique

♠ **87532** Herpes virus-6, amplified probe technique

♠ **87533** Herpes virus-6, quantification

♠ **87534** HIV-1, direct probe technique

♠ **87535** HIV-1, amplified probe technique

♠ **87536** HIV-1, quantification

♠ **87537** HIV-2, direct probe technique

♠ **87538** HIV-2, amplified probe technique

♠ **87539** HIV-2, quantification

♠ **87540** Legionella pneumophila, direct probe technique

♠ **87541** Legionella pneumophila, amplified probe technique

♠ **87542** Legionella pneumophila, quantification

♠ **87550** Mycobacteria species, direct probe technique

♠ **87551** Mycobacteria species, amplified probe technique

♠ **87552** Mycobacteria species, quantification

♠ **87555** Mycobacteria tuberculosis, direct probe technique

♠ **87556** Mycobacteria tuberculosis, amplified probe technique

♠ **87557** Mycobacteria tuberculosis, quantification

♠ **87560** Mycobacteria avium-intracellulare, direct probe technique

♠ **87561** Mycobacteria avium-intracellulare, amplified probe technique

♠ **87562** Mycobacteria avium-intracellulare, quantification

♠ **87580** Mycoplasma pneumoniae, direct probe technique

♠ **87581** Mycoplasma pneumoniae, amplified probe technique

♠ **87582** Mycoplasma pneumoniae, quantification

♠ **87590** Neisseria gonorrhoeae, direct probe technique

♠ **87591** Neisseria gonorrhoeae, amplified probe technique

♠ **87592** Neisseria gonorrhoeae, quantification

♠ **87620** papillomavirus, human, direct probe technique

➲ *CPT Assistant* Feb 02:10

♠ **87621** papillomavirus, human, amplified probe technique

♠ **87622** papillomavirus, human, quantification

♠ **87650** Streptococcus, group A, direct probe technique

♠ 87651 Streptococcus, group A, amplified probe technique

♠ 87652 Streptococcus, group A, quantification

♠ 87660 Trichomonas vaginalis, direct probe technique
➲ *CPT Changes: An Insider's View* 2004

♠ 87797 Infectious agent detection by nucleic acid (DNA or RNA), not otherwise specified; direct probe technique, each organism
➲ *CPT Assistant* Nov 97:34, Nov 01:10, Apr 03:9; *CPT Changes: An Insider's View* 2001

♠ 87798 amplified probe technique, each organism
➲ *CPT Assistant* Nov 97:34, Nov 01:10, Apr 03:9; *CPT Changes: An Insider's View* 2001

♠ 87799 quantification, each organism
➲ *CPT Assistant* Nov 97:34; *CPT Changes: An Insider's View* 2001

♠ 87800 Infectious agent detection by nucleic acid (DNA or RNA), multiple organisms; direct probe(s) technique
➲ *CPT Assistant* Nov 97:34, Nov 01:10, Apr 03:9; *CPT Changes: An Insider's View* 2001

♠ 87801 amplified probe(s) technique
➲ *CPT Assistant* Apr 03:9; *CPT Changes: An Insider's View* 2001

♠ 87802 Infectious agent antigen detection by immunoassay with direct optical observation; Streptococcus, group B
➲ *CPT Changes: An Insider's View* 2002

♠ 87803 Clostridium difficile toxin A
➲ *CPT Changes: An Insider's View* 2002

♠ 87804 Influenza
➲ *CPT Changes: An Insider's View* 2002

♠● 87807 respiratory syncytial virus
➲ *CPT Changes: An Insider's View* 2005

♠ 87810 Infectious agent detection by immunoassay with direct optical observation; Chlamydia trachomatis
➲ *CPT Assistant* Nov 97:34, Jan 98:6

♠ 87850 Neisseria gonorrhoeae
➲ *CPT Assistant* Nov 97:34, Jan 98:6

♠ 87880 Streptococcus, group A
➲ *CPT Assistant* Nov 97:34, Jan 98:6, Dec 98:8

♠ 87899 not otherwise specified
➲ *CPT Assistant* Jun 01:11

♠ 87901 Infectious agent genotype analysis by nucleic acid (DNA or RNA); HIV 1, reverse transcriptase and protease
➲ *CPT Changes: An Insider's View* 2001, 2002

(For infectious agent drug susceptibility phenotype prediction for HIV-1, use Category III code 0023T)

♠ 87902 Hepatitis C virus
➲ *CPT Changes: An Insider's View* 2002

♠ 87903 Infectious agent phenotype analysis by nucleic acid (DNA or RNA) with drug resistance tissue culture analysis, HIV 1; first through 10 drugs tested
➲ *CPT Assistant* Apr 04:15; *CPT Changes: An Insider's View* 2001, 2002

♠+ 87904 each additional 1 through 5 drugs tested (List separately in addition to code for primary procedure)
➲ *CPT Assistant* Apr 04:15; *CPT Changes: An Insider's View* 2001, 2002

(Use 87904 in conjunction with 87903)

♠ 87999 Unlisted microbiology procedure

Anatomic Pathology

Postmortem Examination

Procedures 88000 through 88099 represent physician services only. Use modifier 90 for outside laboratory services.

☐ 88000 Necropsy (autopsy), gross examination only; without CNS

☐ 88005 with brain

☐ 88007 with brain and spinal cord

☐ 88012 infant with brain

☐ 88014 stillborn or newborn with brain

☐ 88016 macerated stillborn

☐ 88020 Necropsy (autopsy), gross and microscopic; without CNS

☐ 88025 with brain

☐ 88027 with brain and spinal cord

☐ 88028 infant with brain

☐ 88029 stillborn or newborn with brain

☐ 88036 Necropsy (autopsy), limited, gross and/or microscopic; regional

☐ 88037 single organ

☐ 88040 Necropsy (autopsy); forensic examination

☐ 88045 coroner's call

☐ 88099 Unlisted necropsy (autopsy) procedure

Cytopathology

(For cervicography, see Category III code 0003T)

(For collection of cytology specimens via mammary duct catheter lavage, report 0045T-0046T)

♣ 88104 Cytopathology, fluids, washings or brushings, except cervical or vaginal; smears with interpretation
➲ *CPT Assistant* Spring 91:6, Fall 94:3

♣ 88106 filter method only with interpretation
➲ *CPT Assistant* Fall 94:3

♣ 88107 smears and filter preparation with interpretation
➲ *CPT Assistant* Fall 94:3

♣ **88108** Cytopathology, concentration technique, smears and interpretation (eg, Saccomanno technique)
➲ *CPT Assistant* Fall 94:3, Nov 97:34, Jan 98:6

(For cervical or vaginal smears, see 88150-88155)

(For gastric intubation with lavage, see 89130-89141, 91055)

(For x-ray localization, use 74340)

♣ **88112** Cytopathology, selective cellular enhancement technique with interpretation (eg, liquid based slide preparation method), except cervical or vaginal
➲ *CPT Changes: An Insider's View* 2004

(Do not report 88112 with 88108)

♣ **88125** Cytopathology, forensic (eg, sperm)

♠ **88130** Sex chromatin identification; Barr bodies

♠ **88140** peripheral blood smear, polymorphonuclear drumsticks
➲ *CPT Assistant* Nov 98:27-28

(For Guard stain, use 88313)

Codes 88141-88155, 88164-88167, 88174-88175 are used to report cervical or vaginal screening by various methods and to report physician interpretation services. Use codes 88150-88154 to report Pap smears that are examined using non-Bethesda reporting. Use codes 88164-88167 to report Pap smears that are examined using the Bethesda System of reporting. Use codes 88142-88143 to report specimens collected in fluid medium with automated thin layer preparation that are examined using any system of reporting (Bethesda or non-Bethesda). Use codes 88174-88175 to report automated screening of specimens collected in fluid medium with automated thin layer preparation that are examined using any system of reporting (Bethesda or non-Bethesda). Within each of these three code families choose the one code that describes the screening method(s) used. Codes 88141 and 88155 should be reported in addition to the screening code chosen when the additional services are provided.

☆+ **88141** Cytopathology, cervical or vaginal (any reporting system), requiring interpretation by physician (List separately in addition to code for technical service)
➲ *CPT Assistant* Nov 97:35, Jan 98:6, Jan 99:11, May 99:6, Nov 99:46, Mar 04:4

(Use 88141 in conjunction with 88142-88154, 88164-88167, 88174-88175)

♠ **88142** Cytopathology, cervical or vaginal (any reporting system), collected in preservative fluid, automated thin layer preparation; manual screening under physician supervision
➲ *CPT Assistant* Nov 97:34-35, Jan 98:6, Nov 98:28, May 99:6, Jul 03:7, Mar 04:4

♠ **88143** with manual screening and rescreening under physician supervision
➲ *CPT Assistant* Nov 97:34-35, Nov 98:28, May 99:6, Jul 03:7, Mar 04:4

(88144 has been deleted)

(88145 has been deleted)

(For automated screening of automated thin layer preparation, see 88174, 88175)

♠ **88147** Cytopathology smears, cervical or vaginal; screening by automated system under physician supervision
➲ *CPT Assistant* Nov 97:35, Nov 98:28, Nov 99:46, Jan 99:1, May 99:6, Mar 04:4

♠ **88148** screening by automated system with manual rescreening under physician supervision
➲ *CPT Assistant* Jan 99:1, May 99:6, Nov 99:46, Mar 04:4; *CPT Changes: An Insider's View* 2000

♠ **88150** Cytopathology, slides, cervical or vaginal; manual screening under physician supervision
➲ *CPT Assistant* Winter 91:19, Nov 97:34-35, Nov 98:28, May 99:6, Mar 04:4

♠ **88152** with manual screening and computer-assisted rescreening under physician supervision
➲ *CPT Assistant* Nov 97:35, Jan 98:6, May 99:6, Mar 04:4

♠ **88153** with manual screening and rescreening under physician supervision
➲ *CPT Assistant* Nov 97:34-35, Nov 98:28, May 99:6, Mar 04:4

♠ **88154** with manual screening and computer-assisted rescreening using cell selection and review under physician supervision
➲ *CPT Assistant* Nov 97:34-35, Nov 98:28, May 99:6, Mar 04:4

♠+ **88155** Cytopathology, slides, cervical or vaginal, definitive hormonal evaluation (eg, maturation index, karyopyknotic index, estrogenic index) (List separately in addition to code(s) for other technical and interpretation services)
➲ *CPT Assistant* Nov 97:35, Nov 98:28, May 99:6, Nov 99:46, Mar 04:4

(Use 88155 in conjunction with 88142-88154, 88164-88167, 88174-88175)

♣ **88160** Cytopathology, smears, any other source; screening and interpretation

♣ **88161** preparation, screening and interpretation
➲ *CPT Assistant* Aug 97:18

♣ **88162** extended study involving over 5 slides and/or multiple stains

(For obtaining specimen, see percutaneous needle biopsy under individual organ in **Surgery**)

(For aerosol collection of sputum, use 89220)

(For special stains, see 88312-88314)

♠ 88164 Cytopathology, slides, cervical or vaginal (the Bethesda System); manual screening under physician supervision
➲ *CPT Assistant* Nov 98:28, May 99:6, Mar 04:4

♠ 88165 with manual screening and rescreening under physician supervision
➲ *CPT Assistant* Nov 98:28, May 99:6, Mar 04:4

♠ 88166 with manual screening and computer-assisted rescreening under physician supervision
➲ *CPT Assistant* Nov 98:28, May 99:6, Mar 04:4

♠ 88167 with manual screening and computer-assisted rescreening using cell selection and review under physician supervision
➲ *CPT Assistant* Nov 98:28, May 99:6, Jul 03:7, Mar 04:4

(88170 has been deleted. To report, see 10021, 10022)

(88171 has been deleted. To report, see 10021, 10022)

♣ 88172 Cytopathology, evaluation of fine needle aspirate; immediate cytohistologic study to determine adequacy of specimen(s)
➲ *CPT Assistant* Fall 93:26, Fall 94:2, Dec 98:8; *CPT Changes: An Insider's View* 2001

♣ 88173 interpretation and report
➲ *CPT Assistant* Fall 93:26, Fall 94:2, Dec 98:8

♠ 88174 Cytopathology, cervical or vaginal (any reporting system), collected in preservative fluid, automated thin layer preparation; screening by automated system, under physician supervision
➲ *CPT Assistant* Jul 03:7, Mar 04:4; *CPT Changes: An Insider's View* 2003

♠ 88175 with screening by automated system and manual rescreening, under physician supervision
➲ *CPT Assistant* Jul 03:7, Mar 04:4; *CPT Changes: An Insider's View* 2003

(For manual screening, see 88142, 88143)

►(88180 has been deleted. To report, see 88182, 88189)◄

♣ 88182 Flow cytometry; cell cycle or DNA analysis

(For tumor morphometry and DNA and ploidy analysis by imaging techniques, use 88358)

♣● 88184 Flow cytometry, cell surface, cytoplasmic, or nuclear marker, technical component only; first marker
➲ *CPT Changes: An Insider's View* 2005

♣+● 88185 each additional marker (List separately in addition to code for first marker)
➲ *CPT Changes: An Insider's View* 2005

►(Report 88185 in conjunction with 88184)◄

♣● 88187 Flow cytometry, interpretation; 2 to 8 markers
➲ *CPT Changes: An Insider's View* 2005

♣● 88188 9 to 15 markers
➲ *CPT Changes: An Insider's View* 2005

♣● 88189 16 or more markers
➲ *CPT Changes: An Insider's View* 2005

♠ 88199 Unlisted cytopathology procedure

(For electron microscopy, see 88348, 88349)

Cytogenetic Studies

►When molecular diagnostic procedures are performed to test for oncologic or inherited disorder, use the appropriate modifier to specify probe type or condition tested. (See **Appendix I**).◄

(For acetylcholinesterase, use 82013)

(For alpha-fetoprotein, serum or amniotic fluid, see 82105, 82106)

(For laser microdissection of cells from tissue sample, see 88380)

♠ 88230 Tissue culture for non-neoplastic disorders; lymphocyte
➲ *CPT Assistant* Nov 98:29, Oct 99:1

♠ 88233 skin or other solid tissue biopsy
➲ *CPT Assistant* Nov 98:29, Oct 99:1

♠ 88235 amniotic fluid or chorionic villus cells
➲ *CPT Assistant* Nov 98:29, Oct 99:1

♠ 88237 Tissue culture for neoplastic disorders; bone marrow, blood cells
➲ *CPT Assistant* Nov 98:29, Oct 99:1

♠ 88239 solid tumor

♠ 88240 Cryopreservation, freezing and storage of cells, each cell line
➲ *CPT Assistant* Nov 98:29, Oct 99:1, Jul 03:7

(For therapeutic cryopreservation and storage, use 38207)

♠ 88241 Thawing and expansion of frozen cells, each aliquot
➲ *CPT Assistant* Nov 98:29, Oct 99:1, Jul 03:7

(For therapeutic thawing of previous harvest, use 38208)

♠ 88245 Chromosome analysis for breakage syndromes; baseline Sister Chromatid Exchange (SCE), 20-25 cells
➲ *CPT Assistant* Nov 98:29, Oct 99:1

♠ 88248 baseline breakage, score 50-100 cells, count 20 cells, 2 karyotypes (eg, for ataxia telangiectasia, Fanconi anemia, fragile X)
➲ *CPT Assistant* Nov 98:29, Oct 99:1

♠ 88249 score 100 cells, clastogen stress (eg, diepoxybutane, mitomycin C, ionizing radiation, UV radiation)
➲ *CPT Assistant* Nov 98:29, Oct 99:1

♠ 88261 Chromosome analysis; count 5 cells, 1 karyotype, with banding
➲ *CPT Assistant* Nov 98:29, Oct 99:1

♠ 88262 count 15-20 cells, 2 karyotypes, with banding
➲ *CPT Assistant* Nov 98:29, Oct 99:1

♠ **88263** count 45 cells for mosaicism, 2 karyotypes, with banding
➲ *CPT Assistant* Nov 98:29, Oct 99:1

♠ **88264** analyze 20-25 cells
➲ *CPT Assistant* Nov 98:29, Oct 99:1

♠ **88267** Chromosome analysis, amniotic fluid or chorionic villus, count 15 cells, 1 karyotype, with banding

♠ **88269** Chromosome analysis, in situ for amniotic fluid cells, count cells from 6-12 colonies, 1 karyotype, with banding

♠ **88271** Molecular cytogenetics; DNA probe, each (eg, FISH)
➲ *CPT Assistant* Nov 98:29, Mar 99:10, Oct 99:1

♠ **88272** chromosomal in situ hybridization, analyze 3-5 cells (eg, for derivatives and markers)
➲ *CPT Assistant* Nov 98:29, Mar 99:10, Oct 99:1

♠ **88273** chromosomal in situ hybridization, analyze 10-30 cells (eg, for microdeletions)
➲ *CPT Assistant* Nov 98:29, Mar 99:10, Oct 99:1

♠ **88274** interphase in situ hybridization, analyze 25-99 cells
➲ *CPT Assistant* Nov 98:29, Mar 99:10, Oct 99:1

♠ **88275** interphase in situ hybridization, analyze 100-300 cells
➲ *CPT Assistant* Nov 98:29, Mar 99:10, Oct 99:1

♠ **88280** Chromosome analysis; additional karyotypes, each study

♠ **88283** additional specialized banding technique (eg, NOR, C-banding)

♠ **88285** additional cells counted, each study

♠ **88289** additional high resolution study
➲ *CPT Assistant* Oct 99:1

♠ **88291** Cytogenetics and molecular cytogenetics, interpretation and report
➲ *CPT Assistant* Nov 98:29, Oct 99:1

♣ **88299** Unlisted cytogenetic study

Surgical Pathology

Services 88300 through 88309 include accession, examination, and reporting. They do not include the services designated in codes 88311 through 88365 and 88399, which are coded in addition when provided.

The unit of service for codes 88300 through 88309 is the specimen.

A specimen is defined as tissue or tissues that is (are) submitted for individual and separate attention, requiring individual examination and pathologic diagnosis. Two or more such specimens from the same patient (eg, separately identified endoscopic biopsies, skin lesions, etc.) are each appropriately assigned an individual code reflective of its proper level of service.

Service code 88300 is used for any specimen that in the opinion of the examining pathologist can be accurately diagnosed without microscopic examination. Service code 88302 is used when gross and microscopic examination is performed on a specimen to confirm identification and the absence of disease. Service codes 88304 through 88309 describe all other specimens requiring gross and microscopic examination, and represent additional ascending levels of physician work. Levels 88302 through 88309 are specifically defined by the assigned specimens.

Any unlisted specimen should be assigned to the code which most closely reflects the physician work involved when compared to other specimens assigned to that code.

♣ **88300** **Level I** - Surgical pathology, gross examination only
➲ *CPT Assistant* Winter 91:18, Sep 00:10

♣ **88302** **Level II** - Surgical pathology, gross and microscopic examination
➲ *CPT Assistant* Winter 91:18, Sep 00:10

Appendix, Incidental

Fallopian Tube, Sterilization

Fingers/Toes, Amputation, Traumatic

Foreskin, Newborn

Hernia Sac, Any Location

Hydrocele Sac

Nerve

Skin, Plastic Repair

Sympathetic Ganglion

Testis, Castration

Vaginal Mucosa, Incidental

Vas Deferens, Sterilization

♣ **88304** **Level III** - Surgical pathology, gross and microscopic examination

Abortion, Induced

Abscess

Aneurysm - Arterial/Ventricular

Anus, Tag

Appendix, Other than Incidental

Artery, Atheromatous Plaque

Bartholin's Gland Cyst

Bone Fragment(s), Other than Pathologic Fracture

Bursa/Synovial Cyst

Carpal Tunnel Tissue

Cartilage, Shavings

Cholesteatoma

Colon, Colostomy Stoma

Conjunctiva - Biopsy/Pterygium

Cornea

Diverticulum - Esophagus/Small Intestine

Dupuytren's Contracture Tissue

Femoral Head, Other than Fracture

Fissure/Fistula

Foreskin, Other than Newborn

Gallbladder

Ganglion Cyst

Hematoma

Hemorrhoids

Hydatid of Morgagni

Intervertebral Disc

Joint, Loose Body

Meniscus

Mucocele, Salivary

Neuroma - Morton's/Traumatic

Pilonidal Cyst/Sinus

Polyps, Inflammatory - Nasal/Sinusoidal

Skin - Cyst/Tag/Debridement

Soft Tissue, Debridement

Soft Tissue, Lipoma

Spermatocele

Tendon/Tendon Sheath

Testicular Appendage

Thrombus or Embolus

Tonsil and/or Adenoids

Varicocele

Vas Deferens, Other than Sterilization

Vein, Varicosity

➲ *CPT Assistant* Spring 91:2, Winter 91:18, Aug 97:18, Sep 00:10; *CPT Changes: An Insider's View* 2002

♣ **88305** **Level IV** - Surgical pathology, gross and microscopic examination

Abortion - Spontaneous/Missed

Artery, Biopsy

Bone Marrow, Biopsy

Bone Exostosis

Brain/Meninges, Other than for Tumor Resection

Breast, Biopsy, Not Requiring Microscopic Evaluation of Surgical Margins

Breast, Reduction Mammoplasty

Bronchus, Biopsy

Cell Block, Any Source

Cervix, Biopsy

Colon, Biopsy

Duodenum, Biopsy

Endocervix, Curettings/Biopsy

Endometrium, Curettings/Biopsy

Esophagus, Biopsy

Extremity, Amputation, Traumatic

Fallopian Tube, Biopsy

Fallopian Tube, Ectopic Pregnancy

Femoral Head, Fracture

Fingers/Toes, Amputation, Non-traumatic

Gingiva/Oral Mucosa, Biopsy

Heart Valve

Joint, Resection

Kidney, Biopsy

Larynx, Biopsy

Leiomyoma(s), Uterine Myomectomy - without Uterus

Lip, Biopsy/Wedge Resection

Lung, Transbronchial Biopsy

Lymph Node, Biopsy

Muscle, Biopsy

Nasal Mucosa, Biopsy

Nasopharynx/Oropharynx, Biopsy

Nerve, Biopsy

Odontogenic/Dental Cyst

Omentum, Biopsy

Ovary with or without Tube, Non-neoplastic

Ovary, Biopsy/Wedge Resection

Parathyroid Gland

Peritoneum, Biopsy

Pituitary Tumor

Placenta, Other than Third Trimester

Pleura/Pericardium - Biopsy/Tissue

Polyp, Cervical/Endometrial

Polyp, Colorectal

Polyp, Stomach/Small Intestine

Prostate, Needle Biopsy

Prostate, TUR

Salivary Gland, Biopsy

Sinus, Paranasal Biopsy

Skin, Other than Cyst/Tag/Debridement/Plastic Repair

Small Intestine, Biopsy

Soft Tissue, Other than Tumor/Mass/Lipoma/Debridement

Spleen

Stomach, Biopsy

Synovium

Testis, Other than Tumor/Biopsy/Castration

Thyroglossal Duct/Brachial Cleft Cyst

Tongue, Biopsy

Tonsil, Biopsy

Trachea, Biopsy

Ureter, Biopsy

Urethra, Biopsy

Urinary Bladder, Biopsy

Uterus, with or without Tubes and Ovaries, for Prolapse

Vagina, Biopsy

Vulva/Labia, Biopsy

➔ *CPT Assistant* Spring 91:6, Winter 91:18, Winter 92:17, Aug 97:18, Jul 98:4, Nov 98:29-30, Jul 00:4, Sep 00:10, Dec 00:15; *CPT Changes: An Insider's View* 2002

♣ **88307** **Level V** - Surgical pathology, gross and microscopic examination

Adrenal, Resection

Bone - Biopsy/Curettings

Bone Fragment(s), Pathologic Fracture

Brain, Biopsy

Brain/Meninges, Tumor Resection

Breast, Excision of Lesion, Requiring Microscopic Evaluation of Surgical Margins

Breast, Mastectomy - Partial/Simple

Cervix, Conization

Colon, Segmental Resection, Other than for Tumor

Extremity, Amputation, Non-traumatic

Eye, Enucleation

Kidney, Partial/Total Nephrectomy

Larynx, Partial/Total Resection

Liver, Biopsy - Needle/Wedge

Liver, Partial Resection

Lung, Wedge Biopsy

Lymph Nodes, Regional Resection

Mediastinum, Mass

Myocardium, Biopsy

Odontogenic Tumor

Ovary with or without Tube, Neoplastic

Pancreas, Biopsy

Placenta, Third Trimester

Prostate, Except Radical Resection

Salivary Gland

Sentinel Lymph Node

Small Intestine, Resection, Other than for Tumor

Soft Tissue Mass (except Lipoma) - Biopsy/Simple Excision

Stomach - Subtotal/Total Resection, Other than for Tumor

Testis, Biopsy

Thymus, Tumor

Thyroid, Total/Lobe

Ureter, Resection

Urinary Bladder, TUR

Uterus, with or without Tubes and Ovaries, Other than Neoplastic/Prolapse

➔ *CPT Assistant* Winter 98:18, Winter 92:18, Jul 98:4, Nov 98:29-30, Jul 00:4, Sep 00:10, Dec 00:15, Dec 03:11; *CPT Changes: An Insider's View* 2001

♣ **88309** **Level VI** - Surgical pathology, gross and microscopic examination

Bone Resection

Breast, Mastectomy - with Regional Lymph Nodes

Colon, Segmental Resection for Tumor

Colon, Total Resection

Esophagus, Partial/Total Resection

Extremity, Disarticulation

Fetus, with Dissection

Larynx, Partial/Total Resection - with Regional Lymph Nodes

Lung - Total/Lobe/Segment Resection

Pancreas, Total/Subtotal Resection

Prostate, Radical Resection

Small Intestine, Resection for Tumor

Soft Tissue Tumor, Extensive Resection

Stomach - Subtotal/Total Resection for Tumor

Testis, Tumor

Tongue/Tonsil - Resection for Tumor

Urinary Bladder, Partial/Total Resection

Uterus, with or without Tubes and Ovaries, Neoplastic

Vulva, Total/Subtotal Resection

➲ *CPT Assistant* Winter 91:2, Winter 91:18, Fall 93:2, 26, Jul 00:4, Sep 00:10, Dec 03:11

(For fine needle aspiration, see 10021, 10022)

(For evaluation of fine needle aspirate, see 88172-88173)

♣+ **88311** Decalcification procedure (List separately in addition to code for surgical pathology examination)

➲ *CPT Assistant* Winter 92:18, Jul 98:4, Jun 02:11

♣+ **88312** Special stains (List separately in addition to code for primary service); Group I for microorganisms (eg, Gridley, acid fast, methenamine silver), each

➲ *CPT Assistant* Jun 02:11; *CPT Changes: An Insider's View* 2004

♣+ **88313** Group II, all other, (eg, iron, trichrome), except immunocytochemistry and immunoperoxidase stains, each

➲ *CPT Assistant* Jun 02:11, Mar 03:22, Nov 03:15

(For immunocytochemistry and immunoperoxidase tissue studies, use 88342)

♣+ **88314** histochemical staining with frozen section(s)

♣ **88318** Determinative histochemistry to identify chemical components (eg, copper, zinc)

♣ **88319** Determinative histochemistry or cytochemistry to identify enzyme constituents, each

♣ **88321** Consultation and report on referred slides prepared elsewhere

➲ *CPT Assistant* Winter 91:19, Apr 97:9, Oct 00:7, Dec 02:10

♣ **88323** Consultation and report on referred material requiring preparation of slides

♣ **88325** Consultation, comprehensive, with review of records and specimens, with report on referred material

➲ *CPT Assistant* Winter 91:19, Apr 97:9

♣ **88329** Pathology consultation during surgery;

➲ *CPT Assistant* Winter 91:19, Apr 97:9, Aug 97:18

♣ **88331** first tissue block, with frozen section(s), single specimen

➲ *CPT Assistant* Spring 91:2, Winter 91:19, Apr 97:12, Aug 97:18, Jul 00:4, Nov 02:5; *CPT Changes: An Insider's View* 2001

♣ **88332** each additional tissue block with frozen section(s)

➲ *CPT Assistant* Winter 91:19, Apr 97:12, Aug 97:18, Jul 00:4

♣ **88342** Immunohistochemistry (including tissue immunoperoxidase), each antibody

➲ *CPT Changes: An Insider's View* 2004

►(Do not report 88342 in conjunction with 88360 or 88361 for the same antibody)◄

(For quantitative or semiquantitative immunohistochemistry, ►see 88360,◄ 88361)

♣ **88346** Immunofluorescent study, each antibody; direct method

♣ **88347** indirect method

♣ **88348** Electron microscopy; diagnostic

♣ **88349** scanning

♣ **88355** Morphometric analysis; skeletal muscle

♣ **88356** nerve

♣ **88358** tumor (eg, DNA ploidy)

➲ *CPT Changes: An Insider's View* 2004

(Do not report 88358 with 88313 unless each procedure is for a different special stain)

♣● **88360** Morphometric analysis, tumor immunohistochemistry (eg, Her-2/neu, estrogen receptor/progesterone receptor), quantitative or semiquantitative, each antibody; manual

➲ *CPT Changes: An Insider's View* 2005

♣▲ **88361** using computer-assisted technology

➲ *CPT Changes: An Insider's View* 2004, 2005

(Do not report ►88360,◄ 88361 with 88342 unless each procedure is for a different antibody)

►(For morphometric analysis, in situ hybridization, see 88367, 88368)◄

(When semi-thin plastic-embedded sections are performed in conjunction with morphometric analysis, only the morphometric analysis should be reported; if performed as an independent procedure, see codes 88300-88309 for surgical pathology.)

♣ **88362** Nerve teasing preparations

♣▲ **88365** In situ hybridization (eg, FISH), each probe

➲ *CPT Changes: An Insider's View* 2005

►(Do not report 88365 in conjunction with 88367, 88368 for the same probe)◄

♣● **88367** Morphometric analysis, in situ hybridization, (quantitative or semi-quantitative) each probe; using computer-assisted technology

➲ *CPT Changes: An Insider's View* 2005

♣● **88368** manual

➲ *CPT Changes: An Insider's View* 2005

♠ **88371** Protein analysis of tissue by Western Blot, with interpretation and report;

♠ **88372** immunological probe for band identification, each

♠ **88380** Microdissection (eg, mechanical, laser capture)

➲ *CPT Assistant* Apr 02:17; *CPT Changes: An Insider's View* 2002

♠ **88399** Unlisted surgical pathology procedure

Transcutaneous Procedures

♠ **88400** Bilirubin, total, transcutaneous

Pathology and Laboratory

Other Procedures

♠ **89050** Cell count, miscellaneous body fluids (eg, cerebrospinal fluid, joint fluid), except blood;

♠ **89051** with differential count

♠ **89055** Leukocyte assessment, fecal, qualitative or semiquantitative

➲ *CPT Assistant* Jul 03:7; *CPT Changes: An Insider's View* 2003, 2004

♠ **89060** Crystal identification by light microscopy with or without polarizing lens analysis, any body fluid (except urine)

♣ **89100** Duodenal intubation and aspiration; single specimen (eg, simple bile study or afferent loop culture) plus appropriate test procedure

♣ **89105** collection of multiple fractional specimens with pancreatic or gallbladder stimulation, single or double lumen tube

(For radiological localization, use 74340)

(For chemical analyses, see **Chemistry,** this section)

(Electrocardiogram, see 93000-93268)

(Esophagus acid perfusion test (Bernstein), see 91030)

♠ **89125** Fat stain, feces, urine, or respiratory secretions

➲ *CPT Changes: An Insider's View* 2001

♣ **89130** Gastric intubation and aspiration, diagnostic, each specimen, for chemical analyses or cytopathology;

♣ **89132** after stimulation

♣ **89135** Gastric intubation, aspiration, and fractional collections (eg, gastric secretory study); one hour

♣ **89136** two hours

♣ **89140** two hours including gastric stimulation (eg, histalog, pentagastrin)

♣ **89141** three hours, including gastric stimulation

(For gastric lavage, therapeutic, use 91105)

(For radiologic localization of gastric tube, use 74340)

(For chemical analyses, see 82926, 82928)

(Joint fluid chemistry, see **Chemistry,** this section)

♠ **89160** Meat fibers, feces

♠ **89190** Nasal smear for eosinophils

(Occult blood, feces, use 82270)

(Paternity tests, use 86910)

♣ **89220** Sputum, obtaining specimen, aerosol induced technique (separate procedure)

➲ *CPT Changes: An Insider's View* 2004

♠ **89225** Starch granules, feces

➲ *CPT Changes: An Insider's View* 2004

♣ **89230** Sweat collection by iontophoresis

➲ *CPT Changes: An Insider's View* 2004

♠ **89235** Water load test

➲ *CPT Changes: An Insider's View* 2004

♠ **89240** Unlisted miscellaneous pathology test

➲ *CPT Changes: An Insider's View* 2004

Reproductive Medicine Procedures

♣ **89250** Culture of oocyte(s)/embryo(s), less than 4 days;

➲ *CPT Assistant* Nov 97:35-36, Jan 98:6, Oct 98:1, Apr 04:1; *CPT Changes: An Insider's View* 2004

♣ **89251** with co-culture of oocyte(s)/embryos

➲ *CPT Assistant* Nov 97:35-36, Jan 98:6, Oct 98:1, Apr 04:1; *CPT Changes: An Insider's View* 2004

(For extended culture of oocyte(s)/embryo(s), see 89272)

(89252 has been deleted. To report, use 89280-89281)

♣ **89253** Assisted embryo hatching, microtechniques (any method)

➲ *CPT Assistant* Apr 04:1

♣ **89254** Oocyte identification from follicular fluid

➲ *CPT Assistant* Nov 97:35-36, Jan 98:6, Oct 98:1, Apr 04:1

♣ **89255** Preparation of embryo for transfer (any method)

➲ *CPT Assistant* Nov 97:35-36, Jan 98:6, Oct 98:1, Nov 98:30, Apr 04:1

(89256 has been deleted. To report, use 89352)

♣ **89257** Sperm identification from aspiration (other than seminal fluid)

➲ *CPT Assistant* Nov 97:35-36, Jan 98:6, Oct 98:1, Nov 98:30, Apr 04:1

(For semen analysis, see 89300-89320)

(For sperm identification from testis tissue, use 89264)

♣ **89258** Cryopreservation; embryo(s)

➲ *CPT Assistant* Nov 97:36, Jan 98:6, Oct 98:1, Apr 04:1; *CPT Changes: An Insider's View* 2004

♣ **89259** sperm

➲ *CPT Assistant* Nov 97:36, Jan 98:6, Oct 98:1, Apr 04:1

(For cryopreservation of reproductive tissue, testicular, use 89335)

(For cryopreservation of reproductive tissue, ovarian, use Category III code 0058T)

(For cryopreservation of oocyte(s), use Category III code 0059T)

♣ **89260** Sperm isolation; simple prep (eg, sperm wash and swim-up) for insemination or diagnosis with semen analysis

➲ *CPT Assistant* Nov 97:36, Jan 98:6, Oct 98:1, Apr 04:1

♣ **89261** complex prep (eg, Percoll gradient, albumin gradient) for insemination or diagnosis with semen analysis

➲ *CPT Assistant* Nov 97:36, Jan 98:6, Oct 98:1, Apr 04:1

(For semen analysis without sperm wash or swim-up, use 89320)

♣ **89264** Sperm identification from testis tissue, fresh or cryopreserved
➲ *CPT Assistant* Nov 98:30, Apr 04:1

(For biopsy of testis, see 54500, 54505)

(For sperm identification from aspiration, use 89257)

(For semen analysis, see 89300-89320)

♣ **89268** Insemination of oocytes
➲ *CPT Assistant* Apr 04:1; *CPT Changes: An Insider's View* 2004

♣ **89272** Extended culture of oocyte(s)/embryo(s), 4-7 days
➲ *CPT Assistant* Apr 04:1; *CPT Changes: An Insider's View* 2004

♣ **89280** Assisted oocyte fertilization, microtechnique; less than or equal to 10 oocytes
➲ *CPT Assistant* Apr 04:1; *CPT Changes: An Insider's View* 2004

♣ **89281** greater than 10 oocytes
➲ *CPT Assistant* Apr 04:1; *CPT Changes: An Insider's View* 2004

♣ **89290** Biopsy, oocyte polar body or embryo blastomere, microtechnique (for pre-implantation genetic diagnosis); less than or equal to 5 embryos
➲ *CPT Assistant* Apr 04:1; *CPT Changes: An Insider's View* 2004

♣ **89291** greater than 5 embryos
➲ *CPT Assistant* Apr 04:1; *CPT Changes: An Insider's View* 2004

♠ **89300** Semen analysis; presence and/or motility of sperm including Huhner test (post coital)
➲ *CPT Assistant* Nov 97:36, Jul 98:10, Oct 98:1, Apr 04:1

♠ **89310** motility and count (not including Huhner test)
➲ *CPT Assistant* Apr 04:1; *CPT Changes: An Insider's View* 2003

♠ **89320** complete (volume, count, motility, and differential)
➲ *CPT Assistant* Apr 04:1

(Skin tests, see 86485-86585 and 95010-95199)

♠ **89321** Semen analysis, presence and/or motility of sperm
➲ *CPT Changes: An Insider's View* 2001

►(To report Hyaluronan binding assay (HBA), use Category III code 0087T)◄

♠ **89325** Sperm antibodies

(For medicolegal identification of sperm, use 88125)

♠ **89329** Sperm evaluation; hamster penetration test

♠ **89330** cervical mucus penetration test, with or without spinnbarkeit test

♣ **89335** Cryopreservation, reproductive tissue, testicular
➲ *CPT Assistant* Apr 04:1; *CPT Changes: An Insider's View* 2004

(For cryopreservation of embryo(s), use 89258. For cryopreservation of sperm, use 89259)

(For cryopreservation of reproductive tissue, ovarian, use Category III code 0058T)

(For cryopreservation of oocyte, use Category III code 0059T)

♣ **89342** Storage, (per year); embryo(s)
➲ *CPT Assistant* Apr 04:1; *CPT Changes: An Insider's View* 2004

♣ **89343** sperm/semen
➲ *CPT Assistant* Apr 04:1; *CPT Changes: An Insider's View* 2004

♣ **89344** reproductive tissue, testicular/ovarian
➲ *CPT Assistant* Apr 04:1; *CPT Changes: An Insider's View* 2004

♣▲ **89346** oocyte(s)
➲ *CPT Assistant* Apr 04:1; *CPT Changes: An Insider's View* 2004

(89350 has been deleted. To report, use 89220)

♣ **89352** Thawing of cryopreserved; embryo(s)
➲ *CPT Assistant* Apr 04:1; *CPT Changes: An Insider's View* 2004

♣ **89353** sperm/semen, each aliquot
➲ *CPT Assistant* Apr 04:1; *CPT Changes: An Insider's View* 2004

♣ **89354** reproductive tissue, testicular/ovarian
➲ *CPT Assistant* Apr 04:1; *CPT Changes: An Insider's View* 2004

(89355 has been deleted. To report, use 89225)

♣ **89356** oocytes, each aliquot
➲ *CPT Assistant* Apr 04:1; *CPT Changes: An Insider's View* 2004

(89360 has been deleted. To report, use 89230)

(89365 has been deleted. To report, use 89235)

(89399 has been deleted. To report, use 89240)

Medicine Guidelines

In addition to the definitions and commonly used terms presented in the **Introduction**, several other items unique to this section on **Medicine** are defined or identified here.

Multiple Procedures

It is appropriate to designate multiple procedures that are rendered on the same date by separate entries. For example: If individual medical psychotherapy (90829) is rendered in addition to subsequent hospital care (eg, 99231), the psychotherapy would be reported separately from the hospital visit. In this instance, both 99231 and 90829 would be reported.

Add-on Codes

Some of the listed procedures are commonly carried out in addition to the primary procedure performed. All add-on codes found in *CPT* are exempt from the multiple procedure concept. They are exempt from the use of modifier 51, as these procedures are not reported as stand-alone codes. These additional or supplemental procedures are designated as "add-on" codes. Add-on codes in *CPT* can be readily identified by specific descriptor nomenclature which includes phrases such as "each additional" or "(List separately in addition to primary procedure)."

Separate Procedures

Some of the procedures or services listed in *CPT* that are commonly carried out as an integral component of a total service or procedure have been identified by the inclusion of the term "separate procedure." The codes designated as "separate procedure" should not be reported in addition to the code for the total procedure or service of which it is considered an integral component.

However, when a procedure or service that is designated as a "separate procedure" is carried out independently or considered to be unrelated or distinct from other procedures/services provided at that time, it may be reported by itself, or in addition to other procedures/services by appending modifier 59 to the specific "separate procedure" code to indicate that the procedure is not considered to be a component of another procedure, but is a distinct, independent procedure. This may represent a different session or patient encounter, different procedure or surgery, different site or organ system, separate incision/excision, separate lesion, or separate injury (or area of injury in extensive injuries).

Subsection Information

Several of the subheadings or subsections have special instructions unique to that section. These special instructions will be presented preceding those procedural terminology listings, referring to that subsection specifically. If there is an "Unlisted Procedure" code number (see section below) for the individual subsection, it will also be shown. Those subsections within the **Medicine** section that have special instructions are as follows:

Immune Globulins 90281-90399
Immunization Administration for Vaccines/Toxoids 90465-90474
Vaccines, Toxoids 90476-90749
Therapeutic or Diagnostic Infusions 90780-90781
Psychiatry 90801-90899
Dialysis 90918-90999
Ophthalmology 92002-92499
Contact Lens Services 92310-92326
Spectacle Services 92340-92396
Otorhinolaryngology 92502-92700
Audiologic Function Tests 92551-92597
Evaluative and Therapeutic Services . 92601-92625
Echocardiography 93303-93350
Cardiac Catheterization 93501-93581
Intracardiac Electrophysiological Procedures/Studies 93600-93662
Peripheral Arterial Disease Rehabilitation 93668
Non-Invasive Vascular Diagnostic Studies 93875-93990
Pulmonary 94010-94799
Allergy and Clinical Immunology . . . 95004-95199
Neurology and Neuromuscular 95805-95999
Neurostimulators, Analysis-Programming 95970-95979
Motion Analysis 96000-96004
Central Nervous System Assessments/Tests 96100-96117
Health and Behavior Assessment/Intervention 96150-96155
Chemotherapy Administration 96400-96549
Dermatological Procedures 96900-96999
Physical Medicine and Rehabilitation 97001-97755
  Modalities 97010-97039
  Constant Attendance 97032-97039

Unlisted Service or Procedure

A service or procedure may be provided that is not listed in this edition of *CPT*. When reporting such a service, the appropriate "Unlisted Procedure" code may be used to indicate the service, identifying it by "Special Report" as discussed on this page. The "Unlisted Procedures" and accompanying codes for **Medicine** are as follows:

⊘ **90399** Unlisted immune globulin
⊘ **90749** Unlisted vaccine/toxoid
90799 Unlisted therapeutic, prophylactic or diagnostic injection
90899 Unlisted psychiatric service or procedure
90999 Unlisted dialysis procedure, inpatient or outpatient
91299 Unlisted diagnostic gastroenterology procedure
92499 Unlisted ophthalmological service or procedure
92700 Unlisted otorhinolaryngological service or procedure
93799 Unlisted cardiovascular service or procedure
94799 Unlisted pulmonary service or procedure
95199 Unlisted allergy/clinical immunologic service or procedure
95999 Unlisted neurological or neuromuscular diagnostic procedure
96549 Unlisted chemotherapy procedure
96999 Unlisted special dermatological service or procedure
97039 Unlisted modality (specify type and time if constant attendance)
97139 Unlisted therapeutic procedure (specify)
97799 Unlisted physical medicine/rehabilitation service or procedure
99199 Unlisted special service, procedure or report
99600 Unlisted home visit service or procedure

Special Report

A service that is rarely provided, unusual, variable, or new may require a special report in determining medical appropriateness of the service. Pertinent information should include an adequate definition or description of the nature, extent, and need for the procedure; and the time, effort, and equipment necessary to provide the service. Additional items which may be included are:

- complexity of symptoms;
- final diagnosis;
- pertinent physical findings;
- diagnostic and therapeutic procedures;
- concurrent problems;
- follow-up care.

Materials Supplied by Physician

Supplies and materials provided by the physician (eg, sterile trays/drugs), over and above those usually included with the procedure(s) rendered are reported separately. List drugs, trays, supplies, and materials provided. Identify as 99070 or specific supply code.

Medicine

Immune Globulins

Codes 90281-90399 identify the immune globulin product only and must be reported in addition to the administration codes 90780-90784 as appropriate. Immune globulin products listed here include broad-spectrum and anti-infective immune globulins, antitoxins, and various isoantibodies.

□⊘ **90281** Immune globulin (Ig), human, for intramuscular use

□⊘ **90283** Immune globulin (IgIV), human, for intravenous use

□⊘ **90287** Botulinum antitoxin, equine, any route

□⊘ **90288** Botulism immune globulin, human, for intravenous use

□⊘ **90291** Cytomegalovirus immune globulin (CMV-IgIV), human, for intravenous use

☆⊘ **90296** Diphtheria antitoxin, equine, any route

□⊘ **90371** Hepatitis B immune globulin (HBIg), human, for intramuscular use

☆⊘ **90375** Rabies immune globulin (RIg), human, for intramuscular and/or subcutaneous use

■⊘ **90376** Rabies immune globulin, heat-treated (RIg-HT), human, for intramuscular and/or subcutaneous use

□⊘ **90378** Respiratory syncytial virus immune globulin (RSV-IgIM), for intramuscular use, 50 mg, each

□⊘ **90379** Respiratory syncytial virus immune globulin (RSV-IgIV), human, for intravenous use

□⊘ **90384** Rho(D) immune globulin (RhIg), human, full-dose, for intramuscular use

☆⊘ **90385** Rho(D) immune globulin (RhIg), human, mini-dose, for intramuscular use

□⊘ **90386** Rho(D) immune globulin (RhIgIV), human, for intravenous use

□⊘ **90389** Tetanus immune globulin (TIg), human, for intramuscular use

■⊘ **90393** Vaccinia immune globulin, human, for intramuscular use

■⊘ **90396** Varicella-zoster immune globulin, human, for intramuscular use

□⊘ **90399** Unlisted immune globulin

Immunization Administration for Vaccines/Toxoids

Codes ►90465◄-90474 must be reported in addition to the vaccine and toxoid code(s) 90476-90749.

►Report codes 90465-90468 only when the physician provides face-to-face counseling of the patient and family during the administration of a vaccine. For immunization administration of any vaccine that is not accompanied by face-to-face physician counseling to the patient/family, report codes 90471-90474.◄

If a significant separately identifiable Evaluation and Management service (eg, office or other outpatient services, preventive medicine services) is performed, the appropriate E/M service code should be reported in addition to the vaccine and toxoid administration codes.

(For allergy testing, see 95004 et seq)

(For skin testing of bacterial, viral, fungal extracts, see 86485-86586)

(For therapeutic or diagnostic injections, see 90782-90799)

☆● **90465** Immunization administration under 8 years of age (includes percutaneous, intradermal, subcutaneous, or intramuscular injections) when the physician counsels the patient/family; first injection (single or combination vaccine/toxoid), per day

➲ *CPT Changes: An Insider's View* 2005

►(Do not report 90465 in conjunction with 90467)◄

☆+● **90466** each additional injection (single or combination vaccine/toxoid), per day (List separately in addition to code for primary procedure)

➲ *CPT Changes: An Insider's View* 2005

►(Use 90466 in conjunction with 90465 or 90467)◄

☆● **90467** Immunization administration under age 8 years (includes intranasal or oral routes of administration) when the physician counsels the patient/family; first administration (single or combination vaccine/toxoid), per day

➲ *CPT Changes: An Insider's View* 2005

►(Do not report 90467 in conjunction with 90465)◄

☆+● **90468** each additional administration (single or combination vaccine/toxoid), per day (List separately in addition to code for primary procedure)

➲ *CPT Changes: An Insider's View* 2005

►(Use 90468 in conjunction with 90465 or 90467)◄

☆▲ **90471** Immunization administration (includes percutaneous, intradermal, subcutaneous, or intramuscular injections); one vaccine (single or combination vaccine/toxoid)

➲ *CPT Changes: An Insider's View* 2005

►(Do not report 90471 in conjunction with 90473)◄

☆✚ **90472** each additional vaccine (single or combination vaccine/toxoid) (List separately in addition to code for primary procedure)

(Use 90472 in conjunction with 90471 ►or 90473◄)

(For administration of immune globulins, use 90780-90784, and see 90281-90399)

(For intravesical administration of BCG vaccine, use 51720, and see 90586)

□ **90473** Immunization administration by intranasal or oral route; one vaccine (single or combination vaccine/toxoid)

►(Do not report 90473 in conjunction with 90471)◄

□✚ **90474** each additional vaccine (single or combination vaccine/toxoid) (List separately in addition to code for primary procedure)

(Use 90474 in conjunction with ►90471 or◄ 90473)

Vaccines, Toxoids

Codes 90476-90748 identify the vaccine product **only.** To report the administration of a vaccine/toxoid, the vaccine/toxoid product codes 90476-90749 must be used in addition to an immunization administration code(s) ►90465-90474◄. Do not append modifier 51 to the vaccine/toxoid product codes 90476-90749.

If a significantly separately identifiable Evaluation and Management service (eg, office or other outpatient services, preventive medicine services) is performed, the appropriate E/M service code should be reported in addition to the vaccine and toxoid administration codes.

To meet the reporting requirements of immunization registries, vaccine distribution programs, and reporting systems (eg, Vaccine Adverse Event Reporting System) the exact vaccine product administered needs to be reported. Multiple codes for a particular vaccine are provided in *CPT* when the schedule (number of doses or timing) differs for two or more products of the same vaccine type (eg, hepatitis A, Hib) or the vaccine product is available in more than one chemical formulation, dosage, or route of administration.

Separate codes are available for combination vaccines (eg, DTP-Hib, DtaP-Hib, HepB-Hib). It is inappropriate to code each component of a combination vaccine separately. If a specific vaccine code is not available, the unlisted procedure code should be reported, until a new code becomes available.

(For immune globulins, see codes 90281-90399, and 90780-90784 for administration of immune globulins)

■⊘ **90476** Adenovirus vaccine, type 4, live, for oral use

☆⊘ **90477** Adenovirus vaccine, type 7, live, for oral use

☆⊘ **90581** Anthrax vaccine, for subcutaneous use

☆⊘ **90585** Bacillus Calmette-Guerin vaccine (BCG) for tuberculosis, live, for percutaneous use

■⊘ **90586** Bacillus Calmette-Guerin vaccine (BCG) for bladder cancer, live, for intravesical use

☆⊘ **90632** Hepatitis A vaccine, adult dosage, for intramuscular use

☆⊘ **90633** Hepatitis A vaccine, pediatric/adolescent dosage-2 dose schedule, for intramuscular use

☆⊘ **90634** Hepatitis A vaccine, pediatric/adolescent dosage-3 dose schedule, for intramuscular use

■⊘ **90636** Hepatitis A and hepatitis B vaccine (HepA-HepB), adult dosage, for intramuscular use

☆⊘ **90645** Hemophilus influenza b vaccine (Hib), HbOC conjugate (4 dose schedule), for intramuscular use

☆⊘ **90646** Hemophilus influenza b vaccine (Hib), PRP-D conjugate, for booster use only, intramuscular use

☆⊘ **90647** Hemophilus influenza b vaccine (Hib), PRP-OMP conjugate (3 dose schedule), for intramuscular use

☆⊘ **90648** Hemophilus influenza b vaccine (Hib), PRP-T conjugate (4 dose schedule), for intramuscular use

✪⊘ **90655** Influenza virus vaccine, split virus, preservative free, for children 6-35 months of age, for intramuscular use

✪⊘● **90656** Influenza virus vaccine, split virus, preservative free, for use in individuals 3 years and above, for intramuscular use

✪⊘ **90657** Influenza virus vaccine, split virus, for children 6-35 months of age, for intramuscular use

➲ *CPT Changes: An Insider's View* 2001

✪⊘ **90658** Influenza virus vaccine, split virus, for use in individuals 3 years of age and above, for intramuscular use

➲ *CPT Changes: An Insider's View* 2001

(90659 has been deleted. To report influenza virus vaccine, split virus, see 90657 or 90658)

□⊘ **90660** Influenza virus vaccine, live, for intranasal use

■⊘ **90665** Lyme disease vaccine, adult dosage, for intramuscular use

□⊘ **90669** Pneumococcal conjugate vaccine, polyvalent, for children under 5 years, for intramuscular use

■⊘ **90675** Rabies vaccine, for intramuscular use

■⊘ **90676** Rabies vaccine, for intradermal use

☆⊘ **90680** Rotavirus vaccine, tetravalent, live, for oral use

☆⊘ **90690** Typhoid vaccine, live, oral

☆⊘ **90691** Typhoid vaccine, Vi capsular polysaccharide (ViCPs), for intramuscular use

☆⊘ **90692** Typhoid vaccine, heat- and phenol-inactivated (H-P), for subcutaneous or intradermal use

☆⊘ **90693** Typhoid vaccine, acetone-killed, dried (AKD), for subcutaneous use (U.S. military)

☆⊘ **90698** Diphtheria, tetanus toxoids, acellular pertussis vaccine, haemophilus influenza Type B, and poliovirus vaccine, inactivated (DTaP - Hib - IPV), for intramuscular use

☆⊘▲ **90700** Diphtheria, tetanus toxoids, and acellular pertussis vaccine (DTaP), for use in individuals younger than 7 years, for intramuscular use

➲ *CPT Assistant* Jan 96:5, Nov 98:31-33, Jan 99:1, Nov 03:13; *CPT Changes: An Insider's View* 2005

☆⊘ **90701** Diphtheria, tetanus toxoids, and whole cell pertussis vaccine (DTP), for intramuscular use

☆⊘ **90702** Diphtheria and tetanus toxoids (DT) adsorbed for use in individuals younger than 7 years, for intramuscular use

☆⊘ **90703** Tetanus toxoid adsorbed, for intramuscular use

☆⊘ **90704** Mumps virus vaccine, live, for subcutaneous use

☆⊘ **90705** Measles virus vaccine, live, for subcutaneous use

☆⊘ **90706** Rubella virus vaccine, live, for subcutaneous use

☆⊘ **90707** Measles, mumps and rubella virus vaccine (MMR), live, for subcutaneous use

☆⊘ **90708** Measles and rubella virus vaccine, live, for subcutaneous use

(90709 has been deleted)

■⊘ **90710** Measles, mumps, rubella, and varicella vaccine (MMRV), live, for subcutaneous use

☆⊘ **90712** Poliovirus vaccine, (any type(s)) (OPV), live, for oral use

☆⊘ **90713** Poliovirus vaccine, inactivated, (IPV), for subcutaneous use

☆⊘ **90715** Tetanus, diphtheria toxoids and acellular pertussis vaccine (TdaP), for use in individuals 7 years or older, for intramuscular use

☆⊘ **90716** Varicella virus vaccine, live, for subcutaneous use

☆⊘ **90717** Yellow fever vaccine, live, for subcutaneous use

☆⊘ **90718** Tetanus and diphtheria toxoids (Td) adsorbed for use in individuals 7 years or older, for intramuscular use

☆⊘ **90719** Diphtheria toxoid, for intramuscular use

☆⊘ **90720** Diphtheria, tetanus toxoids, and whole cell pertussis vaccine and Hemophilus influenza B vaccine (DTP-Hib), for intramuscular use

☆⊘ **90721** Diphtheria, tetanus toxoids, and acellular pertussis vaccine and Hemophilus influenza B vaccine (DtaP-Hib), for intramuscular use

□⊘ **90723** Diphtheria, tetanus toxoids, acellular pertussis vaccine, Hepatitis B, and poliovirus vaccine, inactivated (DtaP-HepB-IPV), for intramuscular use

➲ *CPT Changes: An Insider's View* 2001

■⊘ **90725** Cholera vaccine for injectable use

☆⊘ **90727** Plague vaccine, for intramuscular use

✪⊘ **90732** Pneumococcal polysaccharide vaccine, 23-valent, adult or immunosuppressed patient dosage, for use in individuals 2 years or older, for subcutaneous or intramuscular use

➲ *CPT Changes: An Insider's View* 2001

☆⊘ **90733** Meningococcal polysaccharide vaccine (any group(s)), for subcutaneous use

☆⊘ **90734** Meningococcal conjugate vaccine, serogroups A, C, Y and W-135 (tetravalent), for intramuscular use

■⊘ **90735** Japanese encephalitis virus vaccine, for subcutaneous use

■⊘ **90740** Hepatitis B vaccine, dialysis or immunosuppressed patient dosage (3 dose schedule), for intramuscular use

➲ *CPT Assistant* Apr 03:25

■⊘ **90743** Hepatitis B vaccine, adolescent (2 dose schedule), for intramuscular use

➲ *CPT Assistant* Apr 03:25

■⊘ **90744** Hepatitis B vaccine, pediatric/adolescent dosage (3 dose schedule), for intramuscular use

➲ *CPT Assistant* Apr 03:25

■⊘ **90746** Hepatitis B vaccine, adult dosage, for intramuscular use

➲ *CPT Assistant* Apr 03:25

■⊘ **90747** Hepatitis B vaccine, dialysis or immunosuppressed patient dosage (4 dose schedule), for intramuscular use

➲ *CPT Assistant* Apr 03:25

□⊘ **90748** Hepatitis B and Hemophilus influenza b vaccine (HepB-Hib), for intramuscular use

☆⊘ **90749** Unlisted vaccine/toxoid

Therapeutic or Diagnostic Infusions (Excludes Chemotherapy)

These procedures encompass prolonged intravenous injections.

These codes require the presence of the physician during the infusion. These codes are not to be used for intradermal, subcutaneous or intramuscular or routine IV drug injections. For these services, see 90782-90788.

These codes may not be used in addition to prolonged services codes.

§ **90780** Intravenous infusion for therapy/diagnosis, administered by physician or under direct supervision of physician; up to one hour

☆✚ **90781** each additional hour, up to eight (8) hours (List separately in addition to code for primary procedure)

(Use 90781 in conjunction with 90780)

Medicine

Therapeutic, Prophylactic or Diagnostic Injections

♣ **90782** Therapeutic, prophylactic or diagnostic injection (specify material injected); subcutaneous or intramuscular
➲ *CPT Assistant* Apr 02:15

(For administration of vaccines/toxoids, see ►90465◄-90472)

♣ **90783** intra-arterial

♣ **90784** intravenous

(90782-90784 do not include injections for allergen immunotherapy. For allergen immunotherapy injections, see 95115-95117)

♣ **90788** Intramuscular injection of antibiotic (specify)

(For chemotherapy administration and infusion services, see 95990, 96408-96414, 96420-96425, 96440, 96450, 96530, 96545, 96549)

♣ **90799** Unlisted therapeutic, prophylactic or diagnostic injection

(For allergy immunizations, see 95004 et seq)

Psychiatry

(For repetitive transcranial magnetic stimulation for treatment of clinical depression, use Category III code 0018T)

Hospital care by the attending physician in treating a psychiatric inpatient or partial hospitalization may be initial or subsequent in nature (see 99221-99233) and may include exchanges with nursing and ancillary personnel. Hospital care services involve a variety of responsibilities unique to the medical management of inpatients, such as physician hospital orders, interpretation of laboratory or other medical diagnostic studies and observations.

Some patients receive hospital evaluation and management services only and others receive evaluation and management services and other procedures. If other procedures such as electroconvulsive therapy or psychotherapy are rendered in addition to hospital evaluation and management services, these should be listed separately (ie, hospital care service plus electroconvulsive therapy or when psychotherapy is done, an appropriate code defining psychotherapy with medical evaluation and management services). Modifier 22 may be used to indicate a more extensive service. Modifier 52 may be used to signify a service that is reduced or less extensive than the usual procedure.

Other evaluation and management services, such as office medical service or other patient encounters, may be described as listed in the section on **Evaluation and Management,** if appropriate.

The evaluation and management services should not be reported separately, when reporting codes 90805, 90807, 90809, 90811, 90813, 90815, 90817, 90819, 90822, 90824, 90827, 90829.

Consultation for psychiatric evaluation of a patient includes examination of a patient and exchange of information with the primary physician and other informants such as nurses or family members, and preparation of a report. These consultation services (99241-99263) are limited to initial or follow-up evaluation and do not involve psychiatric treatment.

Psychiatric Diagnostic or Evaluative Interview Procedures

Psychiatric diagnostic interview examination includes a history, mental status, and a disposition, and may include communication with family or other sources, ordering and medical interpretation of laboratory or other medical diagnostic studies. In certain circumstances other informants will be seen in lieu of the patient.

Interactive psychiatric diagnostic interview examination is typically furnished to children. It involves the use of physical aids and non-verbal communication to overcome barriers to therapeutic interaction between the clinician and a patient who has not yet developed, or has lost, either the expressive language communication skills to explain his/her symptoms and response to treatment, or the receptive communication skills to understand the clinician if he/she were to use ordinary adult language for communication.

❖ **90801** Psychiatric diagnostic interview examination
➲ *CPT Assistant* Apr 03:14

❖ **90802** Interactive psychiatric diagnostic interview examination using play equipment, physical devices, language interpreter, or other mechanisms of communication
➲ *CPT Assistant* Apr 03:14

Psychiatric Therapeutic Procedures

Psychotherapy is the treatment for mental illness and behavioral disturbances in which the clinician establishes a professional contract with the patient and, through definitive therapeutic communication, attempts to alleviate the emotional disturbances, reverse or change maladaptive patterns of behavior, and encourage personality growth and development. The codes for reporting psychotherapy are divided into two broad categories: Interactive Psychotherapy; and Insight Oriented, Behavior Modifying and/or Supportive Psychotherapy.

Interactive psychotherapy is typically furnished to children. It involves the use of physical aids and non-verbal communication to overcome barriers to therapeutic interaction between the clinician and a patient who has not yet developed, or has lost, either the expressive language communication skills to explain his/her symptoms and response to treatment, or the receptive communication skills to understand the clinician if he/she were to use ordinary adult language for communication.

Insight oriented, behavior modifying and/or supportive psychotherapy refers to the development of insight or affective understanding, the use of behavior modification techniques, the use of supportive interactions, the use of cognitive discussion of reality, or any combination of the above to provide therapeutic change.

Some patients receive psychotherapy only and others receive psychotherapy and medical evaluation and management services. These evaluation and management services involve a variety of responsibilities unique to the medical management of psychiatric patients, such as medical diagnostic evaluation (eg, evaluation of comorbid medical conditions, drug interactions, and physical examinations), drug management when indicated, physician orders, interpretation of laboratory or other medical diagnostic studies and observations.

In reporting psychotherapy, the appropriate code is chosen on the basis of the type of psychotherapy (interactive using non-verbal techniques versus insight oriented, behavior modifying and/or supportive using verbal techniques), the place of service (office versus inpatient), the face-to-face time spent with the patient during psychotherapy, and whether evaluation and management services are furnished on the same date of service as psychotherapy.

To report medical evaluation and management services furnished on a day when psychotherapy is not provided, select the appropriate code from the **Evaluation and Management Services Guidelines.**

Office or Other Outpatient Facility

Insight Oriented, Behavior Modifying and/or Supportive Psychotherapy

❖ **90804** Individual psychotherapy, insight oriented, behavior modifying and/or supportive, in an office or outpatient facility, approximately 20 to 30 minutes face-to-face with the patient;

❖ **90805** with medical evaluation and management services

❖ **90806** Individual psychotherapy, insight oriented, behavior modifying and/or supportive, in an office or outpatient facility, approximately 45 to 50 minutes face-to-face with the patient;

➲ *CPT Assistant* Sep 03:4

❖ **90807** with medical evaluation and management services

❖ **90808** Individual psychotherapy, insight oriented, behavior modifying and/or supportive, in an office or outpatient facility, approximately 75 to 80 minutes face-to-face with the patient;

❖ **90809** with medical evaluation and management services

Interactive Psychotherapy

❖ **90810** Individual psychotherapy, interactive, using play equipment, physical devices, language interpreter, or other mechanisms of non-verbal communication, in an office or outpatient facility, approximately 20 to 30 minutes face-to-face with the patient;

❖ **90811** with medical evaluation and management services

❖ **90812** Individual psychotherapy, interactive, using play equipment, physical devices, language interpreter, or other mechanisms of non-verbal communication, in an office or outpatient facility, approximately 45 to 50 minutes face-to-face with the patient;

❖ **90813** with medical evaluation and management services

❖ **90814** Individual psychotherapy, interactive, using play equipment, physical devices, language interpreter, or other mechanisms of non-verbal communication, in an office or outpatient facility, approximately 75 to 80 minutes face-to-face with the patient;

❖ **90815** with medical evaluation and management services

Inpatient Hospital, Partial Hospital or Residential Care Facility

Insight Oriented, Behavior Modifying and/or Supportive Psychotherapy

❖ **90816** Individual psychotherapy, insight oriented, behavior modifying and/or supportive, in an inpatient hospital, partial hospital or residential care setting, approximately 20 to 30 minutes face-to-face with the patient;

❖ **90817** with medical evaluation and management services

➲ *CPT Assistant* Apr 03:13

❖ **90818** Individual psychotherapy, insight oriented, behavior modifying and/or supportive, in an inpatient hospital, partial hospital or residential care setting, approximately 45 to 50 minutes face-to-face with the patient;

➲ *CPT Assistant* Apr 03:14

❖ **90819** with medical evaluation and management services

➲ *CPT Assistant* Apr 03:13

❖ **90821** Individual psychotherapy, insight oriented, behavior modifying and/or supportive, in an inpatient hospital, partial hospital or residential care setting, approximately 75 to 80 minutes face-to-face with the patient;

➲ *CPT Assistant* Apr 03:14

❖ **90822** with medical evaluation and management services

➲ *CPT Assistant* Apr 03:13

Interactive Psychotherapy

❖ **90823** Individual psychotherapy, interactive, using play equipment, physical devices, language interpreter, or other mechanisms of non-verbal communication, in an inpatient hospital, partial hospital or residential care setting, approximately 20 to 30 minutes face-to-face with the patient;
➲ *CPT Assistant* Apr 03:14

❖ **90824** with medical evaluation and management services
➲ *CPT Assistant* Apr 03:13

❖ **90826** Individual psychotherapy, interactive, using play equipment, physical devices, language interpreter, or other mechanisms of non-verbal communication, in an inpatient hospital, partial hospital or residential care setting, approximately 45 to 50 minutes face-to-face with the patient;
➲ *CPT Assistant* Apr 03:14

❖ **90827** with medical evaluation and management services
➲ *CPT Assistant* Apr 03:13

❖ **90828** Individual psychotherapy, interactive, using play equipment, physical devices, language interpreter, or other mechanisms of non-verbal communication, in an inpatient hospital, partial hospital or residential care setting, approximately 75 to 80 minutes face-to-face with the patient;
➲ *CPT Assistant* Apr 03:14

❖ **90829** with medical evaluation and management services
➲ *CPT Assistant* Apr 03:13

Other Psychotherapy

❖ **90845** Psychoanalysis

❖ **90846** Family psychotherapy (without the patient present)
➲ *CPT Assistant* Apr 03:14

❖ **90847** Family psychotherapy (conjoint psychotherapy) (with patient present)
➲ *CPT Assistant* Apr 03:14

❖ **90849** Multiple-family group psychotherapy

❖ **90853** Group psychotherapy (other than of a multiple-family group)
➲ *CPT Assistant* Apr 03:14

❖ **90857** Interactive group psychotherapy
➲ *CPT Assistant* Apr 03:14

Other Psychiatric Services or Procedures

♣ **90862** Pharmacologic management, including prescription, use, and review of medication with no more than minimal medical psychotherapy

❖ **90865** Narcosynthesis for psychiatric diagnostic and therapeutic purposes (eg, sodium amobarbital (Amytal) interview)

❖ **90870** Electroconvulsive therapy (includes necessary monitoring); single seizure

☐ **90871** multiple seizures, per day

☐ **90875** Individual psychophysiological therapy incorporating biofeedback training by any modality (face-to-face with the patient), with psychotherapy (eg, insight oriented, behavior modifying or supportive psychotherapy); approximately 20-30 minutes
➲ *CPT Assistant* Apr 03:13, Aug 03:10, Sep 03:12

☐ **90876** approximately 45-50 minutes
➲ *CPT Assistant* Apr 03:13, Aug 03:10, Sep 03:12

❖ **90880** Hypnotherapy

☐ **90882** Environmental intervention for medical management purposes on a psychiatric patient's behalf with agencies, employers, or institutions

☆ **90885** Psychiatric evaluation of hospital records, other psychiatric reports, psychometric and/or projective tests, and other accumulated data for medical diagnostic purposes

☆ **90887** Interpretation or explanation of results of psychiatric, other medical examinations and procedures, or other accumulated data to family or other responsible persons, or advising them how to assist patient

☆ **90889** Preparation of report of patient's psychiatric status, history, treatment, or progress (other than for legal or consultative purposes) for other physicians, agencies, or insurance carriers

❖ **90899** Unlisted psychiatric service or procedure

Biofeedback

(For psychophysiological therapy incorporating biofeedback training, see 90875, 90876)

♠ **90901** Biofeedback training by any modality

❖ **90911** Biofeedback training, perineal muscles, anorectal or urethral sphincter, including EMG and/or manometry

(For incontinence treatment by pulsed magnetic neuromodulation, use Category III code 0029T)

►(For testing of rectal sensation, tone and compliance, use 91120)◄

Dialysis

Codes 90918-90921 are reported ONCE per month to distinguish age-specific services related to the patient's end-stage renal disease (ESRD) performed in an outpatient setting. ESRD-related physician services include establishment of a dialyzing cycle, outpatient evaluation and management of the dialysis visits, telephone calls, and patient management during the dialysis, provided during a full month. These codes are not used if the physician also submits hospitalization codes during the month.

Codes 90918-90921 describe a full month of ESRD-related services provided in an outpatient setting. For ESRD and non-ESRD dialysis services performed in an inpatient setting, and for non-ESRD dialysis services performed in an outpatient setting, see 90935-90937 and 90945-90947.

Evaluation and management services unrelated to ESRD services that cannot be performed during the dialysis session may be reported separately.

Codes 90922-90925 are reported when outpatient ESRD-related services are not performed consecutively during an entire full month (eg, when the patient spends part of the month as a hospital inpatient, or when the outpatient ESRD-related services are initiated after the first of the month). The appropriate age-related code from this series (90922-90925) is reported daily less the days of hospitalization. For reporting purposes, each month is considered 30 days.

Example:

Outpatient ESRD-related services are initiated on July 1 for a 57-year-old male. On July 11, he is admitted to the hospital as an inpatient and is discharged on July 27.

In this example, code 90925 should be reported for each day outside of the inpatient hospitalization (30 days/month less 17 days/hospitalization = 13 days). Report inpatient E/M services as appropriate. Dialysis procedures rendered during the hospitalization (July 11-27) should be reported as appropriate (90935-90937, 90945-90947).

End Stage Renal Disease Services

□ **90918** End stage renal disease (ESRD) related services per full month; for patients under two years of age to include monitoring for the adequacy of nutrition, assessment of growth and development, and counseling of parents
➲ *CPT Assistant* May 00:8

□ **90919** for patients between two and eleven years of age to include monitoring for the adequacy of nutrition, assessment of growth and development, and counseling of parents
➲ *CPT Assistant* May 00:8

□ **90920** for patients between twelve and nineteen years of age to include monitoring for the adequacy of nutrition, assessment of growth and development, and counseling of parents
➲ *CPT Assistant* May 00:8

□ **90921** for patients twenty years of age and over
➲ *CPT Assistant* May 00:8

□ **90922** End stage renal disease (ESRD) related services (less than full month), per day; for patients under two years of age
➲ *CPT Assistant* May 00:8

□ **90923** for patients between two and eleven years of age
➲ *CPT Assistant* May 00:8

□ **90924** for patients between twelve and nineteen years of age
➲ *CPT Assistant* May 00:8

□ **90925** for patients twenty years of age and over
➲ *CPT Assistant* May 00:8

Hemodialysis

Codes 90935, 90937 are reported to describe the hemodialysis procedure with all evaluation and management services related to the patient's renal disease on the day of the hemodialysis procedure. These codes are used for inpatient ESRD and non-ESRD procedures or for outpatient non-ESRD dialysis services. Code 90935 is reported if only one evaluation of the patient is required related to that hemodialysis procedure. Code 90937 is reported when patient re-evaluation(s) is required during a hemodialysis procedure. Utilize modifier 25 with Evaluation and Management codes for separately identifiable services unrelated to the dialysis procedure or renal failure which cannot be rendered during the dialysis session.

(For home visit hemodialysis services performed by a non-physician health care professional, use 99512)

(For cannula declotting, see 36831, 36833, 36860, 36861)

(For declotting of implanted vascular access device or catheter by thrombolytic agent, use 36550)

(For collection of blood specimen from a partially or completely implantable venous access device, use 36540)

(For prolonged physician attendance, see 99354-99360)

❖ **90935** Hemodialysis procedure with single physician evaluation

□ **90937** Hemodialysis procedure requiring repeated evaluation(s) with or without substantial revision of dialysis prescription

☆ **90939** Hemodialysis access flow study to determine blood flow in grafts and arteriovenous fistulae by an indicator dilution method, hook-up; transcutaneous measurement and disconnection

☆ **90940** measurement and disconnection

(For duplex scan of hemodialysis access, use 93990)

Medicine

Miscellaneous Dialysis Procedures

Codes 90945, 90947 describe dialysis procedures other than hemodialysis (eg, peritoneal dialysis, hemofiltration or continuous renal replacement therapies), and all evaluation and management services related to the patient's renal disease on the day of the procedure. Code 90945 is reported if only one evaluation of the patient is required related to that procedure. Code 90947 is reported when patient re-evaluation(s) is required during a procedure. Utilize modifier 25 with Evaluation and Management codes for separately identifiable services unrelated to the procedure or the renal failure which cannot be rendered during the dialysis session.

(For insertion of intraperitoneal cannula or catheter, see 49420, 49421)

(For prolonged physician attendance, see 99354-99360)

❖ **90945** Dialysis procedure other than hemodialysis (eg, peritoneal dialysis, hemofiltration, or other continuous renal replacement therapies), with single physician evaluation

➲ *CPT Assistant* Jan 03:22; *CPT Changes: An Insider's View* 2001

(For home infusion of peritoneal dialysis, use 99601, 99602)

☐ **90947** Dialysis procedure other than hemodialysis (eg, peritoneal dialysis, hemofiltration, or other continuous renal replacement therapies) requiring repeated physician evaluations, with or without substantial revision of dialysis prescription

➲ *CPT Assistant* May 00:8

✣ **90989** Dialysis training, patient, including helper where applicable, any mode, completed course

➲ *CPT Assistant* May 00:8

✣ **90993** Dialysis training, patient, including helper where applicable, any mode, course not completed, per training session

➲ *CPT Assistant* May 00:8

☐ **90997** Hemoperfusion (eg, with activated charcoal or resin)

➲ *CPT Assistant* May 00:8

✣ **90999** Unlisted dialysis procedure, inpatient or outpatient

➲ *CPT Assistant* May 00:8

Gastroenterology

(For duodenal intubation and aspiration, see 89100-89105)

(For gastrointestinal radiologic procedures, see 74210-74363)

(For esophagoscopy procedures, see 43200-43228; upper GI endoscopy 43234-43259; endoscopy, small intestine and stomal 44360-44393; proctosigmoidoscopy 45300-45321; sigmoidoscopy 45330-45339; colonoscopy 45355-45385; anoscopy 46600-46615)

♣ **91000** Esophageal intubation and collection of washings for cytology, including preparation of specimens (separate procedure)

♣ **91010** Esophageal motility (manometric study of the esophagus and/or gastroesophageal junction) study;

♣ **91011** with mecholyl or similar stimulant

♣ **91012** with acid perfusion studies

♣ **91020** Gastric motility (manometric) studies

♣ **91030** Esophagus, acid perfusion (Bernstein) test for esophagitis

►(91032 and 91033 have been deleted. To report, see 91034, 91035)◄

♣● **91034** Esophagus, gastroesophageal reflux test; with nasal catheter pH electrode(s) placement, recording, analysis and interpretation

➲ *CPT Changes: An Insider's View* 2005

❖● **91035** with mucosal attached telemetry pH electrode placement, recording, analysis and interpretation

➲ *CPT Changes: An Insider's View* 2005

♣● **91037** Esophageal function test, gastroesophageal reflux test with nasal catheter intraluminal impedance electrode(s) placement, recording, analysis and interpretation;

➲ *CPT Changes: An Insider's View* 2005

♣● **91038** prolonged (greater than 1 hour, up to 24 hours)

➲ *CPT Changes: An Insider's View* 2005

♣● **91040** Esophageal balloon distension provocation study

➲ *CPT Changes: An Insider's View* 2005

►(For balloon dilatation with endoscopy, see 43220, 43249, 43456, or 43458)◄

♣ **91052** Gastric analysis test with injection of stimulant of gastric secretion (eg, histamine, insulin, pentagastrin, calcium and secretin)

(For gastric biopsy by capsule, peroral, via tube, one or more specimens, use 43600)

(For gastric laboratory procedures, see also 89130-89141)

♣ **91055** Gastric intubation, washings, and preparing slides for cytology (separate procedure)

(For gastric lavage, therapeutic, use 91105)

♣ **91060** Gastric saline load test

(For biopsy by capsule, small intestine, per oral, via tube (one or more specimens), use 44100)

♣▲ **91065** Breath hydrogen test (eg, for detection of lactase deficiency), fructose intolerance, bacterial overgrowth, or oro-cecal gastrointestinal transit)

➲ *CPT Changes: An Insider's View* 2005

►(For H. pylori breath test analysis, use 83013 for non-radioactive (C-13) isotope or 78268 for radioactive (C-14) isotope)◄

♣ **91100** Intestinal bleeding tube, passage, positioning and monitoring

♣ 91105 Gastric intubation, and aspiration or lavage for treatment (eg, for ingested poisons)

(For cholangiography, see 47500, 74320)

(For abdominal paracentesis, see 49080, 49081; with instillation of medication, see 96440, 96445)

(For peritoneoscopy, use 49320; with biopsy, use 49321)

(For peritoneoscopy and guided transhepatic cholangiography, use 47560; with biopsy, use 47561)

(For splenoportography, see 38200, 75810)

§ 91110 Gastrointestinal tract imaging, intraluminal (eg, capsule endoscopy), esophagus through ileum, with physician interpretation and report

(Visualization of the colon is not reported separately)

(Append modifier 52 if the ileum is not visualized)

§● 91120 Rectal sensation, tone, and compliance test (ie, response to graded balloon distention)

➔ *CPT Changes: An Insider's View* 2005

►(For biofeedback training, use 90911)◄

►(For anorectal manometry, use 91122)◄

§ 91122 Anorectal manometry

☆ 91123 Pulsed irrigation of fecal impaction

Gastric Physiology

♣ 91132 Electrogastrography, diagnostic, transcutaneous;

♣ 91133 with provocative testing

➔ *CPT Changes: An Insider's View* 2001

Other Procedures

♣ 91299 Unlisted diagnostic gastroenterology procedure

Ophthalmology

(For surgical procedures, see **Surgery,** Eye and Ocular Adnexa, 65091 et seq)

Definitions

Intermediate ophthalmological services describes an evaluation of a new or existing condition complicated with a new diagnostic or management problem not necessarily relating to the primary diagnosis, including history, general medical observation, external ocular and adnexal examination and other diagnostic procedures as indicated; may include the use of mydriasis for ophthalmoscopy.

For example:

a. Review of history, external examination, ophthalmoscopy, biomicroscopy for an acute complicated condition (eg, iritis) not requiring comprehensive ophthalmological services.

b. Review of interval history, external examination, ophthalmoscopy, biomicroscopy and tonometry in established patient with known cataract not requiring comprehensive ophthalmological services.

Comprehensive ophthalmological services describes a general evaluation of the complete visual system. The comprehensive services constitute a single service entity but need not be performed at one session. The service includes history, general medical observation, external and ophthalmoscopic examinations, gross visual fields and basic sensorimotor examination. It often includes, as indicated: biomicroscopy, examination with cycloplegia or mydriasis and tonometry. It always includes initiation of diagnostic and treatment programs.

Intermediate and comprehensive ophthalmological services constitute integrated services in which medical decision making cannot be separated from the examining techniques used. Itemization of service components, such as slit lamp examination, keratometry, routine ophthalmoscopy, retinoscopy, tonometry, or motor evaluation is not applicable.

For example:

The comprehensive services required for diagnosis and treatment of a patient with symptoms indicating possible disease of the visual system, such as glaucoma, cataract or retinal disease, or to rule out disease of the visual system, new or established patient.

Initiation of diagnostic and treatment program includes the prescription of medication, and arranging for special ophthalmological diagnostic or treatment services, consultations, laboratory procedures and radiological services.

Special ophthalmological services describes services in which a special evaluation of part of the visual system is made, which goes beyond the services included under general ophthalmological services, or in which special treatment is given. Special ophthalmological services may be reported in addition to the general ophthalmological services or evaluation and management services.

For example:

Fluorescein angioscopy, quantitative visual field examination, refraction or extended color vision examination (such as Nagel's anomaloscope) should be separately reported.

Prescription of lenses, when required, is included in 92015. It includes specification of lens type (monofocal, bifocal, other), lens power, axis, prism, absorptive factor, impact resistance, and other factors.

Interpretation and report by the physician is an integral part of special ophthalmological services where indicated. Technical procedures (which may or may not be performed by the physician personally) are often part of the service, but should not be mistaken to constitute the service itself.

Medicine

General Ophthalmological Services

New Patient

Solely for the purposes of distinguishing between new and established patients, **professional services** are those face-to-face services rendered by a physician and reported by a specific code(s). A new patient is one who has not received any professional services from the physician or another physician of the same specialty who belongs to the same group practice within the past three years.

✶➧ **92002** Ophthalmological services: medical examination and evaluation with initiation of diagnostic and treatment program; intermediate, new patient
➲ *CPT Assistant* Feb 97:6, May 03:13

✶➧ **92004** comprehensive, new patient, one or more visits
➲ *CPT Assistant* Feb 97:6, May 03:13

Established Patient

Solely for the purposes of distinguishing between new and established patients, **professional services** are those face-to-face services rendered by a physician and reported by a specific code(s). An established patient is one who has received professional services from the physician or another physician of the same specialty who belongs to the same group practice within the past three years.

✶➧ **92012** Ophthalmological services: medical examination and evaluation, with initiation or continuation of diagnostic and treatment program; intermediate, established patient
➲ *CPT Assistant* Feb 97:6, May 03:13

✶➧ **92014** comprehensive, established patient, one or more visits
➲ *CPT Assistant* Feb 97:6, May 03:13

(For surgical procedures, see **Surgery,** Eye and Ocular Adnexa, 65091 et seq)

Special Ophthalmological Services

□ **92015** Determination of refractive state

§ **92018** Ophthalmological examination and evaluation, under general anesthesia, with or without manipulation of globe for passive range of motion or other manipulation to facilitate diagnostic examination; complete
➲ *CPT Assistant* Feb 97:6

§ **92019** limited
➲ *CPT Assistant* Feb 97:6

✶❖ **92020** Gonioscopy (separate procedure)
➲ *CPT Assistant* Feb 97:6

(For gonioscopy under general anesthesia, use 92018)

✶❖ **92060** Sensorimotor examination with multiple measurements of ocular deviation (eg, restrictive or paretic muscle with diplopia) with interpretation and report (separate procedure)
➲ *CPT Assistant* Feb 97:6

✶❖ **92065** Orthoptic and/or pleoptic training, with continuing medical direction and evaluation
➲ *CPT Assistant* Feb 97:6

☆ **92070** Fitting of contact lens for treatment of disease, including supply of lens
➲ *CPT Assistant* Feb 97:6

✶❖ **92081** Visual field examination, unilateral or bilateral, with interpretation and report; limited examination (eg, tangent screen, Autoplot, arc perimeter, or single stimulus level automated test, such as Octopus 3 or 7 equivalent)
➲ *CPT Assistant* Feb 97:6

✶❖ **92082** intermediate examination (eg, at least 2 isopters on Goldmann perimeter, or semiquantitative, automated suprathreshold screening program, Humphrey suprathreshold automatic diagnostic test, Octopus program 33)
➲ *CPT Assistant* Feb 97:6

✶❖ **92083** extended examination (eg, Goldmann visual fields with at least 3 isopters plotted and static determination within the central 30°, or quantitative, automated threshold perimetry, Octopus program G-1, 32 or 42, Humphrey visual field analyzer full threshold programs 30-2, 24-2, or 30/60-2)
➲ *CPT Assistant* Feb 97:6

(Gross visual field testing (eg, confrontation testing) is a part of general ophthalmological services and is not reported separately)

✶☆ **92100** Serial tonometry (separate procedure) with multiple measurements of intraocular pressure over an extended time period with interpretation and report, same day (eg, diurnal curve or medical treatment of acute elevation of intraocular pressure)
➲ *CPT Assistant* Feb 97:6

✶❖ **92120** Tonography with interpretation and report, recording indentation tonometer method or perilimbal suction method
➲ *CPT Assistant* Feb 97:6

✶❖ **92130** Tonography with water provocation
➲ *CPT Assistant* Feb 97:6

+❖ **92135** Scanning computerized ophthalmic diagnostic imaging (eg, scanning laser) with interpretation and report, unilateral
➲ *CPT Assistant* May 03:16

✶❖ **92136** Ophthalmic biometry by partial coherence interferometry with intraocular lens power calculation
➲ *CPT Changes: An Insider's View* 2002

✶❖ **92140** Provocative tests for glaucoma, with interpretation and report, without tonography
➲ *CPT Assistant* Feb 97:6

Ophthalmoscopy

Routine ophthalmoscopy is part of general and special ophthalmologic services whenever indicated. It is a non-itemized service and is not reported separately.

+❖ **92225** Ophthalmoscopy, extended, with retinal drawing (eg, for retinal detachment, melanoma), with interpretation and report; initial
➲ *CPT Assistant* Feb 97:6

+❖ **92226** subsequent
➲ *CPT Assistant* Feb 97:6

✶§ **92230** Fluorescein angioscopy with interpretation and report
➲ *CPT Assistant* Feb 97:6

+❖ **92235** Fluorescein angiography (includes multiframe imaging) with interpretation and report
➲ *CPT Assistant* Feb 97:6

+❖ **92240** Indocyanine-green angiography (includes multiframe imaging) with interpretation and report

✶❖ **92250** Fundus photography with interpretation and report
➲ *CPT Assistant* Feb 97:6

✶❖ **92260** Ophthalmodynamometry
➲ *CPT Assistant* Feb 97:6

(For ophthalmoscopy under general anesthesia, use 92018)

Other Specialized Services

✶❖ **92265** Needle oculoelectromyography, one or more extraocular muscles, one or both eyes, with interpretation and report
➲ *CPT Assistant* Feb 97:6

+❖ **92270** Electro-oculography with interpretation and report
➲ *CPT Assistant* Feb 97:6

+❖ **92275** Electroretinography with interpretation and report
➲ *CPT Assistant* May 03:13, Mar 04:9, Apr 04:14

(For electronystagmography for vestibular function studies, see 92541 et seq)

(For ophthalmic echography (diagnostic ultrasound), see 76511-76529)

✶❖ **92283** Color vision examination, extended, eg, anomaloscope or equivalent
➲ *CPT Assistant* Feb 97:6

(Color vision testing with pseudoisochromatic plates (such as HRR or Ishihara) is not reported separately. It is included in the appropriate general or ophthalmological service, or 99172)

✶❖ **92284** Dark adaptation examination with interpretation and report
➲ *CPT Assistant* Feb 97:6

+❖ **92285** External ocular photography with interpretation and report for documentation of medical progress (eg, close-up photography, slit lamp photography, goniophotography, stereo-photography)
➲ *CPT Assistant* Feb 97:6

+❖ **92286** Special anterior segment photography with interpretation and report; with specular endothelial microscopy and cell count
➲ *CPT Assistant* Feb 97:6

+❖ **92287** with fluorescein angiography
➲ *CPT Assistant* Feb 97:6

Contact Lens Services

The prescription of contact lens includes specification of optical and physical characteristics (such as power, size, curvature, flexibility, gas-permeability). It is NOT a part of the general ophthalmological services.

The fitting of contact lens includes instruction and training of the wearer and incidental revision of the lens during the training period.

Follow-up of successfully fitted extended wear lenses is reported as part of a general ophthalmological service (92012 et seq).

The supply of contact lenses may be reported as part of the service of fitting. It may also be reported separately by using 92391 or 92396 and modifier 26 for the service of fitting without supply.

(For therapeutic or surgical use of contact lens, see 68340, 92070)

☐ **92310** Prescription of optical and physical characteristics of and fitting of contact lens, with medical supervision of adaptation; corneal lens, both eyes, except for aphakia

(For prescription and fitting of one eye, add modifier 52)

⌘♣ **92311** corneal lens for aphakia, one eye
➲ *CPT Assistant* Feb 97:6

✶♣ **92312** corneal lens for aphakia, both eyes
➲ *CPT Assistant* Feb 97:6

+♣ **92313** corneoscleral lens
➲ *CPT Assistant* Feb 97:6

☐ **92314** Prescription of optical and physical characteristics of contact lens, with medical supervision of adaptation and direction of fitting by independent technician; corneal lens, both eyes except for aphakia

(For prescription and fitting of one eye, add modifier 52)

⌘♣ **92315** corneal lens for aphakia, one eye
➲ *CPT Assistant* Feb 97:7

✶♣ **92316** corneal lens for aphakia, both eyes
➲ *CPT Assistant* Feb 97:7

♣ **92317** corneoscleral lens
➲ *CPT Assistant* Feb 97:7

♣ **92325** Modification of contact lens (separate procedure), with medical supervision of adaptation
➲ *CPT Assistant* Feb 97:7

♣ **92326** Replacement of contact lens
➲ *CPT Assistant* Feb 97:7

Ocular Prosthetics, Artificial Eye

❖ **92330** Prescription, fitting, and supply of ocular prosthesis (artificial eye), with medical supervision of adaptation
➲ *CPT Assistant* Feb 97:7

(If supply is not included, use modifier 26; to report supply separately, use 92393)

☆ **92335** Prescription of ocular prosthesis (artificial eye) and direction of fitting and supply by independent technician, with medical supervision of adaptation
➲ *CPT Assistant* Feb 97:7

Spectacle Services (Including Prosthesis for Aphakia)

Prescription of lenses, when required, is included in 92015 Determination of refractive state. It includes specification of lens type (monofocal, bifocal, other), lens power, axis, prism, absorptive factor, impact resistance, and other factors.

Fitting of spectacles is a separate service; when provided by the physician, it is reported as indicated by 92340-92371.

Fitting includes measurement of anatomical facial characteristics, the writing of laboratory specifications, and the final adjustment of the spectacles to the visual axes and anatomical topography. Presence of physician is not required.

Supply of materials is a separate service component; it is not part of the service of fitting spectacles.

☐ **92340** Fitting of spectacles, except for aphakia; monofocal

☐ **92341** bifocal

☐ **92342** multifocal, other than bifocal

♣ **92352** Fitting of spectacle prosthesis for aphakia; monofocal
➲ *CPT Assistant* Feb 97:7

♣ **92353** multifocal
➲ *CPT Assistant* Feb 97:7

♣ **92354** Fitting of spectacle mounted low vision aid; single element system
➲ *CPT Assistant* Feb 97:7

♣ **92355** telescopic or other compound lens system
➲ *CPT Assistant* Feb 97:7

♣ **92358** Prosthesis service for aphakia, temporary (disposable or loan, including materials)
➲ *CPT Assistant* Feb 97:7

☐ **92370** Repair and refitting spectacles; except for aphakia

♣ **92371** spectacle prosthesis for aphakia
➲ *CPT Assistant* Feb 97:7

Supply of Materials

☐ **92390** Supply of spectacles, except prosthesis for aphakia and low vision aids

☐ **92391** Supply of contact lenses, except prosthesis for aphakia

(For supply of contact lenses reported as part of the service of fitting, see 92310-92313)

(For replacement of contact lens, use 92326)

☐ **92392** Supply of low vision aids (A low vision aid is any lens or device used to aid or improve visual function in a person whose vision cannot be normalized by conventional spectacle correction. Includes reading additions up to 4D.)

☐ **92393** Supply of ocular prosthesis (artificial eye)

(For supply reported as part of the service of fitting, use 92330)

☐ **92395** Supply of permanent prosthesis for aphakia; spectacles

(For temporary spectacle correction, use 92358)

☐ **92396** contact lenses

(For supply reported as part of the service of fitting, see 92311, 92312)

(Use 99070 for the supply of other materials, drugs, trays, etc.)

Other Procedures

❖ **92499** Unlisted ophthalmological service or procedure
➲ *CPT Assistant* Feb 97:7

Special Otorhinolaryngologic Services

Diagnostic or treatment procedures usually included in a comprehensive otorhinolaryngologic evaluation or office visit, are reported as an integrated medical service, using appropriate descriptors from the 99201 series. Itemization of component procedures (eg, otoscopy, rhinoscopy, tuning fork test) does not apply.

Special otorhinolaryngologic services are those diagnostic and treatment services not usually included in a comprehensive otorhinolaryngologic evaluation or office visit. These services are reported separately, using codes 92502-92700.

All services include medical diagnostic evaluation. Technical procedures (which may or may not be performed by the physician personally) are often part of the service, but should not be mistaken to constitute the service itself.

(For laryngoscopy with stroboscopy, use 31579)

§ **92502** Otolaryngologic examination under general anesthesia

☆ **92504** Binocular microscopy (separate diagnostic procedure)

♠ **92506** Evaluation of speech, language, voice, communication, auditory processing, and/or aural rehabilitation status

♠ **92507** Treatment of speech, language, voice, communication, and/or auditory processing disorder (includes aural rehabilitation); individual

♠ **92508** group, two or more individuals

□ **92510** Aural rehabilitation following cochlear implant (includes evaluation of aural rehabilitation status and hearing, therapeutic services) with or without speech processor programming

§ **92511** Nasopharyngoscopy with endoscope (separate procedure)

♣ **92512** Nasal function studies (eg, rhinomanometry)

♣ **92516** Facial nerve function studies (eg, electroneuronography)

♣ **92520** Laryngeal function studies

(92525 has been deleted. To report, see 92610-92611 for specific evaluation)

♠ **92526** Treatment of swallowing dysfunction and/or oral function for feeding

Vestibular Function Tests, With Observation and Evaluation by Physician, Without Electrical Recording

☆ **92531** Spontaneous nystagmus, including gaze

☆ **92532** Positional nystagmus test

☆ **92533** Caloric vestibular test, each irrigation (binaural, bithermal stimulation constitutes four tests)

☆ **92534** Optokinetic nystagmus test
➲ *CPT Changes: An Insider's View* 2002

Vestibular Function Tests, With Recording (eg, ENG, PENG), and Medical Diagnostic Evaluation

♣ **92541** Spontaneous nystagmus test, including gaze and fixation nystagmus, with recording

♣ **92542** Positional nystagmus test, minimum of 4 positions, with recording

♣ **92543** Caloric vestibular test, each irrigation (binaural, bithermal stimulation constitutes four tests), with recording

♣ **92544** Optokinetic nystagmus test, bidirectional, foveal or peripheral stimulation, with recording

♣ **92545** Oscillating tracking test, with recording

♣ **92546** Sinusoidal vertical axis rotational testing

♣+ **92547** Use of vertical electrodes (List separately in addition to code for primary procedure)

(Use 92547 in conjunction with 92541-92546)

(For unlisted vestibular tests, use 92700)

♣ **92548** Computerized dynamic posturography

Audiologic Function Tests With Medical Diagnostic Evaluation

The audiometric tests listed below imply the use of calibrated electronic equipment. Other hearing tests (such as whispered voice, tuning fork) are considered part of the general otorhinolaryngologic services and are not reported separately. All services include testing of both ears. Use modifier 52 if a test is applied to one ear instead of to two ears. All codes (except 92559) apply to testing of individuals; for testing of groups, use 92559 and specify test(s) used.

(For evaluation of speech, language and/or hearing problems through observation and assessment of performance, use 92506)

□ **92551** Screening test, pure tone, air only

♣ **92552** Pure tone audiometry (threshold); air only

♣ **92553** air and bone
➲ *CPT Assistant* Apr 03:9

♣ **92555** Speech audiometry threshold;
➲ *CPT Assistant* Apr 03:9

♣ **92556** with speech recognition
➲ *CPT Assistant* Apr 03:9

♣ **92557** Comprehensive audiometry threshold evaluation and speech recognition (92553 and 92556 combined)
➲ *CPT Assistant* Apr 03:9

(For hearing aid evaluation and selection, see 92590-92595)

□ **92559** Audiometric testing of groups
➲ *CPT Assistant* Apr 03:9

□ **92560** Bekesy audiometry; screening
➲ *CPT Assistant* Apr 03:9

♣ **92561** diagnostic
➲ *CPT Assistant* Apr 03:9

♣ **92562** Loudness balance test, alternate binaural or monaural
➲ *CPT Assistant* Apr 03:9

♣ **92563** Tone decay test
➲ *CPT Assistant* Apr 03:9

♣ **92564** Short increment sensitivity index (SISI)
➲ *CPT Assistant* Apr 03:9

♣ 92565 Stenger test, pure tone
➲ *CPT Assistant* Apr 03:9

♣ 92567 Tympanometry (impedance testing)
➲ *CPT Assistant* Apr 03:9

♣ 92568 Acoustic reflex testing
➲ *CPT Assistant* Apr 03:9

♣ 92569 Acoustic reflex decay test
➲ *CPT Assistant* Apr 03:9

♣ 92571 Filtered speech test
➲ *CPT Assistant* Apr 03:9

♣ 92572 Staggered spondaic word test
➲ *CPT Assistant* Apr 03:9

♣ 92573 Lombard test
➲ *CPT Assistant* Apr 03:9

♣ 92575 Sensorineural acuity level test
➲ *CPT Assistant* Apr 03:9

♣ 92576 Synthetic sentence identification test
➲ *CPT Assistant* Apr 03:9

♣ 92577 Stenger test, speech
➲ *CPT Assistant* Apr 03:9

♣ 92579 Visual reinforcement audiometry (VRA)
➲ *CPT Assistant* Apr 03:9

♣ 92582 Conditioning play audiometry
➲ *CPT Assistant* Apr 03:9

♣ 92583 Select picture audiometry
➲ *CPT Assistant* Apr 03:9

♣ 92584 Electrocochleography
➲ *CPT Assistant* Apr 03:9

❖ 92585 Auditory evoked potentials for evoked response audiometry and/or testing of the central nervous system; comprehensive
➲ *CPT Assistant* Apr 03:9

❖ 92586 limited
➲ *CPT Assistant* Apr 03:9

♣ 92587 Evoked otoacoustic emissions; limited (single stimulus level, either transient or distortion products)
➲ *CPT Assistant* Apr 03:9

♣ 92588 comprehensive or diagnostic evaluation (comparison of transient and/or distortion product otoacoustic emissions at multiple levels and frequencies)
➲ *CPT Assistant* Apr 03:9

►(92589 has been deleted)◄

►(For central auditory function evaluation, see 92620, 92621)◄

□ 92590 Hearing aid examination and selection; monaural
➲ *CPT Assistant* Apr 03:9

□ 92591 binaural
➲ *CPT Assistant* Apr 03:9

□ 92592 Hearing aid check; monaural
➲ *CPT Assistant* Apr 03:9

□ 92593 binaural
➲ *CPT Assistant* Apr 03:9

□ 92594 Electroacoustic evaluation for hearing aid; monaural
➲ *CPT Assistant* Apr 03:9

□ 92595 binaural
➲ *CPT Assistant* Apr 03:9

♣ 92596 Ear protector attenuation measurements
➲ *CPT Assistant* Apr 03:9

♠ 92597 Evaluation for use and/or fitting of voice prosthetic device to supplement oral speech
➲ *CPT Assistant* Apr 03:9

(To report augmentative and alternative communication device services, see 92605, 92607, 92608)

(92598 has been deleted)

(92599 has been deleted. To report use 92700)

Evaluative and Therapeutic Services

Codes 92601 and 92603 describe post-operative analysis and fitting of previously placed external devices, connection to the cochlear implant, and programming of the stimulator. Codes 92602 and 92604 describe subsequent sessions for measurements and adjustment of the external transmitter and re-programming of the internal stimulator.

(For placement of cochlear implant, use 69930)

♣ 92601 Diagnostic analysis of cochlear implant, patient under 7 years of age; with programming
➲ *CPT Changes: An Insider's View* 2003

♣ 92602 subsequent reprogramming
➲ *CPT Changes: An Insider's View* 2003

(Do not report 92602 in addition to 92601)

(For aural rehabilitation services following cochlear implant, including evaluation of rehabilitation status, use 92510)

♣ 92603 Diagnostic analysis of cochlear implant, age 7 years or older; with programming
➲ *CPT Changes: An Insider's View* 2003

♣ 92604 subsequent reprogramming
➲ *CPT Changes: An Insider's View* 2003

(Do not report 92604 in addition to 92603)

♠ 92605 Evaluation for prescription of non-speech-generating augmentative and alternative communication device
➲ *CPT Changes: An Insider's View* 2003

♠ 92606 Therapeutic service(s) for the use of non-speech-generating device, including programming and modification
➲ *CPT Changes: An Insider's View* 2003

♠ **92607** Evaluation for prescription for speech-generating augmentative and alternative communication device, face-to-face with the patient; first hour
➲ *CPT Changes: An Insider's View* 2003

(For evaluation for prescription of a non-speech-generating device, use 92605)

♠+ **92608** each additional 30 minutes (List separately in addition to code for primary procedure)
➲ *CPT Changes: An Insider's View* 2003

(Use 92608 in conjunction with 92607)

♠ **92609** Therapeutic services for the use of speech-generating device, including programming and modification
➲ *CPT Changes: An Insider's View* 2003

(For therapeutic service(s) for the use of a non-speech-generating device, use 92606)

♠ **92610** Evaluation of oral and pharyngeal swallowing function
➲ *CPT Changes: An Insider's View* 2003

(For motion fluoroscopic evaluation of swallowing function, use 92611)

(For flexible endoscopic examination, use 92612-92617)

♠ **92611** Motion fluoroscopic evaluation of swallowing function by cine or video recording
➲ *CPT Changes: An Insider's View* 2003

(For radiological supervision and interpretation, use 74230)

(For evaluation of oral and pharyngeal swallowing function, use 92610)

(For flexible fiberoptic diagnostic laryngoscopy, use 31575. Do not report 31575 in conjunction with 92612-92617)

♠ **92612** Flexible fiberoptic endoscopic evaluation of swallowing by cine or video recording;

(If flexible fiberoptic or endoscopic evaluation of swallowing is performed without cine or video recording, use 92700)

☐ **92613** physician interpretation and report only

(To report an evaluation of oral and pharyngeal swallowing function, use 92610)

(To report motion fluoroscopic evaluation of swallowing function, use 92611)

♠ **92614** Flexible fiberoptic endoscopic evaluation, laryngeal sensory testing by cine or video recording;
➲ *CPT Changes: An Insider's View* 2003

(If flexible fiberoptic or endoscopic evaluation of swallowing is performed without cine or video recording, use 92700)

☐ **92615** physician interpretation and report only

♠ **92616** Flexible fiberoptic endoscopic evaluation of swallowing and laryngeal sensory testing by cine or video recording;
➲ *CPT Changes: An Insider's View* 2003

(If flexible fiberoptic or endoscopic evaluation of swallowing is performed without cine or video recording, use 92700)

☐ **92617** physician interpretation and report only
➲ *CPT Changes: An Insider's View* 2003

♣● **92620** Evaluation of central auditory function, with report; initial 60 minutes
➲ *CPT Changes: An Insider's View* 2005

☆● **92621** each additional 15 minutes
➲ *CPT Changes: An Insider's View* 2005

►(Do not report 92620, 92621 in conjunction with 92506)◄

♣● **92625** Assessment of tinnitus (includes pitch, loudness matching, and masking)
➲ *CPT Changes: An Insider's View* 2005

►(Do not report 92625 in conjunction with 92562)◄

►(For unilateral assessment, use modifier 52)◄

Other Procedures

♣ **92700** Unlisted otorhinolaryngological service or procedure

Cardiovascular

Therapeutic Services

(For non-surgical septal reduction therapy (eg, alcohol ablation), use Category III code 0024T)

❖ **92950** Cardiopulmonary resuscitation (eg, in cardiac arrest)

(See also critical care services, 99291, 99292)

❖⊙ **92953** Temporary transcutaneous pacing

(For physician direction of ambulance or rescue personnel outside the hospital, use 99288)

❖⊙ **92960** Cardioversion, elective, electrical conversion of arrhythmia; external
➲ *CPT Changes: An Insider's View* 2000

❖⊙ **92961** internal (separate procedure)
➲ *CPT Changes: An Insider's View* 2000

(Do not report 92961 in addition to codes 93662, 93618-93624, 93631, 93640-93642, 93650-93652, 93741-93744)

✿ **92970** Cardioassist-method of circulatory assist; internal

✿ **92971** external

(For balloon atrial-septostomy, use 92992)

(For placement of catheters for use in circulatory assist devices such as intra-aortic balloon pump, use 33970)

Medicine

§⊙✚ **92973** Percutaneous transluminal coronary thrombectomy (List separately in addition to code for primary procedure)
➲ *CPT Changes: An Insider's View* 2002

(Use 92973 in conjunction with 92980, 92982)

§⊙✚ **92974** Transcatheter placement of radiation delivery device for subsequent coronary intravascular brachytherapy (List separately in addition to code for primary procedure)
➲ *CPT Changes: An Insider's View* 2002

(Use 92974 in conjunction with 92980, 92982, 92995, 93508)

(For intravascular radioelement application, see 77781-77784)

✿⊙ **92975** Thrombolysis, coronary; by intracoronary infusion, including selective coronary angiography

§ **92977** by intravenous infusion

(For thrombolysis of vessels other than coronary, see 37201, 75896)

(For cerebral thrombolysis, use 37195)

❖⊙✚ **92978** Intravascular ultrasound (coronary vessel or graft) during diagnostic evaluation and/or therapeutic intervention including imaging supervision, interpretation and report; initial vessel (List separately in addition to code for primary procedure)
➲ *CPT Changes: An Insider's View* 2000

❖⊙✚ **92979** each additional vessel (List separately in addition to code for primary procedure)
➲ *CPT Changes: An Insider's View* 2000

(Use 92979 in conjunction with 92978)

(Intravascular ultrasound services include all transducer manipulations and repositioning within the specific vessel being examined, both before and after therapeutic intervention (eg, stent placement))

§⊙ **92980** Transcatheter placement of an intracoronary stent(s), percutaneous, with or without other therapeutic intervention, any method; single vessel
➲ *CPT Assistant* Sep 97: 5, Nov 98:41, May 00:2

§⊙✚ **92981** each additional vessel (List separately in addition to code for primary procedure)
➲ *CPT Assistant* Sep 97:5, Nov 98:41, May 00:2

(Use 92981 in conjunction with 92980)

►(Codes 92980, 92981 are used to report coronary artery stenting. Coronary angioplasty (92982, 92984) or atherectomy (92995, 92996), in the same artery, is considered part of the stenting procedure and is not reported separately. Codes 92973 (percutaneous transluminal coronary thombectomy), 92974 (coronary brachytherapy) and 92978, 92979 (intravascular ultrasound) are add-on codes for reporting procedures performed in addition to coronary stenting, atherectomy, and angioplasty and are not included in the "therapeutic interventions" in 92980)◄

(To report additional vessels treated by angioplasty or atherectomy only during the same session, see 92984, 92996)

(To report transcatheter placement of radiation delivery device for coronary intravascular brachytherapy, use 92974)

(For intravascular radioelement application, see 77781-77784)

§⊙ **92982** Percutaneous transluminal coronary balloon angioplasty; single vessel
➲ *CPT Assistant* Sep 97:5, Nov 98:41, May 00:2

§⊙✚ **92984** each additional vessel (List separately in addition to code for primary procedure)

(Use 92984 in conjunction with 92980, 92982, 92995)

(For stent placement following completion of angioplasty or atherectomy, see 92980, 92981)

(To report transcatheter placement of radiation delivery device for coronary intravascular brachytherapy, use 92974)

(For intravascular radioelement application, see 77781-77784)

§⊙ **92986** Percutaneous balloon valvuloplasty; aortic valve
➲ *CPT Assistant* Jan 03:16

§⊙ **92987** mitral valve
➲ *CPT Assistant* Jan 03:16

§ **92990** pulmonary valve
➲ *CPT Assistant* Jan 03:16

✿ **92992** Atrial septectomy or septostomy; transvenous method, balloon (eg, Rashkind type) (includes cardiac catheterization)

✿ **92993** blade method (Park septostomy) (includes cardiac catheterization)

§⊙ **92995** Percutaneous transluminal coronary atherectomy, by mechanical or other method, with or without balloon angioplasty; single vessel
➲ *CPT Assistant* Sep 97:5, Nov 98:41, May 00:2

§⊙✚ **92996** each additional vessel (List separately in addition to code for primary procedure)
➲ *CPT Assistant* Sep 97:5, Nov 98:41, May 00:2

(Use 92996 in conjunction with 92980, 92982, 92995)

(For stent placement following completion of angioplasty or atherectomy, see 92980, 92981)

(To report additional vessels treated by angioplasty only during the same session, use 92984)

§ **92997** Percutaneous transluminal pulmonary artery balloon angioplasty; single vessel
➲ *CPT Assistant* Jan 03:16

§✚ **92998** each additional vessel (List separately in addition to code for primary procedure)
➲ *CPT Assistant* Jan 03:16

(Use 92998 in conjunction with 92997)

Cardiography

(For echocardiography, see 93303-93350)

✣ **93000** Electrocardiogram, routine ECG with at least 12 leads; with interpretation and report

❖ **93005** tracing only, without interpretation and report

♠ **93010** interpretation and report only

(For ECG monitoring, see 99354-99360)

☆ **93012** Telephonic transmission of post-symptom electrocardiogram rhythm strip(s), 24-hour attended monitoring, per 30 day period of time; tracing only

✣ **93014** physician review with interpretation and report only

✣ **93015** Cardiovascular stress test using maximal or submaximal treadmill or bicycle exercise, continuous electrocardiographic monitoring, and/or pharmacological stress; with physician supervision, with interpretation and report

✣ **93016** physician supervision only, without interpretation and report

♣ **93017** tracing only, without interpretation and report

✣ **93018** interpretation and report only

♣ **93024** Ergonovine provocation test

♣ **93025** Microvolt T-wave alternans for assessment of ventricular arrhythmias

✣ **93040** Rhythm ECG, one to three leads; with interpretation and report

❖ **93041** tracing only without interpretation and report

✣ **93042** interpretation and report only

✣ **93224** Electrocardiographic monitoring for 24 hours by continuous original ECG waveform recording and storage, with visual superimposition scanning; includes recording, scanning analysis with report, physician review and interpretation

♣ **93225** recording (includes hook-up, recording, and disconnection)

♣ **93226** scanning analysis with report

✣ **93227** physician review and interpretation

✣ **93230** Electrocardiographic monitoring for 24 hours by continuous original ECG waveform recording and storage without superimposition scanning utilizing a device capable of producing a full miniaturized printout; includes recording, microprocessor-based analysis with report, physician review and interpretation

♣ **93231** recording (includes hook-up, recording, and disconnection)

♣ **93232** microprocessor-based analysis with report

✣ **93233** physician review and interpretation

✣ **93235** Electrocardiographic monitoring for 24 hours by continuous computerized monitoring and non-continuous recording, and real-time data analysis utilizing a device capable of producing intermittent full-sized waveform tracings, possibly patient activated; includes monitoring and real-time data analysis with report, physician review and interpretation

♣ **93236** monitoring and real-time data analysis with report

✣ **93237** physician review and interpretation

✣ **93268** Patient demand single or multiple event recording with presymptom memory loop, 24-hour attended monitoring, per 30 day period of time; includes transmission, physician review and interpretation

♣ **93270** recording (includes hook-up, recording, and disconnection)

♣ **93271** monitoring, receipt of transmissions, and analysis

✣ **93272** physician review and interpretation only

(For postsymptom recording, see 93012, 93014)

(For implanted patient activated cardiac event recording, see 33282, 93727)

❖ **93278** Signal-averaged electrocardiography (SAECG), with or without ECG

(For interpretation and report only, use 93278 with modifier 26)

(For unlisted cardiographic procedure, use 93799)

Echocardiography

Echocardiography includes obtaining ultrasonic signals from the heart and great arteries, with two-dimensional image and/or Doppler ultrasonic signal documentation, and interpretation and report. When interpretation is performed separately use modifier 26.

►Echocardiography is an ultrasound examination of the cardiac chambers and valves, the adjacent great vessels, and the pericardium. A complete transthoracic echocardiogram (93307) is a comprehensive procedure that includes 2-dimensional and selected M-mode examination of the left and right atria, left and right ventricles, the aortic, mitral, and tricuspid valves, the pericardium, and adjacent portions of the aorta. These structures are assessed using multiple views as required to obtain a complete functional and anatomic evaluation, and appropriate measurements are obtained and recorded. Despite significant effort, identification and measurement of some structures may not always be possible. In such instances, the reason that an element could not be visualized must be documented. Additional structures that may be visualized (eg, pulmonary veins, pulmonary artery, pulmonic valve, inferior vena cava) would be included as part of the service.◄

►A follow-up or limited echocardiographic study (93308) is an examination that does not evaluate or document the attempt to evaluate all the structures that comprise the complete echocardiographic exam. This is typically performed in follow-up of a complete echocardiographic examination when a repeat complete exam is unnecessary due to the more focused clinical concern. In some emergent clinical situations, a limited echocardiographic study may be performed primarily.◄

►Report of an echocardiographic study, whether complete or limited, includes an interpretation of all obtained information, documentation of all clinically relevant findings including quantitative measurements obtained, plus a description of any recognized abnormalities. Pertinent images, videotape, and/or digital data are archived for permanent storage and are available for subsequent review. Use of echocardiography not meeting these criteria is not separately reportable.◄

►Use of ultrasound, without thorough evaluation of organ(s) or anatomic region, image documentation and final, written report, is not separately reportable.◄

(For fetal echocardiography, see 76825-76828)

❖ **93303** Transthoracic echocardiography for congenital cardiac anomalies; complete

❖ **93304** follow-up or limited study

❖ **93307** Echocardiography, transthoracic, real-time with image documentation (2D) with or without M-mode recording; complete

❖ **93308** follow-up or limited study

❖⊙ **93312** Echocardiography, transesophageal, real time with image documentation (2D) (with or without M-mode recording); including probe placement, image acquisition, interpretation and report

❖⊙ **93313** placement of transesophageal probe only

☆⊙ **93314** image acquisition, interpretation and report only

❖⊙ **93315** Transesophageal echocardiography for congenital cardiac anomalies; including probe placement, image acquisition, interpretation and report

❖⊙ **93316** placement of transesophageal probe only

☆⊙ **93317** image acquisition, interpretation and report only

❖⊙ **93318** Echocardiography, transesophageal (TEE) for monitoring purposes, including probe placement, real time 2-dimensional image acquisition and interpretation leading to ongoing (continuous) assessment of (dynamically changing) cardiac pumping function and to therapeutic measures on an immediate time basis

➲ *CPT Changes: An Insider's View* 2001

❖+ **93320** Doppler echocardiography, pulsed wave and/or continuous wave with spectral display (List separately in addition to codes for echocardiographic imaging); complete

(Use 93320 in conjunction with 93303, 93304, 93307, 93308, 93312, 93314, 93315, 93317, 93350)

❖+ **93321** follow-up or limited study (List separately in addition to codes for echocardiographic imaging)

(Use 93321 in conjunction with 93303, 93304, 93307, 93308, 93312, 93314, 93315, 93317, 93350)

❖+ **93325** Doppler echocardiography color flow velocity mapping (List separately in addition to codes for echocardiography)

(Use 93325 in conjunction with 76825, 76826, 76827, 76828, 93303, 93304, 93307, 93308, 93312, 93314, 93315, 93317, 93320, 93321, 93350)

❖ **93350** Echocardiography, transthoracic, real-time with image documentation (2D), with or without M-mode recording, during rest and cardiovascular stress test using treadmill, bicycle exercise and/or pharmacologically induced stress, with interpretation and report

(The appropriate stress testing code from the 93015-93018 series should be reported in addition to 93350 to capture the exercise stress portion of the study)

Cardiac Catheterization

Cardiac catheterization is a diagnostic medical procedure which includes introduction, positioning and repositioning of catheter(s), when necessary, recording of intracardiac and intravascular pressure, obtaining blood samples for measurement of blood gases or dilution curves and cardiac output measurements (Fick or other method, with or without rest and exercise and/or studies) with or without electrode catheter placement, final evaluation and report of procedure. When selective injection procedures are performed without a preceding cardiac catheterization, these services should be reported using codes in the Vascular Injection Procedures section, 36011-36015 and 36215-36218.

When coronary artery, arterial coronary conduit or venous bypass graft angiography is performed without concomitant left heart cardiac catheterization, use 93508. Injection procedures 93539, 93540, 93544, and 93545 represent separate identifiable services and may be reported in conjunction with one another in addition to 93508, as appropriate. To report imaging supervision, interpretation and report in conjunction with 93508, use 93556.

Modifier 51 should not be appended to 93501-93533, 93539-93556.

§⊙⊘ **93501** Right heart catheterization

(For bundle of His recording, use 93600)

§⊘ **93503** Insertion and placement of flow directed catheter (eg, Swan-Ganz) for monitoring purposes

(For subsequent monitoring, see 99356-99357)

§⊙⊘ **93505** Endomyocardial biopsy

Medicine

§⊙⊘ **93508** Catheter placement in coronary artery(s), arterial coronary conduit(s), and/or venous coronary bypass graft(s) for coronary angiography without concomitant left heart catheterization

(93508 is to be used only when left heart catheterization 93510, 93511, 93524, 93526 is not performed)

(93508 is to be used only once per procedure)

(To report transcatheter placement of radiation delivery device for coronary intravascular brachytherapy, use 92974)

(For intravascular radioelement application, see 77781-77784)

§⊙⊘ **93510** Left heart catheterization, retrograde, from the brachial artery, axillary artery or femoral artery; percutaneous

§⊙⊘ **93511** by cutdown

§⊙⊘ **93514** Left heart catheterization by left ventricular puncture

§⊙⊘ **93524** Combined transseptal and retrograde left heart catheterization

§⊙⊘ **93526** Combined right heart catheterization and retrograde left heart catheterization

§⊙⊘ **93527** Combined right heart catheterization and transseptal left heart catheterization through intact septum (with or without retrograde left heart catheterization)

§⊙⊘ **93528** Combined right heart catheterization with left ventricular puncture (with or without retrograde left heart catheterization)

§⊙⊘ **93529** Combined right heart catheterization and left heart catheterization through existing septal opening (with or without retrograde left heart catheterization)

§⊙⊘ **93530** Right heart catheterization, for congenital cardiac anomalies

§⊘ **93531** Combined right heart catheterization and retrograde left heart catheterization, for congenital cardiac anomalies

§⊘ **93532** Combined right heart catheterization and transseptal left heart catheterization through intact septum with or without retrograde left heart catheterization, for congenital cardiac anomalies

§⊘ **93533** Combined right heart catheterization and transseptal left heart catheterization through existing septal opening, with or without retrograde left heart catheterization, for congenital cardiac anomalies

(When injection procedures are performed in conjunction with cardiac catheterization, these services do not include introduction of catheters but do include repositioning of catheters when necessary and use of automatic power injectors. Injection procedures 93539-93545 represent separate identifiable services and may be coded in conjunction with one another when appropriate. The technical details of angiography, supervision of filming and processing, interpretation and report are not included. To report imaging supervision, interpretation and report, use 93555 and/or 93556. Modifier 51 should not be appended to 93539-93556.)

☆⊙⊘ **93539** Injection procedure during cardiac catheterization; for selective opacification of arterial conduits (eg, internal mammary), whether native or used for bypass

☆⊙⊘ **93540** for selective opacification of aortocoronary venous bypass grafts, one or more coronary arteries

☆⊙⊘ **93541** for pulmonary angiography

☆⊙⊘ **93542** for selective right ventricular or right atrial angiography

☆⊙⊘ **93543** for selective left ventricular or left atrial angiography

☆⊙⊘ **93544** for aortography

☆⊙⊘ **93545** for selective coronary angiography (injection of radiopaque material may be by hand)

(To report imaging supervision and interpretation, use 93555)

☆⊙⊘ **93555** Imaging supervision, interpretation and report for injection procedure(s) during cardiac catheterization; ventricular and/or atrial angiography

☆⊙⊘ **93556** pulmonary angiography, aortography, and/or selective coronary angiography including venous bypass grafts and arterial conduits (whether native or used in bypass)

(Codes 93561 and 93562 are not to be used with cardiac catheterization codes)

☆⊙ **93561** Indicator dilution studies such as dye or thermal dilution, including arterial and/or venous catheterization; with cardiac output measurement (separate procedure)

☆⊙ **93562** subsequent measurement of cardiac output

(For radioisotope method of cardiac output, see 78472, 78473, or 78481)

❖⊙+ **93571** Intravascular Doppler velocity and/or pressure derived coronary flow reserve measurement (coronary vessel or graft) during coronary angiography including pharmacologically induced stress; initial vessel (List separately in addition to code for primary procedure)

❖⊙+ **93572** each additional vessel (List separately in addition to code for primary procedure)

(Intravascular distal coronary blood flow velocity measurements include all Doppler transducer manipulations and repositioning within the specific vessel being examined, during coronary angiography or therapeutic intervention (eg, angioplasty))

(For unlisted cardiac catheterization procedure, use 93799)

Repair of Septal Defect

§ **93580** Percutaneous transcatheter closure of congenital interatrial communication (ie, Fontan fenestration, atrial septal defect) with implant

➔ *CPT Changes: An Insider's View* 2003

(Percutaneous transcatheter closure of atrial septal defect includes a right heart catheterization procedure. Code 93580 includes injection of contrast for atrial and ventricular angiograms. Codes 93501, 93529-93533, 93539, 93543, 93555 should not be reported separately in addition to code 93580)

§ **93581** Percutaneous transcatheter closure of a congenital ventricular septal defect with implant

➔ *CPT Changes: An Insider's View* 2003

(Percutaneous transcatheter closure of ventricular septal defect includes a right heart catheterization procedure. Code 93581 includes injection of contrast for atrial and ventricular angiograms. Codes 93501, 93529-93533, 93539, 93543, 93555 should not be reported separately in addition to code 93581)

(For echocardiographic services performed in addition to 93580, 93581, see 93303-93317, 93662 as appropriate)

Intracardiac Electrophysiological Procedures/Studies

Intracardiac electrophysiologic studies (EPS) are an invasive diagnostic medical procedure which include the insertion and repositioning of electrode catheters, recording of electrograms before and during pacing or programmed stimulation of multiple locations in the heart, analysis of recorded information, and report of the procedure. Electrophysiologic studies are most often performed with two or more electrode catheters. In many circumstances, patients with arrhythmias are evaluated and treated at the same encounter. In this situation, a diagnostic *electrophysiologic study* is performed, induced tachycardia(s) are *mapped*, and on the basis of the diagnostic and mapping information, the tissue is *ablated*. Electrophysiologic study(ies), mapping, and ablation represent distinctly different procedures, requiring individual reporting whether performed on the same or subsequent dates.

Definitions

***Arrhythmia Induction*:** In most electrophysiologic studies, an attempt is made to induce arrhythmia(s) from single or multiple sites within the heart. Arrhythmia induction is achieved by performing pacing at different rates, programmed stimulation (introduction of critically timed electrical impulses), and other techniques. Because arrhythmia induction occurs via the same catheter(s) inserted for the electrophysiologic study(ies), catheter insertion and temporary pacemaker codes are not additionally reported. Codes 93600-93603, 93610-93612 and 93618 are used to describe unusual situations where there may be recording, pacing or an attempt at arrhythmia induction from only one site in the heart. Code 93619 describes only evaluation of the sinus node, atrioventricular node and His-Purkinje conduction system, without arrhythmia induction. Codes 93620-93624 and 93640-93642 all include recording, pacing and attempted arrhythmia induction from one or more site(s) in the heart.

***Mapping*:** Mapping is a distinct procedure performed in addition to a diagnostic electrophysiologic procedure and should be separately reported using 93609 or 93613. Do not report standard mapping (93609) in addition to 3-D mapping (93613). When a tachycardia is induced, the site of tachycardia origination or its electrical path through the heart is often defined by mapping. Mapping creates a multidimensional depiction of a tachycardia by recording multiple electrograms obtained sequentially or simultaneously from multiple catheter sites in the heart. Depending upon the technique, certain types of mapping catheters may be repositioned from point-to-point within the heart, allowing sequential recording from the various sites to construct maps. Other types of mapping catheters allow mapping without a point-to-point technique by allowing simultaneous recording from many electrodes on the same catheter and computer-assisted three dimensional reconstruction of the tachycardia activation sequence.

***Ablation*:** Once the part of the heart involved in the tachycardia is localized, the tachycardia may be treated by ablation (the delivery of a radiofrequency energy to the area to selectively destroy cardiac tissue). Ablation procedures (93651-93652) may be performed: independently on a date subsequent to a diagnostic electrophysiologic study and mapping; or, at the time a diagnostic electrophysiologic study, tachycardia(s) induction and mapping is performed. When an electrophysiologic study, mapping, and ablation are performed on the same date, each procedure should be separately reported. In reporting catheter ablation, 93651 and/or 93652 should be reported once to describe ablation of cardiac arrhythmias, regardless of the number of arrhythmias ablated.

Modifier 51 should not be appended to 93600-93660.

§⊘ **93600** Bundle of His recording

§⊘ **93602** Intra-atrial recording

§⊘ **93603** Right ventricular recording

§⊙✚ **93609** Intraventricular and/or intra-atrial mapping of tachycardia site(s) with catheter manipulation to record from multiple sites to identify origin of tachycardia (List separately in addition to code for primary procedure)

➔ *CPT Changes: An Insider's View* 2002

(Use 93609 in conjunction with 93620, 93651, 93652)

(Do not report 93609 in addition to 93613)

Medicine

§⊘ **93610** Intra-atrial pacing

§⊘ **93612** Intraventricular pacing

(Do not report 93612 in conjunction with 93620-93622)

§⊙✚ **93613** Intracardiac electrophysiologic 3-dimensional mapping (List separately in addition to code for primary procedure)

➔ *CPT Changes: An Insider's View* 2002

(Use 93613 in conjunction with 93620, 93651, 93652)

(Do not report 93613 in addition to 93609)

§⊙⊘ **93615** Esophageal recording of atrial electrogram with or without ventricular electrogram(s);

§⊙⊘ **93616** with pacing

§⊙⊘ **93618** Induction of arrhythmia by electrical pacing

(For intracardiac phonocardiogram, use 93799)

§⊙⊘ **93619** Comprehensive electrophysiologic evaluation with right atrial pacing and recording, right ventricular pacing and recording, His bundle recording, including insertion and repositioning of multiple electrode catheters, without induction or attempted induction of arrhythmia

➔ *CPT Changes: An Insider's View* 2002

(Do not report 93619 in conjunction with 93600, 93602, 93610, 93612, 93618, or 93620-93622)

§⊙⊘ **93620** Comprehensive electrophysiologic evaluation including insertion and repositioning of multiple electrode catheters with induction or attempted induction of arrhythmia; with right atrial pacing and recording, right ventricular pacing and recording, His bundle recording

➔ *CPT Changes: An Insider's View* 2002, 2003

(Do not report 93620 in conjunction with 93600, 93602, 93610, 93612, 93618 or 93619)

§⊙✚ **93621** with left atrial pacing and recording from coronary sinus or left atrium (List separately in addition to code for primary procedure)

➔ *CPT Changes: An Insider's View* 2002

(Use 93621 in conjunction with 93620)

§⊙✚ **93622** with left ventricular pacing and recording (List separately in addition to code for primary procedure)

➔ *CPT Changes: An Insider's View* 2002

(Use 93622 in conjunction with 93620)

§✚ **93623** Programmed stimulation and pacing after intravenous drug infusion (List separately in addition to code for primary procedure)

(Use 93623 in conjunction with 93619, 93620)

❖⊙⊘ **93624** Electrophysiologic follow-up study with pacing and recording to test effectiveness of therapy, including induction or attempted induction of arrhythmia

§⊘ **93631** Intra-operative epicardial and endocardial pacing and mapping to localize the site of tachycardia or zone of slow conduction for surgical correction

❖⊙⊘ **93640** Electrophysiologic evaluation of single or dual chamber pacing cardioverter-defibrillator leads including defibrillation threshold evaluation (induction of arrhythmia, evaluation of sensing and pacing for arrhythmia termination) at time of initial implantation or replacement;

➔ *CPT Changes: An Insider's View* 2000

❖⊙⊘ **93641** with testing of single or dual chamber pacing cardioverter-defibrillator pulse generator

➔ *CPT Changes: An Insider's View* 2000

(For subsequent or periodic electronic analysis and/or reprogramming of single or dual chamber pacing cardioverter-defibrillators, see 93642, 93741-93744)

❖⊙⊘ **93642** Electrophysiologic evaluation of single or dual chamber pacing cardioverter-defibrillator (includes defibrillation threshold evaluation, induction of arrhythmia, evaluation of sensing and pacing for arrhythmia termination, and programming or reprogramming of sensing or therapeutic parameters)

➔ *CPT Changes: An Insider's View* 2000

§⊙⊘ **93650** Intracardiac catheter ablation of atrioventricular node function, atrioventricular conduction for creation of complete heart block, with or without temporary pacemaker placement

§⊙⊘ **93651** Intracardiac catheter ablation of arrhythmogenic focus; for treatment of supraventricular tachycardia by ablation of fast or slow atrioventricular pathways, accessory atrioventricular connections or other atrial foci, singly or in combination

§⊙⊘ **93652** for treatment of ventricular tachycardia

❖⊘ **93660** Evaluation of cardiovascular function with tilt table evaluation, with continuous ECG monitoring and intermittent blood pressure monitoring, with or without pharmacological intervention

(For testing of autonomic nervous system function, see 95921-95923)

❖✚ **93662** Intracardiac echocardiography during therapeutic/diagnostic intervention, including imaging supervision and interpretation (List separately in addition to code for primary procedure)

➔ *CPT Changes: An Insider's View* 2001

(Use 93662 in conjunction with 93580, 93581, 93621, 93622, 93651, or 93652, as appropriate)

(Do not report 92961 in addition to 93662)

Peripheral Arterial Disease Rehabilitation

Peripheral arterial disease (PAD) rehabilitative physical exercise consists of a series of sessions, lasting 45-60 minutes per session, involving use of either a motorized treadmill or a track to permit each patient to achieve symptom-limited claudication. Each session is supervised by an exercise physiologist or nurse. The supervising provider monitors the individual patient's claudication threshold and other cardiovascular limitations for adjustment of workload. During this supervised rehabilitation program, the development of new arrhythmias, symptoms that might suggest angina or the continued inability of the patient to progress to an adequate level of exercise may require physician review and examination of the patient. These physician services would be separately reported with an appropriate level E/M service code.

□ **93668** Peripheral arterial disease (PAD) rehabilitation, per session

Other Vascular Studies

(For arterial cannulization and recording of direct arterial pressure, use 36620)

(For radiographic injection procedures, see 36000-36299)

(For vascular cannulization for hemodialysis, see 36800-36821)

(For chemotherapy for malignant disease, see 96408-96549)

(For penile plethysmography, use 54240)

❖ **93701** Bioimpedance, thoracic, electrical
➲ *CPT Changes: An Insider's View* 2002

✤ **93720** Plethysmography, total body; with interpretation and report

♣ **93721** tracing only, without interpretation and report

✤ **93722** interpretation and report only

(For regional plethysmography, see 93875-93931)

❖ **93724** Electronic analysis of antitachycardia pacemaker system (includes electrocardiographic recording, programming of device, induction and termination of tachycardia via implanted pacemaker, and interpretation of recordings)

❖ **93727** Electronic analysis of implantable loop recorder (ILR) system (includes retrieval of recorded and stored ECG data, physician review and interpretation of retrieved ECG data and reprogramming)

❖ **93731** Electronic analysis of dual-chamber pacemaker system (includes evaluation of programmable parameters at rest and during activity where applicable, using electrocardiographic recording and interpretation of recordings at rest and during exercise, analysis of event markers and device response); without reprogramming

❖ **93732** with reprogramming

❖ **93733** Electronic analysis of dual chamber internal pacemaker system (may include rate, pulse amplitude and duration, configuration of wave form, and/or testing of sensory function of pacemaker), telephonic analysis

❖ **93734** Electronic analysis of single chamber pacemaker system (includes evaluation of programmable parameters at rest and during activity where applicable, using electrocardiographic recording and interpretation of recordings at rest and during exercise, analysis of event markers and device response); without reprogramming

❖ **93735** with reprogramming

❖ **93736** Electronic analysis of single chamber internal pacemaker system (may include rate, pulse amplitude and duration, configuration of wave form, and/or testing of sensory function of pacemaker), telephonic analysis

♣ **93740** Temperature gradient studies

❖▲ **93741** Electronic analysis of pacing cardioverter-defibrillator (includes interrogation, evaluation of pulse generator status, evaluation of programmable parameters at rest and during activity where applicable, using electrocardiographic recording and interpretation of recordings at rest and during exercise, analysis of event markers and device response); single chamber or wearable cardioverter-defibrillator system, without reprogramming
➲ *CPT Changes: An Insider's View* 2000

►(Do not report 93741 in conjunction with 93745)◄

❖▲ **93742** single chamber or wearable cardioverter-defibrillator system, with reprogramming
➲ *CPT Changes: An Insider's View* 2000

►(Do not report 93742 in conjunction with 93745)◄

❖ **93743** dual chamber, without reprogramming
➲ *CPT Changes: An Insider's View* 2000

❖ **93744** dual chamber, with reprogramming
➲ *CPT Changes: An Insider's View* 2000

❖● **93745** Initial set-up and programming by a physician of wearable cardioverter-defibrillator includes initial programming of system, establishing baseline electronic ECG, transmission of data to data repository, patient instruction in wearing system and patient reporting of problems or events
➲ *CPT Changes: An Insider's View* 2005

►(Do not report 93745 in conjunction with 93741, 93742)◄

□ **93760** Thermogram; cephalic

□ **93762** peripheral

✰ **93770** Determination of venous pressure

(For central venous cannulization see 36555-36556, 36500)

□ **93784** Ambulatory blood pressure monitoring, utilizing a system such as magnetic tape and/or computer disk, for 24 hours or longer; including recording, scanning analysis, interpretation and report

♣ **93786** recording only

♣ **93788** scanning analysis with report

✤ **93790** physician review with interpretation and report

Other Procedures

❖ **93797** Physician services for outpatient cardiac rehabilitation; without continuous ECG monitoring (per session)

❖ **93798** with continuous ECG monitoring (per session)

❖ **93799** Unlisted cardiovascular service or procedure

Medicine

Non-Invasive Vascular Diagnostic Studies

Vascular studies include patient care required to perform the studies, supervision of the studies and interpretation of study results with copies for patient records of hard copy output with analysis of all data, including bidirectional vascular flow or imaging when provided.

The use of a simple hand-held or other Doppler device that does not produce hard copy output, or that produces a record that does not permit analysis of bidirectional vascular flow, is considered to be part of the physical examination of the vascular system and is not separately reported.

Duplex scan (eg, 93880, 93882) describes an ultrasonic scanning procedure for characterizing the pattern and direction of blood flow in arteries or veins with the production of real time images integrating B-mode two-dimensional vascular structure with spectral and/or color flow Doppler mapping or imaging.

Non-invasive physiologic studies are performed using equipment separate and distinct from the duplex scanner. Codes 93875, 93965, 93922, 93923, and 93924 describe the evaluation of non-imaging physiologic recordings of pressures, Doppler analysis of bi-directional blood flow, plethysmography, and/or oxygen tension measurements appropriate for the anatomic area studied.

Cerebrovascular Arterial Studies

►A complete transcranial Doppler (TCD) study (93886) includes ultrasound evaluation of the right and left anterior circulation territories and the posterior circulation territory (to include vertebral arteries and basilar artery). In a limited TCD study (93888) there is ultrasound evaluation of two or fewer of these territories. For TCD, ultrasound evaluation is a reasonable and concerted attempt to identify arterial signals through an acoustic window.◄

✶❖ **93875** Non-invasive physiologic studies of extracranial arteries, complete bilateral study (eg, periorbital flow direction with arterial compression, ocular pneumoplethysmography, Doppler ultrasound spectral analysis)

✶❖ **93880** Duplex scan of extracranial arteries; complete bilateral study

⌘❖ **93882** unilateral or limited study

❖ **93886** Transcranial Doppler study of the intracranial arteries; complete study

❖ **93888** limited study

❖● **93890** vasoreactivity study

❖● **93892** emboli detection without intravenous microbubble injection

❖● **93893** emboli detection with intravenous microbubble injection

►(Do not report 93890-93893 in conjunction with 93888)◄

Extremity Arterial Studies (Including Digits)

✶❖ **93922** Non-invasive physiologic studies of upper or lower extremity arteries, single level, bilateral (eg, ankle/brachial indices, Doppler waveform analysis, volume plethysmography, transcutaneous oxygen tension measurement)

✶❖ **93923** Non-invasive physiologic studies of upper or lower extremity arteries, multiple levels or with provocative functional maneuvers, complete bilateral study (eg, segmental blood pressure measurements, segmental Doppler waveform analysis, segmental volume plethysmography, segmental transcutaneous oxygen tension measurements, measurements with postural provocative tests, measurements with reactive hyperemia)

✶❖ **93924** Non-invasive physiologic studies of lower extremity arteries, at rest and following treadmill stress testing, complete bilateral study

✶❖ **93925** Duplex scan of lower extremity arteries or arterial bypass grafts; complete bilateral study

⌘❖ **93926** unilateral or limited study

✶❖ **93930** Duplex scan of upper extremity arteries or arterial bypass grafts; complete bilateral study

⌘❖ **93931** unilateral or limited study

Extremity Venous Studies (Including Digits)

✶❖ **93965** Non-invasive physiologic studies of extremity veins, complete bilateral study (eg, Doppler waveform analysis with responses to compression and other maneuvers, phleborheography, impedance plethysmography)

✶❖ **93970** Duplex scan of extremity veins including responses to compression and other maneuvers; complete bilateral study

⌘❖ **93971** unilateral or limited study

Visceral and Penile Vascular Studies

❖ **93975** Duplex scan of arterial inflow and venous outflow of abdominal, pelvic, scrotal contents and/or retroperitoneal organs; complete study

❖ **93976** limited study

✶❖ **93978** Duplex scan of aorta, inferior vena cava, iliac vasculature, or bypass grafts; complete study

⌘❖ **93979** unilateral or limited study

❖ **93980** Duplex scan of arterial inflow and venous outflow of penile vessels; complete study

❖ **93981** follow-up or limited study

Extremity Arterial-Venous Studies

❖ **93990** Duplex scan of hemodialysis access (including arterial inflow, body of access and venous outflow)

(For measurement of hemodialysis access flow using indicator dilution methods, use 90940)

Pulmonary

Codes 94010-94799 include laboratory procedure(s) and interpretation of test results. If a separate identifiable Evaluation and Management service is performed, the appropriate E/M service code should be reported in addition to 94010-94799.

♣ **94010** Spirometry, including graphic record, total and timed vital capacity, expiratory flow rate measurement(s), with or without maximal voluntary ventilation

♣ **94014** Patient-initiated spirometric recording per 30-day period of time; includes reinforced education, transmission of spirometric tracing, data capture, analysis of transmitted data, periodic recalibration and physician review and interpretation
➲ *CPT Changes: An Insider's View* 2000

♣ **94015** recording (includes hook-up, reinforced education, data transmission, data capture, trend analysis, and periodic recalibration)

♠ **94016** physician review and interpretation only

♣▲ **94060** Bronchodilation responsiveness, spirometry as in 94010, pre- and post-bronchodilator administration

►(Report bronchodilator supply separately with 99070 or appropriate supply code)◄

(For prolonged exercise test for bronchospasm with pre- and post-spirometry, use 94620)

♣▲ **94070** Bronchospasm provocation evaluation, multiple spirometric determinations as in 94010, with administered agents (eg, antigen(s), cold air, methacholine)

►(Report antigen(s) administration separately with 99070 or appropriate supply code)◄

♣ **94150** Vital capacity, total (separate procedure)

♣ **94200** Maximum breathing capacity, maximal voluntary ventilation

♣ **94240** Functional residual capacity or residual volume: helium method, nitrogen open circuit method, or other method

♣ **94250** Expired gas collection, quantitative, single procedure (separate procedure)

♣ **94260** Thoracic gas volume

(For plethysmography, see 93720-93722)

♣ **94350** Determination of maldistribution of inspired gas: multiple breath nitrogen washout curve including alveolar nitrogen or helium equilibration time

♣ **94360** Determination of resistance to airflow, oscillatory or plethysmographic methods

♣ **94370** Determination of airway closing volume, single breath tests

♣ **94375** Respiratory flow volume loop

♣ **94400** Breathing response to CO_2 (CO_2 response curve)

♣ **94450** Breathing response to hypoxia (hypoxia response curve)

►(For high altitude simulation test (HAST), see 94452, 94453)◄

♣● **94452** High altitude simulation test (HAST), with physician interpretation and report;
➲ *CPT Changes: An Insider's View* 2005

►(For obtaining arterial blood gases, use 36600)◄

►(Do not report 94452 in conjunction with 94453, 94760, 94761)◄

♣● **94453** with supplemental oxygen titration
➲ *CPT Changes: An Insider's View* 2005

►(For obtaining arterial blood gases, use 36600)◄

►(Do not report 94453 in conjunction with 94452, 94760, 94761)◄

♣ **94620** Pulmonary stress testing; simple (eg, prolonged exercise test for bronchospasm with pre- and post-spirometry)

♣ **94621** complex (including measurements of CO_2 production, O_2 uptake, and electrocardiographic recordings)

❖ **94640** Pressurized or nonpressurized inhalation treatment for acute airway obstruction or for sputum induction for diagnostic purposes (eg, with an aerosol generator, nebulizer, metered dose inhaler or intermittent positive pressure breathing (IPPB) device)
➲ *CPT Changes: An Insider's View* 2003

(For more than one inhalation treatment performed on the same date, append modifier 76)

❖ **94642** Aerosol inhalation of pentamidine for pneumocystis carinii pneumonia treatment or prophylaxis

(94650, 94651, 94652 have been deleted)

❖ **94656** Ventilation assist and management, initiation of pressure or volume preset ventilators for assisted or controlled breathing; first day

❖ **94657** subsequent days

❖ **94660** Continuous positive airway pressure ventilation (CPAP), initiation and management

❖ **94662** Continuous negative pressure ventilation (CNP), initiation and management

❖ **94664** Demonstration and/or evaluation of patient utilization of an aerosol generator, nebulizer, metered dose inhaler or IPPB device

(94664 can be reported one time only per day of service)

(94665 has been deleted)

❖ **94667** Manipulation chest wall, such as cupping, percussing, and vibration to facilitate lung function; initial demonstration and/or evaluation

❖ **94668** subsequent

♣ **94680** Oxygen uptake, expired gas analysis; rest and exercise, direct, simple

♣ **94681** including CO_2 output, percentage oxygen extracted

♣ **94690** rest, indirect (separate procedure)

(For single arterial puncture, use 36600)

♣ **94720** Carbon monoxide diffusing capacity (eg, single breath, steady state)

➲ *CPT Changes: An Insider's View* 2002

♣ **94725** Membrane diffusion capacity

♣ **94750** Pulmonary compliance study (eg, plethysmography, volume and pressure measurements)

➲ *CPT Changes: An Insider's View* 2002

☆ **94760** Noninvasive ear or pulse oximetry for oxygen saturation; single determination

(For blood gases, see 82803-82810)

☆ **94761** multiple determinations (eg, during exercise)

☆ **94762** by continuous overnight monitoring (separate procedure)

♣ **94770** Carbon dioxide, expired gas determination by infrared analyzer

(For bronchoscopy, see 31622-31656)

(For placement of flow directed catheter, use 93503)

(For venipuncture, use 36410)

(For central venous catheter placement, see 36555-36556)

(For arterial puncture, use 36600)

(For arterial catheterization, use 36620)

(For thoracentesis, use 32000)

(For phlebotomy, therapeutic, use 99195)

(For lung biopsy, needle, use 32405)

(For intubation, orotracheal or nasotracheal, use 31500)

♣ **94772** Circadian respiratory pattern recording (pediatric pneumogram), 12 to 24 hour continuous recording, infant

(Separate procedure codes for electromyograms, EEG, ECG, and recordings of respiration are excluded when 94772 is reported)

♣ **94799** Unlisted pulmonary service or procedure

Allergy and Clinical Immunology

Definitions

Allergy sensitivity tests describe the performance and evaluation of selective cutaneous and mucous membrane tests in correlation with the history, physical examination, and other observations of the patient. The number of tests performed should be judicious and dependent upon the history, physical findings, and clinical judgment. All patients should not necessarily receive the same tests nor the same number of sensitivity tests.

Immunotherapy (desensitization, hyposensitization) is the parenteral administration of allergenic extracts as antigens at periodic intervals, usually on an increasing dosage scale to a dosage which is maintained as maintenance therapy. Indications for immunotherapy are determined by appropriate diagnostic procedures coordinated with clinical judgment and knowledge of the natural history of allergic diseases.

Other therapy: for medical conferences on the use of mechanical and electronic devices (precipitators, air conditioners, air filters, humidifiers, dehumidifiers), climatotherapy, physical therapy, occupational and recreational therapy, see **Evaluation and Management** section.

Allergy Testing

♣ **95004** Percutaneous tests (scratch, puncture, prick) with allergenic extracts, immediate type reaction, specify number of tests

♣ **95010** Percutaneous tests (scratch, puncture, prick) sequential and incremental, with drugs, biologicals or venoms, immediate type reaction, specify number of tests

♣ **95015** Intracutaneous (intradermal) tests, sequential and incremental, with drugs, biologicals, or venoms, immediate type reaction, specify number of tests

➲ *CPT Changes: An Insider's View* 2003

♣ **95024** Intracutaneous (intradermal) tests with allergenic extracts, immediate type reaction, specify number of tests

➲ *CPT Changes: An Insider's View* 2003

♣ **95027** Intracutaneous (intradermal) tests, sequential and incremental, with allergenic extracts for airborne allergens, immediate type reaction, specify number of tests

➲ *CPT Changes: An Insider's View* 2003

♣ **95028** Intracutaneous (intradermal) tests with allergenic extracts, delayed type reaction, including reading, specify number of tests

➲ *CPT Changes: An Insider's View* 2003

♣ **95044** Patch or application test(s) (specify number of tests)

♣ **95052** Photo patch test(s) (specify number of tests)

♣ 95056 Photo tests

♣ 95060 Ophthalmic mucous membrane tests

♣ 95065 Direct nasal mucous membrane test

♣ 95070 Inhalation bronchial challenge testing (not including necessary pulmonary function tests); with histamine, methacholine, or similar compounds

♣ 95071 with antigens or gases, specify

(For pulmonary function tests, see 94060, 94070)

♣ 95075 Ingestion challenge test (sequential and incremental ingestion of test items, eg, food, drug or other substance such as metabisulfite)

♣ 95078 Provocative testing (eg, Rinkel test)

(For allergy laboratory tests, see 86000-86999)

(For intravenous therapy for severe or intractable allergic disease, see 90780, 90781, 90784)

Allergen Immunotherapy

Codes 95115-95199 include the professional services necessary for allergen immunotherapy. Office visit codes may be used in addition to allergen immunotherapy if other identifiable services are provided at that time.

♣ 95115 Professional services for allergen immunotherapy not including provision of allergenic extracts; single injection

♣ 95117 two or more injections

✤ 95120 Professional services for allergen immunotherapy in prescribing physicians office or institution, including provision of allergenic extract; single injection

✤ 95125 two or more injections

✤ 95130 single stinging insect venom

✤ 95131 two stinging insect venoms

✤ 95132 three stinging insect venoms

✤ 95133 four stinging insect venoms

✤ 95134 five stinging insect venoms

♣ 95144 Professional services for the supervision of preparation and provision of antigens for allergen immunotherapy, single dose vial(s) (specify number of vials)

(A single dose vial contains a single dose of antigen administered in one injection)

♣ 95145 Professional services for the supervision of preparation and provision of antigens for allergen immunotherapy (specify number of doses); single stinging insect venom

♣ 95146 two single stinging insect venoms

♣ 95147 three single stinging insect venoms

♣ 95148 four single stinging insect venoms

♣ 95149 five single stinging insect venoms

♣ 95165 Professional services for the supervision of preparation and provision of antigens for allergen immunotherapy; single or multiple antigens (specify number of doses)

➲ *CPT Changes: An Insider's View* 2002

♣ 95170 whole body extract of biting insect or other arthropod (specify number of doses)

(For allergy immunotherapy reporting, a dose is the amount of antigen(s) administered in a single injection from a multiple dose vial)

♣ 95180 Rapid desensitization procedure, each hour (eg, insulin, penicillin, equine serum)

♣ 95199 Unlisted allergy/clinical immunologic service or procedure

(For skin testing of bacterial, viral, fungal extracts, see 95028, 86485-86586)

(For special reports on allergy patients, use 99080)

(For testing procedures such as radioallergosorbent testing (RAST), rat mast cell technique (RMCT), mast cell degranulation test (MCDT), lymphocytic transformation test (LTT), leukocyte histamine release (LHR), migration inhibitory factor test (MIF), transfer factor test (TFT), nitroblue tetrazolium dye test (NTD), see Immunology section in **Pathology** or use 95199)

Endocrinology

♣ 95250 Glucose monitoring for up to 72 hours by continuous recording and storage of glucose values from interstitial tissue fluid via a subcutaneous sensor (includes hook-up, calibration, patient initiation and training, recording, disconnection, downloading with printout of data)

➲ *CPT Changes: An Insider's View* 2002

(Do not report 95250 in conjunction with 99091)

(To report physician review, interpretation and written report associated with code 95250, see **Evaluation and Management** services codes)

Neurology and Neuromuscular Procedures

Neurologic services are typically consultative, and any of the levels of consultation (99241-99263) may be appropriate.

In addition, services and skills outlined under **Evaluation and Management** levels of service appropriate to neurologic illnesses should be reported similarly.

The EEG, autonomic function, evoked potential, ►reflex tests, EMG, NCV, and MEG◄ services (95812-95829 and ►95860-95967◄) include recording, interpretation by a physician, and report. For interpretation only, use modifier 26.

(For repetitive transcranial magnetic stimulation for treatment of clinical depression, use Category III code 0018T)

(Do not report codes 95860-95875 in addition to 96000-96004)

Sleep Testing

Sleep studies and polysomnography refer to the continuous and simultaneous monitoring and recording of various physiological and pathophysiological parameters of sleep for 6 or more hours with physician review, interpretation and report. The studies are performed to diagnose a variety of sleep disorders and to evaluate a patient's response to therapies such as nasal continuous positive airway pressure (NCPAP). Polysomnography is distinguished from sleep studies by the inclusion of sleep staging which is defined to include a 1-4 lead electroencephalogram (EEG), an electro-oculogram (EOG), and a submental electromyogram (EMG). Additional parameters of sleep include: 1) ECG; 2) airflow; 3) ventilation and respiratory effort; 4) gas exchange by oximetry, transcutaneous monitoring, or end tidal gas analysis; 5) extremity muscle activity, motor activity-movement; 6) extended EEG monitoring; 7) penile tumescence; 8) gastroesophageal reflux; 9) continuous blood pressure monitoring; 10) snoring; 11) body positions; etc.

The sleep services (95805-95811) include recording, interpretation and report. For interpretation only, use modifier 26.

For a study to be reported as polysomnography, sleep must be recorded and staged.

(Report with modifier 52 if less than 6 hours of recording or in other cases of reduced services as appropriate)

(For unattended sleep study, use 95806)

❖ **95805** Multiple sleep latency or maintenance of wakefulness testing, recording, analysis and interpretation of physiological measurements of sleep during multiple trials to assess sleepiness

❖ **95806** Sleep study, simultaneous recording of ventilation, respiratory effort, ECG or heart rate, and oxygen saturation, unattended by a technologist

❖ **95807** Sleep study, simultaneous recording of ventilation, respiratory effort, ECG or heart rate, and oxygen saturation, attended by a technologist

❖ **95808** Polysomnography; sleep staging with 1-3 additional parameters of sleep, attended by a technologist

❖ **95810** sleep staging with 4 or more additional parameters of sleep, attended by a technologist

❖ **95811** sleep staging with 4 or more additional parameters of sleep, with initiation of continuous positive airway pressure therapy or bilevel ventilation, attended by a technologist

Routine Electroencephalography (EEG)

EEG codes 95812-95822 include hyperventilation and/or photic stimulation when appropriate. Routine EEG codes 95816-95822 include 20 to 40 minutes of recording. Extended EEG codes 95812-95813 include reporting times longer than 40 minutes.

❖ **95812** Electroencephalogram (EEG) extended monitoring; 41-60 minutes
➲ *CPT Changes: An Insider's View* 2003

❖ **95813** greater than one hour

❖ **95816** Electroencephalogram (EEG); including recording awake and drowsy
➲ *CPT Changes: An Insider's View* 2000, 2003

❖ **95819** including recording awake and asleep
➲ *CPT Changes: An Insider's View* 2000, 2003

❖ **95822** recording in coma or sleep only
➲ *CPT Changes: An Insider's View* 2003

❖ **95824** cerebral death evaluation only

❖ **95827** all night recording
➲ *CPT Changes: An Insider's View* 2003

(For 24-hour EEG monitoring, see 95950-95953 or 95956)

(For EEG during nonintracranial surgery, use 95955)

(For Wada test, use 95958)

(For digital analysis of EEG, use 95957)

❖ **95829** Electrocorticogram at surgery (separate procedure)

✢ **95830** Insertion by physician of sphenoidal electrodes for electroencephalographic (EEG) recording

Muscle and Range of Motion Testing

♠ **95831** Muscle testing, manual (separate procedure) with report; extremity (excluding hand) or trunk
➲ *CPT Changes: An Insider's View* 2000

♠ **95832** hand, with or without comparison with normal side

♠ **95833** total evaluation of body, excluding hands

♠ **95834** total evaluation of body, including hands

♠ **95851** Range of motion measurements and report (separate procedure); each extremity (excluding hand) or each trunk section (spine)

♠ **95852** hand, with or without comparison with normal side

❖ **95857** Tensilon test for myasthenia gravis;

❖ **95858** with electromyographic recording

Electromyography and Nerve Conduction Tests

❖ **95860** Needle electromyography; one extremity with or without related paraspinal areas
➲ *CPT Changes: An Insider's View* 2003

❖ **95861** two extremities with or without related paraspinal areas
➲ *CPT Changes: An Insider's View* 2003

(For dynamic electromyography performed during motion analysis studies, see 96002-96003)

❖ **95863** three extremities with or without related paraspinal areas
➲ *CPT Changes: An Insider's View* 2003

❖ **95864** four extremities with or without related paraspinal areas
➲ *CPT Changes: An Insider's View* 2003

⌘❖ **95867** cranial nerve supplied muscle(s), unilateral
➲ *CPT Changes: An Insider's View* 2003

✶❖ **95868** cranial nerve supplied muscles, bilateral
➲ *CPT Changes: An Insider's View* 2003

❖ **95869** thoracic paraspinal muscles (excluding T1 or T12)
➲ *CPT Changes: An Insider's View* 2003

❖ **95870** limited study of muscles in one extremity or non-limb (axial) muscles (unilateral or bilateral), other than thoracic paraspinal, cranial nerve supplied muscles, or sphincters
➲ *CPT Changes: An Insider's View* 2000

(To report a complete study of the extremities, see 95860-95864)

(For anal or urethral sphincter, detrusor, urethra, perineum musculature, see 51785-51792)

(For eye muscles, use 92265)

❖ **95872** Needle electromyography using single fiber electrode, with quantitative measurement of jitter, blocking and/or fiber density, any/all sites of each muscle studied

❖ **95875** Ischemic limb exercise test with serial specimen(s) acquisition for muscle(s) metabolite(s)

❖⊘ **95900** Nerve conduction, amplitude and latency/velocity study, each nerve; motor, without F-wave study
➲ *CPT Changes: An Insider's View* 2000

❖⊘ **95903** motor, with F-wave study

❖⊘ **95904** sensory
➲ *CPT Changes: An Insider's View* 2002

(Report 95900, 95903, and/or 95904 only once when multiple sites on the same nerve are stimulated or recorded)

Intraoperative Neurophysiology

❖✚ **95920** Intraoperative neurophysiology testing, per hour (List separately in addition to code for primary procedure)

(Use 95920 in conjunction with the study performed, 92585, 95822, 95860, 95861, 95867, 95868, ►95870,◄ 95900, 95904, 95925►-◄95937.)

(Code 95920 describes ongoing electrophysiologic testing and monitoring performed during surgical procedures. Code 95920 is reported per hour of service, and includes only the ongoing electrophysiologic monitoring time distinct from performance of specific type(s) of baseline electrophysiologic study(s) (95860, 95861, 95867, 95868, ►95870,◄ 95900, 95904, ►95928, 95929,◄ 95933►-◄95937) or interpretation of specific type(s) of baseline electrophysiologic study(s) (92585, 95822, ►95870, 95925-95928, 95929, 95930◄). The time spent performing or interpreting the baseline electrophysiologic study(s) should not be counted as intraoperative monitoring, but represents separately reportable procedures. Code 95920 should be used once per hour even if multiple electrophysiologic studies are performed. The baseline electrophysiologic study(s) should be used once per operative session.)

(For electrocorticography, use 95829)

(For intraoperative EEG during nonintracranial surgery, use 95955)

(For intraoperative functional cortical or subcortical mapping, see 95961-95962)

(For intraoperative neurostimulator programming and analysis, see 95970-95975)

Autonomic Function Tests

❖ **95921** Testing of autonomic nervous system function; cardiovagal innervation (parasympathetic function), including two or more of the following: heart rate response to deep breathing with recorded R-R interval, Valsalva ratio, and 30:15 ratio

❖ **95922** vasomotor adrenergic innervation (sympathetic adrenergic function), including beat-to-beat blood pressure and R-R interval changes during Valsalva maneuver and at least five minutes of passive tilt

❖ **95923** sudomotor, including one or more of the following: quantitative sudomotor axon reflex test (QSART), silastic sweat imprint, thermoregulatory sweat test, and changes in sympathetic skin potential

Evoked Potentials and Reflex Tests

✶❖ **95925** Short-latency somatosensory evoked potential study, stimulation of any/all peripheral nerves or skin sites, recording from the central nervous system; in upper limbs

✶❖ **95926** in lower limbs

❖ **95927** in the trunk or head

(To report a unilateral study, use modifier 52)

(For auditory evoked potentials, use 92585)

❖● 95928 Central motor evoked potential study (transcranial motor stimulation); upper limbs
➲ *CPT Changes: An Insider's View* 2005

❖● 95929 lower limbs
➲ *CPT Changes: An Insider's View* 2005

✶❖ 95930 Visual evoked potential (VEP) testing central nervous system, checkerboard or flash

❖ 95933 Orbicularis oculi (blink) reflex, by electrodiagnostic testing

♦❖ 95934 H-reflex, amplitude and latency study; record gastrocnemius/soleus muscle

♦❖ 95936 record muscle other than gastrocnemius/soleus muscle

(To report a bilateral study, use modifier 50)

❖ 95937 Neuromuscular junction testing (repetitive stimulation, paired stimuli), each nerve, any one method

Special EEG Tests

❖ 95950 Monitoring for identification and lateralization of cerebral seizure focus, electroencephalographic (eg, 8 channel EEG) recording and interpretation, each 24 hours

❖ 95951 Monitoring for localization of cerebral seizure focus by cable or radio, 16 or more channel telemetry, combined electroencephalographic (EEG) and video recording and interpretation (eg, for presurgical localization), each 24 hours

❖ 95953 Monitoring for localization of cerebral seizure focus by computerized portable 16 or more channel EEG, electroencephalographic (EEG) recording and interpretation, each 24 hours

❖ 95954 Pharmacological or physical activation requiring physician attendance during EEG recording of activation phase (eg, thiopental activation test)

❖ 95955 Electroencephalogram (EEG) during nonintracranial surgery (eg, carotid surgery)

❖ 95956 Monitoring for localization of cerebral seizure focus by cable or radio, 16 or more channel telemetry, electroencephalographic (EEG) recording and interpretation, each 24 hours

❖ 95957 Digital analysis of electroencephalogram (EEG) (eg, for epileptic spike analysis)

❖ 95958 Wada activation test for hemispheric function, including electroencephalographic (EEG) monitoring

❖ 95961 Functional cortical and subcortical mapping by stimulation and/or recording of electrodes on brain surface, or of depth electrodes, to provoke seizures or identify vital brain structures; initial hour of physician attendance
➲ *CPT Changes: An Insider's View* 2000

❖+ 95962 each additional hour of physician attendance (List separately in addition to code for primary procedure)

(Use 95962 in conjunction with 95961)

❖ 95965 Magnetoencephalography (MEG), recording and analysis; for spontaneous brain magnetic activity (eg, epileptic cerebral cortex localization)
➲ *CPT Changes: An Insider's View* 2002

❖ 95966 for evoked magnetic fields, single modality (eg, sensory, motor, language, or visual cortex localization)
➲ *CPT Changes: An Insider's View* 2002

❖+ 95967 for evoked magnetic fields, each additional modality (eg, sensory, motor, language, or visual cortex localization) (List separately in addition to code for primary procedure)
➲ *CPT Changes: An Insider's View* 2002

(Use 95967 in conjunction with 95966)

(For electroencephalography performed in addition to magnetoencephalography, see 95812-95827)

(For somatosensory evoked potentials, auditory evoked potentials, and visual evoked potentials performed in addition to magnetic evoked field responses, see 92585, 95925, 95926, and/or 95930)

(For computerized tomography performed in addition to magnetoencephalography, see 70450-70470, 70496)

(For magnetic resonance imaging performed in addition to magnetoencephalography, see 70551-70553)

Neurostimulators, Analysis-Programming

A simple neurostimulator pulse generator/transmitter (95970, 95971) is one capable of affecting 3 or fewer of the following: pulse amplitude, pulse duration, pulse frequency, 8 or more electrode contacts, cycling, stimulation train duration, train spacing, number of programs, number of channels, alternating electrode polarities, dose time (stimulation parameters changing in time periods of minutes including dose lockout times), more than 1 clinical feature (eg, rigidity, dyskinesia, tremor). A complex neurostimulator pulse generator/transmitter (95970-95975) is one capable of affecting more than 3 of the above.

Code 95970 describes subsequent electronic analysis of a previously-implanted simple or complex brain, spinal cord, or peripheral neurostimulator pulse generator system, without reprogramming. Code 95971 describes intraoperative or subsequent electronic analysis of an implanted simple spinal cord or peripheral (ie, peripheral nerve, autonomic nerve, neuromuscular) neurostimulator pulse generator system, with programming. Codes 95972 and 95973 describe intraoperative (at initial insertion/revision) or subsequent electronic analysis of an implanted complex spinal cord or peripheral (except cranial nerve) neurostimulator pulse generator system, with programming. Codes 95974 and 95975 describe intraoperative (at initial insertion/revision) or subsequent electronic analysis of an implanted complex cranial nerve neurostimulator pulse generator system, with programming. ►Codes 95978 and 95979 describe initial or subsequent electronic analysis of an implanted brain neurostimulator pulse generator system, with programming.◄

(For insertion of neurostimulator pulse generator, see 61885, 63685, 63688, 64590)

(For revision or removal of neurostimulator pulse generator or receiver, see 61888, 63688, 64595)

(For implantation of neurostimulator electrodes, see 61850-61875, 63650-63655, 64553-64580. For revision or removal of neurostimulator electrodes, see 61880, 63660, 64585)

❖ **95970** Electronic analysis of implanted neurostimulator pulse generator system (eg, rate, pulse amplitude and duration, configuration of wave form, battery status, electrode selectability, output modulation, cycling, impedance and patient compliance measurements); simple or complex brain, spinal cord, or peripheral (ie, cranial nerve, peripheral nerve, autonomic nerve, neuromuscular) neurostimulator pulse generator/transmitter, without reprogramming
➲ *CPT Changes: An Insider's View* 2000

❖▲ **95971** simple spinal cord, or peripheral (ie, peripheral nerve, autonomic nerve, neuromuscular) neurostimulator pulse generator/transmitter, with intraoperative or subsequent programming
➲ *CPT Changes: An Insider's View* 2000

❖▲ **95972** complex spinal cord, or peripheral (except cranial nerve) neurostimulator pulse generator/transmitter, with intraoperative or subsequent programming, first hour
➲ *CPT Changes: An Insider's View* 2000

❖+▲ **95973** complex spinal cord, or peripheral (except cranial nerve) neurostimulator pulse generator/transmitter, with intraoperative or subsequent programming, each additional 30 minutes after first hour (List separately in addition to code for primary procedure)
➲ *CPT Changes: An Insider's View* 2000

(Use 95973 in conjunction with 95972)

❖ **95974** complex cranial nerve neurostimulator pulse generator/transmitter, with intraoperative or subsequent programming, with or without nerve interface testing, first hour

❖+ **95975** complex cranial nerve neurostimulator pulse generator/transmitter, with intraoperative or subsequent programming, each additional 30 minutes after first hour (List separately in addition to code for primary procedure)

(Use 95975 in conjunction with 95974)

❖● **95978** Electronic analysis of implanted neurostimulator pulse generator system (eg, rate, pulse amplitude and duration, battery status, electrode selectability and polarity, impedance and patient compliance measurements), complex deep brain neurostimulator pulse generator/transmitter, with initial or subsequent programming; first hour
➲ *CPT Changes: An Insider's View* 2005

❖+● **95979** each additional 30 minutes after first hour (List separately in addition to code for primary procedure)
➲ *CPT Changes: An Insider's View* 2005

►(Use 95979 in conjunction with 95978)◄

Other Procedures

§ **95990** Refilling and maintenance of implantable pump or reservoir for drug delivery, spinal (intrathecal, epidural) or brain (intraventricular);
➲ *CPT Changes: An Insider's View* 2003

(For analysis and/or reprogramming of implantable infusion pump, see 62367-62368)

(For refill and maintenance of implanted infusion pump or reservoir for systemic drug therapy (eg, chemotherapy or insulin, use 96530)

§ **95991** administered by physician
➲ *CPT Changes: An Insider's View* 2004

❖ **95999** Unlisted neurological or neuromuscular diagnostic procedure

Motion Analysis

Codes 96000-96004 describe services performed as part of a major therapeutic or diagnostic decision making process. Motion analysis is performed in a dedicated motion analysis laboratory (ie, a facility capable of performing videotaping from the front, back and both sides, computerized 3-D kinematics, 3-D kinetics, and dynamic electromyography). Code 96000 may include 3-D kinetics and stride characteristics. Codes 96002-96003 describe dynamic electromyography.

Code 96004 should only be reported once regardless of the number of study(ies) reviewed/interpreted.

(For performance of needle electromyography procedures, see 95860-95875)

(For gait training, use 97116)

✶❖ **96000** Comprehensive computer-based motion analysis by video-taping and 3-D kinematics;
➲ *CPT Changes: An Insider's View* 2002

✶❖ **96001** with dynamic plantar pressure measurements during walking
➲ *CPT Changes: An Insider's View* 2002

✶❖ **96002** Dynamic surface electromyography, during walking or other functional activities, 1-12 muscles
➲ *CPT Changes: An Insider's View* 2002

Medicine

✶❖ **96003** Dynamic fine wire electromyography, during walking or other functional activities, 1 muscle
➲ *CPT Changes: An Insider's View* 2002

(Do not report 96002, 96003 in conjunction with 95860-►95864, 95869-95872◄)

✶□ **96004** Physician review and interpretation of comprehensive computer based motion analysis, dynamic plantar pressure measurements, dynamic surface electromyography during walking or other functional activities, and dynamic fine wire electromyography, with written report

Central Nervous System Assessments/Tests (eg, Neuro-Cognitive, Mental Status, Speech Testing)

The following codes are used to report the services provided during testing of the cognitive function of the central nervous system. The testing of cognitive processes, visual motor responses, and abstractive abilities is accomplished by the combination of several types of testing procedures. It is expected that the administration of these tests will generate material that will be formulated into a report.

(For development of cognitive skills, see 97532, 97533)

♣ **96100** Psychological testing (includes psychodiagnostic assessment of personality, psychopathology, emotionality, intellectual abilities, eg, WAIS-R, Rorschach, MMPI) with interpretation and report, per hour
➲ *CPT Assistant* Apr 03:14

♠ **96105** Assessment of aphasia (includes assessment of expressive and receptive speech and language function, language comprehension, speech production ability, reading, spelling, writing, eg, by Boston Diagnostic Aphasia Examination) with interpretation and report, per hour

♣ **96110** Developmental testing; limited (eg, Developmental Screening Test II, Early Language Milestone Screen), with interpretation and report

♣▲ **96111** extended (includes assessment of motor, language, social, adaptive and/or cognitive functioning by standardized developmental instruments) with interpretation and report

♣ **96115** Neurobehavioral status exam (clinical assessment of thinking, reasoning and judgment, eg, acquired knowledge, attention, memory, visual spatial abilities, language functions, planning) with interpretation and report, per hour
➲ *CPT Assistant* Apr 03:14

(For mini-mental status examination performed by a physician, see **Evaluation and Management** services codes)

♣ **96117** Neuropsychological testing battery (eg, Halstead-Reitan, Luria, WAIS-R) with interpretation and report, per hour
➲ *CPT Assistant* Apr 03:14

Health and Behavior Assessment/Intervention

Health and behavior assessment procedures are used to identify the psychological, behavioral, emotional, cognitive, and social factors important to the prevention, treatment, or management of physical health problems.

The focus of the assessment is not on mental health but on the biopsychosocial factors important to physical health problems and treatments. The focus of the intervention is to improve the patient's health and well-being utilizing cognitive, behavioral, social, and/or psychophysiological procedures designed to ameliorate specific disease-related problems.

Codes 96150-96155 describe services offered to patients who present with established illnesses or symptoms, who are not diagnosed with mental illness, and may benefit from evaluations that focus on the biopsychosocial factors related to the patient's physical health status. These services do not represent preventive medicine counseling and risk factor reduction interventions.

For patients that require psychiatric services (90801-90899) as well as health and behavior assessment/intervention (96150-96155), report the predominant service performed. Do not report 96150-96155 in conjunction with 90801-90899 on the same date.

Evaluation and Management services codes (including **Preventive Medicine, Individual Counseling** codes 99401-99404, and **Preventive Medicine, Group Counseling** codes 99411-99412), should not be reported on the same day.

(For health and behavior assessment and/or intervention performed by a physician, see **Evaluation and Management** or **Preventive Medicine** services codes)

❖ **96150** Health and behavior assessment (eg, health-focused clinical interview, behavioral observations, psychophysiological monitoring, health-oriented questionnaires), each 15 minutes face-to-face with the patient; initial assessment
➲ *CPT Changes: An Insider's View* 2002

❖ **96151** re-assessment
➲ *CPT Changes: An Insider's View* 2002

❖ **96152** Health and behavior intervention, each 15 minutes, face-to-face; individual
➲ *CPT Changes: An Insider's View* 2002

❖ **96153** group (2 or more patients)
➲ *CPT Changes: An Insider's View* 2002

❖ **96154** family (with the patient present)
➲ *CPT Changes: An Insider's View* 2002

☐ **96155** family (without the patient present)
➲ *CPT Changes: An Insider's View* 2002

Chemotherapy Administration

Codes 96400-96549 are independent of the patient's visit.

If a significant separately identifiable Evaluation and Management service is performed, the appropriate E/M service code should be reported in addition to 96400-96549.

Either may occur independently on any date of service, or they may occur sequentially on the same day.

Preparation of chemotherapy agent(s) is included in the service for administration of the agent.

Regional (isolation) chemotherapy perfusion should be reported using the codes for arterial infusion (96420-96425). Placement of the intra-arterial catheter should be reported using the appropriate code from the **Cardiovascular Surgery** section. Placement of arterial and venous cannula(s) for extracorporeal circulation via a membrane oxygenator perfusion pump should be reported using 36823. Code 36823 includes dose calculation and administration of the chemotherapy agent by injection into the perfusate. Do not report 96408-96425 in conjunction with 36823.

Report separate codes for each parenteral method of administration employed when chemotherapy is administered by different techniques. Medications (eg, antibiotics, steroidal agents, antiemetics, narcotics, analgesics, biological agents) administered independently or sequentially as supportive management of chemotherapy administration, should be separately reported using 90780-90788, as appropriate.

❖ **96400** Chemotherapy administration, subcutaneous or intramuscular, with or without local anesthesia

❖ **96405** Chemotherapy administration, intralesional; up to and including 7 lesions

❖ **96406** more than 7 lesions

❖ **96408** Chemotherapy administration, intravenous; push technique

❖ **96410** infusion technique, up to one hour

☆+ **96412** infusion technique, one to 8 hours, each additional hour (List separately in addition to code for primary procedure)

(Use 96412 in conjunction with 96410)

❖ **96414** infusion technique, initiation of prolonged infusion (more than 8 hours), requiring the use of a portable or implantable pump

(For refilling and maintenance of a portable pump or an implantable infusion pump or reservoir for drug delivery, see 96520, 96530)

❖ **96420** Chemotherapy administration, intra-arterial; push technique

❖ **96422** infusion technique, up to one hour

☆+ **96423** infusion technique, one to 8 hours, each additional hour (List separately in addition to code for primary procedure)

(Use 96423 in conjunction with 96422)

(For regional chemotherapy perfusion via membrane oxygenator perfusion pump to an extremity, use 36823)

❖ **96425** infusion technique, initiation of prolonged infusion (more than 8 hours), requiring the use of a portable or implantable pump

(For refilling and maintenance of a portable pump or an implantable infusion pump or reservoir for drug delivery, see 96520, 96530)

❖ **96440** Chemotherapy administration into pleural cavity, requiring and including thoracentesis

❖ **96445** Chemotherapy administration into peritoneal cavity, requiring and including peritoneocentesis

❖ **96450** Chemotherapy administration, into CNS (eg, intrathecal), requiring and including spinal puncture

(For intravesical (bladder) chemotherapy administration, use 51720)

(For insertion of subarachnoid catheter and reservoir for infusion of drug, see 62350, 62351, 62360-62362; for insertion of intraventricular catheter and reservoir, see 61210, 61215)

§ **96520** Refilling and maintenance of portable pump

§ **96530** Refilling and maintenance of implantable pump or reservoir for drug delivery, systemic (eg, intravenous, intra-arterial)
➲ *CPT Changes: An Insider's View* 2003

(For refilling and maintenance of an implantable infusion pump for spinal or brain drug infusion, use 95990)

(For collection of blood specimen from a completely implantable venous access device, use 36540)

❖ **96542** Chemotherapy injection, subarachnoid or intraventricular via subcutaneous reservoir, single or multiple agents

☆ **96545** Provision of chemotherapy agent

(For radioactive isotope therapy, ►use 79005◄)

❖ **96549** Unlisted chemotherapy procedure

Photodynamic Therapy

(To report ocular photodynamic therapy, use 67221)

§ **96567** Photodynamic therapy by external application of light to destroy premalignant and/or malignant lesions of the skin and adjacent mucosa (eg, lip) by activation of photosensitive drug(s), each phototherapy exposure session
➔ *CPT Changes: An Insider's View* 2002

§+ **96570** Photodynamic therapy by endoscopic application of light to ablate abnormal tissue via activation of photosensitive drug(s); first 30 minutes (List separately in addition to code for endoscopy or bronchoscopy procedures of lung and esophagus)
➔ *CPT Changes: An Insider's View* 2000

§+ **96571** each additional 15 minutes (List separately in addition to code for endoscopy or bronchoscopy procedures of lung and esophagus)
➔ *CPT Changes: An Insider's View* 2000

(96570, 96571 are to be used in addition to bronchoscopy, endoscopy codes)

(Use 96570, 96571 in conjunction with 31641, 43228 as appropriate)

Special Dermatological Procedures

Dermatologic services are typically consultative, and any of the five levels of consultation (99241-99263) may be appropriate.

In addition, services and skills outlined under **Evaluation and Management** levels of service appropriate to dermatologic illnesses should be coded similarly.

(For whole body photography, see Category III code 0044T, 0045T)

(For intralesional injections, see 11900, 11901)

(For Tzanck smear, use 87207)

❖ **96900** Actinotherapy (ultraviolet light)

☆ **96902** Microscopic examination of hairs plucked or clipped by the examiner (excluding hair collected by the patient) to determine telogen and anagen counts, or structural hair shaft abnormality

❖ **96910** Photochemotherapy; tar and ultraviolet B (Goeckerman treatment) or petrolatum and ultraviolet B

❖ **96912** psoralens and ultraviolet A (PUVA)

❖ **96913** Photochemotherapy (Goeckerman and/or PUVA) for severe photoresponsive dermatoses requiring at least four to eight hours of care under direct supervision of the physician (includes application of medication and dressings)

§ **96920** Laser treatment for inflammatory skin disease (psoriasis); total area less than 250 sq cm
➔ *CPT Changes: An Insider's View* 2003

§ **96921** 250 sq cm to 500 sq cm
➔ *CPT Changes: An Insider's View* 2003

§ **96922** over 500 sq cm
➔ *CPT Changes: An Insider's View* 2003

§ **96999** Unlisted special dermatological service or procedure

Physical Medicine and Rehabilitation

►Codes 97001-97755 should be used to report each distinct procedure performed. Do not append modifier 51 to 97001-97755.◄

(For muscle testing, range of joint motion, electromyography, see 95831 et seq)

(For biofeedback training by EMG, use 90901)

(For transcutaneous nerve stimulation (TNS), use 64550)

♠ **97001** Physical therapy evaluation

♠ **97002** Physical therapy re-evaluation

♠ **97003** Occupational therapy evaluation

♠ **97004** Occupational therapy re-evaluation

☐ **97005** Athletic training evaluation

☐ **97006** Athletic training re-evaluation

Modalities

Any physical agent applied to produce therapeutic changes to biologic tissue; includes but not limited to thermal, acoustic, light, mechanical, or electric energy.

Supervised

The application of a modality that does not require direct (one-on-one) patient contact by the provider.

♠ **97010** Application of a modality to one or more areas; hot or cold packs

♠ **97012** traction, mechanical

☐ **97014** electrical stimulation (unattended)

(For acupuncture with electrical stimulation, ►see 97813, 97814◄)

♠ **97016** vasopneumatic devices

♠ **97018** paraffin bath

♠ **97020** microwave

♠ **97022** whirlpool

Medicine

♠ **97024** diathermy

♠ **97026** infrared

♠ **97028** ultraviolet

Constant Attendance

The application of a modality that requires direct (one-on-one) patient contact by the provider.

♠ **97032** Application of a modality to one or more areas; electrical stimulation (manual), each 15 minutes

♠ **97033** iontophoresis, each 15 minutes

♠ **97034** contrast baths, each 15 minutes

♠ **97035** ultrasound, each 15 minutes

♠ **97036** Hubbard tank, each 15 minutes

♠ **97039** Unlisted modality (specify type and time if constant attendance)

Therapeutic Procedures

A manner of effecting change through the application of clinical skills and/or services that attempt to improve function.

Physician or therapist required to have direct (one-on-one) patient contact.

♠ **97110** Therapeutic procedure, one or more areas, each 15 minutes; therapeutic exercises to develop strength and endurance, range of motion and flexibility

♠ **97112** neuromuscular reeducation of movement, balance, coordination, kinesthetic sense, posture, and/or proprioception for sitting and/or standing activities

➲ *CPT Changes: An Insider's View* 2002

♠ **97113** aquatic therapy with therapeutic exercises

♠ **97116** gait training (includes stair climbing)

(Use 96000-96003 to report comprehensive gait and motion analysis procedures)

♠ **97124** massage, including effleurage, petrissage and/or tapotement (stroking, compression, percussion)

(For myofascial release, use 97140)

♠ **97139** Unlisted therapeutic procedure (specify)

♠ **97140** Manual therapy techniques (eg, mobilization/manipulation, manual lymphatic drainage, manual traction), one or more regions, each 15 minutes

♠ **97150** Therapeutic procedure(s), group (2 or more individuals)

(Report 97150 for each member of group)

(Group therapy procedures involve constant attendance of the physician or therapist, but by definition do not require one-on-one patient contact by the physician or therapist)

(For manipulation under general anesthesia, see appropriate anatomic section in **Musculoskeletal System**)

(For osteopathic manipulative treatment (OMT), see 98925-98929)

♠ **97504** Orthotic(s) fitting and training, upper extremity(ies), lower extremity(ies), and/or trunk, each 15 minutes

➲ *CPT Changes: An Insider's View* 2002

(Code 97504 should not be reported with 97116)

(For casting and strapping of fracture, injury or dislocation, see 29000, 29590)

♠ **97520** Prosthetic training, upper and/or lower extremities, each 15 minutes

♠ **97530** Therapeutic activities, direct (one-on-one) patient contact by the provider (use of dynamic activities to improve functional performance), each 15 minutes

♠ **97532** Development of cognitive skills to improve attention, memory, problem solving, (includes compensatory training), direct (one-on-one) patient contact by the provider, each 15 minutes

➲ *CPT Changes: An Insider's View* 2001

♠ **97533** Sensory integrative techniques to enhance sensory processing and promote adaptive responses to environmental demands, direct (one-on-one) patient contact by the provider, each 15 minutes

➲ *CPT Changes: An Insider's View* 2001

♠ **97535** Self-care/home management training (eg, activities of daily living (ADL) and compensatory training, meal preparation, safety procedures, and instructions in use of assistive technology devices/adaptive equipment) direct one-on-one contact by provider, each 15 minutes

➲ *CPT Changes: An Insider's View* 2002

♠ **97537** Community/work reintegration training (eg, shopping, transportation, money management, avocational activities and/or work environment/modification analysis, work task analysis, use of assistive technology device/adaptive equipment), direct one-on-one contact by provider, each 15 minutes

➲ *CPT Changes: An Insider's View* 2004

(For wheelchair management/propulsion training, use 97542)

♠ **97542** Wheelchair management/propulsion training, each 15 minutes

♠ **97545** Work hardening/conditioning; initial 2 hours

♠+ **97546** each additional hour (List separately in addition to code for primary procedure)

(Use 97546 in conjunction with 97545)

Active Wound Care Management

Active wound care procedures are performed to ►remove devitalized and/or necrotic tissue and◄ promote healing. ►Provider is required to have direct (one-on-one) patient contact.◄

(Do not report ►97597◄-97602 in conjunction with 11040-11044)

♠● **97597** Removal of devitalized tissue from wound(s), selective debridement, without anesthesia (eg, high pressure waterjet with/without suction, sharp selective debridement with scissors, scalpel and forceps), with or without topical application(s), wound assessment, and instruction(s) for ongoing care, may include use of a whirlpool, per session; total wound(s) surface area less than or equal to 20 square centimeters

➲ *CPT Changes: An Insider's View* 2005

♠● **97598** total wound(s) surface area greater than 20 square centimeters

➲ *CPT Changes: An Insider's View* 2005

►(97601 has been deleted. To report, use 97597, 97598)◄

♠ **97602** Removal of devitalized tissue from wound(s), non-selective debridement, without anesthesia (eg, wet-to-moist dressings, enzymatic, abrasion), including topical application(s), wound assessment, and instruction(s) for ongoing care, per session

➲ *CPT Assistant* Apr 03:15; *CPT Changes: An Insider's View* 2001

♠● **97605** Negative pressure wound therapy (eg, vacuum assisted drainage collection), including topical application(s), wound assessment, and instruction(s) for ongoing care, per session; total wound(s) surface area less than or equal to 50 square centimeters

♠● **97606** total wound(s) surface area greater than 50 square centimeters

Tests and Measurements

Requires direct one-on-one patient contact.

(For muscle testing, manual or electrical, joint range of motion, electromyography or nerve velocity determination, see 95831-95904)

♠ **97703** Checkout for orthotic/prosthetic use, established patient, each 15 minutes

♠ **97750** Physical performance test or measurement (eg, musculoskeletal, functional capacity), with written report, each 15 minutes

♠ **97755** Assistive technology assessment (eg, to restore, augment or compensate for existing function, optimize functional tasks and/or maximize environmental accessibility), direct one-on-one contact by provider, with written report, each 15 minutes

➲ *CPT Changes: An Insider's View* 2004

(To report augmentative and alternative communication devices, use 92605 or 92607)

Other Procedures

(For extracorporeal shock wave musculoskeletal therapy, use Category III code 0019T)

►(97780 has been deleted. To report, see 97810, 97811)◄

►(97781 has been deleted. To report, see 97813, 97814)◄

♠ **97799** Unlisted physical medicine/rehabilitation service or procedure

➲ *CPT Assistant* Apr 03:13

Medical Nutrition Therapy

♠ **97802** Medical nutrition therapy; initial assessment and intervention, individual, face-to-face with the patient, each 15 minutes

➲ *CPT Assistant* Apr 03:10; *CPT Changes: An Insider's View* 2001

♠ **97803** re-assessment and intervention, individual, face-to-face with the patient, each 15 minutes

➲ *CPT Assistant* Apr 03:10; *CPT Changes: An Insider's View* 2001

♠ **97804** group (2 or more individual(s)), each 30 minutes

➲ *CPT Assistant* Apr 03:10; *CPT Changes: An Insider's View* 2001

(For medical nutrition therapy assessment and/or intervention performed by a physician, see **Evaluation and Management** or **Preventive Medicine** service codes)

►Acupuncture◄

►Acupuncture is reported based on 15 minute increments of personal (face-to-face) contact with the patient, not the duration of acupuncture needle(s) placement.◄

►If no electrical stimulation is used during a 15 minute increment, use 97810, 97811. If electrical stimulation of any needle is used during a 15 minute increment, use 97813, 97814.◄

✣● **97810** Acupuncture, one or more needles; without electrical stimulation, initial 15 minutes of personal one-on-one contact with the patient

➲ *CPT Changes: An Insider's View* 2005

✣+● **97811** each additional 15 minutes of personal one-on-one contact with the patient, with re-insertion of needle(s) (List separately in addition to code for primary procedure)

➲ *CPT Changes: An Insider's View* 2005

►(Use 97811 in conjunction with 97810)◄

►(Do not report 97810, 97811 in conjunction with 97813 or 97814)◄

Medicine

►(Evaluation and Management services may be reported separately, using modifier 25, if the patient's condition requires a significant separately identifiable E/M service, above and beyond the usual preservice and postservice work associated with the acupuncture services. The time of the E/M service is not included in the time of the acupuncture service.)◄

✣● **97813** Acupuncture, one or more needles; with electrical stimulation, initial 15 minutes of personal one-on-one contact with the patient

➔ *CPT Changes: An Insider's View* 2005

✣+● **97814** each additional 15 minutes of personal one-on-one contact with the patient, with re-insertion of needle(s) (List separately in addition to code for primary procedure)

➔ *CPT Changes: An Insider's View* 2005

►(Use 97814 in conjunction with 97813)◄

► (Do not report 97813, 97814 in conjunction with 97810 or 97811)◄

►(Evaluation and Management services may be reported separately, using modifier 25, if the patient's condition requires a significant separately identifiable E/M service, above and beyond the usual preservice and postservice work associated with the acupuncture services. The time of the E/M service is not included in the time of the acupuncture service.)◄

Osteopathic Manipulative Treatment

Osteopathic manipulative treatment is a form of manual treatment applied by a physician to eliminate or alleviate somatic dysfunction and related disorders. This treatment may be accomplished by a variety of techniques.

Evaluation and Management services may be reported separately if, using modifier 25, the patient's condition requires a significant separately identifiable E/M service, above and beyond the usual preservice and postservice work associated with the procedure. The E/M service may be caused or prompted by the same symptoms or condition for which the OMT service was provided. As such, different diagnoses are not required for the reporting of the OMT and E/M service on the same date.

Body regions referred to are: head region; cervical region; thoracic region; lumbar region; sacral region; pelvic region; lower extremities; upper extremities; rib cage region; abdomen and viscera region.

❖ **98925** Osteopathic manipulative treatment (OMT); one to two body regions involved

❖ **98926** three to four body regions involved

❖ **98927** five to six body regions involved

❖ **98928** seven to eight body regions involved

❖ **98929** nine to ten body regions involved

Chiropractic Manipulative Treatment

Chiropractic manipulative treatment (CMT) is a form of manual treatment to influence joint and neurophysiological function. This treatment may be accomplished using a variety of techniques.

The chiropractic manipulative treatment codes include a pre-manipulation patient assessment. Additional Evaluation and Management services may be reported separately using modifier 25, if the patient's condition requires a significant separately identifiable E/M service, above and beyond the usual preservice and postservice work associated with the procedure. The E/M service may be caused or prompted by the same symptoms or condition for which the CMT service was provided. As such, different diagnoses are not required for the reporting of the CMT and E/M service on the same date.

For purposes of CMT, the five spinal regions referred to are: cervical region (includes atlanto-occipital joint); thoracic region (includes costovertebral and costotransverse joints); lumbar region; sacral region; and pelvic (sacro-iliac joint) region. The five extraspinal regions referred to are: head (including temporomandibular joint, excluding atlanto-occipital) region; lower extremities; upper extremities; rib cage (excluding costotransverse and costovertebral joints) and abdomen.

❖ **98940** Chiropractic manipulative treatment (CMT); spinal, one to two regions

❖ **98941** spinal, three to four regions

❖ **98942** spinal, five regions

☐ **98943** extraspinal, one or more regions

Special Services, Procedures and Reports

The procedures with code numbers 99000 through 99091 provide the reporting physician or other qualified healthcare professional with the means of identifying the completion of special reports and services that are an adjunct to the basic services rendered. The specific number assigned indicates the special circumstances under which a basic procedure is performed.

Code 99091 should be reported no more than once in a 30-day period to include the physician or health care provider time involved with data accession, review and interpretation, modification of care plan as necessary (including communication to patient and/or caregiver), and associated documentation.

If the services described by 99091 are provided on the same day the patient presents for an E/M service, these services should be considered part of the E/M service and not separately reported.

Do not report 99091 if it occurs within 30 days of care plan oversight services 99374-99380. Do not report 99091 if other more specific CPT codes exist (eg, 93014, 93227, 93233, 93272 for cardiographic services; 95250 for continuous glucose monitoring). Do not report 99091 for transfer and interpretation of data from hospital or clinical laboratory computers.

Miscellaneous Services

99000 Handling and/or conveyance of specimen for transfer from the physician's office to a laboratory

99001 Handling and/or conveyance of specimen for transfer from the patient in other than a physician's office to a laboratory (distance may be indicated)

99002 Handling, conveyance, and/or any other service in connection with the implementation of an order involving devices (eg, designing, fitting, packaging, handling, delivery or mailing) when devices such as orthotics, protectives, prosthetics are fabricated by an outside laboratory or shop but which items have been designed, and are to be fitted and adjusted by the attending physician

(For routine collection of venous blood, use 36415)

99024 Postoperative follow-up visit, normally included in the surgical package, to indicate that an evaluation and management service was performed during a postoperative period for a reason(s) related to the original procedure

(As a component of a surgical "package," see **Surgery Guidelines**)

(99025 has been deleted)

□ **99026** Hospital mandated on call service; in-hospital, each hour

□ **99027** out-of-hospital, each hour

(For physician standby services requiring prolonged physician attendance, use 99360, as appropriate. Time spent performing separately reportable procedure(s) or service(s) should not be included in the time reported as mandated on call service)

99050 Services requested after posted office hours in addition to basic service

99052 Services requested between 10:00 PM and 8:00 AM in addition to basic service

99054 Services requested on Sundays and holidays in addition to basic service

99056 Services provided at request of patient in a location other than physician's office which are normally provided in the office

99058 Office services provided on an emergency basis

99070 Supplies and materials (except spectacles), provided by the physician over and above those usually included with the office visit or other services rendered (list drugs, trays, supplies, or materials provided)

(For spectacles, see 92390-92395)

99071 Educational supplies, such as books, tapes, and pamphlets, provided by the physician for the patient's education at cost to physician

□ **99075** Medical testimony

☆ **99078** Physician educational services rendered to patients in a group setting (eg, prenatal, obesity, or diabetic instructions)

99080 Special reports such as insurance forms, more than the information conveyed in the usual medical communications or standard reporting form

(Do not report 99080 in conjunction with 99455, 99456 for the completion of Workmen's Compensation forms)

99082 Unusual travel (eg, transportation and escort of patient)

99090 Analysis of clinical data stored in computers (eg, ECGs, blood pressures, hematologic data)

(For physician/health care professional collection and interpretation of physiologic data stored/transmitted by patient/caregiver, see 99091)

(Do not report 99090 if other more specific CPT codes exist, eg, 93014, 93227, 93233, 93272 for cardiographic services; 95250 for continuous glucose monitoring, 97750 for musculoskeletal function testing)

□ **99091** Collection and interpretation of physiologic data (eg, ECG, blood pressure, glucose monitoring) digitally stored and/or transmitted by the patient and/or caregiver to the physician or other qualified health care professional, requiring a minimum of 30 minutes of time

Qualifying Circumstances for Anesthesia

(For explanation of these services, see **Anesthesia Guidelines**)

+ **99100** Anesthesia for patient of extreme age, under 1 year and over 70 (List separately in addition to code for primary anesthesia procedure)

(For procedure performed on infants less than 1 year of age at time of surgery, see 00326, 00834, 00836)

+ **99116** Anesthesia complicated by utilization of total body hypothermia (List separately in addition to code for primary anesthesia procedure)

+ **99135** Anesthesia complicated by utilization of controlled hypotension (List separately in addition to code for primary anesthesia procedure)

✣✚ **99140** Anesthesia complicated by emergency conditions (specify) (List separately in addition to code for primary anesthesia procedure)

(An emergency is defined as existing when delay in treatment of the patient would lead to a significant increase in the threat to life or body part.)

Sedation With or Without Analgesia (Conscious Sedation)

Sedation with or without analgesia (conscious sedation) is used to achieve a medically controlled state of depressed consciousness while maintaining the patient's airway, protective reflexes and ability to respond to stimulation or verbal commands. Conscious sedation includes performance and documentation of pre- and post-sedation evaluations of the patient, administration of the sedation and/or analgesic agent(s), and monitoring of cardiorespiratory function (ie, pulse oximetry, cardiorespiratory monitor, and blood pressure). The use of these codes requires the presence of an independent trained observer to assist the physician in monitoring the patient's level of consciousness and physiological status.

(If the sedation with or without analgesia (conscious sedation) is administered in support of a procedure provided by another physician, see **Anesthesia** section)

☆⊘ **99141** Sedation with or without analgesia (conscious sedation); intravenous, intramuscular or inhalation

(94760-94762 may not be reported in addition to 99141)

☆⊘ **99142** oral, rectal and/or intranasal

(94760-94762 may not be reported in addition to 99142)

Other Services and Procedures

§ **99170** Anogenital examination with colposcopic magnification in childhood for suspected trauma

(For conscious sedation, use 99141, 99142)

□ **99172** Visual function screening, automated or semi-automated bilateral quantitative determination of visual acuity, ocular alignment, color vision by pseudoisochromatic plates, and field of vision (may include all or some screening of the determination(s) for contrast sensitivity, vision under glare)

(This service must employ graduated visual acuity stimuli that allow a quantitative determination of visual acuity (eg, Snellen chart). This service may not be used in addition to a general ophthalmological service or an E/M service)

(Do not report 99172 in conjunction with 99173)

□ **99173** Screening test of visual acuity, quantitative, bilateral

(The screening test used must employ graduated visual acuity stimuli that allow a quantitative estimate of visual acuity (eg, Snellen chart). Other identifiable services unrelated to this screening test provided at the same time may be reported separately (eg, preventive medicine services). When acuity is measured as part of a general ophthalmological service or of an E/M service of the eye, it is a diagnostic examination and not a screening test.)

(Do not report 99173 in conjunction with 99172)

☆ **99175** Ipecac or similar administration for individual emesis and continued observation until stomach adequately emptied of poison

(For diagnostic intubation, see 82926-82928, 89130-89141)

(For gastric lavage for diagnostic purposes, see 91055)

✣ **99183** Physician attendance and supervision of hyperbaric oxygen therapy, per session

(Evaluation and Management services and/or procedures (eg, wound debridement) provided in a hyperbaric oxygen treatment facility in conjunction with a hyperbaric oxygen therapy session should be reported separately)

☆ **99185** Hypothermia; regional

☆ **99186** total body

✿ **99190** Assembly and operation of pump with oxygenator or heat exchanger (with or without ECG and/or pressure monitoring); each hour

✿ **99191** 3/4 hour

✿ **99192** 1/2 hour

♣ **99195** Phlebotomy, therapeutic (separate procedure)

✣ **99199** Unlisted special service, procedure or report

Home Health Procedures/Services

These codes are used by non-physician health care professionals. Physicians should utilize the home visit codes 99341-99350, and utilize CPT codes other than 99500-99600 for any additional procedure/service provided to a patient living in a residence.

The following codes are used to report services provided in a patient's residence (including assisted living apartments, group homes, non-traditional private homes, custodial care facilities, or schools).

Health care professionals who are authorized to use Evaluation and Management Home Visit codes (99341-99350) may report 99500-99600 in addition to 99341-99350 if both services are performed. Evaluation and Management services may be reported separately, using modifier 25, if the patient's condition requires a significant separately identifiable E/M service, above and beyond the home health service(s)/procedure(s) codes 99500-99600.

☐ **99500** Home visit for prenatal monitoring and assessment to include fetal heart rate, non-stress test, uterine monitoring, and gestational diabetes monitoring

☐ **99501** Home visit for postnatal assessment and follow-up care

☐ **99502** Home visit for newborn care and assessment

☐ **99503** Home visit for respiratory therapy care (eg, bronchodilator, oxygen therapy, respiratory assessment, apnea evaluation)

☐ **99504** Home visit for mechanical ventilation care

☐ **99505** Home visit for stoma care and maintenance including colostomy and cystostomy

☐ **99506** Home visit for intramuscular injections

☐ **99507** Home visit for care and maintenance of catheter(s) (eg, urinary, drainage, and enteral)

(99508 has been deleted. To report see 95806-95811)

☐ **99509** Home visit for assistance with activities of daily living and personal care

(To report self-care/home management training, see 97535)

(To report home medical nutrition assessment and intervention services, see 97802-97804)

(To report home speech therapy services, see 92507-92508)

☐ **99510** Home visit for individual, family, or marriage counseling

☐ **99511** Home visit for fecal impaction management and enema administration

☐ **99512** Home visit for hemodialysis

(For home infusion of peritoneal dialysis, use 99601, 99602)

(99551-99569 have been deleted. To report, see 99601-99602)

☐ **99600** Unlisted home visit service or procedure

Home Infusion Procedures/Services

☐ **99601** Home infusion/specialty drug administration, per visit (up to 2 hours);

☐✚ **99602** each additional hour (List separately in addition to code for primary procedure)

(Use 99602 in conjunction with 99601)

Notes

Category II Codes

The following section of *Current Procedural Terminology (CPT)* contains a set of supplemental tracking codes that can be used for performance measurement. ►It is anticipated that the use of Category II◄ codes for performance measurement will decrease the need for record abstraction and chart review, and thereby minimize administrative burden on physicians, ►other health care professionals, hospitals, and entities seeking to measure the quality of patient care. These codes are intended to facilitate data collection about the quality of care rendered by coding certain services and test results that support nationally established performance measures and that have an evidence base as contributing to quality patient care.◄

The use of these codes is optional. The codes are not required for correct coding and may not be used as a substitute for Category I codes.

►These codes describe clinical components that may be typically included in evaluation and management services or other clinical services and, therefore, do not have a relative value associated with them. Category II codes may also describe results from laboratory tests and procedures, select processes intended to address patient safety practices, or services reflecting compliance with state or federal law.◄

►Category II codes described in this section make use of an alphabetical character as the 5th character in the string (ie, 4 digits followed by the letter **F**). These digits are not intended to reflect the placement of the code in the regular (Category I) part of *CPT*. To promote understanding of these codes and their associated measures, users are referred to Appendix H, which contains information about the measures and their origins. CPT Category II codes are arranged according to the following categories derived from standard clinical documentation format:◄

►Composite Measures .... To begin with 0001F (no measures at this time)◄

►Patient Management .... 0500F-0503F◄

►Patient History .... 1000F-1002F◄

►Physical Examination .... 2000F◄

►Diagnostic/Screening Processes or Results 3000F (no codes at this time)◄

►Therapeutic, Preventive or Other Interventions .... 4000F-4011F◄

►Follow-up or Other Outcomes To begin with 5000F (no codes at this time)◄

►Patient Safety To begin with 6000F (no codes at this time)◄

►Cross-references to the measures associated with each Category II code and their origins are included for reference in Appendix H. Users should review the complete measure(s) associated with each code prior to implementing its use.◄

►Category II codes are reviewed by the Performance Measures Advisory Group (PMAG), an advisory body to the CPT Editorial Panel and the CPT/HCPAC Advisory Committee. The PMAG is comprised of performance measurement experts representing the Agency for Healthcare Research and Quality (AHRQ), the American Medical Association (AMA), the Centers for Medicare and Medicaid Services (CMS), the Joint Commission on Accreditation of Healthcare Organizations (JCAHO), the National Committee for Quality Assurance (NCQA), and the Physician Consortium for Performance Improvement. The PMAG may seek additional expertise and/or input from other national health care organizations, as necessary, for the development of Category II codes. These may include national medical specialty societies, other national health care professional associations, accrediting bodies, and federal regulatory agencies.◄

►Category II codes are published biannually: January 1 and July 1. The most current listing, along with guidelines and forms for submitting code change proposals for Category II codes, may be accessed on the Internet at http://www.ama-assn.org/go/cpt.◄

►(0001F has been deleted. To report, use 2000F)◄

►(0002F has been deleted. To report, use 1000F)◄

►(0003F has been deleted. To report, use 1001F)◄

►(0004F has been deleted. To report, use 4000F)◄

►(0005F has been deleted. To report, use 4001F)◄

►(0006F has been deleted. To report, use 4002F)◄

►(0007F has been deleted. To report, use 4006F)◄

►(0008F has been deleted. To report, use 4009F)◄

►(0009F has been deleted. To report, use 1002F)◄

►(0010F has been deleted)◄

►(0011F has been deleted. To report, use 4011F)◄

►Composite Measures◄

►Composite measures codes combine several measures grouped within a single code descriptor to facilitate reporting for a clinical condition when all components are met. If only some of the components are met, or if services are provided in addition to those included in the composite code, they may be reported individually using the corresponding CPT Category II codes for those services.◄

►No measures at this time.◄

►Patient Management◄

►Patient management codes describe utilization measures or measures of patient care provided for specific clinical purposes (eg, prenatal care, pre- and post-surgical care).◄

□● **0500F** Initial prenatal care visit (report at first prenatal encounter with health care professional providing obstetrical care. Report also date of visit and, in a separate field, the date of the last menstrual period - LMP)[2]

□● **0501F** Prenatal flow sheet documented in medical record by first prenatal visit (documentation includes at minimum blood pressure, weight, urine protein, uterine size, fetal heart tones, and estimated date of delivery). Report also: date of visit and, in a separate field, the date of the last menstrual period - LMP (Note: If reporting 0501F Prenatal flow sheet, it is not necessary to report 0500F Initial prenatal care visit)[1]

□● **0502F** Subsequent prenatal care visit

[Excludes: patients who are seen for a condition unrelated to pregnancy or prenatal care (eg, an upper respiratory infection; patients seen for consultation only, not for continuing care)]

□● **0503F** Postpartum care visit[2]

►Patient History◄

►Patient history codes describe measures for select aspects of patient history or review of systems.◄

□● **1000F** Tobacco use, smoking, assessed[1]

□● **1001F** Tobacco use, non-smoking, assessed[1]

□● **1002F** Anginal symptoms and level of activity, assessed[1]

►Physical Examination◄

►Physical examination codes describe aspects of physical examination or clinical assessment.◄

□● **2000F** Blood pressure, measured[1]

►Diagnostic/Screening Processes or Results◄

►Diagnostic/screening processes or results codes describe results of tests ordered (clinical laboratory tests, radiological or other procedural examinations).◄

►No codes at this timc.◄

►Therapeutic, Preventive or Other Interventions◄

►Therapeutic, preventive or other interventions codes describe pharmacologic, procedural, or behavioral therapies, including preventive services such as patient education and counseling.◄

□● **4000F** Tobacco use cessation intervention, counseling[1]

□● **4001F** Tobacco use cessation intervention, pharmacologic therapy[1]

□● **4002F** Statin therapy, prescribed[1]

□● **4006F** Beta-blocker therapy, prescribed[1]

□● **4009F** Angiotensin converting enzyme (ACE) inhibitor therapy, prescribed[1]

□● **4011F** Oral antiplatelet therapy, prescribed (eg, aspirin, clopidogrel/Plavix, or combination of aspirin and dipyridamole/Aggrenox)[1]

►Follow-up or Other Outcomes◄

►Follow-up or other outcomes codes describe review and communication of test results to patients, patient satisfaction or experience with care, patient functional status, and patient morbidity and mortality.◄

►No codes at this time.◄

►Patient Safety◄

►Patient safety codes that describe patient safety practices.◄

►No codes at this time.◄

Category II Codes

►Footnotes◄

►[1] Physician Consortium for Perfomance Improvement, www.ama-assn.org/go/quality◄

►[2] National Committee on Quality Assurance (NCQA), Health Employer Data Information Set (HEDIS®), www.ncqa.org◄

Category III Codes

The following section contains a set of temporary codes for emerging technology, services, and procedures. Category III codes will allow data collection for these services/procedures. Use of unlisted codes does not offer the opportunity for the collection of specific data. If a Category III code is available, this code must be reported instead of a Category I unlisted code. This is an activity that is critically important in the evaluation of health care delivery and the formation of public and private policy. The use of the codes in this section will allow physicians and other qualified health care professionals, insurers, health services researchers, and health policy experts to identify emerging technology, services, and procedures for clinical efficacy, utilization and outcomes.

The inclusion of a service or procedure in this section neither implies nor endorses clinical efficacy, safety or the applicability to clinical practice. The codes in this section do not conform to the usual requirements for CPT Category I codes established by the Editorial Panel. For Category I codes, the Panel requires that the service/procedure be performed by many health care professionals in clinical practice in multiple locations and that FDA approval, as appropriate, has already been received. The nature of emerging technology, services, and procedures is such that these requirements may not be met. For these reasons, temporary codes for emerging technology, services, and procedures have been placed in a separate section of the *CPT* book and the codes are differentiated from Category I CPT codes by the use of alphanumeric characters.

Services/procedures described in this section make use of alphanumeric characters. These codes have an alpha character as the 5th character in the string, preceded by four digits. The digits are not intended to reflect the placement of the code in the Category I section of CPT nomenclature. Codes in this section may or may not eventually receive a Category I CPT code. In either case, a given Category III code will be archived after five years of its inception unless it is demonstrated that a temporary code is still needed. New codes in this section are released semi-annually via the AMA/CPT internet site, to expedite dissemination for reporting. The full set of temporary codes for emerging technology, services, and procedures are published annually in the *CPT* book. Go to www.ama-assn.org/go/cpt for the most current listing.

►(0001T has been deleted. To report, use 34803)◄

(0002T has been deleted. To report, use 34805)

❖ **0003T** Cervicography

➲ *CPT Assistant* Jan 02:6, Jan 03:4; *CPT Changes: An Insider's View* 2002

►(0005T-0007T have been deleted. To report, see 0075T, 0076T)◄

§ **0008T** Upper gastrointestinal endoscopy including esophagus, stomach, and either the duodenum and/or jejunum as appropriate, with suturing of the esophagogastric junction

➲ *CPT Assistant* Jan 02:6, Jan 03:4; *CPT Changes: An Insider's View* 2002

►(0009T has been deleted. To report, use 58356)◄

♠ **0010T** Tuberculosis test, cell mediated immunity measurement of gamma interferon antigen response

➲ *CPT Assistant* Jan 02:6; *CPT Changes: An Insider's View* 2002

►(0012T has been deleted. To report, use 29866)◄

►(0013T has been deleted. To report, see 29867, 27415)◄

►(0014T has been deleted. To report, use 29868)◄

♦§ **0016T** Destruction of localized lesion of choroid (eg, choroidal neovascularization), transpupillary thermotherapy

➲ *CPT Changes: An Insider's View* 2002

♦□ **0017T** Destruction of macular drusen, photocoagulation

➲ *CPT Changes: An Insider's View* 2002

❖ **0018T** Delivery of high power, focal magnetic pulses for direct stimulation to cortical neurons

➲ *CPT Assistant* Jan 03:4; *CPT Changes: An Insider's View* 2002

□ **0019T** Extracorporeal shock wave therapy; involving musculoskeletal system

➲ *CPT Changes: An Insider's View* 2002

✣ **0020T** involving plantar fascia

➲ *CPT Changes: An Insider's View* 2002

✿ **0021T** Insertion of transcervical or transvaginal fetal oximetry sensor

➲ *CPT Changes: An Insider's View* 2002

♠ **0023T** Infectious agent drug susceptibility phenotype prediction using genotypic comparison to known genotypic/phenotypic database, HIV 1

➲ *CPT Changes: An Insider's View* 2002

✿ **0024T** Non-surgical septal reduction therapy (eg, alcohol ablation), for hypertrophic obstructive cardiomyopathy, with coronary arteriograms, with or without temporary pacemaker

➲ *CPT Assistant* Jan 03:4; *CPT Changes: An Insider's View* 2002

(0025T has been deleted. To report, use 76514)

♠ **0026T** Lipoprotein, direct measurement, intermediate density lipoproteins (IDL) (remnant lipoproteins)

➲ *CPT Changes: An Insider's View* 2002

§ **0027T** Endoscopic lysis of epidural adhesions with direct visualization using mechanical means (eg, spinal endoscopic catheter system) or solution injection (eg, normal saline) including radiologic localization and epidurography
➲ *CPT Assistant* Jan 03:4; *CPT Changes: An Insider's View* 2003

(For diagnostic epidurography, use 64999)

☆ **0028T** Dual energy x-ray absorptiometry (DEXA) body composition study, one or more sites
➲ *CPT Changes: An Insider's View* 2003

♠ **0029T** Treatment(s) for incontinence, pulsed magnetic neuromodulation, per day
➲ *CPT Changes: An Insider's View* 2003

♠ **0030T** Antiprothrombin (phospholipid cofactor) antibody, each Ig class
➲ *CPT Changes: An Insider's View* 2003

☆ **0031T** Speculoscopy;
➲ *CPT Changes: An Insider's View* 2003

☆ **0032T** with directed sampling
➲ *CPT Changes: An Insider's View* 2003

✿ **0033T** Endovascular repair of descending thoracic aortic aneurysm, pseudoaneurysm or dissection; involving coverage of left subclavian artery origin, initial endoprosthesis
➲ *CPT Changes: An Insider's View* 2003

(For radiological supervision and interpretation, use 0038T)

✿ **0034T** not involving coverage of left subclavian artery origin, initial endoprosthesis
➲ *CPT Changes: An Insider's View* 2003

(For radiological supervision and interpretation, use 0039T)

✿ **0035T** Placement of proximal or distal extension prosthesis for endovascular repair of descending thoracic aortic aneurysm, pseudoaneurysm or dissection; initial extension
➲ *CPT Changes: An Insider's View* 2003

(For radiological supervision and interpretation, use 0040T)

(Do not report 0034T and 0035T when placement of extension converts repair to cover left subclavian origin, use only 0033T)

✿+ **0036T** each additional extension (List separately in addition to code for primary procedure)
➲ *CPT Changes: An Insider's View* 2003

(Use 0036T in conjunction with 0035T)

(For radiological supervision and interpretation, use 0040T)

♦✿ **0037T** Open subclavian to carotid artery transposition performed in conjunction with endovascular thoracic aneurysm repair, by neck incision, unilateral
➲ *CPT Changes: An Insider's View* 2003

(For bilateral procedure, use modifier 50)

(Do not report 0037T in addition to 35694)

✿ **0038T** Endovascular repair of descending thoracic aortic aneurysm, pseudoaneurysm or dissection involving coverage of left subclavian artery origin, initial endoprosthesis, radiological supervision and interpretation
➲ *CPT Changes: An Insider's View* 2003

(For implantation of endovascular graft, use 0033T)

✿ **0039T** Endovascular repair of descending thoracic aortic aneurysm, pseudoaneurysm or dissection not involving coverage of left subclavian artery origin, initial endoprosthesis, radiological supervision and interpretation
➲ *CPT Changes: An Insider's View* 2003

(For implantation of endovascular graft, use 0034T)

✿ **0040T** Placement of proximal or distal extension prosthesis for endovascular repair of descending thoracic aortic aneurysm, pseudoaneurysm or dissection, each extension, radiological supervision and interpretation
➲ *CPT Changes: An Insider's View* 2003

(For implantation of endovascular graft extensions, see 0035T, 0036T)

♠ **0041T** Urinalysis infectious agent detection, semi-quantitative analysis of volatile compounds
➲ *CPT Changes: An Insider's View* 2003

☆ **0042T** Cerebral perfusion analysis using computed tomography with contrast administration, including post-processing of parametric maps with determination of cerebral blood flow, cerebral blood volume, and mean transit time
➲ *CPT Changes: An Insider's View* 2003

♠ **0043T** Carbon monoxide, expired gas analysis (eg, $ETCO_c$/hemolysis breath test)
➲ *CPT Changes: An Insider's View* 2003

☆ **0044T** Whole body integumentary photography, at request of a physician, for monitoring of high-risk patients; with dysplastic nevus syndrome or familial melanoma
➲ *CPT Changes: An Insider's View* 2003, 2004

☆ **0045T** with history of dysplastic nevi or personal history of melanoma
➲ *CPT Changes: An Insider's View* 2004

§ **0046T** Catheter lavage of a mammary duct(s) for collection of cytology specimen(s), in high risk individuals (GAIL risk scoring or prior personal history of breast cancer), each breast; single duct
➲ *CPT Changes: An Insider's View* 2004

§ **0047T** each additional duct
➲ *CPT Changes: An Insider's View* 2004

Category III Codes

✿ **0048T** Implantation of a ventricular assist device, extracorporeal, percutaneous transseptal access, single or dual cannulation
➲ *CPT Changes: An Insider's View* 2004

✿+ **0049T** Prolonged extracorporeal percutaneous transseptal ventricular assist device, greater than 24 hours, each subsequent 24 hour period (List separately in addition to code for primary procedure)
➲ *CPT Changes: An Insider's View* 2004

(Use 0049T in conjunction with 0048T)

✿ **0050T** Removal of a ventricular assist device, extracorporeal, percutaneous transseptal access, single or dual cannulation
➲ *CPT Changes: An Insider's View* 2004

✿ **0051T** Implantation of a total replacement heart system (artificial heart) with recipient cardiectomy
➲ *CPT Changes: An Insider's View* 2004

(For implantation of heart assist or ventricular assist device, see 33975, 33976)

✿ **0052T** Replacement or repair of thoracic unit of a total replacement heart system (artificial heart)
➲ *CPT Changes: An Insider's View* 2004

(For replacement or repair of other implantable components in a total replacement heart system (artificial heart), use 0053T)

✿ **0053T** Replacement or repair of implantable component or components of total replacement heart system (artificial heart), excluding thoracic unit
➲ *CPT Changes: An Insider's View* 2004

(For replacement or repair of a thoracic unit of a total replacement heart system (artificial heart), use 0052T)

⚘+ **0054T** Computer-assisted musculoskeletal surgical navigational orthopedic procedure, with image-guidance based on fluoroscopic images (List separately in addition to code for primary procedure)
➲ *CPT Changes: An Insider's View* 2004

⚘+▲ **0055T** Computer-assisted musculoskeletal surgical navigational orthopedic procedure, with image-guidance based on CT/MRI images (List separately in addition to code for primary procedure)
➲ *CPT Changes: An Insider's View* 2004

►(When CT and MRI are both performed, report 0055T only once)◄

⚘+ **0056T** Computer assisted musculoskeletal surgical navigational orthopedic procedure, image-less (List separately in addition to code for primary procedure)
➲ *CPT Changes: An Insider's View* 2004

►(0057T has been deleted. To report, use 43257)◄

♣ **0058T** Cryopreservation; reproductive tissue, ovarian
➲ *CPT Changes: An Insider's View* 2004

♣ **0059T** oocyte(s)
➲ *CPT Changes: An Insider's View* 2004

(For cryopreservation of embryo(s), sperm and testicular reproductive tissue, see 89258, 89259, 89335)

⚘ **0060T** Electrical impedance scan of the breast, bilateral (risk assessment device for breast cancer)
➲ *CPT Changes: An Insider's View* 2004

⚘ **0061T** Destruction/reduction of malignant breast tumor including breast carcinoma cells in the margins, microwave phased array thermotherapy, disposable catheter with combined temperature monitoring probe and microwave sensor, externally applied microwave energy, including interstitial placement of sensor
➲ *CPT Changes: An Insider's View* 2004

(For imaging guidance performed in conjunction with 0061T, see 76942, 76986)

§● **0062T** Percutaneous intradiscal annuloplasty, any method, unilateral or bilateral including fluoroscopic guidance; single level

§+● **0063T** one or more additional levels (List separately in addition to 0062T for primary procedure)

►(For CT or MRI guidance and localization for needle placement and annuloplasty in conjunction with 0062T, 0063T, see 76360, 76393)◄

♠● **0064T** Spectroscopy, expired gas analysis (eg, nitric oxide/carbon dioxide test)

♠● **0065T** Ocular photoscreening, with interpretation and report, bilateral

►(Do not report 0065T in conjunction with 99172 or 99173)◄

□● **0066T** Computed tomographic (CT) colonography (ie, virtual colonoscopy); screening

❖● **0067T** diagnostic

►(Do not report 0066T or 0067T in conjunction with 72192-72194, 74150-74170, 76375)◄

⚘+● **0068T** Acoustic heart sound recording and computer analysis; with interpretation and report (List separately in addition to codes for electrocardiography)

►(Use 0068T in conjunction with 93000)◄

☆+● **0069T** acoustic heart sound recording and computer analysis only (List separately in addition to codes for electrocardiography)

►(Use 0069T in conjunction with 93005)◄

☆+● **0070T** interpretation and report only (List separately in addition to codes for electrocardiography)

►(Use 0070T in conjunction with 93010)◄

§● **0071T** Focused ultrasound ablation of uterine leiomyomata, including MR guidance; total leiomyomata volume less than 200 cc of tissue

§● **0072T** total leiomyomata volume greater or equal to 200 cc of tissue

►(Do not report 0071T, 0072T in conjunction with 51702 or 76394)◄

✣● **0073T** Compensator-based beam modulation treatment delivery of inverse planned treatment using three or more high resolution (milled or cast) compensator convergent beam modulated fields, per treatment session

►(For treatment planning, use 77301)◄

►(Do not report 0073T in conjunction with 77401-77416, 77418)◄

►Online Medical Evaluation◄

►An online medical evaluation is a type of Evaluation and Management (E/M) service provided by a physician or qualified health care professional to a patient using internet resources in response to the patient's online inquiry. Reportable services involve the physician's personal timely response to the patient's inquiry and must involve permanent storage (electronic or hard copy) of the encounter. This service should not be reported for patient contacts (eg, telephone calls) considered to be pre-service or post-service work for other E/M or non E/M services. A reportable service would encompass the sum of communication (eg, related telephone calls, prescription provision, laboratory orders) pertaining to the online patient encounter or problem(s).◄

□● **0074T** Online evaluation and management service, per encounter, provided by a physician, using the Internet or similar electronic communications network, in response to a patient's request, established patient

✿● **0075T** Transcatheter placement of extracranial vertebral or intrathoracic carotid artery stent(s), including radiologic supervision and interpretation, percutaneous; initial vessel

✿+● **0076T** each additional vessel (List separately in addition to code for primary procedure)

►(Use 0076T in conjunction with 0075T)◄

►(When the ipsilateral extracranial vertebral or intrathoracic carotid arteriogram (including imaging and selective catheterization) confirms the need for stenting, then 0075T and 0076T include all ipsilateral extracranial vertebral or intrathoracic selective carotid catheterization, all diagnostic imaging for ipsilateral extracranial vertebral or intrathoracic carotid artery stenting, and all related radiologic supervision and interpretation. If stenting is not indicated, then the appropriate codes for selective catheterization and imaging should be reported in lieu of code 0075T or 0076T.)◄

✿● **0077T** Implanting and securing cerebral thermal perfusion probe, including twist drill or burr hole, to measure absolute cerebral tissue perfusion

►(0078T-0081T should be reported in accordance with the Endovascular Abdominal Aneurysm Repair guidelines established for 34800-34826)◄

✿● **0078T** Endovascular repair of abdominal aortic aneurysm, pseudoaneurysm or dissection, abdominal aorta involving visceral vessels (superior mesenteric, celiac or renal), using fenestrated modular bifurcated prosthesis (two docking limbs)

►(Do not report 0078T in conjunction with 34800-34805, 35081, 35102, 35452, 35454, 35472, 37205-37208)◄

►(Report 0078T in conjunction with 35454, 37205-37208 when these procedures are performed outside the target zone of the endoprosthesis)◄

✿+● **0079T** Placement of visceral extension prosthesis for endovascular repair of abdominal aortic aneurysm involving visceral vessels, each visceral branch (List separately in addition to code for primary procedure)

►(Use 0079T in conjunction with 0078T)◄

►(Do not report 0079T in conjunction with 34800-34805, 35081, 35102, 35452, 35454, 35472, 37205-37208)◄

►(Report 0079T in conjunction with 35454, 37205-37208 when these procedures are performed outside the target zone of the endoprosthesis)◄

✿● **0080T** Endovascular repair of abdominal aortic aneurysm, pseudoaneurysm or dissection, abdominal aorta involving visceral vessels (superior mesenteric, celiac or renal), using fenestrated modular bifurcated prosthesis (two docking limbs), radiological supervision and interpretation

►(Do not report 0080T in conjunction with 34800-34805, 35081, 35102, 35452, 35454, 35472, 37205-37208)◄

►(Report 0080T in conjunction with 35454, 37205-37208 when these procedures are performed outside the target zone of the endoprosthesis)◄

✿+● **0081T** Placement of visceral extension prosthesis for endovascular repair of abdominal aortic aneurysm involving visceral vessels, each visceral branch, radiological supervision and interpretation (List separately in addition to code for primary procedure)

►(Use 0081T in conjunction with 0080T)◄

►(Do not report 0081T in conjunction with 34800-34805, 35081, 35102, 35452, 35454, 35472, 37205-37208)◄

►(Report 0081T in conjunction with 35454, 37205-37208 when these procedures are performed outside the target zone of the endoprosthesis)◄

✣● **0082T** Stereotactic body radiation therapy, treatment delivery, one or more treatment areas, per day

►(Do not report 0082T in conjunction with 77401-77416, 77418)◄

☆● **0083T** Stereotactic body radiation therapy, treatment management, per day

►(Do not report 0083T in conjunction with 77427-77432)◄

§● **0084T** Insertion of a temporary prostatic urethral stent

♣● **0085T** Breath test for heart transplant rejection

☆● **0086T** Left ventricular filling pressure indirect measurement by computerized calibration of the arterial waveform response to Valsalva maneuver

♣● **0087T** Sperm evaluation, Hyaluronan binding assay

§● **0088T** Submucosal radiofrequency tissue volume reduction of tongue base, one or more sites, per session (ie, for treatment of obstructive sleep apnea syndrome)

Notes

Appendix A

Modifiers

This list includes all of the modifiers applicable to *CPT 2005* codes.

21 Prolonged Evaluation and Management Services: When the face-to-face or floor/unit service(s) provided is prolonged or otherwise greater than that usually required for the highest level of evaluation and management service within a given category, it may be identified by adding modifier 21 to the evaluation and management code number. A report may also be appropriate.

22 Unusual Procedural Services: When the service(s) provided is greater than that usually required for the listed procedure, it may be identified by adding modifier 22 to the usual procedure number. A report may also be appropriate.

23 Unusual Anesthesia: Occasionally, a procedure, which usually requires either no anesthesia or local anesthesia, because of unusual circumstances must be done under general anesthesia. This circumstance may be reported by adding modifier 23 to the procedure code of the basic service.

24 Unrelated Evaluation and Management Service by the Same Physician During a Postoperative Period: The physician may need to indicate that an evaluation and management service was performed during a postoperative period for a reason(s) unrelated to the original procedure. This circumstance may be reported by adding modifier 24 to the appropriate level of E/M service.

25 Significant, Separately Identifiable Evaluation and Management Service by the Same Physician on the Same Day of the Procedure or Other Service: The physician may need to indicate that on the day a procedure or service identified by a CPT code was performed, the patient's condition required a significant, separately identifiable E/M service above and beyond the other service provided or beyond the usual preoperative and postoperative care associated with the procedure that was performed. The E/M service may be prompted by the symptom or condition for which the procedure and/or service was provided. As such, different diagnoses are not required for reporting of the E/M services on the same date. This circumstance may be reported by adding modifier 25 to the appropriate level of E/M service. **Note:** This modifier is not used to report an E/M service that resulted in a decision to perform surgery. See modifier 57.

26 Professional Component: Certain procedures are a combination of a physician component and a technical component. When the physician component is reported separately, the service may be identified by adding modifier 26 to the usual procedure number.

32 Mandated Services: Services related to *mandated* consultation and/or related services (eg, PRO, third party payer, governmental, legislative or regulatory requirement) may be identified by adding modifier 32 to the basic procedure.

47 Anesthesia by Surgeon: Regional or general anesthesia provided by the surgeon may be reported by adding modifier 47 to the basic service. (This does not include local anesthesia.) **Note:** Modifier 47 would not be used as a modifier for the anesthesia procedures.

50 Bilateral Procedure: Unless otherwise identified in the listings, bilateral procedures that are performed at the same operative session, should be identified by adding modifier 50 to the appropriate five digit code.

51 Multiple Procedures: When multiple procedures, other than E/M services, are performed at the same session by the same provider, the primary procedure or service may be reported as listed. The additional procedure(s) or service(s) may be identified by appending modifier 51 to the additional procedure or service code(s). **Note:** This modifier should not be appended to designated "add-on" codes (see Appendix D).

52 Reduced Services: Under certain circumstances a service or procedure is partially reduced or eliminated at the physician's discretion. Under these circumstances the service provided can be identified by its usual procedure number and the addition of modifier 52, signifying that the service is reduced. This provides a means of reporting reduced services without disturbing the identification of the basic service. **Note:** For hospital outpatient reporting of a previously scheduled procedure/service that is partially reduced or cancelled as a result of extenuating circumstances or those that threaten the well-being of the patient prior to or after administration of anesthesia, see modifiers 73 and 74 (see modifiers approved for ASC hospital outpatient use).

53 Discontinued Procedure: Under certain circumstances, the physician may elect to terminate a surgical or diagnostic procedure. Due to extenuating circumstances or those that threaten the well being of the patient, it may be necessary to indicate that a surgical or diagnostic procedure was started but discontinued. This circumstance may be reported by adding modifier 53 to the code reported by the physician for the discontinued procedure. **Note:** This modifier is not used to report the elective cancellation of a procedure prior to the patient's anesthesia induction and/or surgical preparation in the operating suite. For outpatient hospital/ambulatory surgery center (ASC) reporting of a previously scheduled procedure/service that is partially reduced or cancelled as a result of extenuating circumstances or those that threaten the well being of the patient prior to or after administration of anesthesia, see modifiers 73 and 74 (see modifiers approved for ASC hospital outpatient use).

54 Surgical Care Only: When one physician performs a surgical procedure and another provides preoperative and/or postoperative management, surgical services may be identified by adding modifier 54 to the usual procedure number.

55 Postoperative Management Only: When one physician performed the postoperative management and another physician performed the surgical procedure, the postoperative component may be identified by adding modifier 55 to the usual procedure number.

56 Preoperative Management Only: When one physician performed the preoperative care and evaluation and another physician performed the surgical procedure, the preoperative component may be identified by adding modifier 56 to the usual procedure number.

57 Decision for Surgery: An evaluation and management service that resulted in the initial decision to perform the surgery may be identified by adding modifier 57 to the appropriate level of E/M service.

58 Staged or Related Procedure or Service by the Same Physician During the Postoperative Period: The physician may need to indicate that the performance of a procedure or service during the postoperative period was: a) planned prospectively at the time of the original procedure (staged); b) more extensive than the original procedure; or c) for therapy following a diagnostic surgical procedure. This circumstance may be reported by adding modifier 58 to the staged or related procedure. **Note:** This modifier is not used to report the treatment of a problem that requires a return to the operating room. See modifier 78.

59 Distinct Procedural Service: Under certain circumstances, the physician may need to indicate that a procedure or service was distinct or independent from other services performed on the same day. Modifier 59 is used to identify procedures/services that are not normally reported together, but are appropriate under the circumstances. This may represent a different session or patient encounter, different procedure or surgery, different site or organ system, separate incision/excision, separate lesion, or separate injury (or area of injury in extensive injuries) not ordinarily encountered or performed on the same day by the same physician. However, when another already established modifier is appropriate it should be used rather than modifier 59. Only if no more descriptive modifier is available, and the use of modifier 59 best explains the circumstances, should modifier 59 be used.

62 Two Surgeons: When two surgeons work together as primary surgeons performing distinct part(s) of a procedure, each surgeon should report his/her distinct operative work by adding modifier 62 to the procedure code and any associated add-on code(s) for that procedure as long as both surgeons continue to work together as primary surgeons. Each surgeon should report the co-surgery once using the same procedure code. If additional procedure(s) (including add-on procedure(s)) are performed during the same surgical session, separate code(s) may also be reported with modifier 62 added. **Note:** If a co-surgeon acts as an assistant in the performance of additional procedure(s) during the same surgical session, those services may be reported using separate procedure code(s) with the modifier 80 or modifier 82 added, as appropriate.

63 Procedure Performed on Infants less than 4 kg: Procedures performed on neonates and infants up to a present body weight of 4 kg may involve significantly increased complexity and physician work commonly associated with these patients. This circumstance may be reported by adding modifier 63 to the procedure number. **Note:** Unless otherwise designated, this modifier may only be appended to procedures/services listed in the 20000-69999 code series. Modifier 63 should not be appended to any CPT codes listed in the **Evaluation and Management Services, Anesthesia, Radiology, Pathology/Laboratory, or Medicine** sections.

66 Surgical Team: Under some circumstances, highly complex procedures (requiring the concomitant services of several physicians, often of different specialties, plus other highly skilled, specially trained personnel, various types of complex equipment) are carried out under the "surgical team" concept. Such circumstances may be identified by each participating physician with the addition of modifier 66 to the basic procedure number used for reporting services.

76 Repeat Procedure by Same Physician: The physician may need to indicate that a procedure or service was repeated subsequent to the original procedure or service. This circumstance may be reported by adding modifier 76 to the repeated procedure/service.

77 Repeat Procedure by Another Physician: The physician may need to indicate that a basic procedure or service performed by another physician had to be repeated. This situation may be reported by adding modifier 77 to the repeated procedure/service.

78 Return to the Operating Room for a Related Procedure During the Postoperative Period: The physician may need to indicate that another procedure was performed during the postoperative period of the initial procedure. When this subsequent procedure is related to the first, and requires the use of the operating room, it may be reported by adding modifier 78 to the related procedure. (For repeat procedures on the same day, see modifier 76.)

79 Unrelated Procedure or Service by the Same Physician During the Postoperative Period: The physician may need to indicate that the performance of a procedure or service during the postoperative period was unrelated to the original procedure. This circumstance may be reported by using modifier 79. (For repeat procedures on the same day, see modifier 76.)

80 Assistant Surgeon: Surgical assistant services may be identified by adding modifier 80 to the usual procedure number(s).

81 Minimum Assistant Surgeon: Minimum surgical assistant services are identified by adding modifier 81 to the usual procedure number.

82 Assistant Surgeon (when qualified resident surgeon not available): The unavailability of a qualified resident surgeon is a prerequisite for use of modifier 82 appended to the usual procedure code number(s).

90 Reference (Outside) Laboratory: When laboratory procedures are performed by a party other than the treating or reporting physician, the procedure may be identified by adding modifier 90 to the usual procedure number.

91 Repeat Clinical Diagnostic Laboratory Test: In the course of treatment of the patient, it may be necessary to repeat the same laboratory test on the same day to obtain subsequent (multiple) test results. Under these circumstances, the laboratory test performed can be identified by its usual procedure number and the addition of modifier 91. **Note:** This modifier may not be used when tests are rerun to confirm initial results; due to testing problems with specimens or equipment; or for any other reason when a normal, one-time, reportable result is all that is required. This modifier may not be used when other code(s) describe a series of test results (eg, glucose tolerance tests, evocative/suppression testing). This modifier may only be used for laboratory test(s) performed more than once on the same day on the same patient.

99 Multiple Modifiers: Under certain circumstances two or more modifiers may be necessary to completely delineate a service. In such situations modifier 99 should be added to the basic procedure, and other applicable modifiers may be listed as part of the description of the service.

Anesthesia Physical Status Modifiers

The Physical Status modifiers are consistent with the American Society of Anesthesiologists ranking of patient physical status, and distinguishing various levels of complexity of the anesthesia service provided. All anesthesia services are reported by use of the anesthesia five-digit procedure code (00100-03108) with the appropriate physical status modifier appended.

Example: 00100-P1

Under certain circumstances, when another established modifier(s) is appropriate, it should be used in addition to the physical status modifier.

Example: 00100-P4-53

Physical Status Modifier P1: A normal healthy patient

Physical Status Modifier P2: A patient with mild systemic disease

Physical Status Modifier P3: A patient with severe systemic disease

Physical Status Modifier P4: A patient with severe systemic disease that is a constant threat to life

Physical Status Modifier P5: A moribund patient who is not expected to survive without the operation

Physical Status Modifier P6: A declared brain-dead patient whose organs are being removed for donor purposes

Modifiers Approved for Ambulatory Surgery Center (ASC) Hospital Outpatient Use

CPT Level I Modifiers

25 Significant, Separately Identifiable Evaluation and Management Service by the Same Physician on the Same Day of the Procedure or Other Service: The physician may need to indicate that on the day a procedure or service identified by a CPT code was performed, the patient's condition required a significant, separately identifiable E/M service above and beyond the other service provided or beyond the usual preoperative and postoperative care associated with the procedure that was performed. The E/M service may be prompted by the symptom or condition for which the procedure and/or service was provided. As such, different diagnoses are not required for reporting of the E/M services on the same date. This circumstance may be reported by adding modifier 25 to the appropriate level of E/M service. **Note:** This modifier is not used to report an E/M service that resulted in a decision to perform surgery. See modifier 57.

27 Multiple Outpatient Hospital E/M Encounters on the Same Date: For hospital outpatient reporting purposes, utilization of hospital resources related to separate and distinct E/M encounters performed in multiple outpatient hospital settings on the same date may be reported by adding modifier 27 to each appropriate level outpatient and/or emergency department E/M code(s). This modifier provides a means of reporting circumstances involving evaluation and management services provided by physician(s) in more than one (multiple) outpatient hospital setting(s) (eg, hospital emergency department, clinic). **Note:** This modifier is not to be used for physician reporting of multiple E/M services performed by the same physician on the same date. For physician reporting of all outpatient evaluation and management services provided by the same physician on the same date and performed in multiple outpatient setting(s) (eg, hospital emergency department, clinic), see **Evaluation and Management, Emergency Department, or Preventive Medicine Services** codes.

50 Bilateral Procedure: Unless otherwise identified in the listings, bilateral procedures that are performed at the same operative session should be identified by adding modifier 50 to the appropriate five digit code.

52 Reduced Services: Under certain circumstances a service or procedure is partially reduced or eliminated at the physician's discretion. Under these circumstances the service provided can be identified by its usual procedure number and the addition of modifier 52, signifying that the service is reduced. This provides a means of reporting reduced services without disturbing the identification of the basic service. **Note:** For hospital outpatient reporting of a previously scheduled procedure/service that is partially reduced or cancelled as a result of extenuating circumstances or those that threaten the well-being of the patient prior to or after administration of anesthesia, see modifiers 73 and 74.

58 Staged or Related Procedure or Service by the Same Physician During the Postoperative Period: The physician may need to indicate that the performance of a procedure or service during the postoperative period was: a) planned prospectively at the time of the original procedure (staged); b) more extensive than the original procedure; or c) for therapy following a diagnostic surgical procedure. This circumstance may be reported by adding modifier 58 to the staged or related procedure. **Note:** This modifier is not used to report the treatment of a problem that requires a return to the operating room. See modifier 78.

59 Distinct Procedural Service: Under certain circumstances, the physician may need to indicate that a procedure or service was distinct or independent from other services performed on the same day. Modifier 59 is used to identify procedures/services that are not normally reported together, but are appropriate under the circumstances. This may represent a different session or patient encounter, different procedure or surgery, different site or organ system, separate incision/excision, separate lesion, or separate injury (or area of injury in extensive injuries) not ordinarily encountered or performed on the same day by the same physician. However, when another already established modifier is appropriate it should be used rather than modifier 59. Only if no more descriptive modifier is available, and the use of modifier 59 best explains the circumstances, should modifier 59 be used.

73 Discontinued Out-Patient Hospital/Ambulatory Surgery Center (ASC) Procedure Prior to the Administration of Anesthesia: Due to extenuating circumstances or those that threaten the well being of the patient, the physician may cancel a surgical or diagnostic procedure subsequent to the patient's surgical preparation (including sedation when provided, and being taken to the room where the procedure is to be performed), but prior to the administration of anesthesia (local, regional block(s) or general). Under these circumstances, the intended service that is prepared for but cancelled can be reported by its usual procedure number and the addition of modifier 73. **Note:** The elective cancellation of a service prior to the administration of anesthesia and/or surgical preparation of the patient should not be reported. For physician reporting of a discontinued procedure, see modifier 53.

74 Discontinued Out-Patient Hospital/Ambulatory Surgery Center (ASC) Procedure After Administration of Anesthesia: Due to extenuating circumstances or those that threaten the well being of the patient, the physician may terminate a surgical or diagnostic procedure after the administration of anesthesia (local, regional block(s), general) or after the procedure was started (incision made, intubation started, scope inserted, etc). Under these circumstances, the procedure started but terminated can be reported by its usual procedure number and the addition of modifier 74. **Note:** The elective cancellation of a service prior to the administration of anesthesia and/or surgical preparation of the patient should not be reported. For physician reporting of a discontinued procedure, see modifier 53.

76 Repeat Procedure by Same Physician: The physician may need to indicate that a procedure or service was repeated subsequent to the original procedure or service. This circumstance may be reported by adding modifier 76 to the repeated procedure/service.

77 Repeat Procedure by Another Physician: The physician may need to indicate that a basic procedure or service performed by another physician had to be repeated. This situation may be reported by adding modifier 77 to the repeated procedure/service.

78 Return to the Operating Room for a Related Procedure During the Postoperative Period: The physician may need to indicate that another procedure was performed during the postoperative period of the initial procedure. When this subsequent procedure is related to the first, and requires the use of the operating room, it may be reported by adding modifier 78 to the related procedure. (For repeat procedures on the same day, see 76.)

79 Unrelated Procedure or Service by the Same Physician During the Postoperative Period: The physician may need to indicate that the performance of a procedure or service during the postoperative period was unrelated to the original procedure. This circumstance may be reported by using modifier 79. (For repeat procedures on the same day, see 76.)

91 Repeat Clinical Diagnostic Laboratory Test: In the course of treatment of the patient, it may be necessary to repeat the same laboratory test on the same day to obtain subsequent (multiple) test results. Under these circumstances, the laboratory test performed can be identified by its usual procedure number and the addition of modifier 91. **Note:** This modifier may not be used when tests are rerun to confirm initial results; due to testing problems with specimens or equipment; or for any other reason when a normal, one-time, reportable result is all that is required. This modifier may not be used when other code(s) describe a series of test results (eg, glucose tolerance tests, evocative/suppression testing). This modifier may only be used for laboratory test(s) performed more than once on the same day on the same patient.

Level II (HCPCS/National) Modifiers

E1 Upper left, eyelid

E2 Lower left, eyelid

E3 Upper right, eyelid

E4 Lower right, eyelid

F1 Left hand, second digit

F2 Left hand, third digit

F3 Left hand, fourth digit

F4 Left hand, fifth digit

F5 Right hand, thumb

F6 Right hand, second digit

F7 Right hand, third digit

F8 Right hand, fourth digit

F9 Right hand, fifth digit

FA Left hand, thumb

LC Left circumflex coronary artery (Hospitals use with codes 92980-92984, 92995, 92996)

LD Left anterior descending coronary artery (Hospitals use with codes 92980-92984, 92995, 92996)

LT Left side (used to identify procedures performed on the left side of the body)

QM Ambulance service provided under arrangement by a provider of services

QN Ambulance service furnished directly by a provider of services

RC Right coronary artery (Hospitals use with codes 92980-92984, 92995, 92996)

RT Right side (used to identify procedures performed on the right side of the body)

T1 Left foot, second digit

T2 Left foot, third digit

T3 Left foot, fourth digit

T4 Left foot, fifth digit

T5 Right foot, great toe

T6 Right foot, second digit

T7 Right foot, third digit

T8 Right foot, fourth digit

T9 Right foot, fifth digit

TA Left foot, great toe

Appendix B

Summary of Additions, Deletions, and Revisions

Appendix B shows the actual changes that were made to the code descriptors. New codes appear with a bullet (●) and are indicated as "Code added." Revised codes are preceded with a triangle (▲). Within revised codes, the deleted language appears with a ~~strikethrough~~, while new text appears underlined. Codes with which conscious sedation would not be separately reported when performed at the same session by the same provider are denoted with the bullseye (⊙).

Revisions to the headings, notes, introductory paragraphs, and cross-references are not included in this Appendix, but are identified in the main text of the book with the "► ◄" symbols and presented in green. Codes listed as "Grammatical change" contain minor revisions that do not alter the original intent of the codes, and therefore are not preceded with a triangle (▲).

Evaluation and Management

▲ 99293 **Initial inpatient pediatric critical care,** ~~31 days up through 24 months of age,~~ per day, for the evaluation and management of a critically ill infant or young child, 29 days through 24 months of age

▲ 99294 **Subsequent inpatient pediatric critical care,** ~~31 days up through 24 months of age,~~ per day, for the evaluation and management of a critically ill infant or young child, 29 days through 24 months of age

▲ 99295 **Initial inpatient neonatal critical care,** per day, for the evaluation and management of a critically ill neonate, 28 ~~30~~ days of age or less

▲ 99296 **Subsequent inpatient neonatal critical care,** per day, for the evaluation and management of a critically ill neonate, 28~~30~~ days of age or less

Anesthesia

● 00561 Code added

Surgery

● 11004 Code added

● 11005 Code added

● 11006 Code added

+● 11008 Code added

▲ 19160 Mastectomy, partial (eg, lumpectomy, tylectomy, quadrantectomy, segmentectomy);

● 19296 Code added

+● 19297 Code added

⊙● 19298 Code added

● 27412 Code added

● 27415 Code added

● 29866 Code added

● 29867 Code added

● 29868 Code added

● 31545 Code added

● 31546 Code added

+⊙● 31620 Code added

▲ 31630 with tracheal/~~or~~bronchial dilation or closed reduction of fracture

▲ 31631 with ~~tracheal dilation and placement of tracheal stent~~placement of tracheal stent(s) (includes tracheal/bronchial dilation as required)

● 31636 Code added

+● 31637 Code added

● 31638 Code added

⊙● 32019 Code added

▲ 32850 Donor pneumonectomy~~(ies)~~ (including cold preservation), from cadaver donor ~~with preparation and maintenance of allograft (cadaver)~~

● 32855 Code added

● 32856 Code added

▲ 33930 Donor cardiectomy-pneumonectomy (including cold preservation)~~, with preparation and maintenance of allograft~~

● 33933 Code added

▲ 33940 Donor cardiectomy (including cold preservation)~~, with preparation and maintenance of allograft~~

● 33944 Code added

● 34803 Code added

~~35161~~ ~~for aneurysm, pseudoaneurysm, and associated occlusive disease, other arteries~~

~~35162~~ ~~for ruptured aneurysm, other arteries~~

~~35582~~ ~~In-situ vein bypass; aortofemoral-popliteal (only femoral-popliteal portion in-situ)~~

● 36475 Code added

+● 36476 Code added

● 36478 Code added

+● 36479 Code added

● 36818 Code added

▲ 37205 Transcatheter placement of an intravascular stent(s), (except ~~non-~~coronary, ~~non-cervical~~ carotid, and vertebral vessel), percutaneous; initial vessel

⊙● 37215 Code added

⊙● 37216 Code added

⊙● 43257 Code added

● 43644 Code added

● 43645 Code added

● 43845 Code added

▲ 43846 Gastric restrictive procedure, with gastric bypass for morbid obesity; with short limb (~~less than 100~~150 cm or less) Roux-en-Y gastroenterostomy

▲ **44132** Donor enterectomy (including cold preservation), open~~, with preparation and maintenance of allograft~~; from cadaver donor

● **44137** Code added

● **44715** Code added

● **44720** Code added

● **44721** Code added

⊙● **45391** Code added

⊙● **45392** Code added

● **46947** Code added

▲ **47133** Donor hepatectomy (including cold preservation), ~~with preparation and maintenance of allograft,~~from cadaver donor

▲ **47140** Donor hepatectomy (including cold preservation), ~~with preparation and maintenance of allograft,~~from living donor; left lateral segment only (segments II and III)

● **47143** Code added

● **47144** Code added

● **47145** Code added

● **47146** Code added

● **47147** Code added

▲ **48550** Donor pancreatectomy (including cold preservation)~~, with preparation and maintenance of allograft from cadaver donor,~~ with or without duodenal segment for transplantation

● **48551** Code added

● **48552** Code added

▲ **50300** Donor nephrectomy (including cold preservation);~~, with preparation and maintenance of allograft,~~ from cadaver donor, unilateral or bilateral

▲ **50320** ~~Donor nephrectomy,~~ open, from living donor~~(excluding preparation and maintenance of allograft)~~

● **50323** Code added

● **50325** Code added

● **50327** Code added

● **50328** Code added

● **50329** Code added

▲ **50360** Renal allotransplantation, implantation of graft; ~~excluding donor and~~without recipient nephrectomy

● **50391** Code added

▲ **50547** donor nephrectomy (including cold preservation), from living donor~~(excluding preparation and maintenance of allograft)~~

~~**50559**~~ ~~with insertion of radioactive substance with or without biopsy and/or fulguration~~

~~**50578**~~ ~~with insertion of radioactive substance, with or without biopsy and/or fulguration~~

~~**50959**~~ ~~with insertion of radioactive substance, with or without biopsy and/or fulguration (not including provision of material)~~

~~**50978**~~ ~~with insertion of radioactive substance, with or without biopsy and/or fulguration (not including provision of material)~~

▲ **52234** Cystourethroscopy, with fulguration (including cryosurgery or laser surgery) and/or resection of; SMALL bladder tumor(s) (0.5 up to 2.0 cm)

~~**52347**~~ ~~Cystourethroscopy with transurethral resection or incision of ejaculatory ducts~~

● **52402** Code added

+● **57267** Code added

▲ **57282** ~~Sacrospinous ligament fixation for prolapse of vagina~~Colpopexy, vaginal; extra-peritoneal approach (sacrospinous, iliococcygeus)

● **57283** Code added

● **58356** Code added

● **58565** Code added

● **58956** Code added

▲ **61885** Insertion or replacement~~Incision and subcutaneous placement~~ of cranial neurostimulator pulse generator or receiver, direct or inductive coupling; with connection to a single electrode array~~Insertion or replacement~~

● **63050** Code added

● **63051** Code added

+● **63295** Code added

▲ **63685** Insertion or replacement ~~Incision and subcutaneous placement~~of spinal neurostimulator pulse generator or receiver, direct or inductive coupling

▲ **64590** Insertion or replacement ~~Incision and subcutaneous placement~~of peripheral neurostimulator pulse generator or receiver, direct or inductive coupling

▲ **66710** cyclophotocoagulation, transscleral

● **66711** Code added

Radiology

▲ **75960** Transcatheter introduction of intravascular stent(s), (except coronary, carotid, and vertebral vessel), percutaneous and/or open, radiological supervision and interpretation, each vessel

▲ **76075** Dual energy x-ray absorptiometry (~~DEXA~~DXA), bone density study, one or more sites; axial skeleton (eg, hips, pelvis, spine)

● **76077** Code added

● **76510** Code added

▲ **76511** ~~Ophthalmic ultrasound, echography, diagnostic;~~quantitative A-scan only~~, with amplitude quantification~~

▲ **76512** ~~contact~~B-scan (with or without ~~simultaneous~~superimposed non-quantitative A-scan)

● **76820** Code added

● **76821** Code added

▲ **76827** Doppler echocardiography, fetal, ~~cardiovascular system,~~ pulsed wave and/or continuous wave with spectral display; complete

▲ **77418** Intensity modulated treatment delivery, single or multiple fields/arcs, via narrow spatially and temporally modulated beams, ~~(eg, binary, dynamic MLC),~~ binary, dynamic MLC, per treatment session

▲ **77750** Infusion or instillation of radioelement solution (includes three months follow-up care)

▲ **78267** Urea breath test, C-14 (isotopic); acquisition for analysis

▲ **78464** tomographic (SPECT), single study (including attenuation correction when performed), at rest or stress (exercise and/or pharmacologic), with or without quantification

▲ **78465** tomographic (SPECT), multiple studies (including attenuation correction when performed), at rest and/or stress (exercise and/or pharmacologic) and redistribution and/or rest injection, with or without quantification

~~78810~~ ~~Tumor imaging, positron emission tomography (PET), metabolic evaluation~~

● 78811 Code added

● 78812 Code added

● 78813 Code added

● 78814 Code added

● 78815 Code added

● 78816 Code added

~~78990~~ ~~Provision of diagnostic radiopharmaceutical(s)~~

~~79000~~ ~~Radiopharmaceutical therapy, hyper thyroidism; initial, including evaluation of patient~~

~~79001~~ ~~subsequent, each therapy~~

● 79005 Code added

~~79020~~ ~~Radiopharmaceutical therapy, thyroid suppression (euthyroid cardiac disease), including evaluation of patient~~

~~79030~~ ~~Radiopharmaceutical ablation of gland for thyroid carcinoma~~

~~79035~~ ~~Radiopharmaceutical therapy for metastases of thyroid carcinoma~~

~~79100~~ ~~Radiopharmaceutical therapy, polycythemia vera, chronic leukemia, each treatment by intravenous injection~~

● 79101 Code added

▲ 79200 Radiopharmaceutical therapy, by ~~I~~intracavitary ~~radioactive colloid therapy~~administration

▲ 79300 Radiopharmaceutical therapy, by ~~I~~interstitial radioactive colloid administration~~therapy~~

~~79400~~ ~~Radiopharmaceutical therapy, nonthyroid, nonhematologic by intravenous injection~~

~~79420~~ ~~Intravascular radiopharmaceutical therapy, particulate~~

▲ 79440 Radiopharmaceutical therapy, by ~~I~~intra-articular ~~radiopharmaceutical therapy~~administration

● 79445 Code added

~~79900~~ ~~Provision of therapeutic radiopharmaceutical(s)~~

▲ 79999 ~~Unlisted r~~Radiopharmaceutical therapy, ~~therapeutic~~unlisted procedure

Pathology and Laboratory

● 82045 Code added

● 82656 Code added

● 83009 Code added

▲ 83013 Helicobacter pylori; breath test analysis for urease activity, non-radioactive isotope (eg, C-13)

▲ 83014 drug administration ~~and sample collection~~

● 83630 Code added

● 84163 Code added

▲ 84165 Protein~~,~~; electrophoretic fractionation and quantitation, serum

● 84166 Code added

▲ 85046 reticulocytes, ~~hemoglobin concentration~~ automated, including one or more cellular parameters (eg, reticulocyte hemoglobin content (CHr), immature reticulocyte fraction (IRF), reticulocyte volume (MRV), RNA content), direct measurement

● 86064 Code added

▲ 86334 Immunofixation electrophoresis; serum

● 86335 Code added

● 86379 Code added

● 86587 Code added

▲ 87046 stool, aerobic, additional pathogens, isolation and presumptive identification of isolates, each plate

● 87807 Code added

~~88180~~ ~~Flow cytometry; each cell surface, cytoplasmic or nuclear marker~~

● 88184 Code added

+● 88185 Code added

● 88187 Code added

● 88188 Code added

● 88189 Code added

● 88360 Code added

▲ 88361 ~~tumor immunohistochemistry (eg, Her-2/neu, estrogen receptor/progesterone receptor), quantitative or semiquantitative~~using computer-assisted technology

▲ 88365 ~~Tissue i~~In situ hybridization (eg, FISH), ~~interpretation and report~~each probe

● 88367 Code added

● 88368 Code added

▲ 89346 oocyte(s)

Medicine

● 90465 Code added

+● 90466 Code added

● 90467 Code added

+● 90468 Code added

▲ 90471 Immunization administration (includes percutaneous, intradermal, subcutaneous, or intramuscular ~~and jet~~ injections); one vaccine (single or combination vaccine/toxoid)

⊘● 90656 Code added

⊘▲ 90700 Diphtheria, tetanus toxoids, and acellular pertussis vaccine (DTaP), for use in individuals younger than ~~seven~~7 years, for intramuscular use

~~91032~~ ~~Esophagus, acid reflux test, with intraluminal pH electrode for detection of gastroesophageal reflux;~~

~~91033~~ ~~prolonged recording~~

● 91034 Code added

● 91035 Code added

● 91037 Code added

● 91038 Code added

● 91040 Code added

▲ 91065 Breath hydrogen test (eg, for detection of lactase deficiency), fructose intolerance, bacterial overgrowth, or oro-cecal gastrointestinal transit)

● 91120 Code added

~~92589~~ ~~Central auditory function test(s) (specify)~~

● **92620** Code added

● **92621** Code added

● **92625** Code added

▲ **93741** Electronic analysis of pacing cardioverter-defibrillator (includes interrogation, evaluation of pulse generator status, evaluation of programmable parameters at rest and during activity where applicable, using electrocardiographic recording and interpretation of recordings at rest and during exercise, analysis of event markers and device response); single chamber or wearable cardioverter-defibrillator system, without reprogramming

▲ **93742** single chamber or wearable cardioverter-defibrillator system, with reprogramming

● **93745** Code added

● **93890** Code added

● **93892** Code added

● **93893** Code added

▲ **94060** ~~Bronchospasm evaluation:~~ Bronchodilation responsiveness, spirometry as in 94010, ~~before and after~~pre- and post-bronchodilator administration ~~(aerosol or parenteral)~~

▲ **94070** ~~Prolonged postexposure evaluation of b~~Bronchospasm ~~with~~ provocation evaluation, multiple spirometric determinations as in 94010, ~~after antigen,~~ with administered agents (eg, antigen(s), cold air, methacholine) ~~or other chemical agent, with subsequent spirometrics~~

● **94452** Code added

● **94453** Code added

● **95928** Code added

● **95929** Code added

▲ **95971** simple ~~brain,~~spinal cord, or peripheral (ie, peripheral nerve, autonomic nerve, neuromuscular) neurostimulator pulse generator/transmitter, with intraoperative or subsequent programming

▲ **95972** complex ~~brain,~~spinal cord, or peripheral (except cranial nerve) neurostimulator pulse generator/transmitter, with intraoperative or subsequent programming, first hour

+▲ **95973** complex ~~brain,~~spinal cord, or peripheral (except cranial nerve) neurostimulator pulse generator/transmitter, with intraoperative or subsequent programming, each additional 30 minutes after first hour (List separately in addition to code for primary procedure)

● **95978** Code added

+● **95979** Code added

▲ **96111** extended (includes assessment of motor, language, social, adaptive and/or cognitive functioning by standardized developmental instruments~~, eg, Bayley Scales of Infant Development~~) with interpretation and report~~, per hour~~

● **97597** Code added

● **97598** Code added

~~**97601**~~ ~~Removal of devitalized tissue from wound(s); selective debridement, without anesthesia (eg, high pressure waterjet, sharp selective debridement with scissors, scalpel and tweezers), including topical application(s), wound assessment, and instruction(s) for ongoing care, per session~~

● **97605** Code added

● **97606** Code added

~~**97780**~~ ~~Acupuncture, one or more needles; without electrical stimulation~~

~~**97781**~~ ~~with electrical stimulation~~

● **97810** Code added

+● **97811** Code added

● **97813** Code added

+● **97814** Code added

Category II Codes

~~**0001F**~~ ~~Blood pressure, measured~~

~~**0002F**~~ ~~Tobacco use, smoking, assessed~~

~~**0003F**~~ ~~Tobacco use, non-smoking, assessed~~

~~**0004F**~~ ~~Tobacco use cessation intervention, counseling, performed~~

~~**0005F**~~ ~~Tobacco use cessation intervention, pharmacologic therapy, prescribed~~

~~**0006F**~~ ~~Statin therapy, prescribed~~

~~**0007F**~~ ~~Beta-blocker therapy, prescribed~~

~~**0008F**~~ ~~ACE inhibitor therapy, prescribed~~

~~**0009F**~~ ~~Anginal symptoms and level of activity, assessed~~

~~**0010F**~~ ~~Anginal symptoms and level of activity, assessed using a standardized instrument (eg, Canadian Cardiovascular Society Classification CCSC System, Seattle Angina Questionnaire SAQ)~~

~~**0011F**~~ ~~Oral antiplatelet therapy; prescribed (eg, aspirin, clopidogrel/Plavix, or combination of aspirin and dipyridamole/Aggrenox)~~

● **0500F** Code added

● **0501F** Code added

● **0502F** Code added

● **0503F** Code added

● **1000F** Code added

● **1001F** Code added

● **1002F** Code added

● **2000F** Code added

● **4000F** Code added

● **4001F** Code added

● **4002F** Code added

● **4006F** Code added

● **4009F** Code added

● **4011F** Code added

Category III Codes

~~**0001T**~~ ~~Endovascular repair of infrarenal abdominal aortic aneurysm or dissection, modular bifurcated prosthesis (two docking limbs)~~

~~**0005T**~~ ~~Transcatheter placement of extracranial cerebrovascular artery stent(s), percutaneous; initial vessel~~

+ ~~**0006T**~~ ~~each additional vessel (List separately in addition to code for primary procedure)~~

~~**0007T**~~ ~~Transcatheter placement of extracranial cerebrovascular artery stent(s), percutaneous, radiological supervision and interpretation, each vessel~~

~~**0009T**~~ ~~Endometrial cryoablation with ultrasonic guidance~~

~~**0012T**~~ ~~Arthroscopy, knee, surgical, implantation of osteochondral graft(s) for treatment of articular surface defect; autografts~~

~~**0013T**~~ ~~allografts~~

~~**0014T**~~ ~~Meniscal transplantation, medial or lateral, knee (any method)~~

+▲ **0055T** Computer-assisted musculoskeletal surgical navigational orthopedic procedure, with image-guidance based on CT/~~and~~MRI images (List separately in addition to code for primary procedure)

~~**0057T**~~ ~~Upper gastrointestinal endoscopy, including esophagus, stomach, and either the duodenum and/or jejunum as appropriate, with delivery of thermal energy to the muscle of the lower esophageal sphincter and/or gastric cardia, for treatment of gastroesophageal reflux disease~~

● **0062T** Code added

+● **0063T** Code added

● **0064T** Code added

● **0065T** Code added

● **0066T** Code added

● **0067T** Code added

+● **0068T** Code added

+● **0069T** Code added

+● **0070T** Code added

● **0071T** Code added

● **0072T** Code added

● **0073T** Code added

● **0074T** Code added

● **0075T** Code added

+● **0076T** Code added

● **0077T** Code added

● **0078T** Code added

+● **0079T** Code added

● **0080T** Code added

+● **0081T** Code added

● **0082T** Code added

● **0083T** Code added

● **0084T** Code added

● **0085T** Code added

● **0086T** Code added

● **0087T** Code added

● **0088T** Code added

Appendix C

Clinical Examples

As described in *CPT 2005*, clinical examples of the CPT codes for Evaluation and Management (E/M) services are intended to be an important element of the coding system. The clinical examples, when used with the E/M descriptors contained in the full text of *CPT*, provide a comprehensive and powerful tool for physicians to report the services provided to their patients.

The American Medical Association is pleased to provide you with these clinical examples for *CPT 2005*. The clinical examples that are provided in this supplement are limited to Office or Other Outpatient Services, Hospital Inpatient Services, Consultations, Critical Care, Prolonged Services and Care Plan Oversight.

These clinical examples do not encompass the entire scope of medical practice. Inclusion or exclusion of any particular specialty group does not infer any judgment of importance or lack thereof; nor does it limit the applicability of the example to any particular specialty.

Of utmost importance is that these clinical examples are just that: examples. A particular patient encounter, depending on the specific circumstances, must be judged by the services provided by the physician for that particular patient. Simply because the patient's complaints, symptoms, or diagnoses match those of a particular clinical example, does not automatically assign that patient encounter to that particular level of service. The three key components (history, examination, and medical decision making) must be met and documented in the medical record to report a particular level of service.

Office or Other Outpatient Services

New Patient

99201 Initial office visit for a 50-year-old male from out-of-town who needs a prescription refill for a nonsteroidal anti-inflammatory drug. (Anesthesiology)

Initial office visit for a 40-year-old female, new patient, requesting information about local pain clinics. (Anesthesiology/Pain Medicine)

Initial office visit for a 10-year-old girl for determination of visual acuity as part of a summer camp physical (does not include determination of refractive error). (Ophthalmology)

Initial office visit for an out-of-town patient requiring topical refill. (Dermatology)

Initial office visit for a 65-year-old male for reassurance about an isolated seborrheic keratosis on upper back. (Plastic Surgery)

Initial office visit for an out-of-state visitor who needs refill of topical steroid to treat lichen planus. (Dermatology)

Initial office visit for an 86-year-old male, out-of-town visitor, who needs prescription refilled for an anal skin preparation that he forgot. (General Surgery/Colon & Rectal Surgery)

Initial office visit for a transient patient with alveolar osteitis for repacking. (Oral & Maxillofacial Surgery)

Initial office visit for a patient with a pedunculated lesion of the neck which is unsightly. (Dermatology)

Initial office visit for a 10-year-old male, for limited subungual hematoma not requiring drainage. (Internal Medicine)

Initial office visit with an out-of-town visitor who needs a prescription refilled because she forgot her hay fever medication. (Allergy & Immunology/Internal Medicine)

Initial office visit with a 9-month-old female with diaper rash. (Pediatrics)

Initial office visit with a 10-year-old male with severe rash and itching for the past 24 hours, positive history for contact with poison oak 48 hours prior to the visit. (Family Medicine)

Initial office visit with a 5-year-old female to remove sutures from simple wound placed by another physician. (Plastic Surgery)

Initial office visit for a 22-year-old male with a small area of sunburn requiring first aid. (Dermatology/Family Medicine/Internal Medicine)

Initial office visit for the evaluation and management of a contusion of a finger. (Orthopaedic Surgery)

99202 Initial office visit for a 13-year-old patient with comedopapular acne of the face unresponsive to over-the-counter medications. (Family Medicine)

Initial office visit for a patient with a clinically benign lesion or nodule of the lower leg which has been present for many years. (Dermatology)

Initial office visit for a patient with a circumscribed patch of dermatitis of the leg. (Dermatology)

Initial office visit for a patient with papulosquamous eruption of elbows. (Dermatology)

Initial office visit for a 9-year-old patient with erythematous, grouped, vesicular eruption of the lip of three days' duration. (Pediatrics)

Initial office visit for an 18-year-old male referred by an orthodontist for advice regarding removal of four wisdom teeth. (Oral & Maxillofacial Surgery)

Initial office visit for a 14-year-old male, who was referred by his orthodontist, for advice on the exposure of impacted maxillary cuspids. (Oral & Maxillofacial Surgery)

Initial office visit for a patient presenting with itching patches on the wrists and ankles. (Dermatology)

Initial office visit for a 30-year-old male for evaluation and discussion of treatment of rhinophyma. (Plastic Surgery)

Initial office visit for a 16-year-old male with severe cystic acne, new patient. (Dermatology)

Initial office evaluation for gradual hearing loss, 58-year-old male, history and physical examination, with interpretation of complete audiogram, air bone, etc. (Otolaryngology)

Initial evaluation and management of recurrent urinary infection in female. (Internal Medicine)

Initial office visit with a 10-year-old girl with history of chronic otitis media and a draining ear. (Pediatrics)

Initial office visit for a 10-year-old female with acute maxillary sinusitis. (Family Medicine)

Initial office visit for a patient with recurring episodes of herpes simplex who has developed a clustering of vesicles on the upper lip. (Internal Medicine)

Initial office visit for a 25-year-old patient with single season allergic rhinitis. (Allergy & Immunology)

Initial office visit to plan transient dialysis for a 56-year-old stable dialysis patient who has accompanying records. (Nephrology)

99203 Initial office visit for a 76-year-old male with a stasis ulcer of three months' duration. (Dermatology)

Initial office visit for a 30-year-old female with pain in the lateral aspect of the forearm. (Physical Medicine & Rehabilitation)

Initial office visit for a 15-year-old patient with a four-year history of moderate comedopapular acne of the face, chest, and back with early scarring. Discussion of use of systemic medication. (Dermatology)

Initial office visit for a patient with papulosquamous eruption of the elbow with pitting of nails and itchy scalp. (Dermatology)

Initial office visit for a 57-year-old female who complains of painful parotid swelling for one week's duration. (Oral & Maxillofacial Surgery)

Initial office visit for a patient with an ulcerated non-healing lesion or nodule on the tip of the nose. (Dermatology)

Initial office visit for a patient with dermatitis of the antecubital and popliteal fossae. (Dermatology)

Initial office visit for a 22-year-old female with irregular menses. (Family Medicine)

Initial office visit for a 50-year-old female with dyspepsia and nausea. (Family Medicine)

Initial office visit for a 53-year-old laborer with degenerative joint disease of the knee with no prior treatment. (Orthopaedic Surgery)

Initial office visit for a 60-year-old male with Dupuytren's contracture of one hand with multiple digit involvement. (Orthopaedic Surgery)

Initial office visit for a 33-year-old male with painless gross hematuria without cystoscopy. (Internal Medicine)

Initial office visit for a 55-year-old female with chronic blepharitis. There is a history of use of many medications. (Ophthalmology)

Initial office visit for an 18-year-old female with a two-day history of acute conjunctivitis. Extensive history of possible exposures, prior normal ocular history, and medication use is obtained. (Ophthalmology)

Initial office visit for a 14-year-old male with unilateral anterior knee pain. (Physical Medicine & Rehabilitation)

Initial office visit of an adult who presents with symptoms of an upper-respiratory infection that has progressed to unilateral purulent nasal discharge and discomfort in the right maxillary teeth. (Otolaryngology, Head & Neck Surgery)

Initial office visit of a 40-year-old female with symptoms of atopic allergies including eye and sinus congestion, often associated with infections. She would like to be tested for allergies. (Otolaryngology, Head & Neck Surgery)

Initial office visit of a 65-year-old with nasal stuffiness. (Otolaryngology, Head & Neck Surgery)

Initial office visit for initial evaluation of a 48-year-old man with recurrent low back pain radiating to the leg. (General Surgery)

Initial office visit for evaluation, diagnosis and management of painless gross hematuria in a new patient, without cystoscopy. (Internal Medicine)

Initial office visit with couple for counseling concerning voluntary vasectomy for sterility. Spent 30 minutes discussing procedure, risks and benefits, and answering questions. (Urology)

Initial office visit of a 49-year-old male with nasal obstruction. Detailed exam with topical anesthesia. (Plastic Surgery)

Initial office visit for evaluation of a 13-year-old female with progressive scoliosis. (Physical Medicine & Rehabilitation)

Initial office visit for a 21-year-old female desiring counseling and evaluation of initiation of contraception. (Family Practice/Internal Medicine/Obstetrics & Gynecology)

Initial office visit for a 49-year-old male presenting with painless blood per rectum associated with bowel movement. (Colon & Rectal Surgery)

Initial office visit for a 19-year-old football player with three-day-old acute knee injury; now with swelling and pain. (Orthopaedic Surgery)

99204 Initial office visit for a 13-year-old female with progressive scoliosis. (Orthopaedic Surgery)

Initial office visit for a 34-year-old female with primary infertility for evaluation and counseling. (Obstetrics & Gynecology)

Initial office visit for a 6-year-old male with multiple upper respiratory infections. (Allergy & Immunology)

Initial office visit for a patient with generalized dermatitis of 80 percent of the body surface area. (Dermatology)

Initial office visit for an adolescent who was referred by school counselor because of repeated skipping school. (Psychiatry)

Initial office visit for a 50-year-old machinist with a generalized eruption. (Dermatology)

Initial office visit for a 45-year-old female who has been abstinent from alcohol and benzodiazepines for three months but complains of headaches, insomnia, and anxiety. (Psychiatry)

Initial office visit for a 60-year-old male with recent change in bowel habits, weight loss, and abdominal pain. (Abdominal Surgery/General Surgery)

Initial office visit for a 50-year-old male with an aortic aneurysm who is considering surgery. (General Surgery)

Initial office visit for a 17-year-old female with depression. (Internal Medicine)

Initial office visit of a 40-year-old with chronic draining ear, imbalance, and probable cholesteatoma. (Otolaryngology, Head & Neck Surgery)

Initial office visit for initial evaluation of a 63-year-old male with chest pain on exertion. (Cardiology/Internal Medicine)

Initial office visit for evaluation of a 70-year-old patient with recent onset of episodic confusion. (Internal Medicine)

Initial office visit for a 7-year-old female with juvenile diabetes mellitus, new to area, past history of hospitalization times three. (Pediatrics)

Initial office visit of a 50-year-old female with progressive solid food dysphagia. (Gastroenterology)

Initial office visit for a 34-year-old patient with primary infertility, including counseling. (Obstetrics & Gynecology)

Initial office visit for evaluation of a 70-year-old female with polyarthralgia. (Rheumatology)

Initial office visit for a patient with papulosquamous eruption involving 60 percent of the cutaneous surface with joint pain. Combinations of topical and systemic treatments discussed. (Dermatology)

99205 Initial office visit for a patient with disseminated lupus erythematosus with kidney disease, edema, purpura, and scarring lesions on the extremities plus cardiac symptoms. (Dermatology/General Surgery/Internal Medicine)

Initial office visit for a 25-year-old female with systemic lupus erythematosus, fever, seizures, and profound thrombocytopenia. (Rheumatology/Allergy & Immunology)

Initial office visit for an adult with multiple cutaneous blisters, denuded secondarily infected ulcerations, oral lesions, weight loss, and increasing weakness refractory to high dose corticosteroid. Initiation of new immunosuppressive therapy. (Dermatology)

Initial office visit for a 28-year-old male with systemic vasculitis and compromised circulation to the limbs. (Rheumatology)

Initial office visit for a 41-year-old female new to the area requesting rheumatologic care, on disability due to scleroderma and recent hospitalization for malignant hypertension. (Rheumatology)

Initial office visit for a 52-year-old female with acute four extremity weakness and shortness of breath one week post-flu vaccination. (Physical Medicine & Rehabilitation)

Initial office visit for a 60-year-old male with previous back surgery; now presents with back and pelvic pain, two-month history of bilateral progressive calf and thigh tightness and weakness when walking, causing several falls. (Orthopaedic Surgery)

Initial office visit for an adolescent referred from ER after making suicide gesture. (Psychiatry)

Initial office visit for a 49-year-old female with a history of headaches and dependence on opioids. She reports weight loss, progressive headache, and depression. (Psychiatry)

Initial office visit for a 50-year-old female with symptoms of rash, swellings, recurrent arthritic complaints, and diarrhea and lymphadenopathy. Patient has had a 25 lb. weight loss and was recently camping in the Amazon. (Allergy & Immunology)

Initial office visit for a 34-year-old uremic Type I diabetic patient referred for ESRD modality assessment and planning. (Nephrology)

Initial office visit for a 75-year-old female with neck and bilateral shoulder pain, brisk deep tendon reflexes, and stress incontinence. (Physical Medicine & Rehabilitation)

Initial office visit for an 8-year-old male with cerebral palsy and spastic quadriparesis. (Physical Medicine & Rehabilitation)

Initial office visit for a 73-year-old male with known prostate malignancy, who presents with severe back pain and a recent onset of lower extremity weakness. (Physical Medicine & Rehabilitation)

Initial office visit for a 38-year-old male with paranoid delusions and a history of alcohol abuse. (Psychiatry)

Initial office visit for a 12-week-old with bilateral hip dislocations and bilateral club feet. (Orthopaedic Surgery)

Initial office visit for a 29-year-old female with acute orbital congestion, eyelid retraction, and bilateral visual loss from optic neuropathy. (Ophthalmology)

Initial office visit for a 70-year-old diabetic patient with progressive visual field loss, advanced optic disc cupping and neovascularization of retina. (Ophthalmology)

Initial office visit for a newly diagnosed Type I diabetic patient. (Endocrinology)

Initial office evaluation of a 65-year-old female with exertional chest pain, intermittent claudication, syncope and a murmur of aortic stenosis. (Cardiology)

Initial office visit for a 73-year-old male with an unexplained 20 lb. weight loss. (Hematology/Oncology)

Initial office evaluation, patient with systemic lupus erythematosus, fever, seizures and profound thrombocytopenia. (Allergy & Immunology/Internal Medicine/Rheumatology)

Initial office evaluation and management of patient with systemic vasculitis and compromised circulation to the limbs. (Rheumatology)

Initial office visit for a 24-year-old homosexual male who has a fever, a cough, and shortness of breath. (Infectious Disease)

Initial outpatient evaluation of a 69-year-old male with severe chronic obstructive pulmonary disease, congestive heart failure, and hypertension. (Family Medicine)

Initial office visit for a 17-year-old female, who is having school problems and has told a friend she is considering suicide. The patient and her family are consulted in regard to treatment options. (Psychiatry)

Initial office visit for a female with severe hirsutism, amenorrhea, weight loss and a desire to have children. (Endocrinology/Obstetrics & Gynecology)

Initial office visit for a 42-year-old male on hypertensive medication, newly arrived to the area, with diastolic blood pressure of 110, history of recurrent calculi, episodic headaches, intermittent chest pain and orthopnea. (Internal Medicine)

Established Patient

99211 Office visit for an 82-year-old female, established patient, for a monthly B12 injection with documented Vitamin B12 deficiency. (Geriatrics/Internal Medicine/Family Medicine)

Office visit for a 50-year-old male, established patient, for removal of uncomplicated facial sutures. (Plastic Surgery)

Office visit for an established patient who lost prescription for lichen planus. Returned for new copy. (Dermatology)

Office visit for an established patient undergoing orthodontics who complains of a wire which is irritating his/her cheek and asks you to check it. (Oral & Maxillofacial Surgery)

Office visit for a 50-year-old female, established patient, seen for her gold injection by the nurse. (Rheumatology)

Office visit for a 73-year-old female, established patient, with pernicious anemia for weekly B12 injection. (Gastroenterology)

Office visit for an established patient for dressing change on a skin biopsy. (Dermatology)

Office visit for a 19-year-old, established patient, for removal of sutures from a two cm. laceration of forehead, which you placed four days ago in ER. (Plastic Surgery)

Office visit of a 20-year-old female, established patient, who receives an allergy vaccine injection and is observed for a reaction by the nurse. (Otolaryngology, Head & Neck Surgery)

Office visit for a 45-year-old male, established patient, with chronic renal failure for the administration of erythropoietin. (Nephrology)

Office visit for an established patient, a Peace Corps enlistee, who requests documentation that third molars have been removed. (Oral & Maxillofacial Surgery)

Office visit for a 69-year-old female, established patient, for partial removal of antibiotic gauze from an infected wound site. (Plastic Surgery)

Office visit for a 9-year-old, established patient, successfully treated for impetigo, requiring release to return to school. (Dermatology/Pediatrics)

Office visit for an established patient requesting a return-to-work certificate for resolving contact dermatitis. (Dermatology)

Office visit for an established patient who is performing glucose monitoring and wants to check accuracy of machine with lab blood glucose by technician who checks accuracy and function of patient machine. (Endocrinology)

Follow-up office visit for a 65-year-old female with a chronic indwelling percutaneous nephrostomy catheter seen for routine pericatheter skin care and dressing change. (Interventional Radiology)

Outpatient visit with 19-year-old male, established patient, for supervised drug screen. (Addiction Medicine)

Office visit with 12-year-old male, established patient, for cursory check of hematoma one day after venipuncture. (Internal Medicine)

Office visit with 31-year-old female, established patient, for return to work certificate. (Anesthesiology)

Office visit for a 42-year-old, established patient, to read tuberculin test results. (Allergy & Immunology)

Office visit for 14-year-old, established patient, to re-dress an abrasion. (Orthopaedic Surgery)

Office visit for a 45-year-old female, established patient, for a blood pressure check. (Obstetrics & Gynecology)

Office visit for a 23-year-old, established patient, for instruction in use of peak flow meter. (Allergy & Immunology)

Office visit for prescription refill for a 35-year-old female, established patient, with schizophrenia who is stable but has run out of neuroleptic and is scheduled to be seen in a week. (Psychiatry)

99212 Office visit for an 11-year-old, established patient, seen in follow-up for mild comedonal acne of the cheeks on topical desquamating agents. (Dermatology/Family Medicine/Pediatrics)

Office visit for a 10-year-old female, established patient, who has been swimming in a lake, now presents with a one-day history of left ear pain with purulent drainage. (Family Medicine)

Office visit of a child, established patient, with chronic secretory otitis media. (Otolaryngology, Head & Neck Surgery)

Office visit for an established patient seen in follow-up of clearing patch of localized contact dermatitis. (Family Medicine/Dermatology)

Office visit for an established patient returning for evaluation of response to treatment of lichen planus on wrists and ankles. (Dermatology)

Office visit for an established patient with tinea pedis being treated with topical therapy. (Dermatology)

Office visit for an established patient with localized erythematous plaque of psoriasis with topical hydration. (Dermatology)

Office visit for a 50-year-old male, established patient, recently seen for acute neck pain, diagnosis of spondylosis, responding to physical therapy and intermittent cervical traction. Returns for evaluation for return to work. (Neurology)

Office visit for an established patient with recurring episodes of herpes simplex who has developed a clustering of vesicles on the upper lip. (Oral & Maxillofacial Surgery)

Evaluation for a 50-year-old male, established patient, who has experienced a recurrence of knee pain after he discontinued NSAID. (Anesthesiology/Pain Medicine)

Office visit for an established patient with an irritated skin tag for reassurance. (Dermatology)

Office visit for a 40-year-old, established patient, who has experienced a systemic allergic reaction following administration of immunotherapy. The dose must be readjusted. (Allergy & Immunology)

Office visit for a 33-year-old, established patient, for contusion and abrasion of lower extremity. (Orthopaedic Surgery)

Office visit for a 22-year-old male, established patient, one month after I & D of "wrestler's ear." (Plastic Surgery)

Office visit for a 21-year-old, established patient, who is seen in follow-up after antibiotic therapy for acute bacterial tonsillitis. (Otolaryngology, Head & Neck Surgery)

Office visit for a 4-year-old, established patient, with tympanostomy tubes, check-up. (Otolaryngology, Head & Neck Surgery)

Office visit for an established patient who has had needle aspiration of a peritonsillar abscess. (Otolaryngology, Head & Neck Surgery)

Follow-up office examination for evaluation and treatment of acute draining ear in a 5-year-old with tympanotomy tubes. (Otolaryngology, Head & Neck Surgery)

Office visit, established patient, 6-year-old with sore throat and headache. (Family Medicine/Pediatrics)

Office evaluation for possible purulent bacterial conjunctivitis with one- to two-day history of redness and discharge, 16-year-old female, established patient. (Pediatrics/Internal Medicine/Family Medicine)

Office visit with a 65-year-old female, established patient, returns for three-week follow-up for resolving severe ankle sprain. (Orthopaedic Surgery)

Office visit, sore throat, fever and fatigue in a 19-year-old college student, established patient. (Internal Medicine)

Office visit with a 33-year-old female, established patient, recently started on treatment for hemorrhoidal complaints, for re-evaluation. (Colon & Rectal Surgery)

Office visit with a 36-year-old male, established patient, for follow-up on effectiveness of medicine management of oral candidiasis. (Oral & Maxillofacial Surgery)

Office visit for a 27-year-old female, established patient, with complaints of vaginal itching. (Obstetrics & Gynecology)

Office visit for a 65-year-old male, established patient, with eruptions on both arms from poison oak exposure. (Allergy & Immunology/Internal Medicine)

99213 Office visit for an established patient with new lesions of lichen planus in spite of topical therapies. (Dermatology)

Office visit for the quarterly follow-up of a 45-year-old male with stable chronic asthma requiring regular drug therapy. (Allergy & Immunology)

Office visit for a 13-year-old, established patient, with comedopapular acne of the face which has shown poor response to topical medication. Discussion of use of systemic medication. (Dermatology)

Office visit for a 62-year-old female, established patient, for follow-up for stable cirrhosis of the liver. (Internal Medicine/Family Medicine)

Office visit for a 3-year-old, established patient, with atopic dermatitis and food hypersensitivity for quarterly follow-up evaluation. The patient is on topical lotions and steroid creams as well as oral antihistamines. (Allergy & Immunology)

Office visit for an 80-year-old female, established patient, to evaluate medical management of osteoarthritis of the temporomandibular joint. (Rheumatology)

Office visit for a 70-year-old female, established patient, one year post excision of basal cell carcinoma of nose with nasolabial flap. Now presents with new suspicious recurrent lesion and suspicious lesion of the back. (Plastic Surgery)

Office visit for a 68-year-old female, established patient, with polymyalgia rheumatic, maintained on chronic low-dose corticosteroid, with no new complaints. (Rheumatology)

Office visit for a 3-year-old female, established patient, for earache and dyshidrosis of feet. (Pediatrics/Family Medicine)

Office visit for an established patient for 18 months post-operative follow-up of TMJ repair. (Oral & Maxillofacial Surgery)

Office visit for a 45-year-old male, established patient, being re-evaluated for recurrent acute prostatitis. (Urology)

Office visit for a 43-year-old male, established patient, with known reflex sympathetic dystrophy. (Anesthesiology)

Office visit for an established patient with an evenly pigmented superficial nodule of leg which is symptomatic. (Dermatology)

Office visit for an established patient with psoriasis involvement of the elbows, pitting of the nails, and itchy scalp. (Dermatology)

Office visit for a 27-year-old male, established patient, with deep follicular and perifollicular inflammation unable to tolerate systemic antibiotics due to GI upset, requires change of systemic medication. (Dermatology)

Office visit for a 16-year-old male, established patient, who is on medication for exercise-induced bronchospasm. (Allergy & Immunology)

Office visit for a 60-year-old, established patient, with chronic essential hypertension on multiple drug regimen, for blood pressure check. (Family Medicine)

Office visit for a 20-year-old male, established patient, for removal of sutures in hand. (Family Medicine)

Office visit for a 58-year-old female, established patient, with unilateral painful bunion. (Orthopaedic Surgery)

Office visit for a 45-year-old female, established patient, with known osteoarthritis and painful swollen knees. (Rheumatology)

Office visit for a 25-year-old female, established patient, complaining of bleeding and heavy menses. (Obstetrics & Gynecology)

Office visit for a 55-year-old male, established patient, with hypertension managed by a beta blocker/thiazide regime; now experiencing mild fatigue. (Nephrology)

Office visit for a 65-year-old female, established patient, with primary glaucoma for interval determination of intraocular pressure and possible adjustment of medication. (Ophthalmology)

Office visit for a 56-year-old man, established patient, with stable exertional angina who complains of new onset of calf pain while walking. (Cardiology)

Office visit for a 63-year-old female, established patient, with rheumatoid arthritis on auranofin and ibuprofen, seen for routine follow-up visit. (Rheumatology)

Office visit for an established patient with Graves' disease, three months post I-131 therapy, who presents with lassitude and malaise. (Endocrinology)

Office visit for the quarterly follow-up of a 63-year-old male, established patient, with chronic myofascial pain syndrome, effectively managed by doxepin, who presents with new onset urinary hesitancy. (Pain Medicine)

Office visit for the biannual follow-up of an established patient with migraine variant having infrequent, intermittent, moderate to severe headaches with nausea and vomiting, which are sometimes effectively managed by ergotamine tartrate and an antiemetic, but occasionally requiring visits to an emergency department. (Pain Medicine)

Office visit for an established patient after discharge from a pain rehabilitation program to review and adjust medication dosage. (Pain Medicine)

Office visit with 55-year-old male, established patient, for management of hypertension, mild fatigue, on beta blocker/thiazide regimen. (Family Medicine/Internal Medicine)

Outpatient visit with 37-year-old male, established patient, who is three years post total colectomy for chronic ulcerative colitis, presents for increased irritation at his stoma. (General Surgery)

Office visit for a 70-year-old diabetic hypertensive established patient with recent change in insulin requirement. (Internal Medicine/Nephrology)

Office visit with 80-year-old female, established patient, for follow-up osteoporosis, status-post compression fractures. (Rheumatology)

Office visit for an established patient with stable cirrhosis of the liver. (Gastroenterology)

Routine, follow-up office evaluation at a three-month interval for a 77-year-old female, established patient, with nodular small cleaved-cell lymphoma. (Hematology/Oncology)

Quarterly follow-up office visit for a 45-year-old male, established patient, with stable chronic asthma, on steroid and bronchodilator therapy. (Pulmonary Medicine)

Office visit for a 50-year-old female, established patient, with insulin-dependent diabetes mellitus and stable coronary artery disease, for monitoring. (Family Medicine/Internal Medicine)

99214 Office visit for an established patient now presenting with generalized dermatitis of 80 percent of the body surface area. (Dermatology)

Office visit for a 32-year-old female, established patient, with new onset right lower quadrant pain. (Family Medicine)

Office visit for reassessment and reassurance/counseling of a 40-year-old female, established patient, who is experiencing increased symptoms while on a pain management treatment program. (Pain Medicine)

Office visit for a 30-year-old, established patient, under management for intractable low back pain, who now presents with new onset right posterior thigh pain. (Pain Medicine)

Office visit for an established patient with frequent intermittent, moderate to severe headaches requiring beta blocker or tricyclic antidepressant prophylaxis, as well as four symptomatic treatments, but who is still experiencing headaches at a frequency of several times a month that are unresponsive to treatment. (Pain Medicine)

Office visit for an established patient with psoriasis with extensive involvement of scalp, trunk, palms, and soles with joint pain. Combinations of topical and systemic treatments discussed and instituted. (Dermatology)

Office visit for a 55-year-old male, established patient, with increasing night pain, limp, and progressive varus of both knees. (Orthopaedic Surgery)

Follow-up visit for a 15-year-old withdrawn patient with four-year history of papulocystic acne of the face, chest, and back with early scarring and poor response to past treatment. Discussion of use of systemic medication. (Dermatology)

Office visit for a 28-year-old male, established patient, with regional enteritis, diarrhea, and low-grade fever. (Internal Medicine)

Office visit for a 25-year-old female, established patient, following recent arthrogram and MR imaging for TMJ pain. (Oral & Maxillofacial Surgery)

Office visit for a 32-year-old female, established patient, with large obstructing stone in left mid-ureter, to discuss management options including urethroscopy with extraction or ESWL. (Urology)

Evaluation for a 28-year-old male, established patient, with new onset of low back pain. (Anesthesiology/Pain Medicine)

Office visit for a 28-year-old female, established patient, with right lower quadrant abdominal pain, fever, and anorexia. (Internal Medicine/Family Medicine)

Office visit for a 45-year-old male, established patient, four months follow-up of L4-5 diskectomy, with persistent incapacitating low back and leg pain. (Orthopaedic Surgery)

Outpatient visit for a 77-year-old male, established patient, with hypertension, presenting with a three-month history of episodic substernal chest pain on exertion. (Cardiology)

Office visit for a 25-year-old female, established patient, for evaluation of progressive saddle nose deformity of unknown etiology. (Plastic Surgery)

Office visit for a 65-year-old male, established patient, with BPH and severe bladder outlet obstruction, to discuss management options such as TURP. (Urology)

Office visit for an adult diabetic established patient with a past history of recurrent sinusitis who presents with a one-week history of double vision. (Otolaryngology, Head & Neck Surgery)

Office visit for an established patient with lichen planus and 60 percent of the cutaneous surface involved, not responsive to systemic steroids, as well as developing symptoms of progressive heartburn and paranoid ideation. (Dermatology)

Office visit for a 52-year-old male, established patient, with a 12-year history of bipolar disorder responding to lithium carbonate and brief psychotherapy. Psychotherapy and prescription provided. (Psychiatry)

Office visit for a 63-year-old female, established patient, with a history of familial polyposis, status post-colectomy with sphincter sparing procedure, who now presents with rectal bleeding and increase in stooling frequency. (General Surgery)

Office visit for a 68-year-old male, established patient, with the sudden onset of multiple flashes and floaters in the right eye due to a posterior vitreous detachment. (Ophthalmology)

Office visit for a 55-year-old female, established patient, on cyclosporin for treatment of resistant, small vessel vasculitis. (Rheumatology)

Follow-up office visit for a 55-year-old male, two months after iliac angioplasty with new onset of contralateral extremity claudication. (Interventional Radiology)

Office visit for a 68-year-old male, established patient, with stable angina, two months post myocardial infarction, who is not tolerating one of his medications. (Cardiology)

Weekly office visit for 5FU therapy for an ambulatory established patient with metastatic colon cancer and increasing shortness of breath. (Hematology/Oncology)

Follow-up office visit for a 60-year-old male, established patient, whose post-traumatic seizures have disappeared on medication and who now raises the question of stopping the medication (Neurology)

Office evaluation on new onset RLQ pain in a 32-year-old woman, established patient. (Urology/General Surgery/Internal Medicine/Family Medicine)

Office evaluation of 28-year-old, established patient, with regional enteritis, diarrhea and low-grade fever. (Family Medicine/Internal Medicine)

Office visit with 50-year-old female, established patient, diabetic, blood sugar controlled by diet. She now complains of frequency of urination and weight loss, blood sugar of 320 and negative ketones on dipstick. (Internal Medicine)

Follow-up office visit for a 45-year-old, established patient, with rheumatoid arthritis on gold, methotrexate, or immunosuppressive therapy. (Rheumatology)

Office visit for a 60-year-old male, established patient, two years post-removal of intracranial meningioma, now with new headaches and visual disturbance. (Neurosurgery)

Office visit for a 68-year-old female, established patient, for routine review and follow-up of non-insulin dependent diabetes, obesity, hypertension and congestive heart failure. Complains of vision difficulties and admits dietary noncompliance. Patient is counseled concerning diet and current medications adjusted. (Family Medicine)

99215 Office visit for an established patient who developed persistent cough, rectal bleeding, weakness, and diarrhea plus pustular infection on skin. Patient on immunosuppressive therapy. (Dermatology)

Office visit for an established patient with disseminated lupus erythematosus, extensive edema of extremities kidney disease, and weakness requiring monitored course on azathioprene, corticosteroid and complicated by acute depression. (Dermatology/Internal Medicine/Rheumatology)

Office visit for an established patient with progressive dermatomyositis and recent onset of fever, nasal speech, and regurgitation of fluids through the nose. (Dermatology)

Office visit for a 28-year-old female, established patient, who is abstinent from previous cocaine dependence, but reports progressive panic attacks and chest pains. (Psychiatry)

Office visit for an established adolescent patient with history of bipolar disorder treated with lithium; seen on urgent basis at family's request because of severe depressive symptoms. (Psychiatry)

Office visit for an established patient having acute migraine with new onset neurological symptoms and whose headaches are unresponsive to previous attempts at management with a combination of preventive and abortive medication. (Pain Medicine)

Office visit for an established patient with exfoliative lichen planus with daily fever spikes, disorientation, and shortness of breath. (Dermatology)

Office visit for a 25-year-old, established patient, two years post-burn with bilateral ectropion, hypertrophic facial burn scars, near absence of left breast, and burn syndactyly of both hands. Discussion of treatment options following examination. (Plastic Surgery)

Office visit for a 6-year-old, established patient, to review newly diagnosed immune deficiency with recommendations for therapy including IV immunoglobulin and chronic antibiotics. (Allergy & Immunology)

Office visit for a 36-year-old, established patient, three months status post-transplant, with new onset of peripheral edema, increased blood pressure, and progressive fatigue. (Nephrology)

Office visit for an established patient with Kaposi's sarcoma who presents with fever and widespread vesicles. (Dermatology)

Office visit for a 27-year-old female, established patient, with bipolar disorder who was stable on lithium carbonate and monthly supportive psychotherapy but now has developed symptoms of hypomania. (Psychiatry)

Office visit for a 25-year-old male, established patient with a history of schizophrenia who has been seen bi-monthly but is complaining of auditory hallucinations. (Psychiatry)

Office visit for a 62-year-old male, established patient, three years post-op abdominal perineal resection, now with a rising carcinoembryonic antigen, weight loss, and pelvic pain. (Abdominal Surgery)

Office visit for a 42-year-old male, established patient, nine months post-op emergency vena cava shunt for variceal bleeding, now presents with complaints of one episode of "dark" bowel movement, weight gain, tightness in abdomen, whites of eyes seem "yellow" and occasional drowsiness after eating hamburgers. (Abdominal Surgery)

Office visit for a 68-year-old male, established patient, with biopsy-proven rectal carcinoma, for evaluation and discussion of treatment options. (General Surgery)

Office visit for a 60-year-old, established patient, with diabetic nephropathy with increasing edema and dyspnea. (Endocrinology)

Office visit with 30-year-old male, established patient for three-month history of fatigue, weight loss, intermittent fever, and presenting with diffuse adenopathy and splenomegaly. (Family Medicine)

Office visit for restaging of an established patient with new lymphadenopathy one year post-therapy for lymphoma. (Hematology/Oncology)

Office visit for evaluation of recent onset syncopal attacks in a 70-year-old woman, established patient. (Internal Medicine)

Follow-up visit, 40-year-old mother of three, established patient, with acute rheumatoid arthritis, anatomical Stage 3, ARA function Class 3 rheumatoid arthritis, and deteriorating function. (Rheumatology)

Office evaluation and discussion of treatment options for a 68-year-old male, established patient, with a biopsy-proven rectal carcinoma. (General Surgery)

Follow-up office visit for a 65-year-old male, established patient, with a fever of recent onset while on outpatient antibiotic therapy for endocarditis. (Infectious Disease)

Office visit for a 75-year-old, established patient, with ALS (amyotrophic lateral sclerosis), who is no longer able to swallow. (Neurology)

Office visit for a 70-year-old female, established patient, with diabetes mellitus and hypertension, presenting with a two-month history of increasing confusion, agitation and short-term memory loss. (Family Medicine/Internal Medicine)

Hospital Inpatient Services

Initial Hospital Care

New or Established Patient

99221 Initial hospital visit following admission for a 42-year-old male for observation following an uncomplicated mandible fracture. (Plastic Surgery/Oral & Maxillofacial Surgery)

Initial hospital visit for a 40-year-old patient with a thrombosed synthetic arteriovenous conduit. (Nephrology)

Initial hospital visit for a healthy 24-year-old male with an acute onset of low back pain following a lifting injury. (Internal Medicine/Anesthesiology/Pain Medicine)

Initial hospital visit for a 69-year-old female with controlled hypertension, scheduled for surgery. (Internal Medicine/Cardiology)

Initial hospital visit for a 24-year-old healthy female with benign tumor of palate. (Oral & Maxillofacial Surgery)

Initial hospital visit for a 14-year-old female with infectious mononucleosis and dehydration. (Internal Medicine)

Initial hospital visit for a 62-year-old female with stable rheumatoid arthritis, admitted for total joint replacement. (Rheumatology)

Initial hospital visit for a 12-year-old patient with a laceration of the upper eyelid, involving the lid margin and superior canaliculus, admitted prior to surgery for IV antibiotic therapy. (Plastic Surgery)

Initial hospital visit for a 69-year-old female with controlled hypertension, scheduled for surgery. (Cardiology)

Hospital admission, examination, and initiation of treatment program for a 67-year-old male with uncomplicated pneumonia who requires IV antibiotic therapy. (Internal Medicine)

Hospital admission for an 18-month-old with 10 percent dehydration. (Pediatrics)

Hospital admission for a 12-year-old with a laceration of the upper eyelid involving the lid margin and superior canaliculus, admitted prior to surgery for IV antibiotic therapy. (Ophthalmology)

Hospital admission for a 32-year-old female with severe flank pain, hematuria and presumed diagnosis of ureteral calculus as determined by Emergency Department physician. (Urology)

Initial hospital visit for a patient with several large venous stasis ulcers not responding to outpatient therapy. (Dermatology)

Initial hospital visit for 21-year-old pregnant patient (nine weeks gestation) with hyperemesis gravidarum. (Obstetrics & Gynecology)

Initial hospital visit for a 73-year-old female with acute pyelonephritis who is otherwise generally healthy. (Geriatrics)

Initial hospital visit for 62-year-old patient with cellulitis of the foot requiring bedrest and intravenous antibiotics. (Orthopaedic Surgery)

99222 Initial hospital visit for a 50-year-old patient with lower quadrant abdominal pain and increased temperature, but without septic picture. (General Surgery/Abdominal Surgery/Colon & Rectal Surgery)

Initial hospital visit for airway management, due to a benign laryngeal mass. (Otolaryngology, Head & Neck Surgery)

Initial hospital visit for a 66-year-old female with an L-2 vertebral compression fracture with acute onset of paralytic ileus; seen in the office two days previously. (Orthopaedic Surgery)

Initial hospital visit and evaluation of a 15-year-old male admitted with peritonsillar abscess or cellulitis requiring intravenous antibiotic therapy. (Otolaryngology, Head & Neck Surgery)

Initial hospital visit for a 42-year-old male with vertebral compression fracture following a motor vehicle accident. (Orthopaedic Surgery)

Initial hospital visit for a patient with generalized atopic dermatitis and secondary infection. (Dermatology)

Initial hospital visit for a 3-year-old patient with high temperature, limp, and painful hip motion of 18 hours' duration. (Pediatrics/Orthopaedic Surgery)

Initial hospital visit for a young adult, presenting with an acute asthma attack unresponsive to outpatient therapy. (Allergy & Immunology)

Initial hospital visit for an 18-year-old male who has suppurative sialoadenitis and dehydration. (Oral & Maxillofacial Surgery)

Initial hospital visit for a 65-year-old female for acute onset of thrombotic cerebrovascular accident with contralateral paralysis and aphasia. (Neurology)

Initial hospital visit for a 50-year-old male chronic paraplegic patient with pain and spasm below the lesion. (Anesthesiology)

Partial hospital admission for an adolescent patient from chaotic blended family, transferred from inpatient setting, for continued treatment to control symptomatic expressions of hostility and depression. (Psychiatry)

Initial hospital visit for a 15-year-old male with acute status asthmaticus, unresponsive to outpatient therapy. (Internal Medicine)

Initial hospital visit for a 61-year-old male with history of previous myocardial infarction, who now complains of chest pain. (Internal Medicine)

Initial hospital visit of a 15-year-old on medications for a sore throat over the last two weeks. The sore throat has worsened and patient now has dysphagia. The exam shows large necrotic tonsils with an adequate airway and small palpable nodes. The initial mono test was negative. (Otolaryngology, Head & Neck Surgery)

Initial hospital evaluation of a 23-year-old allergy patient admitted with eyelid edema and pain on fifth day of oral antibiotic therapy. (Otolaryngology, Head & Neck Surgery)

Hospital admission, young adult patient, failed previous therapy and now presents in acute asthmatic attack. (Family Medicine/Allergy & Immunology)

Hospital admission of a 62-year-old smoker, established patient, with bronchitis in acute respiratory distress. (Internal Medicine/Pulmonary Medicine)

Hospital admission, examination, and initiation of a treatment program for a 65-year-old female with new onset of right-sided paralysis and aphasia. (Neurology)

Hospital admission for a 50-year-old with left lower quadrant abdominal pain and increased temperature, but without septic picture. (General Surgery)

Hospital admission, examination, and initiation of treatment program for a 66-year-old chronic hemodialysis patient with fever and a new pulmonary infiltrate. (Nephrology)

Hospital admission for an 8-year-old febrile patient with chronic sinusitis and severe headache, unresponsive to oral antibiotics. (Allergy & Immunology)

Hospital admission for a 40-year-old male with submaxillary cellulitis and trismus from infected lower molar. (Oral & Maxillofacial Surgery)

99223 Initial hospital visit for a 45-year-old female, who has a history of rheumatic fever as a child and now has anemia, fever, and congestive heart failure. (Cardiology)

Initial hospital visit for a 50-year-old male with acute chest pain and diagnostic electrocardiographic changes of an acute anterior myocardial infarction. (Cardiology/Family Medicine/Internal Medicine)

Initial hospital visit of a 75-year-old with progressive stridor and dysphagia with history of cancer of the larynx treated by radiation therapy in the past. Exam shows a large recurrent tumor of the glottis with a mass in the neck. (Otolaryngology, Head & Neck Surgery)

Initial hospital visit for a 70-year-old male admitted with chest pain, complete heart block, and congestive heart failure. (Cardiology)

Initial hospital visit for an 82-year-old male who presents with syncope, chest pain, and ventricular arrhythmias. (Cardiology)

Initial hospital visit for a 75-year-old male with history of arteriosclerotic coronary vascular disease, who is severely dehydrated, disoriented, and experiencing auditory hallucinations. (Psychiatry)

Initial hospital visit for a 70-year-old male with alcohol and sedative-hypnotic dependence, admitted by family for severe withdrawal, hypertension, and diabetes mellitus. (Psychiatry)

Initial hospital visit for a persistently suicidal latency-aged child whose parents have requested admission to provide safety during evaluation, but are anxious about separation from her. (Psychiatry)

Initial psychiatric visit for an adolescent patient without previous psychiatric history, who was transferred from the medical ICU after a significant overdose. (Psychiatry)

Initial hospital visit for a 35-year-old female with severe systemic lupus erythematosus on corticosteroid and cyclophosphamide, with new onset of fever, chills, rash, and chest pain. (Rheumatology)

Initial hospital visit for a 52-year-old male with known rheumatic heart disease who presents with anasarca, hypertension, and history of alcohol abuse. (Cardiology)

Initial hospital visit for a 55-year-old female with a history of congenital heart disease; now presents with cyanosis. (Cardiology)

Initial hospital visit for a psychotic, hostile, violently combative adolescent, involuntarily committed, for seclusion and restraint in order to provide for safety on unit. (Psychiatry)

Initial hospital visit for a now subdued and sullen teenage male with six-month history of declining school performance, increasing self-endangerment, and resistance of parental expectations, including running away past weekend after physical fight with father. (Psychiatry)

Initial partial hospital admission for a 17-year-old female with history of borderline mental retardation who has developed auditory hallucinations. Parents are known to abuse alcohol, and Child Protective Services is investigating allegations of sexual abuse of a younger sibling. (Psychiatry)

Initial hospital visit of a 67-year old male admitted with a large neck mass, dysphagia, and history of myocardial infarction three months before. (Otolaryngology, Head & Neck Surgery)

Initial hospital visit for a patient with suspected cerebrospinal fluid rhinorrhea which developed two weeks after head injury. (Otolaryngology, Head & Neck Surgery)

Initial hospital visit for a 25-year-old female with history of poly-substance abuse and psychiatric disorder. The patient appears to be psychotic with markedly elevated vital signs. (Psychiatry)

Initial hospital visit for a 70-year-old male with cutaneous T-cell lymphoma who has developed fever and lymphadenopathy. (Internal Medicine)

Initial hospital visit for a 62-year-old female with known coronary artery disease, for evaluation of increasing edema, dyspnea on exertion, confusion, and sudden onset of fever with productive cough. (Internal Medicine)

Initial hospital visit for a 3-year-old female with 36-hour history of sore throat and high fever; now with sudden onset of lethargy, irritability, photophobia, and nuchal rigidity. (Pediatrics)

Initial hospital visit for a 26-year-old female for evaluation of severe facial fractures (LeFort's II/III). (Plastic Surgery)

Initial hospital visit for a 55-year-old female for bilateral mandibular fractures resulting in flail mandible and airway obstruction. (Plastic Surgery)

Initial hospital visit for a 71-year-old patient with a red painful eye four days following uncomplicated cataract surgery due to endophthalmitis. (Ophthalmology)

Initial hospital visit for a 45-year-old patient involved in a motor vehicle accident who suffered a perforating corneoscleral laceration with loss of vision. (Ophthalmology)

Initial hospital visit for a 58-year-old male who has Ludwig's angina and progressive airway compromise. (Oral & Maxillofacial Surgery)

Initial hospital visit for a patient with generalized systemic sclerosis, receiving immunosuppressive therapy because of recent onset of cough, fever, and inability to swallow. (Dermatology)

Initial hospital visit for an 82-year-old male who presents with syncope, chest pain, and ventricular arrhythmias. (Cardiology)

Initial hospital visit for a 62-year-old male with history of previous myocardial infarction, comes in with recurrent, sustained ventricular tachycardia. (Cardiology)

Initial hospital visit for a chronic dialysis patient with infected PTFE fistula, septicemia, and shock. (Nephrology)

Initial hospital visit for a 1-year-old male, victim of child abuse, with central nervous system depression, skull fracture, and retinal hemorrhage. (Family Medicine/Neurology)

Initial hospital visit for a 25-year-old female with recent C4-5 quadriplegia, admitted for rehabilitation. (Physical Medicine & Rehabilitation)

Initial hospital visit for an 18-year-old male, post-traumatic brain injury with multiple impairment. (Physical Medicine & Rehabilitation)

Initial partial hospital admission for 16-year-old male, sullen and subdued, with six-month history of declining school performance, increasing self-endangerment, and resistance to parental expectations. (Psychiatry)

Initial hospital visit for a 16-year-old primigravida at 32 weeks gestation with severe hypertension (200/110), thrombocytopenia, and headache. (Obstetrics & Gynecology)

Initial hospital visit for a 49-year-old male with cirrhosis of liver with hematemesis, hepatic encephalopathy, and fever. (Gastroenterology)

Initial hospital visit for a 55-year-old female in chronic pain who has attempted suicide. (Psychiatry)

Initial hospital visit for a 70-year-old male, with multiple organ system disease, admitted with history of being aneuric and septic for 24 hours prior to admission. (Urology)

Initial hospital visit for a 3-year-old female with 36-hour history of sore throat and high fever, now with sudden onset of lethargy, irritability, photophobia, and nuchal rigidity. (Internal Medicine)

Initial hospital visit for a 78-year-old male, transfers from nursing home with dysuria and pyuria, increasing confusion, and high fever. (Internal Medicine)

Initial hospital visit for a 1-day-old male with cyanosis, respiratory distress, and tachypnea. (Cardiology)

Initial hospital visit for a 3-year-old female with recurrent tachycardia and syncope. (Cardiology)

Initial hospital visit for a thyrotoxic patient who presents with fever, atrial fibrillation, and delirium. (Endocrinology)

Initial hospital visit for a 50-year-old Type I diabetic who presents with diabetic ketoacidosis with fever and obtundation. (Endocrinology)

Initial hospital visit for a 40-year-old female with anatomical stage 3, ARA functional class 3 rheumatoid arthritis on methotrexate, corticosteroid, and nonsteroidal anti-inflammatory drugs. Patient presents with severe arthritis flare, new oral ulcers, abdominal pain, and leukopenia. (Rheumatology)

Initial hospital exam of a pediatric patient with high fever and proptosis. (Otolaryngology, Head & Neck Surgery)

Initial hospital visit for a 25-year-old patient admitted for the first time to the rehab unit, with recent C-4-5 quadriplegia. (Physical Medicine & Rehabilitation)

Hospital admission, examination, and initiation of treatment program for a previously unknown 58-year-old male who presents with acute chest pain (Cardiology)

Hospital admission, examination, and initiation of induction chemotherapy for a 42-year-old patient with newly diagnosed acute myelogenous leukemia. (Hematology/Oncology)

Hospital admission following a motor vehicle accident of a 24-year-old male with fracture dislocation of C5-6; neurologically intact. (Neurosurgery)

Hospital admission for a 78-year-old female with left lower lobe pneumonia and a history of coronary artery disease, congestive heart failure, osteoarthritis and gout. (Family Medicine)

Hospital admission, examination, and initiation of treatment program for a 65-year-old immunosuppressed male with confusion, fever, and a headache. (Infectious Disease)

Hospital admission for a 9-year-old with vomiting, dehydration, fever, tachypnea and an admitting diagnosis of diabetic ketoacidosis. (Pediatrics)

Initial hospital visit for a 65-year-old male who presents with acute myocardial infarction, oliguria, hypotension, and altered state of consciousness. (Cardiology)

Initial hospital visit for a hostile/resistant adolescent patient who is severely depressed and involved in poly-substance abuse. Patient is experiencing significant conflict in his chaotic family situation and was suspended from school following an attack on a teacher with a baseball bat. (Psychiatry)

Initial hospital visit for 89-year-old female with fulminant hepatic failure and encephalopathy. (Gastroenterology)

Initial hospital visit for a 42-year-old female with rapidly progressing scleroderma, malignant hypertension, digital infarcts, and oligurea. (Rheumatology)

Subsequent Hospital Care

99231 Subsequent hospital visit for a 65-year-old female, post-open reduction and internal fixation of a fracture. (Physical Medicine & Rehabilitation)

Subsequent hospital visit for a 33-year-old patient with pelvic pain who is responding to pain medication and observation. (Obstetrics & Gynecology)

Subsequent hospital visit for a 21-year-old female with hyperemesis who has responded well to intravenous fluids. (Obstetrics & Gynecology)

Subsequent hospital visit to re-evaluate post-op pain and titrate patient-controlled analgesia for a 27-year-old female. (Anesthesiology)

Follow-up hospital visit for a 35-year-old female, status post-epidural analgesia. (Anesthesiology/Pain Medicine)

Subsequent hospital visit for a 56-year-old male, post-gastrectomy, for maintenance of analgesia using an intravenous dilaudid infusion. (Anesthesiology)

Subsequent hospital visit for a 4-year-old on day three receiving medication for uncomplicated pneumonia. (Allergy & Immunology)

Subsequent hospital visit for a 30-year-old female with urticaria which has stabilized with medication. (Allergy & Immunology)

Subsequent hospital visit for a 76-year-old male with venous stasis ulcers. (Dermatology)

Subsequent hospital visit for a 24-year-old female with otitis externa, seen two days before in consultation, now to have otic wick removal. (Otolaryngology, Head & Neck Surgery)

Subsequent hospital visit for a 27-year-old with acute labyrinthitis. (Otolaryngology, Head & Neck Surgery)

Subsequent hospital visit for a 10-year-old male admitted for lobar pneumonia with vomiting and dehydration; is becoming afebrile and tolerating oral fluids. (Family Medicine/Pediatrics)

Subsequent hospital visit for a 62-year-old patient with resolving cellulitis of the foot. (Orthopaedic Surgery)

Subsequent hospital visit for a 25-year-old male admitted for supra-ventricular tachycardia and converted on medical therapy. (Cardiology)

Subsequent hospital visit for a 27-year-old male two days after open reduction and internal fixation for malar complex fracture. (Plastic Surgery)

Subsequent hospital visit for a 76-year-old male with venous stasis ulcers. (Geriatrics)

Subsequent hospital visit for a 67-year-old female admitted three days ago with bleeding gastric ulcer; now stable. (Gastroenterology)

Subsequent hospital visit for stable 33-year-old male, status post-lower gastrointestinal bleeding. (General Surgery/Gastroenterology)

Subsequent hospital visit for a 29-year-old auto mechanic with effort thrombosis of left upper extremity. (General Surgery)

Subsequent hospital visit for a 14-year-old female in middle phase of inpatient treatment, who is now behaviorally stable and making satisfactory progress in treatment. (Psychiatry)

Subsequent hospital visit for an 18-year-old male with uncomplicated asthma who is clinically stable. (Allergy & Immunology)

Subsequent hospital visit for a 55-year-old male with rheumatoid arthritis, two days following an uncomplicated total joint replacement. (Rheumatology)

Subsequent hospital visit for a 60-year-old dialysis patient with an access infection, now afebrile on antibiotic. (Nephrology)

Subsequent hospital visit for a 36-year-old female with stable post-rhinoplasty epistaxis. (Plastic Surgery)

Subsequent hospital visit for a 66-year-old female with L-2 vertebral compression fracture with resolving ileus. (Orthopaedic Surgery)

Subsequent hospital visit for a patient with peritonsillar abscess. (Otolaryngology, Head & Neck Surgery)

Subsequent hospital visit for an 18-year-old female responding to intravenous antibiotic therapy for ear or sinus infection. (Otolaryngology, Head & Neck Surgery)

Subsequent hospital visit for a 70-year-old male admitted with congestive heart failure who has responded to therapy. (Cardiology)

Follow-up hospital visit for a 32-year-old female with left ureteral calculus; being followed in anticipation of spontaneous passage. (Urology)

Subsequent hospital visit for a 4-year-old female, admitted for acute gastroenteritis and dehydration, requiring IV hydration; now stable. (Family Medicine)

Subsequent hospital visit for a 50-year-old Type II diabetic who is clinically stable and without complications requiring regulation of a single dose of insulin daily. (Endocrinology)

Subsequent hospital visit to reassesses the status of a 65-year-old patient post-open reduction and internal fixation of hip fracture, on the rehab unit. (Physical Medicine & Rehabilitation)

Subsequent hospital visit for a 78-year-old male with cholangiocarcinoma managed by biliary drainage. (Interventional Radiology)

Subsequent hospital visit for a 50-year-old male with uncomplicated myocardial infarction who is clinically stable and without chest pain. (Family Medicine/Cardiology/Internal Medicine)

Subsequent hospital visit for a stable 72-year-old lung cancer patient undergoing a five-day course of infusion chemotherapy. (Hematology/Oncology)

Subsequent hospital visit, two days post admission for a 65-year-old male with a CVA (cerebral vascular accident) and left hemiparesis, who is clinically stable. (Neurology/Physical Medicine and Rehabilitation)

Subsequent hospital visit for now stable, 33-year-old male, status post lower gastrointestinal bleeding. (General Surgery)

Subsequent visit on third day of hospitalization for a 60-year-old female recovering from an uncomplicated pneumonia. (Infectious Disease/Internal Medicine/Pulmonary Medicine)

Subsequent hospital visit for a 3-year-old patient in traction for a congenital dislocation of the hip. (Orthopaedic Surgery)

Subsequent hospital visit for a 4-year-old female, admitted for acute gastroenteritis and dehydration, requiring IV hydration; now stable. (Family Medicine/Internal Medicine)

Subsequent hospital visit for 50-year-old female with resolving uncomplicated acute pancreatitis. (Gastroenterology)

99232 Subsequent hospital visit for a patient with venous stasis ulcers who developed fever and red streaks adjacent to the ulcer. (Dermatology/Internal Medicine/Family Medicine)

Subsequent hospital visit for a 66-year-old male for dressing changes and observation. Patient has had a myocutaneous flap to close a pharyngeal fistula and now has a low-grade fever. (Plastic Surgery)

Subsequent hospital visit for a 54-year-old female admitted for myocardial infarction, but who is now having frequent premature ventricular contractions. (Internal Medicine)

Subsequent hospital visit for an 80-year-old patient with a pelvic rim fracture, inability to walk, and severe pain; now 36 hours post-injury, experiencing urinary retention. (Orthopaedic Surgery)

Subsequent hospital visit for a 17-year-old female with fever, pharyngitis, and airway obstruction, who after 48 hours develops a maculopapular rash. (Pediatrics/Family Medicine)

Follow-up hospital visit for a 32-year-old patient admitted the previous day for corneal ulcer. (Dermatology)

Follow-up visit for a 67-year-old male with congestive heart failure who has responded to antibiotics and diuretics, and has now developed a monoarthropathy. (Internal Medicine)

Follow-up hospital visit for a 58-year-old male receiving continuous opioids who is experiencing severe nausea and vomiting. (Pain Medicine)

Subsequent hospital visit for a patient after an auto accident who is slow to respond to ambulation training. (Physical Medicine & Rehabilitation)

Subsequent hospital visit for a 14-year-old with unstable bronchial asthma complicated by pneumonia. (Allergy & Immunology)

Subsequent hospital visit for a 50-year-old diabetic, hypertensive male with back pain not responding to conservative inpatient management with continued radiation of pain to the lower left extremity. (Orthopaedic Surgery)

Subsequent hospital visit for a 37-year-old female on day five of antibiotics for bacterial endocarditis, who still has low-grade fever. (Cardiology)

Subsequent hospital visit for a 54-year-old patient, post MI (myocardial infarction), who is out of the CCU (coronary care unit) but is now having frequent premature ventricular contractions on telemetry. (Cardiology/Internal Medicine)

Subsequent hospital visit for a patient with neutropenia, a fever responding to antibiotics, and continued slow gastrointestinal bleeding on platelet support. (Hematology/Oncology)

Subsequent hospital visit for a 50-year-old male admitted two days ago for sub-acute renal allograft rejection. (Nephrology)

Subsequent hospital visit for a 35-year-old drug addict, not responding to initial antibiotic therapy for pyelonephritis. (Urology)

Subsequent hospital visit of an 81-year-old male with abdominal distention, nausea, and vomiting. (General Surgery)

Subsequent hospital care for a 62-year-old female with congestive heart failure, who remains dyspneic and febrile. (Internal Medicine)

Subsequent hospital visit for a 73-year-old female with recently diagnosed lung cancer, who complains of unsteady gait. (Pulmonary Medicine)

Subsequent hospital visit for a 20-month-old male with bacterial meningitis treated one week with antibiotic therapy; has now developed a temperature of 101.0. (Pediatrics)

Subsequent hospital visit for 13-year-old male admitted with left lower quadrant abdominal pain and fever, not responding to therapy. (General Surgery)

Subsequent hospital visit for a 65-year-old male with hemiplegia and painful paretic shoulder. (Physical Medicine & Rehabilitation)

99233 Subsequent hospital visit for a 38-year-old male, quadriplegic with acute autonomic hyperreflexia, who is not responsive to initial care. (Physical Medicine & Rehabilitation)

Follow-up hospital visit for a teenage female who continues to experience severely disruptive, violent and life-threatening symptoms in a complicated multi-system illness. Family/social circumstances also a contributing factor. (Psychiatry)

Subsequent hospital visit for a 42-year-old female with progressive systemic sclerosis (scleroderma), renal failure on dialysis, congestive heart failure, cardiac arrhythmias, and digital ulcers. (Allergy & Immunology)

Subsequent hospital visit for a 50-year-old diabetic, hypertensive male with nonresponding back pain and radiating pain to the lower left extremity, who develops chest pain, cough, and bloody sputum. (Orthopaedic Surgery)

Subsequent hospital visit for a 64-year-old female, status post-abdominal aortic aneurysm resection, with non-responsive coagulopathy, who has now developed lower GI bleeding. (Abdominal Surgery/Colon & Rectal Surgery/General Surgery)

Follow-up hospital care of a patient with pansinusitis infection complicated by a brain abscess and asthma; no response to current treatment. (Otolaryngology, Head & Neck Surgery)

Subsequent hospital visit for a patient with a laryngeal neoplasm who develops airway compromise, suspected metastasis. (Otolaryngology, Head & Neck Surgery)

Subsequent hospital visit for a 49-year-old male with significant rectal bleeding, etiology undetermined, not responding to treatment. (Abdominal Surgery/General Surgery/Colon & Rectal Surgery)

Subsequent hospital visit for a 50-year-old male, post-aortocoronary bypass surgery; now develops hypotension and oliguria. (Cardiology)

Subsequent hospital visit for an adolescent patient who is violent, unsafe, and noncompliant, with multiple expectations for participation in treatment plan and behavior on the treatment unit. (Psychiatry)

Subsequent hospital visit for an 18-year-old male being treated for presumed PCP psychosis. Patient is still moderately symptomatic with auditory hallucinations and is insisting on signing out against medical advice. (Psychiatry)

Subsequent hospital visit for an 8-year-old female with caustic ingestion, who now has fever, dyspnea, and dropping hemoglobin. (Gastroenterology)

Follow-up hospital visit for a chronic renal failure patient on dialysis who develops chest pain and shortness of breath and a new onset pericardial friction rub. (Nephrology)

Subsequent hospital visit for a 44-year-old patient with electrical burns to the left arm with ascending infection. (Orthopaedic Surgery)

Subsequent hospital visit for a patient with systemic sclerosis who has aspirated and is short of breath. (Dermatology)

Subsequent hospital visit for a 65-year-old female, status post-op resection of abdominal aortic aneurysm, with suspected ischemic bowel. (General Surgery)

Subsequent hospital visit for a 50-year-old male, post-aortocoronary bypass surgery, now develops hypotension and oliguria. (Cardiology)

Subsequent hospital visit for a 65-year-old male, following an acute myocardial infarction, who complains of shortness of breath and new chest pain. (Cardiology)

Subsequent hospital visit for a 65-year-old female with rheumatoid arthritis (stage 3, class 3) admitted for urosepsis. On the third hospital day, chest pain, dyspnea and fever develop. (Rheumatology)

Follow-up hospital care of a pediatric case with stridor, laryngomalacia, established tracheostomy, complicated by multiple medical problems in PICU. (Otolaryngology, Head & Neck Surgery)

Subsequent hospital visit for a 60-year-old female, four days post uncomplicated inferior myocardial infarction who has developed severe chest pain, dyspnea, diaphoresis and nausea. (Family Medicine)

Subsequent hospital visit for a patient with AML (acute myelogenous leukemia), fever, elevated white count and uric acid undergoing induction chemotherapy. (Hematology/Oncology)

Subsequent hospital visit for a 38-year-old quadriplegic male with acute autonomic hyperreflexia, who is not responsive to initial care. (Physical Medicine & Rehabilitation)

Subsequent hospital visit for a 65-year-old female post-op resection of abdominal aortic aneurysm, with suspected ischemic bowel. (General Surgery)

Subsequent hospital visit for a 60-year-old female with persistent leukocytosis and a fever seven days after a sigmoid colon resection for carcinoma. (Infectious Disease)

Subsequent hospital visit for a chronic renal failure patient on dialysis, who develops chest pain, shortness of breath and new onset of pericardial friction rub. (Nephrology)

Subsequent hospital visit for a 65-year-old male with acute myocardial infarction who now demonstrates complete heart block and congestive heart failure. (Cardiology)

Subsequent hospital visit for a 25-year-old female with hypertension and systemic lupus erythematosus, admitted for fever and respiratory distress. On the third hospital day, the patient presented with purpuric skin lesions and acute renal failure. (Allergy & Immunology)

Subsequent hospital visit for a 55-year-old male with severe chronic obstructive pulmonary disease and bronchospasm; initially admitted for acute respiratory distress requiring ventilatory support in the ICU. The patient was stabilized, extubated and transferred to the floor, but has now developed acute fever, dyspnea, left lower lobe rhonchi and laboratory evidence of carbon dioxide retention and hypoxemia. (Family Medicine/Internal Medicine)

Subsequent hospital visit for 46-year-old female, known liver cirrhosis patient, with recent upper gastrointestinal hemorrhage from varices; now with worsening ascites and encephalopathy. (Gastroenterology)

Subsequent hospital visit for 62-year-old female admitted with acute subarachnoid hemorrhage, negative cerebral arteriogram, increased lethargy and hemiparesis with fever. (Neurosurgery)

Consultations

Office or Other Outpatient Consultations

New or Established Patient

99241 Initial office consultation for a 40-year-old female in pain from blister on lip following a cold. (Oral & Maxillofacial Surgery)

Initial office consultation for a 62-year-old construction worker with olecranon bursitis. (Orthopaedic Surgery)

Office consultation with 25-year-old postpartum female with severe symptomatic hemorrhoids. (Colon & Rectal Surgery)

Office consultation with 58-year-old male, referred for follow-up of creatinine level and evaluation of obstructive uropathy, relieved two months ago. (Nephrology)

Office consultation for 30-year-old female tennis player with sprain or contusion of the forearm. (Orthopaedic Surgery)

Office consultation for a 45-year-old male, requested by his internist, with asymptomatic torus palatinus requiring no further treatment. (Oral & Maxillofacial Surgery)

99242 Initial office consultation for a 20-year-old male with acute upper respiratory tract symptoms. (Allergy & Immunology)

Initial office consultation for a 29-year-old soccer player with painful proximal thigh/groin injury. (Orthopaedic Surgery)

Initial office consultation for a 66-year-old female with wrist and hand pain, numbness of finger tips, suspected median nerve compression by carpal tunnel syndrome. (Plastic Surgery)

Initial office consultation for a patient with a solitary lesion of discoid lupus erythematosus on left cheek to rule out malignancy or self-induced lesion. (Dermatology)

Office consultation for management of systolic hypertension in a 70-year-old male scheduled for elective prostate resection. (Geriatrics)

Office consultation with 27-year-old female, with old amputation, for evaluation of existing above-knee prosthesis. (Physical Medicine & Rehabilitation)

Office consultation with 66-year-old female with wrist and hand pain, and finger numbness, secondary to suspected carpal tunnel syndrome. (Orthopaedic Surgery)

Office consultation for 61-year-old female, recently on antibiotic therapy, now with diarrhea and leukocytosis. (Abdominal Surgery)

Office consultation for a patient with papulosquamous eruption of elbow with pitting of nails and itchy scalp. (Dermatology)

Office consultation for a 30 year old female with single season allergic rhinitis. (Allergy & Immunology)

99243 Initial office consultation for a 60-year-old male with avascular necrosis of the left femoral head with increasing pain. (Orthopaedic Surgery)

Office consultation for a 31-year-old woman complaining of palpitations and chest pains. Her internist had described a mild systolic click. (Cardiology)

Office consultation for a 65-year-old female with persistent bronchitis. (Infectious Disease)

Office consultation for a 65-year-old man with chronic low-back pain radiating to the leg. (Neurosurgery)

Office consultation for 23-year-old female with Crohn's disease not responding to therapy. (Abdominal Surgery/Colon & Rectal Surgery)

Office consultation for 25-year-old patient with symptomatic knee pain and swelling, with torn anterior cruciate ligament and/or torn meniscus. (Orthopaedic Surgery)

Office consultation for a 67-year-old patient with osteoporosis and mandibular atrophy with regard to reconstructive alternatives. (Oral & Maxillofacial Surgery)

Office consultation for 39-year-old patient referred at a perimenopausal age for irregular menses and menopausal symptoms. (Obstetrics & Gynecology)

99244 Initial office consultation for a 28-year-old male, HIV+, with a recent change in visual acuity. (Ophthalmology)

Initial office consultation for a 15-year-old male with failing grades, suspected drug abuse. (Pediatrics)

Initial office consultation for a 36-year-old factory worker, status four months post-occupational low back injury and requires management of intractable low back pain. (Pain Medicine)

Initial office consultation for a 45-year-old female with a history of chronic arthralgia of TMJ and associated myalgia and sudden progressive symptomatology over last two to three months. (Oral & Maxillofacial Surgery)

Initial office consultation for evaluation of a 70-year-old male with appetite loss and diminished energy. (Psychiatry)

Initial office consultation for an elementary school-aged patient, referred by pediatrician, with multiple systematic complaints and recent onset of behavioral discontrol. (Psychiatry)

Initial office consultation for a 23-year-old female with developmental facial skeletal anomaly and subsequent abnormal relationship of jaw(s) to cranial base. (Oral & Maxillofacial Surgery)

Initial office consultation for a 45-year-old myopic patient with a one-week history of floaters and a partial retinal detachment. (Ophthalmology)

Initial office consultation for a 65-year-old female with moderate dementia, mild unsteadiness, back pain fatigue on ambulation, intermittent urinary incontinence. (Neurosurgery)

Initial office consultation for a 33-year-old female referred by endocrinologist with amenorrhea and galactorrhea, for evaluation of pituitary tumor. (Neurosurgery)

Initial office consultation for a 34-year-old male with new onset nephrotic syndrome. (Nephrology)

Initial office consultation for a 39-year-old female with intractable chest wall pain secondary to metastatic breast cancer. (Anesthesiology/Pain Medicine)

Initial office consultation for a patient with multiple giant tumors of jaws. (Oral & Maxillofacial Surgery)

Initial office consultation for a patient with a failed total hip replacement with loosening and pain upon walking. (Orthopaedic Surgery)

Initial office consultation for a 60-year-old female with three-year history of intermittent tic-like unilateral facial pain; now constant pain for six weeks without relief by adequate carbamazepine dosage. (Neurosurgery)

Initial office consultation for a 45-year-old male heavy construction worker with prior lumbar disk surgery two years earlier; now gradually recurring low back and unilateral leg pain for three months, unable to work for two weeks. (Neurosurgery)

Initial office consultation of a patient who presents with a 30-year history of smoking and right neck mass. (Otolaryngology, Head & Neck Surgery)

Office consultation with 38-year-old female, with inflammatory bowel disease, who now presents with right lower quadrant pain and suspected intra-abdominal abscess. (General Surgery/Colon & Rectal Surgery)

Office consultation with 72-year-old male with esophageal carcinoma, symptoms of dysphagia and reflux. (Thoracic Surgery)

Office consultation for discussion of treatment options for a 40-year-old female with a two-centimeter adenocarcinoma of the breast. (Radiation Oncology)

Office consultation for young patient referred by pediatrician because of patient's short attention span, easy distractibility and hyperactivity. (Psychiatry)

Office consultation for 66-year-old female, history of colon resection for adenocarcinoma six years earlier, now with severe mid-back pain; x-rays showing osteoporosis and multiple vertebral compression fractures. (Neurosurgery)

Office consultation for a patient with chronic pelvic inflammatory disease who now has left lower quadrant pain with a palpable pelvic mass. (Obstetrics & Gynecology)

Office consultation for a patient with long-standing psoriasis with acute onset of erythroderma, pustular lesions, chills and fever. Combinations of topical and systemic treatments discussed and instituted. (Dermatology)

99245 Initial office consultation for a 35-year-old multiple-trauma male patient with complex pelvic fractures, for evaluation and formulation of management plan. (Orthopaedic Surgery)

Initial emergency room consultation for 10-year-old male in status epilepticus, recent closed head injury, information about medication not available. (Neurosurgery)

Initial emergency room consultation for a 23-year-old patient with severe abdominal pain, guarding, febrile, and unstable vital signs. (Obstetrics & Gynecology)

Office consultation for a 67-year-old female longstanding uncontrolled diabetic who presents with retinopathy, nephropathy, and a foot ulcer. (Endocrinology)

Office consultation for a 37-year-old male for initial evaluation and management of Cushing's disease. (Endocrinology)

Office consultation for a 60-year-old male who presents with thyrotoxicosis, exophthalmos, frequent premature ventricular contractions and congestive heart failure. (Endocrinology)

Initial office consultation for a 36-year-old patient, one year status post occupational herniated cervical disk treated by laminectomy, requiring management of multiple sites of intractable pain, depression, and narcotic dependence. (Pain Medicine)

Office consultation for a 58-year-old man with a history of MI and CHF who complains of the recent onset of rest angina and shortness of breath. The patient has a systolic blood pressure of 90mmHG and is in Class IV heart failure. (Cardiology)

Emergency room consultation for a 1-year-old with a three-day history of fever with increasing respiratory distress who is thought to have cardiac tamponade by the ER physician. (Cardiology)

Office consultation in the emergency room for a 25-year-old male with severe, acute, closed head injury. (Neurosurgery)

Office consultation for a 23-year-old female with Stage II A Hodgkins disease with positive supraclavicular and mediastinal nodes. (Radiation Oncology)

Office consultation for a 27-year-old juvenile diabetic patient with severe diabetic retinopathy, gastric atony, nephrotic syndrome and progressive renal failure, now with a serum creatinine of 2.7, and a blood pressure of 170/114. (Nephrology)

Office consultation for independent medical evaluation of a patient with a history of complicated low back and neck problems with previous multiple failed back surgeries. (Orthopaedic Surgery)

Office consultation for an adolescent referred by pediatrician for recent onset of violent and self-injurious behavior. (Psychiatry)

Office consultation for a 6-year-old male for evaluation of severe muscle and joint pain and a diffuse rash. Patient well until 4-6 weeks earlier, when he developed arthralgia, myalgias, and a fever of 102 for one week. (Rheumatology)

Initial Inpatient Consultations

New or Established Patient

99251 Initial hospital consultation for a 27-year-old female with fractured incisor post-intubation. (Oral & Maxillofacial Surgery)

Initial hospital consultation for an orthopaedic patient on IV antibiotics who has developed an apparent candida infection of the oral cavity. (Oral & Maxillofacial Surgery)

Initial inpatient consultation for a 30-year-old female complaining of vaginal itching, post orthopaedic surgery. (Obstetrics & Gynecology)

Initial inpatient consultation for a 36-year-old male on orthopaedic service with complaint of localized dental pain. (Oral & Maxillofacial Surgery)

99252 Initial hospital consultation for a 45-year-old male, previously abstinent alcoholic, who relapsed and was admitted for management of gastritis. The patient readily accepts the need for further treatment. (Addiction Medicine)

Initial hospital consultation for a 35-year-old dialysis patient with episodic oral ulcerations. (Oral & Maxillofacial Surgery)

Initial inpatient preoperative consultation for a 43-year-old woman with cholecystitis and well-controlled hypertension. (Cardiology)

Initial inpatient consultation for recommendation of antibiotic prophylaxis for a patient with a synthetic heart valve who will undergo urologic surgery. (Internal Medicine)

Initial inpatient consultation for possible drug induced skin eruption in 50-year-old male. (Dermatology)

Preoperative inpatient consultation for evaluation of hypertension in a 60-year-old male who will undergo a cholecystectomy. Patient had a normal annual check-up in your office four months ago. (Internal Medicine)

Initial inpatient consultation for 66-year-old patient with wrist and hand pain and finger numbness, secondary to carpal tunnel syndrome. (Orthopaedic Surgery/Plastic Surgery)

Initial inpatient consultation for a 66-year-old male smoker referred for pain management immediately status post-biliary tract surgery done via sub-costal incision. (Anesthesiology/Pain Medicine)

99253 Initial hospital consultation for a 50-year-old female with incapacitating knee pain due to generalized rheumatoid arthritis. (Orthopaedic Surgery)

Initial hospital consultation for a 60-year-old male with avascular necrosis of the left femoral heel with increasing pain. (Orthopaedic Surgery)

Initial hospital consultation for a 45-year-old female with compound mandibular fracture and concurrent head, abdominal and/or orthopaedic injuries. (Oral & Maxillofacial Surgery)

Initial hospital consultation for a 22-year-old female, paraplegic, to evaluate wrist and hand pain. (Orthopaedic Surgery)

Initial hospital consultation for a 40-year-old male with 10-day history of incapacitating unilateral sciatica, unable to walk now, not improved by bed rest. (Neurosurgery)

Initial hospital consultation, requested by pediatrician, for treatment recommendations for a patient admitted with persistent inability to walk following soft tissue injury to ankle. (Physiatry)

Initial hospital consultation for a 27-year-old previously healthy male who vomited during IV sedation and may have aspirated gastric contents. (Anesthesiology)

Initial hospital consultation for a 33-year-old female, post-abdominal surgery, who now has a fever. (Internal Medicine)

Initial inpatient consultation for a 57-year-old male, post lower endoscopy, for evaluation of abdominal pain and fever. (General Surgery)

Initial inpatient consultation for rehabilitation of a 73-year-old female one week after surgical management of a hip fracture. (Physical Medicine & Rehabilitation)

Initial inpatient consultation for diagnosis/management of fever following abdominal surgery. (Internal Medicine)

Initial inpatient consultation for a 35-year-old female with a fever and pulmonary infiltrate following cesarean section. (Pulmonary Medicine)

Initial inpatient consultation for a 42-year-old non-diabetic patient, post-op cholecystectomy, now with an acute urinary tract infection. (Nephrology)

Initial inpatient consultation for 53-year-old female with moderate uncomplicated pancreatitis. (Gastroenterology)

Initial inpatient consultation for 45-year-old patient with chronic neck pain with radicular pain of the left arm. (Orthopaedic Surgery)

Initial inpatient consultation for 8-year-old patient with new onset of seizures who has a normal examination and previous history. (Neurology)

99254 Initial hospital consultation for a 15-year-old patient with painless swelling of proximal humerus with lytic lesion by x-ray. (Orthopaedic Surgery)

Initial hospital consultation for evaluation of a 29-year-old female with a diffusely positive medical review of systems and history of multiple surgeries. (Psychiatry)

Initial hospital consultation for a 70-year-old diabetic female with gangrene of the foot. (Orthopaedic Surgery)

Initial inpatient consultation for a 47-year-old female with progressive pulmonary infiltrate, hypoxemia, and diminished urine output. (Anesthesiology)

Initial hospital consultation for a 13-month-old with spasmodic cough, respiratory distress, and fever. (Allergy & Immunology)

Initial hospital consultation for a patient with failed total hip replacement with loosening and pain upon walking. (Orthopaedic Surgery)

Initial hospital consultation for a 62-year-old female with metastatic breast cancer to the femoral neck and thoracic vertebra. (Orthopaedic Surgery)

Initial hospital consultation for a 39-year-old female with nephrolithiasis requiring extensive opioid analgesics, whose vital signs are now elevated. She initially denied any drug use, but today gives history of multiple substance abuse, including opioids and prior treatment for a personality disorder. (Psychiatry)

Initial hospital consultation for a 70-year-old female without previous psychiatric history, who is now experiencing nocturnal confusion and visual hallucinations following hip replacement surgery. (Psychiatry)

Initial inpatient consultation for evaluation of a 63-year-old in the ICU with diabetes and chronic renal failure who develops acute respiratory distress syndrome 36 hours after a mitral valve replacement. (Anesthesiology)

Initial inpatient consultation for a 66-year-old female with enlarged supraclavicular lymph nodes, found on biopsy to be malignant. (Hematology/Oncology)

Initial inpatient consultation for a 43-year-old female for evaluation of sudden painful visual loss, optic neuritis and episodic paresthesia. (Ophthalmology)

Initial inpatient consultation for evaluation of a 71-year-old male with hyponatremia (serum sodium 114) who was admitted to the hospital with pneumonia. (Nephrology)

Initial inpatient consultation for a 72-year-old male with emergency admission for possible bowel obstruction. (Internal Medicine/General Surgery)

Initial inpatient consultation for a 35-year-old female with fever, swollen joints, and rash of one-week duration. (Rheumatology)

99255 Initial inpatient consultation for a 76-year-old female with massive, life-threatening gastrointestinal hemorrhage and chest pain. (Gastroenterology)

Initial inpatient consultation for a 75-year-old female, admitted to intensive care with acute respiratory distress syndrome, who is hypersensitive, has a moderate metabolic acidosis, and a rising serum creatinine. (Nephrology)

Initial hospital consultation for patient with a history of complicated low back pain and neck problems with previous multiple failed back surgeries. (Orthopaedic Surgery/Neurosurgery)

Initial hospital consultation for a 66-year-old female, two days post-abdominal aneurysm repair, with oliguria and hypertension of one-day duration. (Nephrology/Internal Medicine)

Initial hospital consultation for a patient with shotgun wound to face with massive facial trauma and airway obstruction. (Oral & Maxillofacial Surgery)

Initial hospital consultation for patient with severe pancreatitis complicated by respiratory insufficiency, acute renal failure, and abscess formation. (General Surgery/Colon & Rectal Surgery)

Initial hospital consultation for a 35-year-old multiple-trauma male patient with complex pelvic fractures to evaluate and formulate management plan. (Orthopaedic Surgery)

Initial inpatient consultation for adolescent patient with fractured femur and pelvis who pulled out IVs and disconnected traction in attempt to elope from hospital. (Psychiatry)

Initial hospital consultation for a 16-year-old primigravida at 32 weeks gestation requested by a family practitioner for evaluation of severe hypertension, thrombocytopenia, and headache. (Obstetrics & Gynecology)

Initial hospital consultation for a 58-year-old insulin-dependent diabetic with multiple antibiotic allergies, now with multiple fascial plane abscesses and airway obstruction. (Oral & Maxillofacial Surgery)

Initial inpatient consultation for a 55-year-old male with known cirrhosis and ascites, now with jaundice, encephalopathy, and massive hematemesis. (Gastroenterology)

Initial hospital consultation for a 25-year-old male, seen in emergency room with severe, closed head injury. (Neurosurgery)

Initial hospital consultation for a 2-day-old male with single ventricle physiology and subaortic obstruction. Family counseling following evaluation for multiple, staged surgical procedures. (Thoracic Surgery)

Initial hospital consultation for a 45-year-old male admitted with subarachnoid hemorrhage and intracranial aneurysm on angiogram. (Neurosurgery)

Initial inpatient consultation for myxedematous patient who is hypoventilating and obtunded. (Endocrinology)

Initial hospital consultation for a 45-year-old patient with widely metastatic lung carcinoma, intractable back pain, and a history that includes substance dependence, NSAID allergy, and two prior laminectomies with fusion for low back pain. (Pain Medicine)

Initial hospital consultation for evaluation of treatment options in a 50-year-old patient with cirrhosis, known peptic ulcer disease, hypotension, encephalopathy, and massive acute upper gastrointestinal bleeding which cannot be localized by endoscopy. (Interventional Radiology)

Initial inpatient consultation in the ICU for a 70-year-old male who experienced a cardiac arrest during surgery and was resuscitated. (Cardiology)

Initial inpatient consultation for a patient with severe pancreatitis complicated by respiratory insufficiency, acute renal failure and abscess formation. (Gastroenterology)

Initial inpatient consultation for a 70-year-old cirrhotic male admitted with ascites, jaundice, encephalopathy, and massive hematemesis. (Gastroenterology)

Initial inpatient consultation in the ICU for a 51-year-old patient who is on a ventilator and has a fever two weeks after a renal transplantation. (Infectious Disease)

Initial inpatient consultation for evaluation and formulation of plan for management of multiple trauma patient with complex pelvic fracture, 35-year-old male. (General Surgery/Orthopaedic Surgery)

Initial inpatient consultation for a 50-year-old male with a history of previous myocardial infarction, now with acute pulmonary edema and hypotension. (Cardiology)

Initial inpatient consultation for 45-year-old male with recent, acute subarachnoid hemorrhage, hesitant speech, mildly confused, drowsy. High risk group for HIV+ status. (Neurosurgery)

Initial inpatient consultation for 36-year-old female referred by her internist to evaluate a patient being followed for abdominal pain and fever. The patient has developed diffuse abdominal pain, guarding, rigidity and increased fever. (Obstetrics & Gynecology)

Follow-up Inpatient Consultations

Established Patient

99261 Follow-up consultation for a 78-year-old female nursing home resident for evaluation of medical management of pruritus ani. (Colon & Rectal Surgery/Geriatrics/General Surgery)

Follow-up hospital consultation on first post-op day for a 64-year-old male who has undergone uneventful CABG. (Anesthesiology)

Follow-up inpatient consultation for a 67-year-old female admitted several days ago for bleeding ulcer; now stable. (Gastroenterology)

Follow-up hospital consultation for a 35-year-old female with history of mitral valve prolapse. (Cardiology)

Follow-up inpatient consultation to complete initial consultation for dental pain after review of radiographs. (Oral & Maxillofacial Surgery)

Follow-up inpatient consultation for evaluation of response to therapy for moniliasis. (Oral & Maxillofacial Surgery)

Follow-up inpatient consultation for a 22-year-old female with recurrent aphthous ulcers. (Oral & Maxillofacial Surgery)

Follow-up hospital consultation for a 37-year-old female to complete review of previously unavailable studies. (Therapeutic Radiology & Oncology)

Follow-up consultation for a highly functional 75-year-old female with urinary incontinence to review preliminary results of diagnostic evaluation. (Geriatrics)

Follow-up inpatient consultation for a 1-week-old premature female with patent ductus arteriosus. The murmur has disappeared. (Cardiology)

Follow-up hospital consultation to review the results of an audiogram. (Otolaryngology, Head & Neck Surgery)

Follow-up inpatient consultation with 35-year-old female with pulmonary embolism post-op cesarean section, now stable, for assessment of response to anticoagulation and recommended adjustment of heparin dose. (Pulmonary Medicine)

Follow-up inpatient consultation for a 74-year-old male whose postoperative facial paralysis after a cholecystectomy is now resolving. (Neurology)

Follow-up inpatient consultation with 67-year-old female, established patient, for review of diagnostic studies ordered at time of first contact. (Internal Medicine)

Follow-up inpatient consultation for 78-year-old female nursing home resident for evaluation of medical management of pruritis ani. (General Surgery/Colon & Rectal Surgery)

Follow-up inpatient consultation for a 36-year-old female two days after spontaneous passage of 3mm stone. (Urology)

Follow-up inpatient consultation for a 94-year-old male nursing home resident for re-evaluation of hemorrhoids following conservative therapy. (Colon & Rectal Surgery/General Surgery/Geriatrics)

Follow-up inpatient consultation for a 50-year-old male, asymptomatic with borderline ECG abnormality, needs preoperative opinion after a thallium exercise perfusion scan. (Cardiology)

99262 Follow-up inpatient consultation for a 6-year-old female, established patient, with endocarditis and changing heart murmur. (Cardiology)

Follow-up inpatient consultation on a 2-year-old male, one day postoperative ventricular septal defect closure with signs of tachycardia. (Cardiology)

Follow-up inpatient consultation for a 63-year-old man, established patient, with moderately severe pulmonary insufficiency, 10 days postoperative coronary artery bypass for unstable angina. Patient has developed severe dyspnea, fever, and a new exudative right pleural effusion. (Cardiology)

Follow-up inpatient consultation for a 67-year-old woman with lung cancer and syndrome of inappropriate secretion of antidiuretic hormone (SIADH) who has had a seizure following intravenous saline. (Endocrinology)

Follow-up inpatient consultation for a 22-year-old female, established patient, with steroid-dependent systemic lupus erythematosus, arthritis, and glomerulonephritis. Patient is re-evaluated for loss of consciousness and chest pain. (Rheumatology)

Follow-up inpatient consultation for a 75-year-old diabetic with fever, chills, a gangrenous heel ulcer, rhonchi, and dyspnea who appears lethargic and tachypneic. (Endocrinology)

Follow-up inpatient consultation for a 30-year-old, established patient, with intractable neck and low back pain, who is excessively sedated after institution of methadone therapy. (Pain Medicine)

Follow-up inpatient consultation for a 65-year-old man with a history of hypertension and MI who is five days post uncomplicated GI procedure with an unremarkable postoperative recovery. He has just been resuscitated from a cardiopulmonary arrest. (Cardiology)

Follow-up inpatient consultation with 72-year-old female, established patient with bullous pemphigoid on combined oral therapy steroids and immunosuppressive to evaluate progress of cutaneous care orders and adjustment of oral/parenteral therapy dosages. (Dermatology)

Follow-up inpatient consultation for a 71-year-old male who has developed a maculopapular skin rash while on antibiotics recommended for an uncomplicated pneumonia. (Infectious Disease)

Follow-up inpatient consultation with 68-year-old, incapacitated male with spinal stenosis and failure to respond to bedrest, analgesics, and PT. (Neurosurgery)

Follow-up inpatient consultation with 51-year-old male for evaluation and determination of the etiology of postoperative hyponatremia following TURP. (Family Medicine)

Follow-up inpatient consultation for re-evaluation of a stroke patient, and development of plan for initial rehabilitation services. (Neurology)

Follow-up inpatient consultation with 45-year-old male, established patient for discussion of CT scan which demonstrates a cavernous hemangioma. (Ophthalmology)

Follow-up inpatient consultation for an asymptomatic 35-year-old Type I diabetic patient with hyperkalemic, hyperchloremia acidosis, to review lab results. (Nephrology)

Follow-up inpatient consultation for an elderly male with a perioperative myocardial infarction requiring adjustment of vasoactive medications. (Anesthesiology)

99263 Follow-up hospital consultation of an AIDS patient admitted with a sore throat who now has enlarging neck mass. (Otolaryngology, Head & Neck Surgery)

Follow-up hospital consultation of a pansinusitis patient with sudden onset of proptosis. (Otolaryngology, Head & Neck Surgery)

Follow-up inpatient consultation for a 53-year-old man with known angina who develops crescendo angina post cholecystectomy. (Cardiology)

Follow-up inpatient consultation with 72-year-old male established patient admitted for management of alcohol withdrawal, now confused and febrile. (Addiction Medicine)

Follow-up inpatient consultation for an HIV+ patient with an increasing fever following 10 days of antibiotic therapy for pneumocystis carinii pneumonia. (Infectious Disease)

Follow-up inpatient consultation with 58-year-old diabetic female, with bacterial endocarditis, continued fever after two weeks of intravenous antibiotic therapy, and new onset ventricular ectopia. (Cardiology)

Follow-up inpatient consultation for a 90-year-old female with urinary incontinence who has a complicated medical history requiring reassessment of multiple medical problems, recommendations for placement, further recommendation for management of incontinence and reevaluation of cognitive status because of competency issues. (Geriatrics/Psychiatry)

Follow-up inpatient consultation for 42-year-old male with persistent gastrointestinal bleeding, etiology undetermined, not responding to conservative therapy of transfusions. (General Surgery/Colon & Rectal Surgery)

Follow-up inpatient consultation for a 62-year-old female with steroid-dependent asthma, diabetes mellitus, thyrotoxicosis, abdominal pain and possible vasculitis. (Rheumatology)

Follow-up inpatient consultation for a 62-year-old male, status post-op acute small bowel obstruction; now with acute renal failure. (Family Medicine)

Emergency Department Services

New or Established Patient

99281 Emergency department visit for a patient for removal of sutures from a well-healed, uncomplicated laceration. (Emergency Medicine)

Emergency department visit for a patient for tetanus toxoid immunization. (Emergency Medicine)

Emergency department visit for a patient with several uncomplicated insect bites. (Emergency Medicine)

99282 Emergency department visit for a 20-year-old student who presents with a painful sunburn with blister formation on the back. (Emergency Medicine)

Emergency department visit for a child presenting with impetigo localized to the face. (Emergency Medicine)

Emergency department visit for a patient with a minor traumatic injury of an extremity with localized pain, swelling, and bruising. (Emergency Medicine)

Emergency department visit for an otherwise healthy patient whose chief complaint is a red, swollen cystic lesion on his/her back. (Emergency Medicine)

Emergency department visit for a patient presenting with a rash on both legs after exposure to poison ivy. (Emergency Medicine)

Emergency department visit for a young adult patient with infected sclera and purulent discharge from both eyes without pain, visual disturbance or history of foreign body in either eye. (Emergency Medicine)

99283 Emergency department visit for a sexually active female complaining of vaginal discharge who is afebrile and denies experiencing abdominal or back pain. (Emergency Medicine)

Emergency department visit for a well-appearing 8-year-old who has a fever, diarrhea and abdominal cramps, is tolerating oral fluids and is not vomiting. (Emergency Medicine)

Emergency department visit for a patient with an inversion ankle injury, who is unable to bear weight on the injured foot and ankle. (Emergency Medicine)

Emergency department visit for a patient who has a complaint of acute pain associated with a suspected foreign body in the painful eye. (Emergency Medicine)

Emergency department visit for a healthy, young adult patient who sustained a blunt head injury with local swelling and bruising without subsequent confusion, loss of consciousness or memory deficit. (Emergency Medicine)

99284 Emergency department visit for a 4-year-old who fell off a bike sustaining a head injury with brief loss of consciousness. (Emergency Medicine)

Emergency department visit for an elderly female who has fallen and is now complaining of pain in her right hip and is unable to walk. (Emergency Medicine)

Emergency department visit for a patient with flank pain and hematuria. (Emergency Medicine)

Emergency department visit for a female presenting with lower abdominal pain and a vaginal discharge. (Emergency Medicine)

99285 Emergency department visit for a patient with a complicated overdose requiring aggressive management to prevent side effects from the ingested materials. (Emergency Medicine)

Emergency department visit for a patient with a new onset of rapid heart rate requiring IV drugs. (Emergency Medicine)

Emergency department visit for a patient exhibiting active, upper gastrointestinal bleeding. (Emergency Medicine)

Emergency department visit for a previously healthy young adult patient who is injured in an automobile accident and is brought to the emergency department immobilized and has symptoms compatible with intra-abdominal injuries or multiple extremity injuries. (Emergency Medicine)

Emergency department visit for a patient with an acute onset of chest pain compatible with symptoms of cardiac ischemia and/or pulmonary embolus. (Emergency Medicine)

Emergency department visit for a patient who presents with a sudden onset of "the worst headache of her life," and complains of a stiff neck, nausea, and inability to concentrate. (Emergency Medicine)

Emergency department visit for a patient with a new onset of a cerebral vascular accident. (Emergency Medicine)

Emergency department visit for acute febrile illness in an adult, associated with shortness of breath and an altered level of alertness. (Emergency Medicine)

Critical Care Services

99291 First hour of critical care of a 65-year-old man with septic shock following relief of ureteral obstruction caused by a stone.

First hour of critical care of a 15-year-old with acute respiratory failure from asthma.

First hour of critical care of a 45-year-old who sustained a liver laceration, cerebral hematoma, flailed chest, and pulmonary contusion after being struck by an automobile.

First hour of critical care of a 65-year-old woman who, following a hysterectomy, suffered a cardiac arrest associated with a pulmonary embolus.

First hour of critical care of a 6-month-old with hypovolemic shock secondary to diarrhea and dehydration.

First hour of critical care of a 3-year-old with respiratory failure secondary to pneumocystis carinii pneumonia.

Comprehensive Nursing Facility Assessments

New or Established Patient

99301 Annual nursing facility history and physical and MDS/RAI evaluation for a two-year nursing facility resident who is an 84-year-old female with multiple chronic health problems, including: stable controlled hypertension, chronic constipation, osteoarthritis, and moderated stable dementia.

Nursing facility visit for an assessment of a resident with non-insulin dependent diabetes, stable angina, and chronic obstructive pulmonary disease (COPD) one year after previous MDS/RAI.

99302 Nursing facility visit one year after previous MDS/RAI to assess an 80-year-old woman with Parkinson's disease, chronic hypertension, and degenerative arthritis. Visit reveals Stage II decubitus.

Nursing facility assessment of a 28-year-old diabetic, male resident with a new Stage IV pressure ulcer on his left lateral malleolus that is unresponsive to treatment, thus triggering the need for a new MDS/RAI and new medical plan of care.

Nursing facility assessment of an 88-year-old male resident with a permanent change in status following a new cerebral vascular accident (CVA) that has triggered the need for a new MDS/RAI and medical plan of care.

Nursing facility visit and assessment to take over the primary care of a 75-year-old diabetic, previously stable, who was on oral hypoglycemic agents, but who now requires initiation of insulin therapy, a new MDS/RAI, and medical plan of care.

Nursing facility visit and assessment for an 81-year-old female resident with dementia, who, under structured guidance and intensive nutritional support has regained significant levels of function in three activities of daily living and is now able to feed and dress herself and ambulate with appliance and who now thus requires a new MDS/RAI and medical plan of care.

99303 Initial nursing facility assessment (MDS/RAI and medical plan of care) of a 72-year-old insulin dependent diabetic amputee with hearing and visual impairments and possible dementia seen in the office the day before and judged to require nursing facility care.

Sub-acute nursing facility assessment of a previously independently living 90-year-old male who suffered a recent cerebral vascular accident (CVA) and is transferred to the hospital sub-acute rehabilitation unit for further rehabilitation supportive services.

Initial nursing facility visit to evaluate a 72-year-old woman found confused and wandering, admitted by Adult Protective Services without a qualifying hospital stay or inpatient diagnostic work. The patient lives alone and has no relatives or significant others in the community.

Nursing facility assessment and creation of medical plan of care upon readmission to the nursing facility of an 82-year-old male who was previously discharged. The patient has just been discharged from the hospital where he had been treated for an acute gastric ulcer bleed associated with transient delirium. The patient returns to the nursing facility debilitated, protein depleted, and with a Stage III coccygeal decubitus.

Subsequent Nursing Facility Care

New or Established Patient

99311 Scheduled follow-up visit for a known 70-year-old stable paraplegic with no status change noted during visit.

Scheduled monthly nursing home visit with a patient who has mild senile dementia, Alzheimers' type, with no change in status, stable hypertension, and who is ambulating with a walker one year past stroke.

Follow-up in skilled nursing facility with a 70-year-old patient following a 10-day treatment of a cellulitis of the foot.

99312 Scheduled follow-up visit to a resident with controlled dementia, hypertension, and diabetes. During visit, patient seems to exhibit flu symptoms.

Scheduled nursing facility visit with an afebrile demented resident who also has a mild cough, requiring no change in the medical plan of care.

Subsequent visit in a skilled nursing facility with a patient who is six months post stroke and now has a fever and mild cough.

Scheduled nursing facility visit for an 84-year-old male with chronic renal insufficiency, on digitalis and diuretics, requiring adjustment of medications and revision of medical plan of care.

Nursing facility visit of a resident with multiple chronic health problems who is six months post stroke and now has a fever and mild cough, to evaluate for possible pneumonia. Requires the development of a new medical plan of care, but not a revised MDS/RAI.

99313 Follow-up nursing facility visit to evaluate the reason for frequent falls by a 90-year-old ataxic resident, and to determine possible need for change in medications and medical care plan.

Re-admission of a 75-year-old man with stroke who was hospitalized with pneumonia for his illness and who returns to the nursing facility with no permanent change in status from his condition prior to hospitalization; no new MDS/RAI is required.

Nursing facility visit with a diabetic resident who has developed Stage II decubitus ulcers with cellulitis, requiring a revision in the medical plan of care.

Nursing facility visit to develop a new plan of care for an amputee with atherosclerosis obliterans who has refused to eat for three days and has developed decreased urinary output.

Nursing facility visit for a 78-year-old resident with chronic atrial fibrillation and a history of heart failure to evaluate an acute confusional state and to revise the medical plan of care.

Unscheduled nursing facility visit for evaluation of a patient with fever and obtundation who is determined not to require hospital admission or new MDS, but who does require workup and revision of medical plan of care.

Prolonged Services

Prolonged Physician Service With Direct (Face-to-Face) Patient Contact

Office or Other Outpatient

99354/ 99355 A 20-year-old female with history of asthma presents with acute bronchospasm and moderate respiratory distress. Initial evaluation shows respiratory rate 30, labored breathing and wheezing heard in all lung fields. Office treatment is initiated which includes intermittent bronchial dilation and subcutaneous epinephrine. Requires intermittent physician face-to-face time with patient over a period of 2-3 hours. (Family Medicine/Internal Medicine)

Inpatient

99356 A 34-year-old primigravida presents to hospital in early labor. Admission history and physical reveals severe preeclampsia. Physician supervises management of preeclampsia, IV magnesium initiation and maintenance, labor augmentation with pitocin, and close maternal-fetal monitoring. Physician face-to-face involvement includes 40 minutes of continuous bedside care until the patient is stable, then is intermittent over several hours until the delivery. (Family Medicine/Internal Medicine/Obstetrics & Gynecology)

Prolonged Physician Service Without Direct Patient (Face-to-Face) Contact

99358/ 99359 A 65-year-old new patient with multiple problems is seen and evaluated. After the visit, the physician requires extensive time to talk with the patient's daughter, to review complex, detailed medical records transferred from previous physicians and to complete a comprehensive treatment plan. This plan also requires the physician to personally initiate and coordinate the care plan with a local home health agency and a dietician. (Family Medicine/Internal Medicine)

Physician Standby Services

99360 A 24-year-old patient is admitted to OB unit attempting VBAC. Fetal monitoring shows increasing fetal distress. Patient's blood pressure is rising and labor progressing slowly. A primary care physician is requested by the OB/GYN to standby in the unit for possible cesarean delivery and neonatal resuscitation. (Family Medicine/Internal Medicine)

Care Plan Oversight Services

99375 First month of care plan oversight for terminal care of a 58-year-old woman with advanced intraabdominal ovarian cancer. Care plan includes home oxygen, diuretics IV for edema and ascites control and pain control management involving IV morphine infusion when progressive ileus occurred. Physician phone contacts with nurse, family, and MSW. Discussion with MSW concerning plans to withdraw supportive measures per patient wishes. Documentation includes review and modification of care plan and certifications from nursing, MSW, pharmacy, and DME. (Family Medicine/Internal Medicine)

Appendix D

Summary of CPT Add-on Codes

This listing is a summary of CPT add-on codes for *CPT 2005*. The codes listed below are identified in *CPT 2005* with a ✚ symbol.

01953
01968
01969
11001
11008
11101
11201
11732
11922
13102
13122
13133
13153
15001
15101
15121
15201
15221
15241
15261
15343
15351
15401
15787
16036
17003
17310
19001
19126
19291
19295
19297
22103
22116
22216
22226
22328
22522
22534
22585
22614
22632
26125
26861
26863
27358
27692
31620
31632
31633
31637
32501
33141
33225
33508
33530
33572
33924
33961
34808
34813
34826
35390
35400
35500
35572
35681
35682
35683
35685
35686
35697
35700
36218
36248
36476
36479
37206
37208
37250
37251
38102
38746
38747
43635
44015
44121
44128
44139
44203
44701
44955
47001
47550
48400
49568
49905
56606
57267
58611
59525
60512
61316
61517
61609
61610
61611
61612
61795
61864
61868
62148
62160
63035
63043
63044
63048
63057
63066
63076
63078
63082
63086
63088
63091
63103
63295
63308
64472
64476
64480
64484
64623
64627
64727
64778
64783
64787
64832
64837
64859
64872
64874
64876
64901
64902
66990
67225
67320
67331
67332
67334
67335
67340
69990
74301
75774
75946
75964
75968
75993
75996
75998
76082
76083
76125
76802
76810
76812
76937
78020
78478
78480
78496
87187
87904
88141
88155
88185
88311
88312
88313
88314
90466
90468
90472
90474
90781
92547
92608
92973
92974
92978
92979
92981
92984
92996
92998
93320
93321
93325
93571
93572
93609
93613
93621
93622
93623
93662
95920
95962
95967
95973
95975
95979
96412
96423
96570
96571
97546
97811
97814
99100
99116
99135
99140
99290
99292
99354
99355
99356
99357
99358
99359
99602
0036T
0049T
0054T
0055T
0056T
0063T
0068T
0069T
0070T
0076T
0079T
0081T

Appendix E

Summary of CPT Codes Exempt from Modifier 51

This listing is a summary of CPT codes that are exempt from the use of modifier 51 but have NOT been designated as CPT add-on procedures/services. The codes listed below are identified in *CPT 2005* with a ⊘ symbol.

17004
17304
17305
17306
17307
20660
20690
20692
20900
20902
20910
20912
20920
20922
20924
20926
20930
20931
20936
20937
20938
20974
20975
22840
22841
22842
22843
22844
22845
22846
22847
22848
22851
31500
32000
32002
32020
33517
33518
33519
33521
33522
33523
35600
36620
36660
38792
44500
44720
44721
47146
47147
48552
50327
50328
50329
61107
61210
62284
90281
90283
90287
90288
90291
90296
90371
90375
90376
90378
90379
90384
90385
90386
90389
90393
90396
90399
90476
90477
90581
90585
90586
90632
90633
90634
90636
90645
90646
90647
90648
90655
90656
90657
90658
90660
90665
90669
90675
90676
90680
90690
90691
90692
90693
90698
90700
90701
90702
90703
90704
90705
90706
90707
90708
90710
90712
90713
90715
90716
90717
90718
90719
90720
90721
90723
90725
90727
90732
90733
90734
90735
90740
90743
90744
90746
90747
90748
90749
93501
93503
93505
93508
93510
93511
93514
93524
93526
93527
93528
93529
93530
93531
93532
93533
93539
93540
93541
93542
93543
93544
93545
93555
93556
93600
93602
93603
93610
93612
93615
93616
93618
93619
93620
93624
93631
93640
93641
93642
93650
93651
93652
93660
95900
95903
95904
99141
99142

Appendix F

Summary of CPT Codes Exempt from Modifier 63

The listing is a summary of CPT codes that are exempt from the use of modifier 63. The codes listed below are additionally identified in *CPT 2005* with the parenthetical instruction "(Do not report modifier 63 in conjunction with ...)"

30545
31520
33401
33403
33450
33472
33502
33503
33505
33506
33610
33611
33619
33647
33670
33690
33694
33730
33732
33735
33736
33750
33755
33762
33778
33786
33918
33919
33922
33960
33961
36415
36420
36450
36460
36510
36660
39503
43313
43314
43520
43831
44055
44126
44127
44128
46070
46705
46715
46716
46730
46735
46740
46742
46744
47700
47701
49215
49491
49492
49495
49496
49600
49605
49606
49610
49611
53025
54000
54150
54160
63700
63702
63704
63706
65820

Appendix G

Summary of CPT Codes which Include Conscious Sedation

The following list of procedures for *CPT 2005* includes conscious sedation as an inherent part of providing the procedure. The codes listed below are identified in *CPT 2005* with a ⊙ symbol. Conscious sedation is defined as moderate sedation/analgesia and is a drug-induced depression of consciousness during which patients respond knowingly and intentionally to verbal commands, either alone or accompanied by light tactile stimulation. No interventions are required to maintain a patent airway, spontaneous ventilation is adequate, and cardiovascular function is usually maintained. Conscious or moderate sedation is not the less intense minimal sedation ("anxiolysis") or the more intense deep sedation/analgesia.

Since these services include conscious sedation, it is not appropriate for the same physician to report both the service and one of the conscious sedation codes (99141 or 99142). It is expected that if conscious sedation is provided to the patient as part of one of these services, it is provided by the same physician who is providing the service. The provision of conscious sedation by the operating physician includes the oversight of personnel who are monitoring the patient.

The inclusion of a procedure on this list does not prevent separate reporting of an associated anesthesia procedure/service (CPT codes 00100-01999) when performed by a physician other than the operating physician or a qualified professional under the responsible supervision of a physician other than the operating physician. In such cases the person providing anesthesia services shall be present for the purpose of continuously monitoring the patient and shall not act as a surgical assistant. When clinical conditions of the patient require such anesthesia services, or in the circumstances when the patient does not require sedation, the operating physician is not required to report the procedure as a reduced service using modifier 52.

19298
20982
31615
31620
31622
31623
31624
31625
31628
31629
31635
31645
31646
31656
31725
32019
32020
32201
33010
33011
33206
33207
33208
33210
33211
33212
33213
33214
33216
33217
33218
33220
33222
33223
33233
33234
33235
33240
33241
33244
33249
35470
35471
35472
35473
35474
35475
35476
36555
36557
36558
36560
36561
36563
36565
36566
36568
36570
36571
36576
36578
36581
36582
36583
36585
36590
36870
37203
37215
37216
43200
43201
43202
43204
43205
43215
43216
43217
43219
43220
43226
43227
43228
43231
43232
43234
43235
43236
43239
43240
43241
43242
43243
43244
43245
43246
43247
43248
43249
43250
43251
43255
43256
43257
43258
43259
43260
43261
43262
43263
43264
43265
43267
43268
43269
43271
43272
43453
43456
43458
44360
44361
44363
44364
44365
44366
44369
44370
44372
44373
44376
44377
44378
44379
44380
44382
44383
44385
44386
44388
44389
44390
44391
44392
44393
44394
44397
44500
44901
45303
45305
45307
45308
45309
45315
45317
45320
45327
45332
45333
45334
45337
45338
45339
45340
45341
45342
45345
45355
45378
45379
45380
45381
45382
45383
45384
45385
45386
45387
45391

45392
47011
48511
49021
49041
49061
50021
58823
66720
77600
77605
77610
77615
92953
92960
92961
92973
92974
92975
92978
92979
92980
92981
92982
92984
92986
92987
92995
92996
93312
93313
93314
93315
93316
93317
93318
93501
93505
93508
93510
93511
93514
93524
93526
93527
93528
93529
93530
93539
93540
93541
93542
93543
93544
93545
93555
93556
93561
93562
93571
93572
93609
93613
93615
93616
93618
93619
93620
93621
93622
93624
93640
93641
93642
93650
93651
93652

Appendix H

Alphabetic Index of Performance Measures by Clinical Condition or Topic

Note: Prior to coding, the user must review the complete description of the code in the Category II section of the CPT coding manual and the complete description of its associated measure by accessing the measure developer's Web site provided in the footnoted reference.

Brief Description of Performance Measure & Source: Title, Numerator, Denominator, Inclusion/Exclusion Criteria	**CPT Code(s)**	**Brief Code Descriptor**
Coronary Artery Disease (CAD)		
Blood Pressure Measurement[1]—Percentage of patients who had a blood pressure measurement during the last office visit **Numerator:** Patients who had a blood pressure measurement during the last office visit **Denominator:** All patients with CAD **Inclusion/Exclusion:** None	**2000F**	Blood pressure measured
Smoking Cessation Evaluation[1]—Percentage of patients evaluated for smoking or other tobacco use **Numerator:** Patients evaluated for smoking or other tobacco use **Denominator:** All patients **Inclusion/Exclusion:** None	**1000F** **1001F**	Tobacco use, smoking, assessed Tobacco use, non-smoking, assessed
Smoking Cessation Intervention[1]—Percentage of patients identified as cigarette smokers who received smoking cessation intervention **Numerator:** Patients identified as smokers or other tobacco users who were offered an intervention for tobacco use cessation, either counseling or pharmacologic therapy during one or more office visits **Denominator:** All patients identified as smokers or other tobacco users **Inclusion/Exclusion:** None	**4000F** **4001F**	Tobacco use cessation counseling Tobacco use cessation intervention, pharmacologic therapy
Drug Therapy for Lowering Cholesterol[1]—Percentage of patients who were prescribed a statin (based on current ACC/AHA guidelines) **Numerator:** Patients who were prescribed a statin **Denominator:** All patients with CAD **Inclusion:** None **Exclusion:** Documentation that a statin was not indicated; documentation of medical or patient reason(s) for not prescribing a statin	**4002F**	Statin therapy prescribed
Beta-blocker Therapy–Prior Myocardial Infarction (MI)[1]—Percentage of CAD patients who also have prior MI who were prescribed beta-blocker therapy **Numerator:** Patients who were prescribed beta-blocker therapy **Denominator:** All patients with CAD **Inclusion:** Patients with prior MI **Exclusion:** Documentation that a beta-blocker was not indicated; documentation of medical or patient reason(s) for not prescribing a beta-blocker	**4006F**	Beta-blocker therapy prescribed
Angiotensin Converting Enzyme (ACE) Inhibitor Therapy[1]—Percentage of CAD patients who also have diabetes and/or left ventricular systolic dysfunction (LVSD) who were prescribed ACE inhibitor therapy **Numerator:** Patients who were prescribed ACE inhibitor therapy **Denominator:** All patients with CAD who also have diabetes and/or LVSD **Inclusion:** Patients with CAD who also have diabetes and/or LVSD, left ventricular ejection fraction (LVEF) < 40% or moderately or severely depressed left ventricular systolic function) (continued)	**4009F**	Angiotensin Converting Enzyme (ACE) inhibitor prescribed

[1]Physician Consortium for Performance Improvement, www.ama-assn.org/go/quality
[2]National Committee on Quality Assurance (NCQA), Health Employer Data Information Set (HEDIS®), www.ncqa.org

Brief Description of Performance Measure & Source: Title, Numerator, Denominator, Inclusion/Exclusion Criteria	CPT Code(s)	Brief Code Descriptor
Exclusion: Documentation that ACE inhibitor was not indicated (eg, patients on angiotensin receptor blockers; documentation of medical or patient reason(s) for not prescribing ACE inhibitor		
Symptom & Activity Assessment[1]—Percentage of CAD patients who were evaluated for both level of activity and anginal symptoms during one or more office visits **Numerator:** Patients who were evaluated for both level of activity and anginal symptoms during one or more office visits **Denominator**—All patients with CAD **Inclusion/Exclusion:** None	**1002F**	Anginal symptoms and level of activity assessed
Antiplatelet Therapy[1]—Percentage of patients who were prescribed antiplatelet therapy **Numerator:** Patients who were prescribed antiplatelet therapy **Denominator:** All patients with CAD **Inclusion:** None **Exclusion:** Documentation that antiplatelet therapy was not indicated; documentation of medical or patient reason(s) for not prescribing a beta-blocker	**4011F**	Oral antiplatelet therapy prescribed
Prenatal-Postpartum Care		
Timeliness of Prenatal Care[2]—Percentage of patients in the denominator who received prenatal care **Numerator:** Number of women in the denominator who received a prenatal care visit as a member of the managed care organization (MCO) in the first trimester or within 42 days of enrollment in the MCO **Denominator:** Women who had live births between November 6th of the year prior to the measurement year and November 5th of the measurement year, who were continuously enrolled at least 43 days prior to delivery through 56 days after delivery **Inclusion/Exclusion Criteria:** None	**0500F**	Initial prenatal care visit
Prenatal Flow Sheet[1]—Percentage of patients in the denominator with a prenatal flow sheet in use by the first physician visit **Numerator:** Percentage of patients in the denominator with a flow sheet in use by the date of the first physician visit, which contains at a minimum: blood pressure, weight, urine protein, uterine size, fetal heart tones, and estimated date of delivery **Denominator:** Pregnant women seen for prenatal care **Exclusion Criteria:** Patients seen for consultation only, not for continuing care	**0501F**	Prenatal flow sheet documented
Frequency of Ongoing Prenatal Care[2]—Percentage of patients in the denominator with expected number of prenatal visits **Numerator:** Number of women in the denominator who had an unduplicated count of less than 21%, 21%-40%, 41%-60%, 61%-80%, or greater than or equal to 81% of the expected number of prenatal care visits, adjusted for the month of pregnancy at time of enrollment and gestational age **Denominator:** Women who had live births during the measurement year **Inclusion/Exclusion Criteria:** MCOs must exclude members for whom a prenatal visit is not indicated	**0502F**	Subsequent prenatal care visit
Postpartum Care[2]—Percentage of patients in the denominator who had a postpartum visit between 21 and 56 days after delivery **Numerator:** Number of women in the denominator who had a postpartum visit on or between 21 days and 56 days after delivery **Denominator:** Women who had live births between November 6th of the year prior to the measurement year and November 5th of the measurement year, who were continuously enrolled at least 43 days prior to delivery through 56 days after delivery **Inclusion/Exclusion:** None	**0503F**	Postpartum care visit

[1]Physician Consortium for Performance Improvement, www.ama-assn.org/go/quality
[2]National Committee on Quality Assurance (NCQA), Health Employer Data Information Set (HEDIS®), www.ncqa.org

Appendix I

Genetic Testing Code Modifiers

This listing of modifiers is intended for reporting with molecular laboratory procedures related to genetic testing. Genetic test modifiers should be used in conjunction with CPT and HCPCS codes to provide diagnostic granularity of service to enable providers to submit complete and precise genetic testing information without altering test descriptors. These modifiers are categorized by mutation. The first (numeric) digit indicates the disease category and the second (alpha) digit denotes gene type. Introductory guidelines in the molecular diagnostic and molecular cytogenetic code sections of CPT provide further guidance in interpretation and application of genetic test modifiers.

Neoplasia (solid tumor)

0A BRCA1 (Hereditary breast/ovarian cancer)

0B BRCA2 (Hereditary breast cancer)

0C Neurofibromin (Neurofibromatosis, type 1)

0D Merlin (Neurofibromatosis, type 2)

0E c-RET (Multiple endocrine neoplasia, types 2A/B, familial medullary thyroid carcinoma)

0F VHL (Von Hippel Lindau disease)

0G SDHD (Hereditary paraganglioma)

0H SDHB (Hereditary paraganglioma)

0I Her-2/neu

0J MLH1 (HNPCC)

0K MSH2 (HNPCC)

0L APC (Hereditary polyposis coli)

0M Rb (Retinoblastoma)

1Z Solid tumor, not otherwise specified

Neoplasia (lymphoid/hematopoetic)

2A AML1 - also ETO (Acute myeloid leukemia)

2B BCR - also ABL (Chronic myeloid, acute lymphoid leukemia)

2C CGF1

2D CBF beta (Leukemia)

2E MML (Leukemia)

2F PML/RAR alpha (Promyelocytic leukemia)

2G TEL (Leukemia)

2H bcl-2 (Lymphoma)

2I bcl-1 (Lymphoma)

2J c-myc (Lymphoma)

2K IgH (Lymphoma/leukemia)

2Z Lymphoid/hematopoetic neoplasia, not otherwise specified

Non-neoplastic hematology/coagulation

3A Factor V (Leiden, others) (Hypercoagulable state)

3B FACC (Fanconi anemia)

3C FACD (Fanconi anemia)

3D Beta globin (Thalassemia)

3E Alpha globin (Thalassemia)

3F MTHFR (Elevated homocysteine)

3G Prothrombin (Factor II, 20210A) (Hypercoagulable state)

3H Factor VIII (Hemophilia A/VWF)

3I Factor IX (Hemophilia B)

3J Beta globin

3Z Non-neoplastic hematology/coagulation, not otherwise specified

Histocompatibility/blood typing

4A HLA-A

4B HLA-B

4C HLA-C

4D HLA-D

4E HLA-DR

4F HLA-DQ

4G HLA-DP

4H Kell

4Z Histocompatibility/blood typing, not otherwise specified

Neurologic, non-neoplastic

5A Aspartoacylase A (Canavan disease)

5B FMR-1 (Fragile X, FRAXA, syndrome)

5C Frataxin (Freidreich's ataxia)

5D Huntington (Huntington's disease)

5E GABRA (Prader Willi-Angelman syndrome)

5F Connexin-26 (GJB2) (Hereditary deafness)

5G Connexin-32 (X-linked Charcot-Marie-Tooth disease)

5H SNRPN (Prader Willi-Angelman syndrome)

5I Ataxin-1 (Spinocerebellar ataxia, type 1)

5J Ataxin-2 (Spinocerebellar ataxia, type 2)

5K Ataxin-3 (Spinocerebellar ataxia, type 3, Machado-Joseph disease)

5L CACNA1A (Spinocerebellar ataxia, type 6)

5M Ataxin-7 (Spinocerebellar ataxia, type 7)

5N PMP-22 (Charcot-Marie-Tooth disease, type 1A)

5O MECP2 (Rett syndrome)

5Z Neurologic, non-neoplastic, not otherwise specified

Muscular, non-neoplastic

6A Dystrophin (Duchenne/Becker muscular dystrophy)

6B DMPK (Myotonic dystrophy, type 1)

6C ZNF-9 (Myotonic dystrophy, type 2)

6D SMN (Autosomal recessive spinal muscular atrophy)

6Z Muscular, not otherwise specified

Metabolic, other

7A Apolipoprotein E (Cardiovascular disease, Alzheimer's disease)

7B Sphingomyelin phosphodiesterase (Nieman-Pick disease)

7C Acid Beta Glucosidase (Gaucher disease)

7D HFE (Hemochromatosis)

7E Hexosaminidase A (Tay-Sachs disease)

7Z Metabolic, other, not otherwise specified

Metabolic, transport

8A CFTR (Cystic fibrosis)

8Z Metabolic, transport, not otherwise specified

Metabolic-pharmacogenetics

9A TPMT (thiopurine methyltransferase) (patients on antimetabolite therapy)

9L Metabolic-pharmacogenetics, not otherwise specified

Dysmorphology

9M FGFR1 (Pfeiffer and Kallmann syndromes)

9N FGFR2 (Crouzon, Jackson-Weiss, Apert, Saethre-Chotzen syndromes)

9O FGFR3 (Achondroplasia, Hypochondroplasia, Thanatophoric dysplasia, types I and II, Crouzon syndrome with acanthosis nigricans, Muencke syndromes)

9P TWIST (Saethre-Chotzen syndrome)

9Q CATCH-22 (22q11 deletion syndromes)

9Z Dysmorphology, not otherwise specified

Appendix J

Summary of 2005 Clinical Ambulatory Payment Classification Groups

This listing is a summary of Level I CPT and Level II Healthcare Common Procedure Coding System (HCPCS) codes representing groups of services comprising the 2005 clinical Ambulatory Payment Classification Groups (APCs). APCs are established and assigned by the Center for Medicare and Medicaid Services (CMS) specifically for the Hospital Outpatient Prospective Payment System (OPPS). An APC group includes those outpatient services having clinical coherence. Because the services within each group are clinically similar and require comparable resources, CMS establishes national payment rates applicable to all the services described within the group. The APC has a separate payment rate that is meant to account for all of the items used in the procedure; therefore, each APC is assigned a relative payment weight, based on the median costs of the services within the APC. Each year, the secretary must review and adjust as necessary the APC groupings, relative payment weights, and adjustments to assure they are consistent with clinical practice. The 2005 APC payment status is not reflected in the following listing, but is available at the CMS web site at **www.cms.hhs.gov**

APC/APC Title	CPT/ HCPCS Code	CPT/ HCPCS Description	APC Status Indicator
0001 Level I Photochemotherapy			S
	96900	Ultraviolet light therapy	
	96910	Photochemotherapy with UV-B	
	96912	Photochemotherapy with UV-A	
0002 Level I Fine Needle Biopsy/Aspiration			T
	10021	Fna w/o image	
	47399	Liver surgery procedure	
0003 Bone Marrow Biopsy/Aspiration			T
	38220	Bone marrow aspiration	
	38221	Bone marrow biopsy	
0004 Level I Needle Biopsy/ Aspiration Except Bone Marrow			T
	19000	Drainage of breast lesion	
	19001	Drain breast lesion add-on	
	20615	Treatment of bone cyst	
	48999	Pancreas surgery procedure	
	54800	Biopsy of epididymis	
	55000	Drainage of hydrocele	
	60001	Aspirate/inject thyroid cyst	
	60100	Biopsy of thyroid	
0005 Level II Needle Biopsy /Aspiration Except Bone Marrow			T
	19100	Bx breast percut w/o image	
	19102	Bx breast percut w/image	
	20206	Needle biopsy, muscle	
	38505	Needle biopsy, lymph nodes	
	42400	Biopsy of salivary gland	
0006 Level I Incision & Drainage			T
	10060	Drainage of skin abscess	
	10061	Drainage of skin abscess	
	10080	Drainage of pilonidal cyst	
	10120	Remove foreign body	
	17999	Skin tissue procedure	
	20000	Incision of abscess	
	20950	Fluid pressure, muscle	
	21725	Revision of neck muscle	
	26010	Drainage of finger abscess	
	69000	Drain external ear lesion	
	69020	Drain outer ear canal lesion	
0007 Level II Incision & Drainage			T
	10081	Drainage of pilonidal cyst	
	10140	Drainage of hematoma/fluid	
	10180	Complex drainage, wound	
	19020	Incision of breast lesion	
	23931	Drainage of arm bursa	
	26011	Drainage of finger abscess	
	27603	Drain lower leg lesion	
	28001	Drainage of bursa of foot	
	51080	Drainage of bladder abscess	
	54015	Drain penis lesion	
	55100	Drainage of scrotum abscess	
	57022	I & D vaginal hematoma, pp	
	57023	I & D vag hematoma, non-OB	
	69005	Drain external ear lesion	
0008 Level III Incision & Drainage			T
	21501	Drain neck/chest lesion	
	23030	Drain shoulder lesion	
	23031	Drain shoulder bursa	
	23930	Drainage of arm lesion	
	27301	Drain thigh/knee lesion	
	38300	Drainage, lymph node lesion	
	38305	Drainage, lymph node lesion	
	54115	Treatment of penis lesion	
0009 Nail Procedures			T
	11719	Trim nail(s)	
	11720	Debride nail, 1-5	
	11721	Debride nail, 6 or more	
	11740	Drain blood from under nail	
	G0127	Trim nail(s)	
	G0247	Routine footcare w LOPS	
0010 Level I Destruction of Lesion			T
	10040	Acne surgery	
	17000	Destroy benign/premal lesion	
	17003	Destroy lesions, 2-14	
	17110	Destruct lesion, 1-14	
	17111	Destruct lesion, 15 or more	
	96999	Dermatological procedure	
0011 Level II Destruction of Lesion			T
	17004	Destroy lesions, 15 or more	
	17106	Destruction of skin lesions	
	17107	Destruction of skin lesions	
	17108	Destruction of skin lesions	

APC/APC Title	CPT/ HCPCS Code	CPT/ HCPCS Description	APC Status Indicator
0012 Level I Debridement & Destruction			T
	11001	Debride infected skin add-on	
	11055	Trim skin lesion	
	11056	Trim skin lesions, 2 to 4	
	11300	Shave skin lesion	
	11301	Shave skin lesion	
	11732	Remove nail plate, add-on	
	11900	Injection into skin lesions	
	11901	Added skin lesions injection	
	15788	Chemical peel, face, epiderm	
	15793	Chemical peel, nonfacial	
	16000	Initial treatment of burn(s)	
	17340	Cryotherapy of skin	
	54056	Cryosurgery, penis lesion(s)	
	69220	Clean out mastoid cavity	
0013 Level II Debridement & Destruction			T
	11057	Trim skin lesions, over 4	
	11200	Removal of skin tags	
	11302	Shave skin lesion	
	11305	Shave skin lesion	
	11306	Shave skin lesion	
	11307	Shave skin lesion	
	11308	Shave skin lesion	
	11310	Shave skin lesion	
	11311	Shave skin lesion	
	11312	Shave skin lesion	
	11730	Removal of nail plate	
	15786	Abrasion, lesion, single	
	15787	Abrasion, lesions, add-on	
	15792	Chemical peel, nonfacial	
	16020	Treatment of burn(s)	
	16025	Treatment of burn(s)	
	17250	Chemical cautery, tissue	
	17271	Destruction of skin lesions	
	17360	Skin peel therapy	
	17380	Hair removal by electrolysis	
	46916	Cryosurgery, anal lesion(s)	
	54050	Destruction, penis lesion(s)	
	96567	Photodynamic tx, skin	
	96920	Laser tx, skin < 250 sq cm	
	96921	Laser tx, skin 250-500 sq cm	
	96922	Laser tx, skin>500 sq cm	
0015 Level III Debridement & Destruction			T
	11000	Debride infected skin	
	11040	Debride skin, partial	
	11041	Debride skin, full	
	11201	Remove skin tags add-on	
	11303	Shave skin lesion	
	11765	Excision of nail fold, toe	
	15789	Chemical peel, face, dermal	
	16030	Treatment of burn(s)	
	17260	Destruction of skin lesions	
	17261	Destruction of skin lesions	
	17262	Destruction of skin lesions	
	17263	Destruction of skin lesions	
	17264	Destruction of skin lesions	
	17270	Destruction of skin lesions	
	17272	Destruction of skin lesions	
	17273	Destruction of skin lesions	
	17280	Destruction of skin lesions	
	17281	Destruction of skin lesions	
	17282	Destruction of skin lesions	
	17283	Destruction of skin lesions	
	17286	Destruction of skin lesions	
	96570	Photodynamic tx, 30 min	
	96571	Photodynamic tx, addl 15 min	
0016 Level IV Debridement & Destruction			T
	11042	Debride skin/tissue	
	11043	Debride tissue/muscle	
	11313	Shave skin lesion	
	15783	Abrasion treatment of skin	
	15810	Salabrasion	
	15811	Salabrasion	
	15850	Removal of sutures	
	15851	Removal of sutures	
	16010	Treatment of burn(s)	
	17266	Destruction of skin lesions	
	17274	Destruction of skin lesions	
	17276	Destruction of skin lesions	
	17284	Destruction of skin lesions	
	46900	Destruction, anal lesion(s)	
0017 Level VI Debridement & Destruction			T
	16015	Treatment of burn(s)	
	46910	Destruction, anal lesion(s)	
	54055	Destruction, penis lesion(s)	
	54057	Laser surg, penis lesion(s)	
	54060	Excision of penis lesion(s)	
	56501	Destroy, vulva lesions, sim	
0018 Biopsy of Skin/Puncture of Lesion			T
	10160	Puncture drainage of lesion	
	11100	Biopsy skin lesion	
	11101	Biopsy, skin add-on	
0019 Level I Excision/ Biopsy			T
	11010	Debride skin, fx	
	11011	Debride skin/muscle, fx	
	11012	Debride skin/muscle/bone, fx	
	11400	Exc tr-ext b9+marg 0.5 < cm	
	11401	Exc tr-ext b9+marg 0.6-1 cm	
	11402	Exc tr-ext b9+marg 1.1-2 cm	
	11440	Exc face-mm b9+marg 0.5 < cm	
	11441	Exc face-mm b9+marg 0.6-1 cm	
	11600	Exc tr-ext mlg+marg 0.5 < cm	
	11601	Exc tr-ext mlg+marg 0.6-1 cm	
	11602	Exc tr-ext mlg+marg 1.1-2 cm	
	11621	Exc h-f-nk-sp mlg+marg 0.6-1	
	11640	Exc face-mm malig+marg 0.5 <	
	11641	Exc face-mm malig+marg 0.6-1	
	11750	Removal of nail bed	
	11755	Biopsy, nail unit	
	11976	Removal of contraceptive cap	
	15781	Abrasion treatment of skin	
	15782	Abrasion treatment of skin	
	15920	Removal of tail bone ulcer	
	15999	Removal of pressure sore	
	20220	Bone biopsy, trocar/needle	
	20520	Removal of foreign body	
	22999	Abdomen surgery procedure	
	24200	Removal of arm foreign body	
	28190	Removal of foot foreign body	
	56605	Biopsy of vulva/perineum	
	56606	Biopsy of vulva/perineum	
	69100	Biopsy of external ear	
0020 Level II Excision/Biopsy			T
	11403	Exc tr-ext b9+marg 2.1-3 cm	
	11420	Exc h-f-nk-sp b9+marg 0.5 <	
	11421	Exc h-f-nk-sp b9+marg 0.6-1	
	11422	Exc h-f-nk-sp b9+marg 1.1-2	
	11423	Exc h-f-nk-sp b9+marg 2.1-3	
	11442	Exc face-mm b9+marg 1.1-2 cm	
	11443	Exc face-mm b9+marg 2.1-3 cm	
	11444	Exc face-mm b9+marg 3.1-4 cm	

APC/APC Title	CPT/ HCPCS Code	CPT/ HCPCS Description	APC Status Indicator
0020 Level II Excision/Biopsy Cont'd.			T
	11603	Exc tr-ext mlg+marg 2.1-3 cm	
	11604	Exc tr-ext mlg+marg 3.1-4 cm	
	11620	Exc h-f-nk-sp mlg+marg 0.5 <	
	11622	Exc h-f-nk-sp mlg+marg 1.1-2	
	11642	Exc face-mm malig+marg 1.1-2	
	11643	Exc face-mm malig+marg 2.1-3	
	20225	Bone biopsy, trocar/needle	
	21920	Biopsy soft tissue of back	
	23330	Remove shoulder foreign body	
	27040	Biopsy of soft tissues	
	27041	Biopsy of soft tissues	
	27086	Remove hip foreign body	
	27613	Biopsy lower leg soft tissue	
	28193	Removal of foot foreign body	
0021 Level III Excision/Biopsy			T
	0046T	Cath lavage, mammary duct(s)	
	0047T	Cath lavage, mammary duct(s)	
	10121	Remove foreign body	
	11404	Exc tr-ext b9+marg 3.1-4 cm	
	11406	Exc tr-ext b9+marg > 4.0 cm	
	11424	Exc h-f-nk-sp b9+marg 3.1-4	
	11606	Exc tr-ext mlg+marg > 4 cm	
	11623	Exc h-f-nk-sp mlg+marg 2.1-3	
	11624	Exc h-f-nk-sp mlg+marg 3.1-4	
	11644	Exc face-mm malig+marg 3.1-4	
	15836	Excise excessive skin tissue	
	15837	Excise excessive skin tissue	
	15838	Excise excessive skin tissue	
	15839	Excise excessive skin tissue	
	19260	Removal of chest wall lesion	
	20200	Muscle biopsy	
	20205	Deep muscle biopsy	
	20670	Removal of support implant	
	21550	Biopsy of neck/chest	
	23000	Removal of calcium deposits	
	23065	Biopsy shoulder tissues	
	23075	Removal of shoulder lesion	
	24065	Biopsy arm/elbow soft tissue	
	24066	Biopsy arm/elbow soft tissue	
	24075	Remove arm/elbow lesion	
	24201	Removal of arm foreign body	
	25065	Biopsy forearm soft tissues	
	25075	Remove forearm lesion subcut	
	26320	Removal of implant from hand	
	27323	Biopsy, thigh soft tissues	
	27618	Remove lower leg lesion	
	28043	Excision of foot lesion	
	28192	Removal of foot foreign body	
	37609	Temporal artery procedure	
	54100	Biopsy of penis	
	69110	Remove external ear, partial	
	69145	Remove ear canal lesion(s)	
0022 Level IV Excision/Biopsy			T
	11426	Exc h-f-nk-sp b9+marg > 4 cm	
	11446	Exc face-mm b9+marg > 4 cm	
	11450	Removal, sweat gland lesion	
	11451	Removal, sweat gland lesion	
	11462	Removal, sweat gland lesion	
	11463	Removal, sweat gland lesion	
	11470	Removal, sweat gland lesion	
	11471	Removal, sweat gland lesion	
	11626	Exc h-f-nk-sp mlg+mar > 4 cm	
	11646	Exc face-mm mlg+marg > 4 cm	
	11752	Remove nail bed/finger tip	
	11770	Removal of pilonidal lesion	
	11771	Removal of pilonidal lesion	
	11772	Removal of pilonidal lesion	
	11971	Remove tissue expander(s)	
	15780	Abrasion treatment of skin	
	15831	Excise excessive skin tissue	
	15832	Excise excessive skin tissue	
	15833	Excise excessive skin tissue	
	15834	Excise excessive skin tissue	
	15931	Remove sacrum pressure sore	
	15933	Remove sacrum pressure sore	
	15940	Remove hip pressure sore	
	15941	Remove hip pressure sore	
	15950	Remove thigh pressure sore	
	15951	Remove thigh pressure sore	
	20240	Bone biopsy, excisional	
	20245	Bone biopsy, excisional	
	20525	Removal of foreign body	
	20680	Removal of support implant	
	21555	Remove lesion, neck/chest	
	21556	Remove lesion, neck/chest	
	21557	Remove tumor, neck/chest	
	21925	Biopsy soft tissue of back	
	21930	Remove lesion, back or flank	
	21935	Remove tumor, back	
	22900	Remove abdominal wall lesion	
	23066	Biopsy shoulder tissues	
	23076	Removal of shoulder lesion	
	23077	Remove tumor of shoulder	
	23331	Remove shoulder foreign body	
	24076	Remove arm/elbow lesion	
	24077	Remove tumor of arm/elbow	
	25066	Biopsy forearm soft tissues	
	25076	Remove forearm lesion deep	
	25077	Remove tumor, forearm/wrist	
	26115	Remove hand lesion subcut	
	26116	Remove hand lesion, deep	
	26117	Remove tumor, hand/finger	
	27047	Remove hip/pelvis lesion	
	27048	Remove hip/pelvis lesion	
	27049	Remove tumor, hip/pelvis	
	27324	Biopsy, thigh soft tissues	
	27327	Removal of thigh lesion	
	27328	Removal of thigh lesion	
	27329	Remove tumor, thigh/knee	
	27372	Removal of foreign body	
	27614	Biopsy lower leg soft tissue	
	27619	Remove lower leg lesion	
	54105	Biopsy of penis	
	60512	Autotransplant parathyroid	
	69205	Clear outer ear canal	
0023 Exploration Penetrating Wound			T
	20100	Explore wound, neck	
	20103	Explore wound, extremity	
0024 Level I Skin Repair			T
	11760	Repair of nail bed	
	11762	Reconstruction of nail bed	
	11920	Correct skin color defects	
	11921	Correct skin color defects	
	11922	Correct skin color defects	
	11950	Therapy for contour defects	
	11951	Therapy for contour defects	
	11952	Therapy for contour defects	
	11954	Therapy for contour defects	
	12001	Repair superficial wound(s)	
	12002	Repair superficial wound(s)	
	12004	Repair superficial wound(s)	
	12005	Repair superficial wound(s)	
	12006	Repair superficial wound(s)	
	12007	Repair superficial wound(s)	
	12011	Repair superficial wound(s)	
	12013	Repair superficial wound(s)	
	12014	Repair superficial wound(s)	

APC/APC Title	CPT/ HCPCS Code	CPT/ HCPCS Description	APC Status Indicator
0024 Level I Skin Repair Cont'd.			T
	12015	Repair superficial wound(s)	
	12016	Repair superficial wound(s)	
	12017	Repair superficial wound(s)	
	12018	Repair superficial wound(s)	
	12020	Closure of split wound	
	12021	Closure of split wound	
	12031	Layer closure of wound(s)	
	12032	Layer closure of wound(s)	
	12034	Layer closure of wound(s)	
	12035	Layer closure of wound(s)	
	12036	Layer closure of wound(s)	
	12041	Layer closure of wound(s)	
	12042	Layer closure of wound(s)	
	12044	Layer closure of wound(s)	
	12045	Layer closure of wound(s)	
	12046	Layer closure of wound(s)	
	12051	Layer closure of wound(s)	
	12052	Layer closure of wound(s)	
	12053	Layer closure of wound(s)	
	12054	Layer closure of wound(s)	
	12055	Layer closure of wound(s)	
	12056	Layer closure of wound(s)	
	13102	Repair wound/lesion add-on	
	13120	Repair of wound or lesion	
	13121	Repair of wound or lesion	
	13122	Repair wound/lesion add-on	
	13131	Repair of wound or lesion	
	13132	Repair of wound or lesion	
	13133	Repair wound/lesion add-on	
	13151	Repair of wound or lesion	
	13153	Repair wound/lesion add-on	
	15342	Cultured skin graft, 25 cm	
	15343	Culture skn graft addl 25 cm	
0025 Level II Skin Repair			T
	12037	Layer closure of wound(s)	
	12047	Layer closure of wound(s)	
	12057	Layer closure of wound(s)	
	13100	Repair of wound or lesion	
	13101	Repair of wound or lesion	
	13150	Repair of wound or lesion	
	13152	Repair of wound or lesion	
	15000	Skin graft	
	15001	Skin graft add-on	
	15050	Skin pinch graft	
	15201	Skin full graft add-on	
	15221	Skin full graft add-on	
	15241	Skin full graft add-on	
	15261	Skin full graft add-on	
	15400	Skin heterograft	
	15401	Skin heterograft add-on	
	15775	Hair transplant punch grafts	
	15776	Hair transplant punch grafts	
	15819	Plastic surgery, neck	
	15835	Excise excessive skin tissue	
	23921	Amputation follow-up surgery	
0027 Level IV Skin Repair			T
	11960	Insert tissue expander(s)	
	11970	Replace tissue expander	
	13160	Late closure of wound	
	14000	Skin tissue rearrangement	
	14001	Skin tissue rearrangement	
	14020	Skin tissue rearrangement	
	14021	Skin tissue rearrangement	
	14040	Skin tissue rearrangement	
	14041	Skin tissue rearrangement	
	14060	Skin tissue rearrangement	
	14061	Skin tissue rearrangement	
	14300	Skin tissue rearrangement	
	14350	Skin tissue rearrangement	
	15100	Skin split graft	
	15101	Skin split graft add-on	
	15120	Skin split graft	
	15121	Skin split graft add-on	
	15200	Skin full graft	
	15220	Skin full graft	
	15240	Skin full graft	
	15260	Skin full graft	
	15351	Skin homograft add-on	
	15570	Form skin pedicle flap	
	15572	Form skin pedicle flap	
	15574	Form skin pedicle flap	
	15576	Form skin pedicle flap	
	15600	Skin graft	
	15610	Skin graft	
	15620	Skin graft	
	15630	Skin graft	
	15650	Transfer skin pedicle flap	
	15732	Muscle-skin graft, head/neck	
	15734	Muscle-skin graft, trunk	
	15736	Muscle-skin graft, arm	
	15738	Muscle-skin graft, leg	
	15740	Island pedicle flap graft	
	15750	Neurovascular pedicle graft	
	15760	Composite skin graft	
	15770	Derma-fat-fascia graft	
	15820	Revision of lower eyelid	
	15821	Revision of lower eyelid	
	15822	Revision of upper eyelid	
	15823	Revision of upper eyelid	
	15824	Removal of forehead wrinkles	
	15825	Removal of neck wrinkles	
	15826	Removal of brow wrinkles	
	15828	Removal of face wrinkles	
	15829	Removal of skin wrinkles	
	15840	Graft for face nerve palsy	
	15841	Graft for face nerve palsy	
	15842	Flap for face nerve palsy	
	15845	Skin and muscle repair, face	
	15876	Suction assisted lipectomy	
	15877	Suction assisted lipectomy	
	15878	Suction assisted lipectomy	
	15879	Suction assisted lipectomy	
	15922	Removal of tail bone ulcer	
	15934	Remove sacrum pressure sore	
	15935	Remove sacrum pressure sore	
	15936	Remove sacrum pressure sore	
	15937	Remove sacrum pressure sore	
	15944	Remove hip pressure sore	
	15945	Remove hip pressure sore	
	15946	Remove hip pressure sore	
	15952	Remove thigh pressure sore	
	15953	Remove thigh pressure sore	
	15956	Remove thigh pressure sore	
	15958	Remove thigh pressure sore	
	20101	Explore wound, chest	
	20102	Explore wound, abdomen	
	20910	Remove cartilage for graft	
	20912	Remove cartilage for graft	
	20920	Removal of fascia for graft	
	20922	Removal of fascia for graft	
	20926	Removal of tissue for graft	
	25929	Amputation follow-up surgery	
	33222	Revise pocket, pacemaker	
	33223	Revise pocket, pacing-defib	
	44312	Revision of ileostomy	
	44340	Revision of colostomy	

APC/APC Title	CPT/ HCPCS Code	CPT/ HCPCS Description	APC Status Indicator
0028 Level I Breast Surgery			T
	19101	Biopsy of breast, open	
	19110	Nipple exploration	
	19112	Excise breast duct fistula	
	19120	Removal of breast lesion	
	19125	Excision, breast lesion	
	19126	Excision, addl breast lesion	
	19140	Removal of breast tissue	
	19160	Removal of breast tissue	
	19350	Breast reconstruction	
	19499	Breast surgery procedure	
0029 Level II Breast Surgery			T
	19180	Removal of breast	
	19182	Removal of breast	
	19316	Suspension of breast	
	19328	Removal of breast implant	
	19330	Removal of implant material	
	19355	Correct inverted nipple(s)	
	19366	Breast reconstruction	
	19370	Surgery of breast capsule	
	19371	Removal of breast capsule	
	19396	Design custom breast implant	
0030 Level III Breast Surgery			T
	19240	Removal of breast	
	19340	Immediate breast prosthesis	
	19380	Revise breast reconstruction	
0032 Insertion of Central Venous/ Arterial Catheter			T
	36557	Insert tunneled CV cath	
	36558	Insert tunneled CV cath	
	36570	Insert tunneled CV cath	
	36571	Insert tunneled CV cath	
	36581	Replace tunneled CV cath	
	36585	Replace tunneled CV cath	
	36640	Insertion catheter, artery	
0033 Partial Hospitalization			P
	G0129	Partial hosp prog service	
	G0176	OPPS/PHP; activity therapy	
	G0177	OPPS/PHP; train & educ serv	
0035 Placement of Arterial or Central Venous Catheter			T
	36420	Vein access cutdown < 1 yr	
	36425	Vein access cutdown > 1 yr	
	37799	Vascular surgery procedure	
0036 Level II Fine Needle Biopsy/Aspiration			T
	10022	Fna w/image	
0037 Level III Needle Biopsy/ Aspiration Except Bone Marrow			T
	44901	Drain app abscess, percut	
	47011	Percut drain, liver lesion	
	48511	Drain pancreatic pseudocyst	
	49021	Drain abdominal abscess	
	49041	Drain, perc, abdom abscess	
	49061	Drain, perc, retroper absc	
	50021	Renal abscess, percut drain	
	54500	Biopsy of testis	
0039 Level I Implantation of Neurostimulator			S
	61885	Implant neurostim one array	
0040 Level II Implantation of Neurostimulator Electrodes			S
	63650	Implant neuroelectrodes	
	64555	Implant neuroelectrodes	
	64560	Implant neuroelectrodes	
	64561	Implant neuroelectrodes	
	64565	Implant neuroelectrodes	
	64575	Implant neuroelectrodes	
	64581	Implant neuroelectrodes	
0041 Level I Arthroscopy			T
	29804	Jaw arthroscopy/surgery	
	29805	Shoulder arthroscopy, dx	
	29819	Shoulder arthroscopy/surgery	
	29820	Shoulder arthroscopy/surgery	
	29821	Shoulder arthroscopy/surgery	
	29822	Shoulder arthroscopy/surgery	
	29823	Shoulder arthroscopy/surgery	
	29825	Shoulder arthroscopy/surgery	
	29830	Elbow arthroscopy	
	29834	Elbow arthroscopy/surgery	
	29835	Elbow arthroscopy/surgery	
	29836	Elbow arthroscopy/surgery	
	29837	Elbow arthroscopy/surgery	
	29838	Elbow arthroscopy/surgery	
	29840	Wrist arthroscopy	
	29843	Wrist arthroscopy/surgery	
	29844	Wrist arthroscopy/surgery	
	29845	Wrist arthroscopy/surgery	
	29846	Wrist arthroscopy/surgery	
	29848	Wrist endoscopy/surgery	
	29850	Knee arthroscopy/surgery	
	29860	Hip arthroscopy, dx	
	29870	Knee arthroscopy, dx	
	29871	Knee arthroscopy/drainage	
	29873	Knee arthroscopy/surgery	
	29874	Knee arthroscopy/surgery	
	29875	Knee arthroscopy/surgery	
	29876	Knee arthroscopy/surgery	
	29877	Knee arthroscopy/surgery	
	29879	Knee arthroscopy/surgery	
	29880	Knee arthroscopy/surgery	
	29881	Knee arthroscopy/surgery	
	29882	Knee arthroscopy/surgery	
	29883	Knee arthroscopy/surgery	
	29884	Knee arthroscopy/surgery	
	29886	Knee arthroscopy/surgery	
	29887	Knee arthroscopy/surgery	
	29891	Ankle arthroscopy/surgery	
	29892	Ankle arthroscopy/surgery	
	29894	Ankle arthroscopy/surgery	
	29895	Ankle arthroscopy/surgery	
	29897	Ankle arthroscopy/surgery	
	29898	Ankle arthroscopy/surgery	
	29999	Arthroscopy of joint	
0042 Level II Arthroscopy			T
	27412	Autochondrocyte implant knee	
	27415	Osteochondral knee allograft	
	29800	Jaw arthroscopy/surgery	
	29806	Shoulder arthroscopy/surgery	
	29807	Shoulder arthroscopy/surgery	
	29824	Shoulder arthroscopy/surgery	
	29826	Shoulder arthroscopy/surgery	
	29827	Arthroscop rotator cuff repr	
	29847	Wrist arthroscopy/surgery	
	29851	Knee arthroscopy/surgery	
	29855	Tibial arthroscopy/surgery	
	29856	Tibial arthroscopy/surgery	

APC/APC Title	CPT/ HCPCS Code	CPT/ HCPCS Description	APC Status Indicator
	29861	Hip arthroscopy/surgery	
	29862	Hip arthroscopy/surgery	
	29863	Hip arthroscopy/surgery	
	29866	Autgrft implnt, knee w/scope	
	29867	Allgrft implnt, knee w/scope	
	29868	Allgrft implnt, knee w/scope	
	29885	Knee arthroscopy/surgery	
	29888	Knee arthroscopy/surgery	
	29889	Knee arthroscopy/surgery	
	29899	Ankle arthroscopy/surgery	
0043 Closed Treatment Fracture Finger/Toe/Trunk			T
	21800	Treatment of rib fracture	
	21820	Treat sternum fracture	
	22305	Treat spine process fracture	
	22310	Treat spine fracture	
	22315	Treat spine fracture	
	22899	Spine surgery procedure	
	23500	Treat clavicle fracture	
	23505	Treat clavicle fracture	
	23520	Treat clavicle dislocation	
	23525	Treat clavicle dislocation	
	23540	Treat clavicle dislocation	
	23545	Treat clavicle dislocation	
	23570	Treat shoulder blade fx	
	23575	Treat shoulder blade fx	
	23600	Treat humerus fracture	
	23605	Treat humerus fracture	
	23620	Treat humerus fracture	
	23625	Treat humerus fracture	
	23650	Treat shoulder dislocation	
	23665	Treat dislocation/fracture	
	23675	Treat dislocation/fracture	
	23929	Shoulder surgery procedure	
	24500	Treat humerus fracture	
	24505	Treat humerus fracture	
	24530	Treat humerus fracture	
	24535	Treat humerus fracture	
	24560	Treat humerus fracture	
	24565	Treat humerus fracture	
	24576	Treat humerus fracture	
	24577	Treat humerus fracture	
	24600	Treat elbow dislocation	
	24620	Treat elbow fracture	
	24640	Treat elbow dislocation	
	24650	Treat radius fracture	
	24655	Treat radius fracture	
	24670	Treat ulnar fracture	
	24675	Treat ulnar fracture	
	24999	Upper arm/elbow surgery	
	25259	Manipulate wrist w/anesthes	
	25500	Treat fracture of radius	
	25505	Treat fracture of radius	
	25520	Treat fracture of radius	
	25530	Treat fracture of ulna	
	25535	Treat fracture of ulna	
	25560	Treat fracture radius & ulna	
	25565	Treat fracture radius & ulna	
	25600	Treat fracture radius/ulna	
	25605	Treat fracture radius/ulna	
	25622	Treat wrist bone fracture	
	25624	Treat wrist bone fracture	
	25630	Treat wrist bone fracture	
	25635	Treat wrist bone fracture	
	25650	Treat wrist bone fracture	
	25660	Treat wrist dislocation	
	25675	Treat wrist dislocation	
	25680	Treat wrist fracture	
	25690	Treat wrist dislocation	
	25999	Forearm or wrist surgery	
	26340	Manipulate finger w/anesth	
	26600	Treat metacarpal fracture	
	26605	Treat metacarpal fracture	
	26607	Treat metacarpal fracture	
	26641	Treat thumb dislocation	
	26645	Treat thumb fracture	
	26670	Treat hand dislocation	
	26675	Treat hand dislocation	
	26700	Treat knuckle dislocation	
	26705	Treat knuckle dislocation	
	26706	Pin knuckle dislocation	
	26720	Treat finger fracture, each	
	26725	Treat finger fracture, each	
	26740	Treat finger fracture, each	
	26742	Treat finger fracture, each	
	26750	Treat finger fracture, each	
	26755	Treat finger fracture, each	
	26770	Treat finger dislocation	
	26989	Hand/finger surgery	
	27193	Treat pelvic ring fracture	
	27200	Treat tail bone fracture	
	27220	Treat hip socket fracture	
	27230	Treat thigh fracture	
	27238	Treat thigh fracture	
	27246	Treat thigh fracture	
	27250	Treat hip dislocation	
	27256	Treat hip dislocation	
	27265	Treat hip dislocation	
	27299	Pelvis/hip joint surgery	
	27500	Treatment of thigh fracture	
	27501	Treatment of thigh fracture	
	27502	Treatment of thigh fracture	
	27503	Treatment of thigh fracture	
	27508	Treatment of thigh fracture	
	27510	Treatment of thigh fracture	
	27516	Treat thigh fx growth plate	
	27517	Treat thigh fx growth plate	
	27520	Treat kneecap fracture	
	27530	Treat knee fracture	
	27532	Treat knee fracture	
	27538	Treat knee fracture(s)	
	27550	Treat knee dislocation	
	27560	Treat kneecap dislocation	
	27599	Leg surgery procedure	
	27750	Treatment of tibia fracture	
	27752	Treatment of tibia fracture	
	27760	Treatment of ankle fracture	
	27762	Treatment of ankle fracture	
	27780	Treatment of fibula fracture	
	27781	Treatment of fibula fracture	
	27786	Treatment of ankle fracture	
	27788	Treatment of ankle fracture	
	27808	Treatment of ankle fracture	
	27810	Treatment of ankle fracture	
	27816	Treatment of ankle fracture	
	27818	Treatment of ankle fracture	
	27824	Treat lower leg fracture	
	27825	Treat lower leg fracture	
	27830	Treat lower leg dislocation	
	27831	Treat lower leg dislocation	
	27840	Treat ankle dislocation	
	27899	Leg/ankle surgery procedure	
	28400	Treatment of heel fracture	
	28405	Treatment of heel fracture	
	28430	Treatment of ankle fracture	
	28435	Treatment of ankle fracture	
	28450	Treat midfoot fracture, each	
	28455	Treat midfoot fracture, each	
	28470	Treat metatarsal fracture	
	28475	Treat metatarsal fracture	
	28490	Treat big toe fracture	
	28495	Treat big toe fracture	
	28510	Treatment of toe fracture	

APC/APC Title	CPT/ HCPCS Code	CPT/ HCPCS Description	APC Status Indicator
0043 Closed Treatment Fracture Finger/Toe/Trunk Cont'd.			T
	28515	Treatment of toe fracture	
	28530	Treat sesamoid bone fracture	
	28540	Treat foot dislocation	
	28570	Treat foot dislocation	
	28575	Treat foot dislocation	
	28600	Treat foot dislocation	
	28605	Treat foot dislocation	
	28630	Treat toe dislocation	
	28660	Treat toe dislocation	
	28899	Foot/toes surgery procedure	
0045 Bone/Joint Manipulation Under Anesthesia			T
	22505	Manipulation of spine	
	23655	Treat shoulder dislocation	
	23700	Fixation of shoulder	
	24300	Manipulate elbow w/anesth	
	24605	Treat elbow dislocation	
	26775	Treat finger dislocation	
	27194	Treat pelvic ring fracture	
	27252	Treat hip dislocation	
	27257	Treat hip dislocation	
	27266	Treat hip dislocation	
	27275	Manipulation of hip joint	
	27552	Treat knee dislocation	
	27562	Treat kneecap dislocation	
	27570	Fixation of knee joint	
	27842	Treat ankle dislocation	
	27860	Fixation of ankle joint	
	28545	Treat foot dislocation	
	28635	Treat toe dislocation	
	28665	Treat toe dislocation	
0046 Open/Percutaneous Treatment Fracture or Dislocation			T
	21336	Treat nasal septal fracture	
	21805	Treatment of rib fracture	
	23515	Treat clavicle fracture	
	23530	Treat clavicle dislocation	
	23532	Treat clavicle dislocation	
	23550	Treat clavicle dislocation	
	23552	Treat clavicle dislocation	
	23585	Treat scapula fracture	
	23615	Treat humerus fracture	
	23616	Treat humerus fracture	
	23630	Treat humerus fracture	
	23660	Treat shoulder dislocation	
	23670	Treat dislocation/fracture	
	23680	Treat dislocation/fracture	
	24515	Treat humerus fracture	
	24516	Treat humerus fracture	
	24538	Treat humerus fracture	
	24545	Treat humerus fracture	
	24546	Treat humerus fracture	
	24566	Treat humerus fracture	
	24575	Treat humerus fracture	
	24579	Treat humerus fracture	
	24582	Treat humerus fracture	
	24586	Treat elbow fracture	
	24587	Treat elbow fracture	
	24615	Treat elbow dislocation	
	24635	Treat elbow fracture	
	24665	Treat radius fracture	
	24666	Treat radius fracture	
	24685	Treat ulnar fracture	
	25515	Treat fracture of radius	
	25525	Treat fracture of radius	
	25526	Treat fracture of radius	
	25545	Treat fracture of ulna	
	25574	Treat fracture radius & ulna	
	25575	Treat fracture radius/ulna	
	25611	Treat fracture radius/ulna	
	25620	Treat fracture radius/ulna	
	25628	Treat wrist bone fracture	
	25645	Treat wrist bone fracture	
	25651	Pin ulnar styloid fracture	
	25652	Treat fracture ulnar styloid	
	25670	Treat wrist dislocation	
	25671	Pin radioulnar dislocation	
	25676	Treat wrist dislocation	
	25685	Treat wrist fracture	
	25695	Treat wrist dislocation	
	26608	Treat metacarpal fracture	
	26615	Treat metacarpal fracture	
	26650	Treat thumb fracture	
	26665	Treat thumb fracture	
	26676	Pin hand dislocation	
	26685	Treat hand dislocation	
	26686	Treat hand dislocation	
	26715	Treat knuckle dislocation	
	26727	Treat finger fracture, each	
	26735	Treat finger fracture, each	
	26746	Treat finger fracture, each	
	26756	Pin finger fracture, each	
	26765	Treat finger fracture, each	
	26776	Pin finger dislocation	
	26785	Treat finger dislocation	
	27202	Treat tail bone fracture	
	27509	Treatment of thigh fracture	
	27524	Treat kneecap fracture	
	27566	Treat kneecap dislocation	
	27615	Remove tumor, lower leg	
	27756	Treatment of tibia fracture	
	27758	Treatment of tibia fracture	
	27759	Treatment of tibia fracture	
	27766	Treatment of ankle fracture	
	27784	Treatment of fibula fracture	
	27792	Treatment of ankle fracture	
	27814	Treatment of ankle fracture	
	27822	Treatment of ankle fracture	
	27823	Treatment of ankle fracture	
	27826	Treat lower leg fracture	
	27827	Treat lower leg fracture	
	27828	Treat lower leg fracture	
	27829	Treat lower leg joint	
	27832	Treat lower leg dislocation	
	27846	Treat ankle dislocation	
	27848	Treat ankle dislocation	
	28406	Treatment of heel fracture	
	28415	Treat heel fracture	
	28420	Treat/graft heel fracture	
	28436	Treatment of ankle fracture	
	28445	Treat ankle fracture	
	28456	Treat midfoot fracture	
	28465	Treat midfoot fracture, each	
	28476	Treat metatarsal fracture	
	28485	Treat metatarsal fracture	
	28496	Treat big toe fracture	
	28505	Treat big toe fracture	
	28525	Treat toe fracture	
	28531	Treat sesamoid bone fracture	
	28546	Treat foot dislocation	
	28555	Repair foot dislocation	
	28576	Treat foot dislocation	
	28585	Repair foot dislocation	
	28606	Treat foot dislocation	
	28615	Repair foot dislocation	
	28636	Treat toe dislocation	
	28645	Repair toe dislocation	
	28666	Treat toe dislocation	
	28675	Repair of toe dislocation	

APC/APC Title	CPT/ HCPCS Code	CPT/ HCPCS Description	APC Status Indicator
0047 Arthroplasty without Prosthesis			T
	24360	Reconstruct elbow joint	
	24365	Reconstruct head of radius	
	25332	Revise wrist joint	
	25447	Repair wrist joint(s)	
	25449	Remove wrist joint implant	
	26530	Revise knuckle joint	
	26535	Revise finger joint	
	27437	Revise kneecap	
	27440	Revision of knee joint	
	27441	Revision of knee joint	
	27442	Revision of knee joint	
	27443	Revision of knee joint	
	27700	Revision of ankle joint	
0048 Level I Arthroplasty with Prosthesis			T
	24362	Reconstruct elbow joint	
	25443	Reconstruct wrist joint	
	25444	Reconstruct wrist joint	
	25445	Reconstruct wrist joint	
	26531	Revise knuckle with implant	
	26536	Revise/implant finger joint	
	27438	Revise kneecap with implant	
0049 Level I Musculoskeletal Procedures Except Hand and Foot			T
	20005	Incision of deep abscess	
	20250	Open bone biopsy	
	20251	Open bone biopsy	
	20650	Insert and remove bone pin	
	20693	Adjust bone fixation device	
	20694	Remove bone fixation device	
	20999	Musculoskeletal surgery	
	21502	Drain chest lesion	
	21700	Revision of neck muscle	
	21720	Revision of neck muscle	
	23035	Drain shoulder bone lesion	
	23100	Biopsy of shoulder joint	
	23140	Removal of bone lesion	
	23935	Drain arm/elbow bone lesion	
	24100	Biopsy elbow joint lining	
	24105	Removal of elbow bursa	
	24110	Remove humerus lesion	
	24120	Remove elbow lesion	
	24310	Revision of arm tendon	
	24332	Tenolysis, triceps	
	24925	Amputation follow-up surgery	
	25000	Incision of tendon sheath	
	25001	Incise flexor carpi radialis	
	25020	Decompress forearm 1 space	
	25028	Drainage of forearm lesion	
	25031	Drainage of forearm bursa	
	25035	Treat forearm bone lesion	
	25085	Incision of wrist capsule	
	25100	Biopsy of wrist joint	
	25110	Remove wrist tendon lesion	
	25115	Remove wrist/forearm lesion	
	25116	Remove wrist/forearm lesion	
	25248	Remove forearm foreign body	
	25295	Release wrist/forearm tendon	
	25907	Amputation follow-up surgery	
	25922	Amputate hand at wrist	
	26990	Drainage of pelvis lesion	
	26991	Drainage of pelvis bursa	
	27000	Incision of hip tendon	
	27050	Biopsy of sacroiliac joint	
	27052	Biopsy of hip joint	
	27060	Removal of ischial bursa	
	27062	Remove femur lesion/bursa	
	27065	Removal of hip bone lesion	
	27087	Remove hip foreign body	
	27305	Incise thigh tendon & fascia	
	27306	Incision of thigh tendon	
	27307	Incision of thigh tendons	
	27340	Removal of kneecap bursa	
	27345	Removal of knee cyst	
	27347	Remove knee cyst	
	27380	Repair of kneecap tendon	
	27381	Repair/graft kneecap tendon	
	27385	Repair of thigh muscle	
	27386	Repair/graft of thigh muscle	
	27390	Incision of thigh tendon	
	27391	Incision of thigh tendons	
	27392	Incision of thigh tendons	
	27496	Decompression of thigh/knee	
	27497	Decompression of thigh/knee	
	27498	Decompression of thigh/knee	
	27499	Decompression of thigh/knee	
	27594	Amputation follow-up surgery	
	27600	Decompression of lower leg	
	27601	Decompression of lower leg	
	27602	Decompression of lower leg	
	27604	Drain lower leg bursa	
	27606	Incision of achilles tendon	
	27607	Treat lower leg bone lesion	
	27630	Removal of tendon lesion	
	27656	Repair leg fascia defect	
	27658	Repair of leg tendon, each	
	27659	Repair of leg tendon, each	
	27664	Repair of leg tendon, each	
	27675	Repair lower leg tendons	
	27704	Removal of ankle implant	
	27707	Incision of fibula	
	27884	Amputation follow-up surgery	
	27892	Decompression of leg	
	27893	Decompression of leg	
	27894	Decompression of leg	
	28002	Treatment of foot infection	
	28003	Treatment of foot infection	
0050 Level II Musculoskeletal Procedures Except Hand and Foot			T
	20690	Apply bone fixation device	
	20692	Apply bone fixation device	
	20900	Removal of bone for graft	
	20902	Removal of bone for graft	
	20924	Removal of tendon for graft	
	21600	Partial removal of rib	
	21610	Partial removal of rib	
	22520	Percut vertebroplasty thor	
	22521	Percut vertebroplasty lumb	
	22522	Percut vertebroplasty addl	
	23040	Exploratory shoulder surgery	
	23044	Exploratory shoulder surgery	
	23101	Shoulder joint surgery	
	23105	Remove shoulder joint lining	
	23106	Incision of collarbone joint	
	23107	Explore treat shoulder joint	
	23145	Removal of bone lesion	
	23146	Removal of bone lesion	
	23150	Removal of humerus lesion	
	23155	Removal of humerus lesion	
	23156	Removal of humerus lesion	
	23170	Remove collar bone lesion	
	23172	Remove shoulder blade lesion	
	23174	Remove humerus lesion	
	23180	Remove collar bone lesion	
	23182	Remove shoulder blade lesion	
	23184	Remove humerus lesion	
	23190	Partial removal of scapula	
	23195	Removal of head of humerus	

APC/APC Title	CPT/ HCPCS Code	CPT/ HCPCS Description	APC Status Indicator
0050 Level II Musculoskeletal Procedures Except Hand and Foot Cont'd.			T
	23400	Fixation of shoulder blade	
	23405	Incision of tendon & muscle	
	23406	Incise tendon(s) & muscle(s)	
	24000	Exploratory elbow surgery	
	24006	Release elbow joint	
	24101	Explore/treat elbow joint	
	24102	Remove elbow joint lining	
	24115	Remove/graft bone lesion	
	24116	Remove/graft bone lesion	
	24125	Remove/graft bone lesion	
	24126	Remove/graft bone lesion	
	24130	Removal of head of radius	
	24134	Removal of arm bone lesion	
	24136	Remove radius bone lesion	
	24138	Remove elbow bone lesion	
	24140	Partial removal of arm bone	
	24145	Partial removal of radius	
	24147	Partial removal of elbow	
	24149	Radical resection of elbow	
	24160	Remove elbow joint implant	
	24164	Remove radius head implant	
	24301	Muscle/tendon transfer	
	24305	Arm tendon lengthening	
	24343	Repr elbow lat ligmnt w/tiss	
	24345	Repr elbow med ligmnt w/tiss	
	24350	Repair of tennis elbow	
	24351	Repair of tennis elbow	
	24352	Repair of tennis elbow	
	24354	Repair of tennis elbow	
	24356	Revision of tennis elbow	
	24400	Revision of humerus	
	24410	Revision of humerus	
	24495	Decompression of forearm	
	25023	Decompress forearm 1 space	
	25024	Decompress forearm 2 spaces	
	25025	Decompress forearm 2 spaces	
	25040	Explore/treat wrist joint	
	25101	Explore/treat wrist joint	
	25105	Remove wrist joint lining	
	25107	Remove wrist joint cartilage	
	25118	Excise wrist tendon sheath	
	25119	Partial removal of ulna	
	25120	Removal of forearm lesion	
	25125	Remove/graft forearm lesion	
	25126	Remove/graft forearm lesion	
	25130	Removal of wrist lesion	
	25135	Remove & graft wrist lesion	
	25136	Remove & graft wrist lesion	
	25145	Remove forearm bone lesion	
	25150	Partial removal of ulna	
	25151	Partial removal of radius	
	25230	Partial removal of radius	
	25240	Partial removal of ulna	
	25250	Removal of wrist prosthesis	
	25251	Removal of wrist prosthesis	
	25260	Repair forearm tendon/muscle	
	25263	Repair forearm tendon/muscle	
	25265	Repair forearm tendon/muscle	
	25270	Repair forearm tendon/muscle	
	25272	Repair forearm tendon/muscle	
	25274	Repair forearm tendon/muscle	
	25275	Repair forearm tendon sheath	
	25280	Revise wrist/forearm tendon	
	25290	Incise wrist/forearm tendon	
	25300	Fusion of tendons at wrist	
	25301	Fusion of tendons at wrist	
	25360	Revision of ulna	
	25365	Revise radius & ulna	
	25390	Shorten radius or ulna	
	25392	Shorten radius & ulna	
	25400	Repair radius or ulna	
	25405	Repair/graft radius or ulna	
	25415	Repair radius & ulna	
	27001	Incision of hip tendon	
	27003	Incision of hip tendon	
	27066	Removal of hip bone lesion	
	27067	Remove/graft hip bone lesion	
	27080	Removal of tail bone	
	27097	Revision of hip tendon	
	27098	Transfer tendon to pelvis	
	27216	Treat pelvic ring fracture	
	27235	Treat thigh fracture	
	27310	Exploration of knee joint	
	27330	Biopsy, knee joint lining	
	27331	Explore/treat knee joint	
	27332	Removal of knee cartilage	
	27333	Removal of knee cartilage	
	27334	Remove knee joint lining	
	27335	Remove knee joint lining	
	27350	Removal of kneecap	
	27355	Remove femur lesion	
	27356	Remove femur lesion/graft	
	27357	Remove femur lesion/graft	
	27358	Remove femur lesion/fixation	
	27360	Partial removal, leg bone(s)	
	27393	Lengthening of thigh tendon	
	27394	Lengthening of thigh tendons	
	27396	Transplant of thigh tendon	
	27403	Repair of knee cartilage	
	27425	Lateral retinacular release	
	27610	Explore/treat ankle joint	
	27612	Exploration of ankle joint	
	27620	Explore/treat ankle joint	
	27625	Remove ankle joint lining	
	27626	Remove ankle joint lining	
	27635	Remove lower leg bone lesion	
	27637	Remove/graft leg bone lesion	
	27638	Remove/graft leg bone lesion	
	27641	Partial removal of fibula	
	27665	Repair of leg tendon, each	
	27676	Repair lower leg tendons	
	27680	Release of lower leg tendon	
	27681	Release of lower leg tendons	
	27685	Revision of lower leg tendon	
	27686	Revise lower leg tendons	
	27687	Revision of calf tendon	
	27695	Repair of ankle ligament	
	27696	Repair of ankle ligaments	
	27698	Repair of ankle ligament	
	27709	Incision of tibia & fibula	
	27730	Repair of tibia epiphysis	
	27732	Repair of fibula epiphysis	
	27734	Repair lower leg epiphyses	
	27740	Repair of leg epiphyses	
	27889	Amputation of foot at ankle	

APC/APC Title	CPT/ HCPCS Code	CPT/ HCPCS Description	APC Status Indicator
0051 Level III Musculoskeletal Procedures Except Hand and Foot			T
	20150	Excise epiphyseal bar	
	21742	Repair stern/nuss w/o scope	
	21743	Repair sternum/nuss w/scope	
	23020	Release shoulder joint	
	23120	Partial removal, collar bone	
	23125	Removal of collar bone	
	23130	Remove shoulder bone, part	
	23395	Muscle transfer, shoulder/arm	
	23415	Release of shoulder ligament	
	23480	Revision of collar bone	
	23485	Revision of collar bone	
	23490	Reinforce clavicle	
	23491	Reinforce shoulder bones	
	23800	Fusion of shoulder joint	
	23802	Fusion of shoulder joint	
	24155	Removal of elbow joint	
	24320	Repair of arm tendon	
	24330	Revision of arm muscles	
	24331	Revision of arm muscles	
	24340	Repair of biceps tendon	
	24341	Repair arm tendon/muscle	
	24342	Repair of ruptured tendon	
	24344	Reconstruct elbow lat ligmnt	
	24346	Reconstruct elbow med ligmnt	
	24420	Revision of humerus	
	24430	Repair of humerus	
	24435	Repair humerus with graft	
	24470	Revision of elbow joint	
	24498	Reinforce humerus	
	24800	Fusion of elbow joint	
	24802	Fusion/graft of elbow joint	
	25310	Transplant forearm tendon	
	25312	Transplant forearm tendon	
	25315	Revise palsy hand tendon(s)	
	25316	Revise palsy hand tendon(s)	
	25320	Repair/revise wrist joint	
	25335	Realignment of hand	
	25337	Reconstruct ulna/radioulnar	
	25350	Revision of radius	
	25355	Revision of radius	
	25370	Revise radius or ulna	
	25375	Revise radius & ulna	
	25391	Lengthen radius or ulna	
	25393	Lengthen radius & ulna	
	25420	Repair/graft radius & ulna	
	25425	Repair/graft radius or ulna	
	25426	Repair/graft radius & ulna	
	25440	Repair/graft wrist bone	
	25450	Revision of wrist joint	
	25455	Revision of wrist joint	
	25490	Reinforce radius	
	25491	Reinforce ulna	
	25492	Reinforce radius and ulna	
	25800	Fusion of wrist joint	
	25805	Fusion/graft of wrist joint	
	25810	Fusion/graft of wrist joint	
	25830	Fusion, radioulnar jnt/ulna	
	27033	Exploration of hip joint	
	27100	Transfer of abdominal muscle	
	27105	Transfer of spinal muscle	
	27110	Transfer of iliopsoas muscle	
	27111	Transfer of iliopsoas muscle	
	27395	Lengthening of thigh tendons	
	27397	Transplants of thigh tendons	
	27400	Revise thigh muscles/tendons	
	27405	Repair of knee ligament	
	27407	Repair of knee ligament	
	27409	Repair of knee ligaments	
	27418	Repair degenerated kneecap	
	27420	Revision of unstable kneecap	
	27422	Revision of unstable kneecap	
	27424	Revision/removal of kneecap	
	27430	Revision of thigh muscles	
	27435	Incision of knee joint	
	27640	Partial removal of tibia	
	27647	Extensive ankle/heel surgery	
	27650	Repair achilles tendon	
	27652	Repair/graft achilles tendon	
	27654	Repair of achilles tendon	
	27690	Revise lower leg tendon	
	27691	Revise lower leg tendon	
	27692	Revise additional leg tendon	
	27705	Incision of tibia	
	27742	Repair of leg epiphyses	
	27745	Reinforce tibia	
	27870	Fusion of ankle joint	
	27871	Fusion of tibiofibular joint	
	C9718	Kyphoplasty, first vertebra	
	C9719	Kyphoplasty, each addl	
0052 Level IV Musculoskeletal Procedures Except Hand and Foot			T
	23397	Muscle transfers	
	23410	Repair of tendon(s)	
	23412	Repair rotator cuff, chronic	
	23420	Repair of shoulder	
	23430	Repair biceps tendon	
	23440	Remove/transplant tendon	
	23450	Repair shoulder capsule	
	23455	Repair shoulder capsule	
	23460	Repair shoulder capsule	
	23462	Repair shoulder capsule	
	23465	Repair shoulder capsule	
	23466	Repair shoulder capsule	
	24150	Extensive humerus surgery	
	24151	Extensive humerus surgery	
	24152	Extensive radius surgery	
	24153	Extensive radius surgery	
	24935	Revision of amputation	
	25170	Extensive forearm surgery	
	27035	Denervation of hip joint	
	27427	Reconstruction, knee	
	27428	Reconstruction, knee	
	27429	Reconstruction, knee	
0053 Level I Hand Musculoskeletal Procedures			T
	25111	Remove wrist tendon lesion	
	25112	Reremove wrist tendon lesion	
	25394	Repair carpal bone, shorten	
	25820	Fusion of hand bones	
	26020	Drain hand tendon sheath	
	26025	Drainage of palm bursa	
	26030	Drainage of palm bursa(s)	
	26034	Treat hand bone lesion	
	26035	Decompress fingers/hand	
	26037	Decompress fingers/hand	
	26055	Incise finger tendon sheath	
	26060	Incision of finger tendon	
	26070	Explore/treat hand joint	
	26075	Explore/treat finger joint	
	26080	Explore/treat finger joint	
	26100	Biopsy hand joint lining	
	26105	Biopsy finger joint lining	
	26110	Biopsy finger joint lining	
	26130	Remove wrist joint lining	
	26140	Revise finger joint, each	
	26145	Tendon excision, palm/finger	
	26160	Remove tendon sheath lesion	
	26170	Removal of palm tendon, each	
	26180	Removal of finger tendon	

APC/APC Title	CPT/ HCPCS Code	CPT/ HCPCS Description	APC Status Indicator
0053 Level I Hand Musculoskeletal Procedures Cont'd.			T
	26185	Remove finger bone	
	26200	Remove hand bone lesion	
	26210	Removal of finger lesion	
	26215	Remove/graft finger lesion	
	26230	Partial removal of hand bone	
	26235	Partial removal, finger bone	
	26236	Partial removal, finger bone	
	26250	Extensive hand surgery	
	26260	Extensive finger surgery	
	26261	Extensive finger surgery	
	26262	Partial removal of finger	
	26410	Repair hand tendon	
	26418	Repair finger tendon	
	26432	Repair finger tendon	
	26433	Repair finger tendon	
	26437	Realignment of tendons	
	26440	Release palm/finger tendon	
	26445	Release hand/finger tendon	
	26450	Incision of palm tendon	
	26455	Incision of finger tendon	
	26460	Incise hand/finger tendon	
	26471	Fusion of finger tendons	
	26474	Fusion of finger tendons	
	26476	Tendon lengthening	
	26477	Tendon shortening	
	26478	Lengthening of hand tendon	
	26479	Shortening of hand tendon	
	26500	Hand tendon reconstruction	
	26508	Release thumb contracture	
	26520	Release knuckle contracture	
	26525	Release finger contracture	
	26540	Repair hand joint	
	26542	Repair hand joint with graft	
	26560	Repair of web finger	
	26587	Reconstruct extra finger	
	26593	Release muscles of hand	
	26951	Amputation of finger/thumb	
	26952	Amputation of finger/thumb	
	29900	Mcp joint arthroscopy, dx	
	29901	Mcp joint arthroscopy, surg	
	29902	Mcp joint arthroscopy, surg	
0054 Level II Hand Musculoskeletal Procedures			T
	25210	Removal of wrist bone	
	25215	Removal of wrist bones	
	25430	Vasc graft into carpal bone	
	25431	Repair nonunion carpal bone	
	25825	Fuse hand bones with graft	
	26040	Release palm contracture	
	26045	Release palm contracture	
	26121	Release palm contracture	
	26123	Release palm contracture	
	26125	Release palm contracture	
	26135	Revise finger joint, each	
	26205	Remove/graft bone lesion	
	26255	Extensive hand surgery	
	26350	Repair finger/hand tendon	
	26352	Repair/graft hand tendon	
	26356	Repair finger/hand tendon	
	26357	Repair finger/hand tendon	
	26358	Repair/graft hand tendon	
	26370	Repair finger/hand tendon	
	26372	Repair/graft hand tendon	
	26373	Repair finger/hand tendon	
	26390	Revise hand/finger tendon	
	26392	Repair/graft hand tendon	
	26412	Repair/graft hand tendon	
	26415	Excision, hand/finger tendon	
	26416	Graft hand or finger tendon	
	26420	Repair/graft finger tendon	
	26426	Repair finger/hand tendon	
	26428	Repair/graft finger tendon	
	26434	Repair/graft finger tendon	
	26442	Release palm & finger tendon	
	26449	Release forearm/hand tendon	
	26480	Transplant hand tendon	
	26483	Transplant/graft hand tendon	
	26485	Transplant palm tendon	
	26489	Transplant/graft palm tendon	
	26490	Revise thumb tendon	
	26492	Tendon transfer with graft	
	26494	Hand tendon/muscle transfer	
	26496	Revise thumb tendon	
	26497	Finger tendon transfer	
	26498	Finger tendon transfer	
	26499	Revision of finger	
	26502	Hand tendon reconstruction	
	26504	Hand tendon reconstruction	
	26510	Thumb tendon transfer	
	26516	Fusion of knuckle joint	
	26517	Fusion of knuckle joints	
	26518	Fusion of knuckle joints	
	26541	Repair hand joint with graft	
	26545	Reconstruct finger joint	
	26546	Repair nonunion hand	
	26548	Reconstruct finger joint	
	26550	Construct thumb replacement	
	26555	Positional change of finger	
	26561	Repair of web finger	
	26562	Repair of web finger	
	26565	Correct metacarpal flaw	
	26567	Correct finger deformity	
	26568	Lengthen metacarpal/finger	
	26580	Repair hand deformity	
	26590	Repair finger deformity	
	26591	Repair muscles of hand	
	26596	Excision constricting tissue	
	26820	Thumb fusion with graft	
	26841	Fusion of thumb	
	26842	Thumb fusion with graft	
	26843	Fusion of hand joint	
	26844	Fusion/graft of hand joint	
	26850	Fusion of knuckle	
	26852	Fusion of knuckle with graft	
	26860	Fusion of finger joint	
	26861	Fusion of finger jnt, add-on	
	26862	Fusion/graft of fingor joint	
	26863	Fuse/graft added joint	
	26910	Amputate metacarpal bone	
	64821	Remove sympathetic nerves	
	64822	Remove sympathetic nerves	
	64823	Remove sympathetic nerves	
0055 Level I Foot Musculoskeletal Procedures			T
	27605	Incision of achilles tendon	
	28005	Treat foot bone lesion	
	28008	Incision of foot fascia	
	28010	Incision of toe tendon	
	28011	Incision of toe tendons	
	28020	Exploration of foot joint	
	28022	Exploration of foot joint	
	28024	Exploration of toe joint	
	28045	Excision of foot lesion	
	28046	Resection of tumor, foot	
	28050	Biopsy of foot joint lining	
	28052	Biopsy of foot joint lining	
	28054	Biopsy of toe joint lining	
	28080	Removal of foot lesion	
	28086	Excise foot tendon sheath	
	28088	Excise foot tendon sheath	

APC/APC Title	CPT/ HCPCS Code	CPT/ HCPCS Description	APC Status Indicator
0055 Level I Foot Musculoskeletal Procedures Cont'd.			T
	28090	Removal of foot lesion	
	28092	Removal of toe lesions	
	28100	Removal of ankle/heel lesion	
	28104	Removal of foot lesion	
	28108	Removal of toe lesions	
	28111	Part removal of metatarsal	
	28112	Part removal of metatarsal	
	28113	Part removal of metatarsal	
	28114	Removal of metatarsal heads	
	28116	Revision of foot	
	28118	Removal of heel bone	
	28119	Removal of heel spur	
	28120	Part removal of ankle/heel	
	28122	Partial removal of foot bone	
	28124	Partial removal of toe	
	28126	Partial removal of toe	
	28130	Removal of ankle bone	
	28140	Removal of metatarsal	
	28150	Removal of toe	
	28153	Partial removal of toe	
	28160	Partial removal of toe	
	28171	Extensive foot surgery	
	28173	Extensive foot surgery	
	28175	Extensive foot surgery	
	28200	Repair of foot tendon	
	28208	Repair of foot tendon	
	28220	Release of foot tendon	
	28222	Release of foot tendons	
	28225	Release of foot tendon	
	28226	Release of foot tendons	
	28230	Incision of foot tendon(s)	
	28232	Incision of toe tendon	
	28234	Incision of foot tendon	
	28240	Release of big toe	
	28270	Release of foot contracture	
	28272	Release of toe joint, each	
	28280	Fusion of toes	
	28285	Repair of hammertoe	
	28286	Repair of hammertoe	
	28310	Revision of big toe	
	28312	Revision of toe	
	28313	Repair deformity of toe	
	28315	Removal of sesamoid bone	
	28340	Resect enlarged toe tissue	
	28341	Resect enlarged toe	
	28755	Fusion of big toe joint	
	28810	Amputation toe & metatarsal	
	28820	Amputation of toe	
	28825	Partial amputation of toe	
	29893	Scope, plantar fasciotomy	
0056 Level II Foot Musculoskeletal Procedures			T
	28060	Partial removal, foot fascia	
	28062	Removal of foot fascia	
	28070	Removal of foot joint lining	
	28072	Removal of foot joint lining	
	28102	Remove/graft foot lesion	
	28103	Remove/graft foot lesion	
	28106	Remove/graft foot lesion	
	28107	Remove/graft foot lesion	
	28110	Part removal of metatarsal	
	28202	Repair/graft of foot tendon	
	28210	Repair/graft of foot tendon	
	28238	Revision of foot tendon	
	28250	Revision of foot fascia	
	28260	Release of midfoot joint	
	28261	Revision of foot tendon	
	28262	Revision of foot and ankle	
	28264	Release of midfoot joint	
	28288	Partial removal of foot bone	
	28289	Repair hallux rigidus	
	28290	Correction of bunion	
	28294	Correction of bunion	
	28296	Correction of bunion	
	28298	Correction of bunion	
	28300	Incision of heel bone	
	28302	Incision of ankle bone	
	28304	Incision of midfoot bones	
	28305	Incise/graft midfoot bones	
	28306	Incision of metatarsal	
	28307	Incision of metatarsal	
	28308	Incision of metatarsal	
	28309	Incision of metatarsals	
	28320	Repair of foot bones	
	28322	Repair of metatarsals	
	28344	Repair extra toe(s)	
	28345	Repair webbed toe(s)	
	28360	Reconstruct cleft foot	
	28705	Fusion of foot bones	
	28715	Fusion of foot bones	
	28725	Fusion of foot bones	
	28730	Fusion of foot bones	
	28735	Fusion of foot bones	
	28737	Revision of foot bones	
	28740	Fusion of foot bones	
	28750	Fusion of big toe joint	
	28760	Fusion of big toe joint	
0057 Bunion Procedures			T
	28292	Correction of bunion	
	28293	Correction of bunion	
	28297	Correction of bunion	
	28299	Correction of bunion	
0058 Level I Strapping and Cast Application			S
	29020	Application of body cast	
	29040	Application of body cast	
	29049	Application of figure eight	
	29058	Application of shoulder cast	
	29105	Apply long arm splint	
	29125	Apply forearm splint	
	29126	Apply forearm splint	
	29130	Application of finger splint	
	29131	Application of finger splint	
	29200	Strapping of chest	
	29220	Strapping of low back	
	29240	Strapping of shoulder	
	29260	Strapping of elbow or wrist	
	29280	Strapping of hand or finger	
	29450	Application of leg cast	
	29505	Application, long leg splint	
	29515	Application lower leg splint	
	29520	Strapping of hip	
	29530	Strapping of knee	
	29540	Strapping of ankle and/or ft	
	29550	Strapping of toes	
	29580	Application of paste boot	
	29590	Application of foot splint	
	29700	Removal/revision of cast	
	29705	Removal/revision of cast	
	29715	Removal/revision of cast	
	29720	Repair of body cast	
	29730	Windowing of cast	
	29740	Wedging of cast	
	29750	Wedging of clubfoot cast	
	29799	Casting/strapping procedure	

APC/APC Title	CPT/ HCPCS Code	CPT/ HCPCS Description	APC Status Indicator
0060 Manipulation Therapy			S
	98925	Osteopathic manipulation	
	98926	Osteopathic manipulation	
	98927	Osteopathic manipulation	
	98928	Osteopathic manipulation	
	98929	Osteopathic manipulation	
	98940	Chiropractic manipulation	
	98941	Chiropractic manipulation	
	98942	Chiropractic manipulation	
0068 CPAP Initiation			S
	94660	Pos airway pressure, CPAP	
0069 Thoracoscopy			T
	32601	Thoracoscopy, diagnostic	
	32602	Thoracoscopy, diagnostic	
	32603	Thoracoscopy, diagnostic	
	32604	Thoracoscopy, diagnostic	
	32605	Thoracoscopy, diagnostic	
	32606	Thoracoscopy, diagnostic	
	39400	Visualization of chest	
0070 Thoracentesis/ Lavage Procedures			T
	32000	Drainage of chest	
	32002	Treatment of collapsed lung	
	32005	Treat lung lining chemically	
	32019	Insert pleural catheter	
	32020	Insertion of chest tube	
	32201	Drain, percut, lung lesion	
	32420	Puncture/clear lung	
	32960	Therapeutic pneumothorax	
	32999	Chest surgery procedure	
	33010	Drainage of heart sac	
	33011	Repeat drainage of heart sac	
	33999	Cardiac surgery procedure	
	49080	Puncture, peritoneal cavity	
	49081	Removal of abdominal fluid	
0071 Level I Endoscopy Upper Airway			T
	31505	Diagnostic laryngoscopy	
	31720	Clearance of airways	
	92511	Nasopharyngoscopy	
0072 Level II Endoscopy Upper Airway			T
	31231	Nasal endoscopy, dx	
	31233	Nasal/sinus endoscopy, dx	
	31511	Remove foreign body, larynx	
	31513	Injection into vocal cord	
	31520	Diagnostic laryngoscopy	
	31575	Diagnostic laryngoscopy	
	31700	Insertion of airway catheter	
0073 Level III Endoscopy Upper Airway			T
	31577	Remove foreign body, larynx	
	31579	Diagnostic laryngoscopy	
	31717	Bronchial brush biopsy	
	31730	Intro, windpipe wire/tube	
0074 Level IV Endoscopy Upper Airway			T
	31235	Nasal/sinus endoscopy, dx	
	31238	Nasal/sinus endoscopy, surg	
	31240	Nasal/sinus endoscopy, surg	
	31510	Laryngoscopy with biopsy	
	31512	Removal of larynx lesion	
	31515	Laryngoscopy for aspiration	
	31525	Diagnostic laryngoscopy	
	31528	Laryngoscopy and dilation	
	31529	Laryngoscopy and dilation	
	31570	Laryngoscopy with injection	
0075 Level V Endoscopy Upper Airway			T
	31237	Nasal/sinus endoscopy, surg	
	31239	Nasal/sinus endoscopy, surg	
	31254	Revision of ethmoid sinus	
	31255	Removal of ethmoid sinus	
	31256	Exploration maxillary sinus	
	31267	Endoscopy, maxillary sinus	
	31276	Sinus endoscopy, surgical	
	31287	Nasal/sinus endoscopy, surg	
	31288	Nasal/sinus endoscopy, surg	
	31292	Nasal/sinus endoscopy, surg	
	31526	Diagnostic laryngoscopy	
	31527	Laryngoscopy for treatment	
	31530	Operative laryngoscopy	
	31531	Operative laryngoscopy	
	31535	Operative laryngoscopy	
	31536	Operative laryngoscopy	
	31540	Operative laryngoscopy	
	31541	Operative laryngoscopy	
	31545	Remove vc lesion w/scope	
	31546	Remove vc lesion scope/graft	
	31560	Operative laryngoscopy	
	31561	Operative laryngoscopy	
	31571	Laryngoscopy with injection	
	31576	Laryngoscopy with biopsy	
	31578	Removal of larynx lesion	
0076 Level I Endoscopy Lower Airway			T
	31615	Visualization of windpipe	
	31622	Dx bronchoscope/wash	
	31623	Dx bronchoscope/brush	
	31624	Dx bronchoscope/lavage	
	31625	Bronchoscopy w/biopsy(s)	
	31628	Bronchoscopy/lung bx, each	
	31629	Bronchoscopy/needle bx, add'l	
	31632	Bronchoscopy/lung bx, add'l	
	31633	Bronchoscopy/needle bx add'l	
	31635	Bronchoscopy w/fb removal	
	31637	Bronchoscopy, stent add-on	
	31643	Diag bronchoscope/catheter	
	31645	Bronchoscopy, clear airways	
	31646	Bronchoscopy, reclear airway	
	31656	Bronchoscopy, inj for xray	
	31899	Airways surgical procedure	
0077 Level I Pulmonary Treatment			S
	94640	Airway inhalation treatment	
	94664	Evaluate pt use of inhaler	
	94667	Chest wall manipulation	
	94668	Chest wall manipulation	
0078 Level II Pulmonary Treatment			S
	94642	Aerosol inhalation treatment	
0079 Ventilation Initiation and Management			S
	94656	Initial ventilator mgmt	
	94657	Continued ventilator mgmt	
	94662	Neg press ventilation, cnp	
0080 Diagnostic Cardiac Catheterization			T
	93501	Right heart catheterization	
	93508	Cath placement, angiography	
	93510	Left heart catheterization	
	93511	Left heart catheterization	
	93514	Left heart catheterization	

APC/APC Title	CPT/ HCPCS Code	CPT/ HCPCS Description	APC Status Indicator
0080 Diagnostic Cardiac Catheterization Cont'd.			T
	93524	Left heart catheterization	
	93526	Rt & Lt heart catheters	
	93527	Rt & Lt heart catheters	
	93528	Rt & Lt heart catheters	
	93529	Rt & Lt heart catheterization	
	93530	Rt heart cath, congenital	
	93531	R & l heart cath, congenital	
	93532	R & l heart cath, congenital	
	93533	R & l heart cath, congenital	
0081 Non-Coronary Angioplasty or Atherectomy			T
	35458	Repair arterial blockage	
	35459	Repair arterial blockage	
	35460	Repair venous blockage	
	35470	Repair arterial blockage	
	35471	Repair arterial blockage	
	35472	Repair arterial blockage	
	35473	Repair arterial blockage	
	35474	Repair arterial blockage	
	35475	Repair arterial blockage	
	35476	Repair venous blockage	
	35484	Atherectomy, open	
	35485	Atherectomy, open	
	35490	Atherectomy, percutaneous	
	35491	Atherectomy, percutaneous	
	35492	Atherectomy, percutaneous	
	35493	Atherectomy, percutaneous	
	35494	Atherectomy, percutaneous	
	35495	Atherectomy, percutaneous	
	61626	Transcath occlusion, nonCNS	
	92997	Pul art balloon repr, percut	
	92998	Pul art balloon repr, percut	
0082 Coronary Atherectomy			T
	92995	Coronary atherectomy	
	92996	Coronary atherectomy add-on	
0083 Coronary Angioplasty and Percutaneous Valvuloplasty			T
	92982	Coronary artery dilation	
	92984	Coronary artery dilation	
	92986	Revision of aortic valve	
	92987	Revision of mitral valve	
	92990	Revision of pulmonary valve	
0084 Level I Electrophysiologic Evaluation			S
	93624	Electrophysiologic study	
	93640	Evaluation heart device	
	93641	Electrophysiology evaluation	
	93642	Electrophysiology evaluation	
0085 Level II Electrophysiologic Evaluation			T
	93619	Electrophysiology evaluation	
	93620	Electrophysiology evaluation	
	93621	Electrophysiology evaluation	
	93622	Electrophysiology evaluation	
0086 Ablate Heart Dysrhythm Focus			T
	93650	Ablate heart dysrhythm focus	
	93651	Ablate heart dysrhythm focus	
	93652	Ablate heart dysrhythm focus	
0087 Cardiac Electrophysiologic Recording/Mapping			T
	93600	Bundle of His recording	
	93602	Intra-atrial recording	
	93603	Right ventricular recording	
	93609	Map tachycardia, add-on	
	93610	Intra-atrial pacing	
	93612	Intraventricular pacing	
	93613	Electrophys map, 3D, add-on	
	93615	Esophageal recording	
	93616	Esophageal recording	
	93618	Heart rhythm pacing	
	93623	Stimulation, pacing heart	
	93631	Heart pacing, mapping	
0088 Thrombectomy			T
	34101	Removal of artery clot	
	34111	Removal of arm artery clot	
	34201	Removal of artery clot	
	34203	Removal of leg artery clot	
	34421	Removal of vein clot	
	34471	Removal of vein clot	
	34490	Removal of vein clot	
	34501	Repair valve, femoral vein	
	34510	Transposition of vein valve	
	34520	Cross-over vein graft	
	34530	Leg vein fusion	
	35188	Repair blood vessel lesion	
	35207	Repair blood vessel lesion	
	35875	Removal of clot in graft	
	35876	Removal of clot in graft	
	35879	Revise graft w/vein	
	35881	Revise graft w/vein	
	36818	AV fuse, uppr arm, cephalic	
	36819	AV fusion/uppr arm vein	
	36820	AV fusion/forearm vein	
	36821	AV fusion direct any site	
	36825	Artery-vein graft	
	36830	Artery-vein graft	
	36831	Open thrombect AV fistula	
	36832	AV fistula revision, open	
	36833	AV fistula revision	
	36834	Repair AV aneurysm	
	36838	Dist revas ligation, hemo	
0089 Insertion/ Replacement of Permanent Pacemaker and Electrodes			T
	33206	Insertion of heart pacemaker	
	33207	Insertion of heart pacemaker	
0090 Insertion/ Replacement of Pacemaker Pulse Generator			T
	33212	Insertion of pulse generator	
0091 Level II Vascular Ligation			T
	30915	Ligation, nasal sinus artery	
	37605	Ligation of neck artery	
	37606	Ligation of neck artery	
	37615	Ligation of neck artery	
	37620	Revision of major vein	
	37650	Revision of major vein	
	37700	Revise leg vein	
	37760	Revision of leg veins	
	37765	Phleb veins – extrem – to 20	
	37766	Phleb veins-extrem 20+	
	37780	Revision of leg vein	
	37785	Ligate/divide/excise vein	

APC/APC Title	CPT/ HCPCS Code	CPT/ HCPCS Description	APC Status Indicator
0092 Level I Vascular Ligation			T
	30920	Ligation, upper jaw artery	
	36475	Endovenous rf, 1st vein	
	36476	Endovenous rf, vein add-on	
	36478	Endovenous laser, 1st vein	
	36479	Endovenous laser vein add-on	
	37500	Endoscopy ligate perf veins	
	37501	Vascular endoscopy procedure	
	37607	Ligation of AV fistula	
	37720	Removal of leg vein	
	37730	Removal of leg veins	
	37735	Removal of leg veins/lesion	
0093 Vascular Reconstruction/ Fistula Repair without Device			T
	35180	Repair blood vessel lesion	
	35184	Repair blood vessel lesion	
	35190	Repair blood vessel lesion	
	35201	Repair blood vessel lesion	
	35206	Repair blood vessel lesion	
	35226	Repair blood vessel lesion	
	35231	Repair blood vessel lesion	
	35236	Repair blood vessel lesion	
	35256	Repair blood vessel lesion	
	35321	Rechanneling of artery	
	35685	Bypass graft patency/patch	
	35686	Bypass graft/AV fist patency	
	35860	Explore limb vessels	
	37565	Ligation of neck vein	
	37600	Ligation of neck artery	
0094 Level I Resuscitation and Cardioversion			S
	31500	Insert emergency airway	
	92950	Heart/lung resuscitation cpr	
	92953	Temporary external pacing	
	99440	Newborn resuscitation	
0095 Cardiac Rehabilitation			S
	93797	Cardiac rehab	
	93798	Cardiac rehab/monitor	
0096 Non-Invasive Vascular Studies			S
	76820	Umbilical artery echo	
	76821	Middle cerebral artery echo	
	93799	Cardiovascular procedure	
	93875	Extracranial study	
	93922	Extremity study	
	93923	Extremity study	
	93924	Extremity study	
	93965	Extremity study	
0097 Cardiac and Ambulatory Blood Pressure Monitoring			X
	93225	ECG monitor/record, 24 hrs	
	93226	ECG monitor/report, 24 hrs	
	93231	ECG monitor/record, 24 hrs	
	93232	ECG monitor/report, 24 hrs	
	93236	ECG monitor/report, 24 hrs	
	93270	ECG recording	
	93271	ECG/monitoring and analysis	
	93786	Ambulatory BP recording	
	93788	Ambulatory BP analysis	
0098 Injection of Sclerosing Solution			T
	36468	Injection(s), spider veins	
	36469	Injection(s), spider veins	
	36470	Injection therapy of vein	
	36471	Injection therapy of veins	
	45520	Treatment of rectal prolapse	
0099 Electrocardiograms			S
	93005	Electrocardiogram, tracing	
	93041	Rhythm ECG, tracing	
	93278	ECG/signal-averaged	
	93701	Bioimpedance, thoracic	
	G0367	EKG tracing for initial prev	
0100 Cardiac Stress Tests			X
	93017	Cardiovascular stress test	
	93024	Cardiac drug stress test	
	93025	Microvolt T-wave assess	
	Q0035	Cardiokymography	
0101 Tilt Table Evaluation			S
	93660	Tilt table evaluation	
0103 Miscellaneous Vascular Procedures			T
	37203	Transcatheter retrieval	
	37209	Exchange arterial catheter	
	93503	Insert/place heart catheter	
	93505	Biopsy of heart lining	
0104 Transcatheter Placement of Intracoronary Stents			T
	92980	Insert intracoronary stent	
	92981	Insert intracoronary stent	
0105 Revision/Removal of Pacemakers, AICD, or Vascular			T
	33215	Reposition pacing-defib lead	
	33226	Reposition l ventric lead	
	33233	Removal of pacemaker system	
	33234	Removal of pacemaker system	
	33235	Removal pacemaker electrode	
	33241	Remove pulse generator	
	33244	Remove eltrd, transven	
	49422	Remove perm cannula/catheter	
	49429	Removal of shunt	
0106 Insertion/ Replacement/Repair of Pacemaker and/or Electrodes			T
	33210	Insertion of heart electrode	
	33211	Insertion of heart electrode	
	33216	Revise eltrd pacing-defib	
	33217	Insert lead pace-defib, dual	
	33218	Repair lead pace-defib, one	
	33220	Repair lead pace-defib, dual	
0107 Insertion of Cardioverter-Defibrillator			T
	G0297	Insert dual chamber/ICD	
	G0298	Insert dual chamber/ICD	
0108 Insertion/ Replacement/Repair of Cardioverter-Defibrillator Leads			T
	G0299	Inser/repos single ICD+leads	
	G0300	Insert reposit lead dual+gen	
0109 Removal of Implanted Devices			T
	33284	Remove pat-active ht record	
	36589	Removal tunneled CV catheter	
	63746	Removal of spinal shunt	
0110 Transfusion			S
	36430	Blood transfusion service	
	36440	Bl push transfuse, 2 yr or <	
	36450	Bl exchange/transfuse, nb	
	36455	Bl exchange/transfuse, non-nb	
	36460	Transfusion service, fetal	
	38999	Blood/lymph system procedure	
	G0267	Bone marrow or PSC harvest	

APC/APC Title	CPT/ HCPCS Code	CPT/ HCPCS Description	APC Status Indicator
0111 Blood Product Exchange			S
	36511	Apheresis WBC	
	36512	Apheresis RBC	
	36513	Apheresis platelets	
	36514	Apheresis plasma	
	36515	Apheresis, adsorp/reinfuse	
	38205	Harvest allogenic stem cells	
	38206	Harvest auto stem cells	
	38230	Bone marrow collection	
	38242	Lymphocyte infuse transplant	
0112 Apheresis, Photopheresis, and Plasmapheresis			S
	36516	Apheresis, selective	
	36522	Photopheresis	
0113 Excision Lymphatic System			T
	38308	Incision of lymph channels	
	38500	Biopsy/removal, lymph nodes	
	38510	Biopsy/removal, lymph nodes	
	38520	Biopsy/removal, lymph nodes	
	38525	Biopsy/removal, lymph nodes	
	38530	Biopsy/removal, lymph nodes	
	38550	Removal, neck/armpit lesion	
	38555	Removal, neck/armpit lesion	
	38700	Removal of lymph nodes, neck	
	38720	Removal of lymph nodes, neck	
	38760	Remove groin lymph nodes	
0114 Thyroid/ Lymphadenectomy Procedures			T
	38542	Explore deep node(s), neck	
	38740	Remove armpit lymph nodes	
	38745	Remove armpit lymph nodes	
	60200	Remove thyroid lesion	
	60210	Partial thyroid excision	
	60212	Parital thyroid excision	
	60220	Partial removal of thyroid	
	60225	Partial removal of thyroid	
	60240	Removal of thyroid	
	60280	Remove thyroid duct lesion	
	60281	Remove thyroid duct lesion	
	60699	Endocrine surgery procedure	
0115 Cannula/Access Device Procedures			T
	35761	Exploration of artery/vein	
	35903	Excision, graft, extremity	
	36560	Insert tunneled CV cath	
	36561	Insert tunneled CV cath	
	36565	Insert tunneled CV cath	
	36582	Replace tunneled CV cath	
	36800	Insertion of cannula	
	36810	Insertion of cannula	
	36815	Insertion of cannula	
	36835	Artery to vein shunt	
	36861	Cannula declotting	
	37204	Transcatheter occlusion	
	49419	Insrt abdom cath for chemotx	
0116 Chemotherapy Administration by Other Technique Except Infusion			S
	96400	Chemotherapy, SQ/IM	
	96405	Intralesional chemo admin	
	96406	Intralesional chemo admin	
	96408	Chemotherapy, push technique	
	96420	Chemotherapy, push technique	
	96440	Chemotherapy, intracavitary	
	96445	Chemotherapy, intracavitary	
	96450	Chemotherapy, into CNS	
	96542	Chemotherapy injection	
	96549	Chemotherapy, unspecified	
0117 Chemotherapy Administration by Infusion Only			S
	96410	Chemotherapy, infusion method	
	96414	Chemo, infuse method add-on	
	96422	Chemotherapy, infusion method	
	96425	Chemotherapy, infusion method	
0119 Implantation of Infusion Pump			T
	36260	Insertion of infusion pump	
	36563	Insert tunneled CV cath	
	36583	Replace tunneled CV cath	
0120 Infusion Therapy Except Chemotherapy			T
	36680	Insert needle, bone cavity	
	90780	IV infusion therapy, 1 hour	
0121 Level I Tube Changes and Repositioning			T
	31502	Change of windpipe airway	
	43760	Change gastrostomy tube	
	43761	Reposition gastrostomy tube	
	44500	Intro, gastrointestinal tube	
	51705	Change of bladder tube	
	62194	Replace/irrigate catheter	
0122 Level II Tube Changes and Repositioning			T
	47525	Change bile duct catheter	
	47530	Revise/reinsert bile tube	
	50398	Change kidney tube	
	50688	Change of ureter tube	
	51710	Change of bladder tube	
	62225	Replace/irrigate catheter	
0123 Bone Marrow Harvesting and Bone Marrow/Stem Cell Transplant			S
	38240	Bone marrow/stem transplant	
	38241	Bone marrow/stem transplant	
0124 Revision of Implanted Infusion Pump			T
	36261	Revision of infusion pump	
	36262	Removal of infusion pump	
0125 Refilling of Infusion Pump			
	95990	Spin/brain pump refil & main	
	95991	Spin/brain pump refil & main	
	96520	Port pump refill & main	
	96530	Syst pump refill & main	
0130 Level I Laparoscopy			T
	38129	Laparoscope proc, spleen	
	38589	Laparoscope proc, lymphatic	
	43289	Laparoscope proc, esoph	
	43659	Laparoscope proc, stom	
	44238	Laparoscope proc, intestine	
	44239	Laparoscope proc, rectum	
	44979	Laparoscope proc, app	
	47379	Laparoscope procedure, liver	
	47560	Laparoscopy w/cholangio	
	47561	Laparo w/cholangio/biopsy	
	47579	Laparoscope proc, biliary	
	49200	Removal of abdominal lesion	
	49320	Diag laparo separate proc	
	49321	Laparoscopy, biopsy	
	49322	Laparoscopy, aspiration	
	49323	Laparo drain lymphocele	
	49329	Laparo proc, abdm/per/oment	
	49659	Laparo proc, hernia repair	
	50541	Laparo ablate renal cyst	
	50544	Laparoscopy, pyeloplasty	

APC/APC Title	CPT/ HCPCS Code	CPT/ HCPCS Description	APC Status Indicator
0130 Level I Laparoscopy Cont'd.			T
	50549	Laparoscope proc, renal	
	50949	Laparoscope proc, ureter	
	54699	Laparoscope proc, testis	
	55559	Laparo proc, spermatic cord	
	57425	Laparoscopy, surg, colpopexy	
	58545	Laparoscopic myomectomy	
	58578	Laparo proc, uterus	
	58679	Laparo proc, oviduct-ovary	
	59898	Laparo proc, ob care/deliver	
	60659	Laparo proc, endocrine	
0131 Level II Laparoscopy			T
	38120	Laparoscopy, splenectomy	
	38570	Laparoscopy, lymph node biop	
	38572	Laparoscopy, lymphadenectomy	
	43653	Laparoscopy, gastrostomy	
	44200	Laparoscopy, enterolysis	
	44201	Laparoscopy, jejunostomy	
	44970	Laparoscopy, appendectomy	
	47370	Laparo ablate liver tumor rf	
	47371	Laparo ablate liver cryosurg	
	47562	Laparoscopic cholecystectomy	
	47563	Laparo cholecystectomy/graph	
	47564	Laparo cholecystectomy/explr	
	49650	Laparo hernia repair initial	
	49651	Laparo hernia repair recur	
	50542	Laparo ablate renal mass	
	50543	Laparo partial nephrectomy	
	50945	Laparoscopy ureterolithotomy	
	50947	Laparo new ureter/bladder	
	50948	Laparo new ureter/bladder	
	51990	Laparo urethral suspension	
	54690	Laparoscopy, orchiectomy	
	55550	Laparo ligate spermatic vein	
	58546	Laparo-myomectomy, complex	
	58552	Laparo-vag hyst incl t/o	
	58553	Laparo-vag hyst, complex	
	58554	Laparo-vag hyst w/t/o, compl	
	58660	Laparoscopy, lysis	
	58661	Laparoscopy, remove adnexa	
	58662	Laparoscopy, excise lesions	
	58670	Laparoscopy, tubal cautery	
	58671	Laparoscopy, tubal block	
	58672	Laparoscopy, fimbrioplasty	
	58673	Laparoscopy, salpingostomy	
	59150	Treat ectopic pregnancy	
	59151	Treat ectopic pregnancy	
0132 Level III Laparoscopy			T
	38571	Laparoscopy, lymphadenectomy	
	43280	Laparoscopy, fundoplasty	
	43651	Laparoscopy, vagus nerve	
	43652	Laparoscopy, vagus nerve	
	44206	Lap part colectomy w/stoma	
	44207	L colectomy/coloproctostomy	
	44208	L colectomy/coloproctostomy	
	51992	Laparo sling operation	
	54692	Laparoscopy, orchiopexy	
	58550	Laparo-asst vag hysterectomy	
0140 Esophageal Dilation without Endoscopy			T
	43450	Dilate esophagus	
	43453	Dilate esophagus	
	43456	Dilate esophagus	
	43458	Dilate esophagus	

APC/APC Title	CPT/ HCPCS Code	CPT/ HCPCS Description	APC Status Indicator
0141 Level I Upper GI Procedures			T
	43200	Esophagus endoscopy	
	43201	Esoph scope w/submucous inj	
	43202	Esophagus endoscopy, biopsy	
	43204	Esoph scope w/sclerosis inj	
	43205	Esophagus endoscopy/ligation	
	43215	Esophagus endoscopy	
	43216	Esophagus endoscopy/lesion	
	43217	Esophagus endoscopy	
	43220	Esoph endoscopy, dilation	
	43226	Esoph endoscopy, dilation	
	43227	Esoph endoscopy, repair	
	43231	Esoph endoscopy w/us exam	
	43232	Esoph endoscopy w/us fn bx	
	43234	Upper GI endoscopy, exam	
	43235	Uppr GI endoscopy, diagnosis	
	43236	Uppr GI scope w/submuc inj	
	43237	Endoscopic us exam, esoph	
	43238	Uppr GI endoscopy w/us fn bx	
	43239	Upper GI endoscopy, biopsy	
	43240	Esoph endoscope w/drain cyst	
	43241	Upper GI endoscopy with tube	
	43242	Uppr GI endoscopy w/us fn bx	
	43243	Upper GI endoscopy & inject	
	43244	Upper GI endoscopy/ligation	
	43245	Uppr GI scope dilate strictr	
	43246	Place gastrostomy tube	
	43247	Operative upper GI endoscopy	
	43248	Uppr GI endoscopy/guide wire	
	43249	Esoph endoscopy, dilation	
	43250	Upper GI endoscopy/tumor	
	43251	Operative upper GI endoscopy	
	43255	Operative upper GI endoscopy	
	43258	Operative upper GI endoscopy	
	43259	Endoscopic ultrasound exam	
	43499	Esophagus surgery procedure	
	43510	Surgical opening of stomach	
	43600	Biopsy of stomach	
	43750	Place gastrostomy tube	
	43831	Place gastrostomy tube	
	43870	Repair stomach opening	
	43999	Stomach surgery procedure	
	44100	Biopsy of bowel	
0142 Small Intestine Endoscopy			T
	44360	Small bowel endoscopy	
	44361	Small bowel endoscopy/biopsy	
	44363	Small bowel endoscopy	
	44364	Small bowel endoscopy	
	44365	Small bowel endoscopy	
	44366	Small bowel endoscopy	
	44369	Small bowel endoscopy	
	44372	Small bowel endoscopy	
	44373	Small bowel endoscopy	
	44376	Small bowel endoscopy	
	44377	Small bowel endoscopy/biopsy	
	44378	Small bowel endoscopy	
	44380	Small bowel endoscopy	
	44382	Small bowel endoscopy	
	44799	Unlisted procedure intestine	
	91110	GI tract capsule endoscopy	
0143 Lower GI Endoscopy			T
	44385	Endoscopy of bowel pouch	
	44386	Endoscopy, bowel pouch/biop	
	44388	Colonoscopy	
	44389	Colonoscopy with biopsy	
	44390	Colonoscopy for foreign body	
	44391	Colonoscopy for bleeding	
	44392	Colonoscopy & polypectomy	
	44393	Colonoscopy, lesion removal	

APC/APC Title	CPT/ HCPCS Code	CPT/ HCPCS Description	APC Status Indicator
0143 Lower GI Endoscopy Cont'd.			T
	44394	Colonoscopy w/snare	
	45355	Surgical colonoscopy	
	45378	Diagnostic colonoscopy	
	45379	Colonoscopy w/fb removal	
	45380	Colonoscopy and biopsy	
	45381	Colonoscope, submucous inj	
	45382	Colonoscopy/control bleeding	
	45383	Lesion removal colonoscopy	
	45384	Lesion remove colonoscopy	
	45385	Lesion removal colonoscopy	
	45386	Colonoscopy dilate stricture	
	45391	Colonoscopy w/endoscope US	
	45392	Colonoscopy w/endoscopic fnb	
0146 Level I Sigmoidoscopy			T
	45300	Proctosigmoidoscopy dx	
	45303	Proctosigmoidoscopy dilate	
	45305	Protosigmoidoscopy w/bx	
	45307	Protosigmoidoscopy fb	
	45330	Diagnostic sigmoidoscopy	
	45331	Sigmoidoscopy and biopsy	
	45332	Sigmoidoscopy w/fb removal	
0147 Level II Sigmoidoscopy			T
	45308	Protosigmoidoscopy removal	
	45309	Protosigmoidoscopy removal	
	45315	Protosigmoidoscopy removal	
	45317	Protosigmoidoscopy bleed	
	45320	Protosigmoidoscopy ablate	
	45321	Protosigmoidoscopy volvul	
	45333	Sigmoidoscopy & polypectomy	
	45334	Sigmoidoscopy for bleeding	
	45335	Sigmoidoscope w/submuc inj	
	45337	Sigmoidoscopy & decompress	
	45338	Sigmoidoscpy w/tumr remove	
	45339	Sigmoidoscpy w/ablate tumr	
	45340	Sig w/balloon dilation	
	45341	Sigmoidoscopy w/ultrasound	
	45342	Sigmoidoscopy w/us guide bx	
	46604	Anoscopy and dilation	
	46606	Anoscopy and biopsy	
	46608	Anoscopy, remove for body	
	46610	Anoscopy, remove lesion	
	46611	Anoscopy	
	46612	Anoscopy, remove lesions	
	46614	Anoscopy, control bleeding	
	46615	Anoscopy	
0148 Level I Anal/ Rectal Procedure			T
	45000	Drainage of pelvic abscess	
	45900	Reduction of rectal prolapse	
	45915	Remove rectal obstruction	
	45999	Rectum surgery procedure	
	46030	Removal of rectal marker	
	46050	Incision of anal abscess	
	46083	Incise external hemorrhoid	
	46221	Ligation of hemorrhoid(s)	
	46320	Removal of hemorrhoid clot	
	46942	Treatment of anal fissure	
	46999	Anus surgery procedure	
0149 Level III Anal/ Rectal Procedure			T
	45100	Biopsy of rectum	
	45150	Excision of rectal stricture	
	45500	Repair of rectum	
	45905	Dilation of anal sphincter	
	45910	Dilation of rectal narrowing	
	46040	Incision of rectal abscess	
	46080	Incision of anal sphincter	
	46210	Removal of anal crypt	
	46220	Removal of anal tag	
	46230	Removal of anal tags	
	46754	Removal of suture from anus	
	46936	Destruction of hemorrhoids	
	46937	Cryotherapy of rectal lesion	
	46940	Treatment of anal fissure	
0150 Level IV Anal/ Rectal Procedure			T
	45108	Removal of anorectal lesion	
	45160	Excision of rectal lesion	
	45170	Excision of rectal lesion	
	45190	Destruction, rectal tumor	
	45505	Repair of rectum	
	45541	Correct rectal prolapse	
	45560	Repair of rectocele	
	46020	Placement of seton	
	46045	Incision of rectal abscess	
	46060	Incision of rectal abscess	
	46200	Removal of anal fissure	
	46211	Removal of anal crypts	
	46250	Hemorrhoidectomy	
	46255	Hemorrhoidectomy	
	46257	Remove hemorrhoids & fissure	
	46258	Remove hemorrhoids & fistula	
	46260	Hemorrhoidectomy	
	46261	Remove hemorrhoids & fissure	
	46262	Remove hemorrhoids & fistula	
	46270	Removal of anal fistula	
	46275	Removal of anal fistula	
	46280	Removal of anal fistula	
	46285	Removal of anal fistula	
	46288	Repair anal fistula	
	46700	Repair of anal stricture	
	46706	Repr of anal fistula w/glue	
	46750	Repair of anal sphincter	
	46753	Reconstruction of anus	
	46760	Repair of anal sphincter	
	46761	Repair of anal sphincter	
	46762	Implant artificial sphincter	
	46938	Cryotherapy of rectal lesion	
	46947	Hemorrhoidopexy by stapling	
0151 Endoscopic Retrograde Cholangio-Pancreatography (ERCP)			T
	43260	Endo cholangiopancreatograph	
	43261	Endo cholangiopancreatograph	
	43262	Endo cholangiopancreatograph	
	43263	Endo cholangiopancreatograph	
	43264	Endo cholangiopancreatograph	
	43265	Endo cholangiopancreatograph	
	43267	Endo cholangiopancreatograph	
	43271	Endo cholangiopancreatograph	
	43272	Endo cholangiopancreatograph	
0152 Level I Percutaneous Abdominal and Biliary Procedures			T
	47490	Incision of gallbladder	
	47510	Insert catheter, bile duct	
	47511	Insert bile duct drain	
	47552	Biliary endoscopy thru skin	
	47553	Biliary endoscopy thru skin	
	47554	Biliary endoscopy thru skin	
	47555	Biliary endoscopy thru skin	
	47556	Biliary endoscopy thru skin	
	47630	Remove bile duct stone	
	47999	Bile tract surgery procedure	
	49423	Exchange drainage catheter	

APC/APC Title	CPT/ HCPCS Code	CPT/ HCPCS Description	APC Status Indicator
0153 Peritoneal and Abdominal Procedures			T
	49085	Remove abdomen foreign body	
	49250	Excision of umbilicus	
	49426	Revise abdomen-venous shunt	
	49999	Abdomen surgery procedure	
0154 Hernia/Hydrocele Procedures			T
	49491	Rpr ing hern premie reduc	
	49492	Rpr ing hern premie, blocked	
	49495	Rpr ing hernia baby, reduc	
	49496	Rpr ing hernia baby, blocked	
	49500	Rpr ing hernia, init, reduce	
	49501	Rpr ing hernia, init blocked	
	49505	Rpr i/hern init reduc>5 yr	
	49507	Rpr i/hern init block>5 yr	
	49520	Rerepair ing hernia, reduce	
	49521	Rerepair ing hernia, blocked	
	49525	Repair ing hernia, sliding	
	49540	Repair lumbar hernia	
	49550	Rpr fem hernia, init, reduce	
	49553	Rpr fem hernia, init blocked	
	49555	Rerepair fem hernia, reduce	
	49557	Rerepair fem hernia, blocked	
	49560	Rpr ventral hern init, reduc	
	49561	Rpr ventral hern init, block	
	49565	Rerepair ventrl hern, reduce	
	49566	Rerepair ventrl hern, block	
	49568	Hernia repair w/mesh	
	49570	Rpr epigastric hern, reduce	
	49572	Rpr epigastric hern, blocked	
	49580	Rpr umbil hern, reduc <5 yr	
	49582	Rpr umbil hern, block < 5 yr	
	49585	Rpr umbil hern, reduc > 5 yr	
	49587	Rpr umbil hern, block > 5 yr	
	49590	Repair spigelian hernia	
	49600	Repair umbilical lesion	
	51500	Removal of bladder cyst	
	54530	Removal of testis	
	54550	Exploration for testis	
	54640	Suspension of testis	
	55040	Removal of hydrocele	
	55041	Removal of hydroceles	
	55535	Revise spermatic cord veins	
	55540	Revise hernia & sperm veins	
	57267	Insert mesh/pelvic flr add-on	
0155 Level II Anal/Rectal Procedure			T
	45005	Drainage of rectal abscess	
	45020	Drainage of rectal abscess	
	46070	Incision of anal septum	
	46500	Injection into hemorrhoid(s)	
	46934	Destruction of hemorrhoids	
	46935	Destruction of hemorrhoids	
	46945	Ligation of hemorrhoids	
	46946	Ligation of hemorrhoids	
0156 Level II Urinary and Anal Procedures			T
	50391	Instll rx agnt into rnal tub	
	51720	Treatment of bladder lesion	
	51725	Simple cystometrogram	
	51726	Complex cystometrogram	
	53600	Dilate urethra stricture	
	54200	Treatment of penis lesion	
	54220	Treatment of penis lesion	
	54450	Preputial stretching	
	91120	Rectal sensation test	
	91122	Anal pressure record	
0157 Colorectal Cancer Screening: Barium Enema			S
	G0106	Colon ca screen; barium enema	
	G0120	Colon ca scrn; barium enema	
0158 Colorectal Cancer Screening: Colonoscopy			T
	G0105	Colorectal scrn; hi risk ind	
	G0121	Colon ca scrn not hi rsk ind	
0159 Colorectal Cancer Screening: Flexible Sigmoidoscopy			S
	G0104	Ca screen; flexi sigmoidscope	
0160 Level I Cystourethroscopy and Other Genitourinary Procedures			T
	50551	Kidney endoscopy	
	50555	Kidney endoscopy & biopsy	
	50562	Renal scope w/tumor resect	
	50570	Kidney endoscopy	
	50572	Kidney endoscopy	
	50574	Kidney endoscopy & biopsy	
	50951	Endoscopy of ureter	
	50953	Endoscopy of ureter	
	50970	Ureter endoscopy	
	50972	Ureter endoscopy & catheter	
	51045	Incise bladder/drain ureter	
	52000	Cystoscopy	
	52001	Cystoscopy, removal of clots	
	52010	Cystoscopy & duct catheter	
	52265	Cystoscopy and treatment	
	52310	Cystoscopy and treatment	
0161 Level II Cystourethroscopy and Other Genitourinary Procedures			T
	50392	Insert kidney drain	
	50393	Insert ureteral tube	
	50395	Create passage to kidney	
	50553	Kidney endoscopy	
	50561	Kidney endoscopy & treatment	
	50576	Kidney endoscopy & treatment	
	50955	Ureter endoscopy & biopsy	
	50957	Ureter endoscopy & treatment	
	50961	Ureter endoscopy & treatment	
	50974	Ureter endoscopy & biopsy	
	50976	Ureter endoscopy & treatment	
	50980	Ureter endoscopy & treatment	
	52005	Cystoscopy & ureter catheter	
	52007	Cystoscopy and biopsy	
	52204	Cystoscopy	
	52260	Cystoscopy and treatment	
	52270	Cystoscopy & revise urethra	
	52275	Cystoscopy & revise urethra	
	52276	Cystoscopy and treatment	
	52281	Cystoscopy and treatment	
	52283	Cystoscopy and treatment	
	52285	Cystoscopy and treatment	
	52290	Cystoscopy and treatment	
	52300	Cystoscopy and treatment	
	52301	Cystoscopy and treatment	
	52305	Cystoscopy and treatment	
	52315	Cystoscopy and treatment	
	52351	Cystouretero & or pyeloscope	
	52510	Dilation prostatic urethra	
	53605	Dilate urethra stricture	

APC/APC Title	CPT/ HCPCS Code	CPT/ HCPCS Description	APC Status Indicator
162 Level III Cystourethroscopy and Other Genitourinary Procedures			T
	50020	Renal abscess, open drain	
	50557	Kidney endoscopy & treatment	
	51020	Incise & treat bladder	
	51030	Incise & treat bladder	
	51040	Incise & drain bladder	
	51050	Removal of bladder stone	
	51065	Remove ureter calculus	
	51520	Removal of bladder lesion	
	51880	Repair of bladder opening	
	52214	Cystoscopy and treatment	
	52224	Cystoscopy and treatment	
	52234	Cystoscopy and treatment	
	52235	Cystoscopy and treatment	
	52240	Cystoscopy and treatment	
	52250	Cystoscopy and radiotracer	
	52277	Cystoscopy and treatment	
	52317	Remove bladder stone	
	52318	Remove bladder stone	
	52320	Cystoscopy and treatment	
	52325	Cystoscopy, stone removal	
	52327	Cystoscopy, inject material	
	52330	Cystoscopy and treatment	
	52332	Cystoscopy and treatment	
	52334	Create passage to kidney	
	52341	Cysto w/ureter stricture tx	
	52342	Cysto w/up stricture tx	
	52343	Cysto w/renal stricture tx	
	52344	Cysto/uretero, stricture tx	
	52345	Cysto/uretero w/up stricture	
	52346	Cystouretero w/renal strict	
	52352	Cystouretro w/stone remove	
	52354	Cystouretero w/biopsy	
	52355	Cystouretero w/excise tumor	
	52400	Cystouretero w/congen repr	
	52402	Cystourethro cut ejacul duct	
	52450	Incision of prostate	
	52500	Revision of bladder neck	
	52606	Control postop bleeding	
	52640	Relieve bladder contracture	
	52700	Drainage of prostate abscess	
	53853	Prostatic water thermother	
	55720	Drainage of prostate abscess	
	55725	Drainage of prostate abscess	
0163 Level IV Cystourethroscopy and Other Genitourinary Procedures			T
	50080	Removal of kidney stone	
	50081	Removal of kidney stone	
	50575	Kidney endoscopy	
	52282	Cystoscopy, implant stent	
	52353	Cystouretero w/lithotripsy	
	52601	Prostatectomy (TURP)	
	52612	Prostatectomy, first stage	
	52614	Prostatectomy, second stage	
	52620	Remove residual prostate	
	52630	Remove prostate regrowth	
	52647	Laser surgery of prostate	
	52648	Laser surgery of prostate	
	55859	Percut/needle insert, pros	
0164 Level I Urinary and Anal Procedures			T
	0084T	Temp prostate urethral stent	
	50396	Measure kidney pressure	
	50686	Measure ureter pressure	
	51000	Drainage of bladder	
	51005	Drainage of bladder	
	51700	Irrigation of bladder	
	51736	Urine flow measurement	
	51741	Electro-uroflowmetry, first	
	51772	Urethra pressure profile	
	51784	Anal/urinary muscle study	
	51785	Anal/urinary muscle study	
	51792	Urinary reflex study	
	51795	Urine voiding pressure study	
	51797	Intraabdominal pressure test	
	53601	Dilate urethra stricture	
	53621	Dilate urethra stricture	
	53660	Dilation of urethra	
	53661	Dilation of urethra	
	53899	Urology surgery procedure	
	54235	Penile injection	
	54240	Penis study	
	54250	Penis study	
	55899	Genital surgery procedure	
0165 Level III Urinary and Anal Procedures			T
	51010	Drainage of bladder	
	53620	Dilate urethra stricture	
	54231	Dynamic cavernosometry	
	55860	Surgical exposure, prostate	
0166 Level I Urethral Procedures			T
	53000	Incision of urethra	
	53010	Incision of urethra	
	53020	Incision of urethra	
	53025	Incision of urethra	
	53060	Drainage of urethra abscess	
	53080	Drainage of urinary leakage	
	53085	Drainage of urinary leakage	
	53200	Biopsy of urethra	
	53215	Removal of urethra	
	53235	Removal of urethra lesion	
	53250	Removal of urethra gland	
	53260	Treatment of urethra lesion	
	53265	Treatment of urethra lesion	
	53275	Repair of urethra defect	
	53460	Revision of urethra	
	53502	Repair of urethra injury	
	53510	Repair of urethra injury	
	53665	Dilation of urethra	
	54000	Slitting of prepuce	
	54001	Slitting of prepuce	
0167 Level III Urethral Procedures			T
	51715	Endoscopic injection/implant	
	53040	Drainage of urethra abscess	
	53270	Removal of urethra gland	
	53442	Remove/revise male sling	
	53505	Repair of urethra injury	
0168 Level II Urethral Procedures			T
	53210	Removal of urethra	
	53220	Treatment of urethra lesion	
	53230	Removal of urethra lesion	
	53240	Surgery for urethra pouch	
	53400	Revise urethra, stage 1	
	53405	Revise urethra, stage 2	
	53410	Reconstruction of urethra	
	53420	Reconstruct urethra, stage 1	
	53425	Reconstruct urethra, stage 2	
	53430	Reconstruction of urethra	
	53431	Reconstruct urethra/bladder	
	53446	Remove uro sphincter	
	53449	Repair uro sphincter	
	53450	Revision of urethra	
	53500	Urethryls, transvag w/ scope	
	53515	Repair of urethra injury	
	53520	Repair of urethra defect	

APC/APC Title	CPT/ HCPCS Code	CPT/ HCPCS Description	APC Status Indicator
0169 Lithotripsy			T
	50590	Fragmenting of kidney stone	
0170 Dialysis			S
	90935	Hemodialysis, one evaluation	
	90945	Dialysis, one evaluation	
	G0257	Unsched dialysis ESRD pt hos	
0180 Circumcision			T
	54150	Circumcision	
	54152	Circumcision	
	54160	Circumcision	
	54161	Circumcision	
	54162	Lysis penil circumcis lesion	
	54163	Repair of circumcision	
	54164	Frenulotomy of penis	
0181 Penile Procedures			T
	37790	Penile venous occlusion	
	54110	Treatment of penis lesion	
	54111	Treat penis lesion, graft	
	54112	Treat penis lesion, graft	
	54120	Partial removal of penis	
	54205	Treatment of penis lesion	
	54300	Revision of penis	
	54304	Revision of penis	
	54308	Reconstruction of urethra	
	54312	Reconstruction of urethra	
	54316	Reconstruction of urethra	
	54318	Reconstruction of urethra	
	54322	Reconstruction of urethra	
	54324	Reconstruction of urethra	
	54326	Reconstruction of urethra	
	54328	Revise penis/urethra	
	54340	Secondary urethral surgery	
	54344	Secondary urethral surgery	
	54348	Secondary urethral surgery	
	54352	Reconstruct urethra/penis	
	54360	Penis plastic surgery	
	54380	Repair penis	
	54385	Repair penis	
	54406	Remove multi-comp penis pros	
	54408	Repair multi-comp penis pros	
	54415	Remove self-contd penis pros	
	54420	Revision of penis	
	54435	Revision of penis	
	54440	Repair of penis	
0183 Testes/ Epididymis Procedures			T
	54505	Biopsy of testis	
	54512	Excise lesion testis	
	54520	Removal of testis	
	54522	Orchiectomy, partial	
	54600	Reduce testis torsion	
	54620	Suspension of testis	
	54660	Revision of testis	
	54670	Repair testis injury	
	54680	Relocation of testis(es)	
	54700	Drainage of scrotum	
	54820	Exploration of epididymis	
	54830	Remove epididymis lesion	
	54840	Remove epididymis lesion	
	54860	Removal of epididymis	
	54861	Removal of epididymis	
	54900	Fusion of spermatic ducts	
	54901	Fusion of spermatic ducts	
	55060	Repair of hydrocele	
	55110	Explore scrotum	
	55120	Removal of scrotum lesion	
	55150	Removal of scrotum	
	55175	Revision of scrotum	
	55180	Revision of scrotum	
	55200	Incision of sperm duct	
	55250	Removal of sperm duct(s)	
	55400	Repair of sperm duct	
	55450	Ligation of sperm duct	
	55500	Removal of hydrocele	
	55520	Removal of sperm cord lesion	
	55530	Revise spermatic cord veins	
	55680	Remove sperm pouch lesion	
0184 Prostate Biopsy			T
	55700	Biopsy of prostate	
	55705	Biopsy of prostate	
0187 Miscellaneous Placement/Repositioning			T
	36555	Insert non-tunnel CV cath	
	36556	Insert non-tunnel CV cath	
	36568	Insert PICC cath	
	36569	Insert PICC cath	
	36575	Repair tunneled CV cath	
	36576	Repair tunneled CV cath	
	36578	Replace tunneled CV cath	
	36580	Replace CVAD cath	
	36584	Replace PICC cath	
	36590	Removal tunneled CV cath	
	36595	Mech remov tunneled CV cath	
	36596	Mech remov tunneled CV cath	
	36597	Reposition venous catheter	
	75940	X-ray placement, vein filter	
	76095	Stereotactic breast biopsy	
0188 Level II Female Reproductive Procedures			T
	56820	Exam of vulva w/scope	
	57160	Insert pessary/other device	
	58100	Biopsy of uterus lining	
0189 Level III Female Reproductive Procedures			T
	56420	Drainage of gland abscess	
	56821	Exam/biopsy of vulva w/scope	
	57180	Treat vaginal bleeding	
	57420	Exam of vagina w/scope	
	57421	Exam/biopsy of vag w/scope	
	57452	Examination of cervix w/scope	
	57454	Bx/curett of cervix w/scope	
	57455	Biopsy of cervix w/scope	
	57456	Endocerv curettage w/scope	
	57505	Endocervical curettage	
	57511	Cryocautery of cervix	
	58301	Remove intrauterine device	
	59200	Insert cervical dilator	
0190 Level I Hysteroscopy			T
	58555	Hysteroscopy, dx, sep proc	
	58558	Hysteroscopy, biopsy	
	58559	Hysteroscopy, lysis	
	58562	Hysteroscopy, remove fb	
	58579	Hysteroscope procedure	
0191 Level I Female Reproductive Procedures			T
	57150	Treat vagina infection	
	57170	Fitting of diaphragm/cap	
	58999	Genital surgery procedure	
	99170	Anogenital exam, child	
	Q0091	Obtaining screen pap smear	
0192 Level IV Female Reproductive Procedures			T
	56405	I & D of vulva/perineum	
	57020	Drainage of pelvic fluid	
	57100	Biopsy of vagina	
	57500	Biopsy of cervix	

APC/APC Title	CPT/ HCPCS Code	CPT/ HCPCS Description	APC Status Indicator
0193 Level V Female Reproductive Procedures			T
	0071T	U/S leiomyomata ablate <200	
	0072T	U/S leiomyomata ablate >200	
	56441	Lysis of labial lesion(s)	
	56720	Incision of hymen	
	57155	Insert uteri tandems/ovoids	
	57460	Bx of cervix w/scope, LEEP	
	57510	Cauterization of cervix	
	57513	Laser surgery of cervix	
	57800	Dilation of cervical canal	
	58346	Insert Heyman uteri capsule	
	58800	Drainage of ovarian cyst(s)	
	58823	Drain pelvic abscess, percut	
	58900	Biopsy of ovary(s)	
	59300	Episiotomy or vaginal repair	
0194 Level VIII Female Reproductive Procedures			T
	56440	Surgery for vulva lesion	
	56700	Partial removal of hymen	
	56740	Remove vagina gland lesion	
	56800	Repair of vagina	
	56805	Repair clitoris	
	56810	Repair of perineum	
	57000	Exploration of vagina	
	57010	Drainage of pelvic abscess	
	57061	Destroy vag lesions, simple	
	57065	Destroy vag lesions, complex	
	57105	Biopsy of vagina	
	57106	Remove vagina wall, partial	
	57130	Remove vagina lesion	
	57135	Remove vagina lesion	
	57200	Repair of vagina	
	57210	Repair vagina/perineum	
	57400	Dilation of vagina	
	57410	Pelvic examination	
	57415	Remove vaginal foreign body	
	57461	Conz of cervix w/scope, LEEP	
	57520	Conization of cervix	
	57700	Revision of cervix	
	57720	Revision of cervix	
	58345	Reopen fallopian tube	
	58615	Occlude fallopian tube(s)	
	58970	Retrieval of oocyte	
	59320	Revision of cervix	
	59409	Obstetrical care	
	59414	Deliver placenta	
	59612	VBAC delivery only	
	59871	Remove cerclage suture	
0195 Level IX Female Reproductive Procedures			T
	56620	Partial removal of vulva	
	56625	Complete removal of vulva	
	57107	Remove vagina tissue, part	
	57109	Vaginectomy partial w/nodes	
	57120	Closure of vagina	
	57230	Repair of urethral lesion	
	57240	Repair bladder & vagina	
	57250	Repair rectum & vagina	
	57260	Repair of vagina	
	57268	Repair of bowel bulge	
	57289	Repair bladder & vagina	
	57291	Construction of vagina	
	57300	Repair rectum-vagina fistula	
	57320	Repair bladder-vagina lesion	
	57330	Repair bladder-vagina lesion	
	57522	Conization of cervix	
	57530	Removal of cervix	
	57550	Removal of residual cervix	
	57555	Remove cervix/repair vagina	
	58145	Myomectomy vag method	
	58350	Reopen fallopian tube	
	58353	Endometr ablate, thermal	
	58600	Division of fallopian tube	
	58770	Create new tubal opening	
	58820	Drain ovary abscess, open	
	58920	Partial removal of ovary(s)	
	58925	Removal of ovarian cyst(s)	
0196 Dilation and Curettage			T
	57820	D & C of residual cervix	
	58120	Dilation and curettage	
	59160	D & C after delivery	
0197 Infertility Procedures			T
	55870	Electroejaculation	
	58321	Artificial insemination	
	58322	Artificial insemination	
	58323	Sperm washing	
	58974	Transfer of embryo	
	58976	Transfer of embryo	
0198 Pregnancy and Neonatal Care Procedures			T
	59000	Amniocentesis, diagnostic	
	59001	Amniocentesis, therapeutic	
	59012	Fetal cord puncture, prenatal	
	59015	Chorion biopsy	
	59020	Fetal contract stress test	
	59025	Fetal non-stress test	
	59030	Fetal scalp blood sample	
	59070	Transabdom amnioinfus w/US	
	59072	Umbilical cord occlud w/US	
	59074	Fetal fluid drainage w/US	
	59076	Fetal shunt placement, w/US	
	59866	Abortion (MPR)	
	59897	Fetal invas px w/US	
	59899	Maternity care procedure	
0200 Level VII Female Reproductive Procedures			T
	59840	Abortion	
	59841	Abortion	
0201 Level VI Female Reproductive Procedures			T
	59812	Treatment of miscarriage	
	59820	Care of miscarriage	
	59821	Treatment of miscarriage	
	59870	Evacuate mole of uterus	
0202 Level X Female Reproductive Procedures			T
	57220	Revision of urethra	
	57265	Extensive repair of vagina	
	57284	Repair paravaginal defect	
	57287	Revise/remove sling repair	
	57288	Repair bladder defect	
	57310	Repair urethrovaginal lesion	
	57556	Remove cervix, repair bowel	
	58356	Endometrial cryoablation	
	58565	Hysteroscopy, sterilization	
0203 Level IV Nerve Injections			T
	0062T	Rep intradisc annulus; 1 lev	
	0063T	Rep intradisc annulus; >1lev	
	62263	Epidural lysis mult sessions	
	62264	Epidural lysis on single day	
	62355	Remove spinal canal catheter	
	64600	Injection treatment of nerve	
	64605	Injection treatment of nerve	

APC/APC Title	CPT/ HCPCS Code	CPT/ HCPCS Description	APC Status Indicator
0203 Level IV Nerve Injections Cont'd.			T
	64610	Injection treatment of nerve	
	64620	Injection treatment of nerve	
	64622	Destr paravertebrl nerve l/s	
	64626	Destr paravertebrl nerve c/t	
	64681	Injection treatment of nerve	
0204 Level I Nerve Injections			T
	20526	Ther injection carpal tunnel	
	20550	Inj tendon sheath/ligament	
	20551	Inj tendon origin/insertion	
	20552	Inject trigger point, 1/2 muscl	
	20553	Inject trigger points,=/> 3	
	20600	Drain/inject, joint/bursa	
	20605	Drain/inject, joint/bursa	
	20610	Drain/inject, joint/bursa	
	20612	Aspirate/Inj ganglion cyst	
	62270	Spinal fluid tap, diagnostic	
	62272	Drain cerebro spinal fluid	
	64400	N block inj, trigeminal	
	64402	N block inj, facial	
	64405	N block inj, occipital	
	64408	N block inj, vagus	
	64413	N block inj, cervical plexus	
	64415	Injection for nerve block	
	64416	N block cont infuse, b plex	
	64417	N block inj, axillary	
	64418	N block inj, suprascapular	
	64420	N block inj, intercost, sng	
	64425	N block inj ilio-ing/hypogi	
	64430	N block inj, pudendal	
	64435	N block inj, paracervical	
	64445	N block inj, sciatic, sng	
	64447	N block inj fem, single	
	64448	N block inj fem, cont inf	
	64449	N block inj, lumbar plexus	
	64450	N block, other peripheral	
	64505	N block, spenopalatine gangl	
	64508	N block, carotid sinus s/p	
	64517	N block inj, hypogas plxs	
	64612	Destroy nerve, face muscle	
	64613	Destroy nerve, spine muscle	
	64614	Destroy nerve, extrem musc	
	64999	Nervous system surgery	
0206 Level II Nerve Injections			T
	61791	Treat trigeminal tract	
	62273	Inject epidural patch	
	64410	N block inj, phrenic	
	64412	N block inj, spinal accessor	
	64421	N block inj, intercost, mlt	
	64446	N blk inj, sciatic, cont inf	
	64472	Inj paravertebral c/t add-on	
	64476	Inj paravertebral l/s add-on	
	64630	Injection treatment of nerve	
	64640	Injection treatment of nerve	
	G0260	Inj for sacroiliac jt anesth	
0207 Level III Nerve Injections			T
	62280	Treat spinal cord lesion	
	62281	Treat spinal cord lesion	
	62282	Treat spinal canal lesion	
	62310	Inject spine c/t	
	62311	Inject spine l/s (cd)	
	62318	Inject spine w/cath, c/t	
	62319	Inject spine w/cath l/s (cd)	
	64470	Inj paravertebral c/t	
	64475	Inj paravertebral l/s	
	64479	Inj foramen epidural c/t	
	64480	Inj foramen epidural add-on	
	64483	Inj foramen epidural l/s	
	64484	Inj foramen epidural add-on	
	64510	N block, stellate ganglion	
	64520	N block, lumbar/thoracic	
	64530	N block inj, celiac plexus	
	64623	Destr paravertebral n add-on	
	64627	Destr paravertebral n add-on	
	64680	Injection treatment of nerve	
0208 Laminotomies and Laminectomies			T
	22100	Remove part of neck vertebra	
	22101	Remove part, thorax vertebra	
	22102	Remove part, lumbar vertebra	
	22103	Remove extra spine segment	
	22222	Revision of thorax spine	
	22612	Lumbar spine fusion	
	22614	Spine fusion, extra segment	
	62351	Implant spinal canal cath	
	63001	Removal of spinal lamina	
	63003	Removal of spinal lamina	
	63005	Removal of spinal lamina	
	63011	Removal of spinal lamina	
	63012	Removal of spinal lamina	
	63015	Removal of spinal lamina	
	63016	Removal of spinal lamina	
	63017	Removal of spinal lamina	
	63020	Neck spine disk surgery	
	63030	Low back disk surgery	
	63035	Spinal disk surgery add-on	
	63040	Laminotomy, single cervical	
	63042	Laminotomy, single lumbar	
	63045	Removal of spinal lamina	
	63046	Removal of spinal lamina	
	63047	Removal of spinal lamina	
	63048	Remove spinal lamina add-on	
	63055	Decompress spinal cord	
	63056	Decompress spinal cord	
	63057	Decompress spine cord add-on	
	63064	Decompress spinal cord	
	63066	Decompress spine cord add-on	
0209 Extended EEG Studies and Sleep Studies, Level II			S
	95805	Multiple sleep latency test	
	95807	Sleep study, attended	
	95808	Polysomnography, 1-3	
	95810	Polysomnography, 4 or more	
	95811	Polysomnography w/CPAP	
	95950	Ambulatory EEG monitoring	
	95951	EEG monitoring/videorecord	
	95953	EEG monitoring/computer	
	95956	EEG monitoring, cable/radio	
0212 Nervous System Injections			T
	61000	Remove cranial cavity fluid	
	61001	Remove cranial cavity fluid	
	61020	Remove brain cavity fluid	
	61026	Injection into brain canal	
	61050	Remove brain canal fluid	
	61055	Injection into brain canal	
	61070	Brain canal shunt procedure	
	62268	Drain spinal cord cyst	
	62292	Injection into disk lesion	
	62294	Injection into spinal artery	
0213 Extended EEG Studies and Sleep Studies, Level I			S
	95806	Sleep study, unattended	
	95812	EEG, 41-60 minutes	
	95813	EEG, over 1 hour	
	95827	EEG, all night recording	
	95955	EEG during surgery	
	95958	EEG monitoring/function test	

APC/APC Title	CPT/ HCPCS Code	CPT/ HCPCS Description	APC Status Indicator
0214 Electroencephalogram			S
	95816	EEG, awake and drowsy	
	95819	EEG, awake and drowsy	
	95822	EEG, coma or sleep only	
	95824	EEG, cerebral death only	
	95829	Surgery electrocorticogram	
	95954	EEG monitoring/giving drugs	
	95957	EEG digital analysis	
0215 Level I Nerve and Muscle Tests			S
	0018T	Transcranial magnetic stimul	
	95858	Tensilon test & myogram	
	95869	Muscle test, thor paraspinal	
	95870	Muscle test, nonparaspinal	
	95875	Limb exercise test	
	95900	Motor nerve conduction test	
	95903	Motor nerve conduction test	
	95904	Sense nerve conduction test	
	95933	Blink reflex test	
	95934	H-reflex test	
	95936	H-reflex test	
	95999	Neurological procedure	
	96003	Dynamic fine wire EMG	
0216 Level III Nerve and Muscle Tests			S
	92585	Auditor evoke potent, compre	
	95920	Intraop nerve test add-on	
	95925	Somatosensory testing	
	95926	Somatosensory testing	
	95927	Somatosensory testing	
	95930	Visual evoked potential test	
	95961	Electrode stimulation, brain	
	95962	Electrode stim, brain add-on	
	96000	Motion analysis, video/3D	
	96001	Motion test w/ft press meas	
0218 Level II Nerve and Muscle Tests			S
	92586	Auditor evoke potent, limit	
	95857	Tensilon test	
	95860	Muscle test, one limb	
	95861	Muscle test, 2 limbs	
	95863	Muscle test, 3 limbs	
	95864	Muscle test, 4 limbs	
	95867	Muscle test cran nerv unilat	
	95868	Muscle test cran nerve bilat	
	95872	Muscle test, one fiber	
	95921	Autonomic nerv function test	
	95922	Autonomic nerv function test	
	95923	Autonomic nerv function test	
	95928	C motor evoked, uppr limbs	
	95929	C motor evoked, lwr limbs	
	95937	Neuromuscular junction test	
	95970	Analyze neurostim, no prog	
	96002	Dynamic surface EMG	
0220 Level I Nerve Procedures			T
	27315	Partial removal, thigh nerve	
	27320	Partial removal, thigh nerve	
	28030	Removal of foot nerve	
	28035	Decompression of tibia nerve	
	61790	Treat trigeminal nerve	
	63600	Remove spinal cord lesion	
	63610	Stimulation of spinal cord	
	63615	Remove lesion of spinal cord	
	64702	Revise finger/toe nerve	
	64704	Revise hand/foot nerve	
	64708	Revise arm/leg nerve	
	64712	Revision of sciatic nerve	
	64713	Revision of arm nerve(s)	
	64714	Revise low back nerve(s)	
	64716	Revision of cranial nerve	
	64718	Revise ulnar nerve at elbow	
	64719	Revise ulnar nerve at wrist	
	64721	Carpal tunnel surgery	
	64722	Relieve pressure on nerve(s)	
	64726	Release foot/toe nerve	
	64727	Internal nerve revision	
	64732	Incision of brow nerve	
	64734	Incision of cheek nerve	
	64736	Incision of chin nerve	
	64738	Incision of jaw nerve	
	64740	Incision of tongue nerve	
	64742	Incision of facial nerve	
	64744	Incise nerve, back of head	
	64746	Incise diaphragm nerve	
	64761	Incision of pelvis nerve	
	64771	Sever cranial nerve	
	64772	Incision of spinal nerve	
	64774	Remove skin nerve lesion	
	64776	Remove digit nerve lesion	
	64778	Digit nerve surgery add-on	
	64782	Remove limb nerve lesion	
	64783	Limb nerve surgery add-on	
	64784	Remove nerve lesion	
	64787	Implant nerve end	
	64788	Remove skin nerve lesion	
	64790	Removal of nerve lesion	
	64795	Biopsy of nerve	
	64802	Remove sympathetic nerves	
	64820	Remove sympathetic nerves	
0221 Level II Nerve Procedures			T
	62287	Percutaneous diskectomy	
	62365	Remove spine infusion device	
	64786	Remove sciatic nerve lesion	
	64792	Removal of nerve lesion	
	64831	Repair of digit nerve	
	64832	Repair nerve add-on	
	64834	Repair of hand or foot nerve	
	64835	Repair of hand or foot nerve	
	64836	Repair of hand or foot nerve	
	64837	Repair nerve add-on	
	64840	Repair of leg nerve	
	64856	Repair/transpose nerve	
	64857	Repair arm/leg nerve	
	64858	Repair sciatic nerve	
	64859	Nerve surgery	
	64861	Repair of arm nerves	
	64862	Repair of low back nerves	
	64864	Repair of facial nerve	
	64865	Repair of facial nerve	
	64870	Fusion of facial/other nerve	
	64872	Subsequent repair of nerve	
	64874	Repair & revise nerve add-on	
	64876	Repair nerve/shorten bone	
	64885	Nerve graft, head or neck	
	64886	Nerve graft, head or neck	
	64890	Nerve graft, hand or foot	
	64891	Nerve graft, hand or foot	
	64892	Nerve graft, arm or leg	
	64893	Nerve graft, arm or leg	
	64895	Nerve graft, hand or foot	
	64896	Nerve graft, hand or foot	
	64897	Nerve graft, arm or leg	
	64898	Nerve graft, arm or leg	
	64901	Nerve graft add-on	
	64902	Nerve graft add-on	
	64905	Nerve pedicle transfer	
	64907	Nerve pedicle transfer	
0222 Implantation of Neurological Device			T
	63685	Insrt/redo spine n generator	
	64590	Insrt/redo perph n generator	

APC/APC Title	CPT/ HCPCS Code	CPT/ HCPCS Description	APC Status Indicator
0223 Implantation or Revision of Pain Management Catheter			T
	62350	Implant spinal canal cath	
0224 Implantation of Reservoir/Pump/Shunt			T
	61215	Insert brain-fluid device	
	62230	Replace/revise brain shunt	
0225 Level I Implantation of Neurostimulator Electrodes			S
	63655	Implant neuroelectrodes	
	64553	Implant neuroelectrodes	
	64573	Implant neuroelectrodes	
	64577	Implant neuroelectrodes	
	64580	Implant neuroelectrodes	
0226 Implantation of Drug Infusion Reservoir			T
	62360	Insert spine infusion device	
0227 Implantation of Drug Infusion Device			T
	62361	Implant spine infusion pump	
	62362	Implant spine infusion pump	
0228 Creation of Lumbar Subarachnoid Shunt			T
	63741	Install spinal shunt	
	63744	Revision of spinal shunt	
0229 Transcatherter Placement of Intravascular Shunts			T
	37205	Transcath IV stent, percut	
	37206	Transcath IV stent/perc addl	
	37207	Transcath IV stent, open	
	37208	Transcath IV stent/open addl	
0230 Level I Eye Tests & Treatments			S
	65430	Corneal smear	
	68200	Treat eyelid by injection	
	68899	Tear duct system surgery	
	92020	Special eye evaluation	
	92060	Special eye evaluation	
	92065	Orthoptic/pleoptic training	
	92081	Visual field examination(s)	
	92082	Visual field examination(s)	
	92083	Visual field examination(s)	
	92120	Tonography & eye evaluation	
	92130	Water provocation tonography	
	92135	Ophthalmic dx imaging	
	92136	Ophthalmic biometry	
	92225	Special eye exam, initial	
	92226	Special eye exam, subsequent	
	92250	Eye exam with photos	
	92260	Ophthalmoscopy/dynamometry	
	92265	Eye muscle evaluation	
	92270	Electro-oculography	
	92283	Color vision examination	
	92285	Eye photography	
	92330	Fitting of artificial eye	
	92499	Eye service or procedure	
	G0117	Glaucoma scrn hgh risk direc	
	G0118	Glaucoma scrn hgh risk direc	
0231 Level III Eye Tests & Treatments			S
	65450	Treatment of corneal lesion	
	67500	Inject/treat eye socket	
	68761	Close tear duct opening	
	68840	Explore/irrigate tear ducts	
	92235	Eye exam with photos	
	92240	ICG angiography	
	92275	Electroretinography	
0232 Level I Anterior Segment Eye Procedures			T
	65286	Repair of eye wound	
	65820	Relieve inner eye pressure	
	66030	Injection treatment of eye	
	66500	Incision of iris	
	66505	Incision of iris	
	66625	Removal of iris	
	66820	Incision, secondary cataract	
	66830	Removal of lens lesion	
	66999	Eye surgery procedure	
	68100	Biopsy of eyelid lining	
0233 Level II Anterior Segment Eye Procedures			T
	65235	Remove foreign body from eye	
	65400	Removal of eye lesion	
	65410	Biopsy of cornea	
	65420	Removal of eye lesion	
	65436	Curette/treat cornea	
	65772	Correction of astigmatism	
	65775	Correction of astigmatism	
	65800	Drainage of eye	
	65805	Drainage of eye	
	65865	Incise inner eye adhesions	
	65880	Incise inner eye adhesions	
	65900	Remove eye lesion	
	66020	Injection treatment of eye	
	66250	Follow-up surgery of eye	
	66700	Destruction, ciliary body	
	66710	Ciliary transscleral therapy	
	66711	Ciliary endoscopic ablation	
	66720	Destruction, ciliary body	
	67880	Revision of eyelid	
	68130	Remove eyelid lining lesion	
	68371	Harvest eye tissue, allograft	
0234 Level III Anterior Segment Eye Procedures			T
	65272	Repair of eye wound	
	65275	Repair of eye wound	
	65426	Removal of eye lesion	
	65810	Drainage of eye	
	65815	Drainage of eye	
	65850	Incision of eye	
	65870	Incise inner eye adhesions	
	65875	Incise inner eye adhesions	
	65920	Remove implant of eye	
	65930	Remove blood clot from eye	
	66130	Remove eye lesion	
	66150	Glaucoma surgery	
	66155	Glaucoma surgery	
	66160	Glaucoma surgery	
	66165	Glaucoma surgery	
	66170	Glaucoma surgery	
	66600	Remove iris and lesion	
	66605	Removal of iris	
	66630	Removal of iris	
	66635	Removal of iris	
	66680	Repair iris & ciliary body	
	66682	Repair iris & ciliary body	
	66740	Destruction, ciliary body	
	66825	Reposition intraocular lens	
	68330	Revise eyelid lining	
	68360	Revise eyelid lining	
	68362	Revise eyelid lining	

APC/APC Title	CPT/ HCPCS Code	CPT/ HCPCS Description	APC Status Indicator
0235 Level I Posterior Segment Eye Procedures			T
	0016T	Thermotx choroid vasc lesion	
	67028	Injection eye drug	
	67101	Repair detached retina	
	67141	Treatment of retina	
	67208	Treatment of retinal lesion	
	67220	Treatment of choroid lesion	
	67221	Ocular photodynamic ther	
	67225	Eye photodynamic ther add-on	
	67227	Treatment of retinal lesion	
	67299	Eye surgery procedure	
	G0186	Dstry eye lesn, fdr vssl tech	
0236 Level II Posterior Segment Eye Procedures			T
	65260	Remove foreign body from eye	
	65265	Remove foreign body from eye	
	65280	Repair of eye wound	
	65285	Repair of eye wound	
	66220	Repair eye lesion	
	67025	Replace eye fluid	
	67030	Incise inner eye strands	
	67110	Repair detached retina	
	67115	Release encircling material	
	67120	Remove eye implant material	
	67121	Remove eye implant material	
	67218	Treatment of retinal lesion	
0237 Level III Posterior Segment Eye Procedures			T
	67005	Partial removal of eye fluid	
	67010	Partial removal of eye fluid	
	67015	Release of eye fluid	
	67027	Implant eye drug system	
	67036	Removal of inner eye fluid	
	67038	Strip retinal membrane	
	67039	Laser treatment of retina	
	67255	Reinforce/graft eye wall	
0238 Level I Repair and Plastic Eye Procedures			T
	67345	Destroy nerve of eye muscle	
	67505	Inject/treat eye socket	
	67515	Inject/treat eye socket	
	67599	Orbit surgery procedure	
	67700	Drainage of eyelid abscess	
	67800	Remove eyelid lesion	
	67805	Remove eyelid lesions	
	67810	Biopsy of eyelid	
	67825	Revise eyelashes	
	67999	Revision of eyelid	
	68399	Eyelid lining surgery	
	68400	Incise/drain tear gland	
	68440	Incise tear duct opening	
	68705	Revise tear duct opening	
0239 Level II Repair and Plastic Eye Procedures			T
	65435	Curette/treat cornea	
	67710	Incision of eyelid	
	67801	Remove eyelid lesions	
	67830	Revise eyelashes	
	67840	Remove eyelid lesion	
	67850	Treat eyelid lesion	
	67875	Closure of eyelid by suture	
	67912	Correction eyelid w/implant	
	67915	Repair eyelid defect	
	68135	Remove eyelid lining lesion	
0240 Level III Repair and Plastic Eye Procedures			T
	65125	Revise ocular implant	
	65175	Removal of ocular implant	
	65270	Repair of eye wound	
	65600	Revision of cornea	
	67250	Reinforce eye wall	
	67415	Aspiration, orbital contents	
	67715	Incision of eyelid fold	
	67808	Remove eyelid lesion(s)	
	67835	Revise eyelashes	
	67882	Revision of eyelid	
	67900	Repair brow defect	
	67901	Repair eyelid defect	
	67902	Repair eyelid defect	
	67903	Repair eyelid defect	
	67904	Repair eyelid defect	
	67906	Repair eyelid defect	
	67908	Repair eyelid defect	
	67909	Revise eyelid defect	
	67911	Revise eyelid defect	
	67914	Repair eyelid defect	
	67916	Repair eyelid defect	
	67917	Repair eyelid defect	
	67921	Repair eyelid defect	
	67922	Repair eyelid defect	
	67923	Repair eyelid defect	
	67924	Repair eyelid defect	
	67930	Repair eyelid wound	
	67935	Repair eyelid wound	
	67950	Revision of eyelid	
	67961	Revision of eyelid	
	67966	Revision of eyelid	
	67975	Reconstruction of eyelid	
	68020	Incise/drain eyelid lining	
	68115	Remove eyelid lining lesion	
	68320	Revise/graft eyelid lining	
	68340	Separate eyelid adhesions	
	68420	Incise/drain tear sac	
	68510	Biopsy of tear gland	
	68525	Biopsy of tear sac	
	68530	Clearance of tear duct	
	68770	Close tear system fistula	
	68811	Probe nasolacrimal duct	
	68815	Probe nasolacrimal duct	
0241 Level IV Repair and Plastic Eye Procedures			T
	65093	Revise eye with implant	
	65130	Insert ocular implant	
	65135	Insert ocular implant	
	65150	Revise ocular implant	
	67400	Explore/biopsy eye socket	
	67405	Explore/drain eye socket	
	67412	Explore/treat eye socket	
	67413	Explore/treat eye socket	
	67560	Revise eye socket implant	
	67971	Reconstruction of eyelid	
	67973	Reconstruction of eyelid	
	67974	Reconstruction of eyelid	
	68326	Revise/graft eyelid lining	
	68328	Revise/graft eyelid lining	
	68335	Revise/graft eyelid lining	
	68500	Removal of tear gland	
	68505	Partial removal, tear gland	
	68520	Removal of tear sac	
	68540	Remove tear gland lesion	
	68700	Repair tear ducts	
	68745	Create tear duct drain	

APC/APC Title	CPT/ HCPCS Code	CPT/ HCPCS Description	APC Status Indicator
0242 Level V Repair and Plastic Eye Procedures			T
	65091	Revise eye	
	65101	Removal of eye	
	65103	Remove eye/insert implant	
	65105	Remove eye/attach implant	
	65110	Removal of eye	
	65112	Remove eye/revise socket	
	65114	Remove eye/revise socket	
	65140	Attach ocular implant	
	65155	Reinsert ocular implant	
	67414	Explr/decompress eye socket	
	67420	Explore/treat eye socket	
	67430	Explore/treat eye socket	
	67440	Explore/drain eye socket	
	67445	Explr/decompress eye socket	
	67450	Explore/biopsy eye socket	
	67550	Insert eye socket implant	
	67570	Decompress optic nerve	
	68325	Revise/graft eyelid lining	
	68550	Remove tear gland lesion	
	68720	Create tear sac drain	
	68750	Create tear duct drain	
0243 Strabismus/ Muscle Procedures			T
	65290	Repair of eye socket wound	
	67311	Revise eye muscle	
	67312	Revise two eye muscles	
	67314	Revise eye muscle	
	67316	Revise two eye muscles	
	67318	Revise eye muscle(s)	
	67320	Revise eye muscle(s) add-on	
	67331	Eye surgery follow-up add-on	
	67332	Rerevise eye muscles add-on	
	67334	Revise eye muscle w/suture	
	67335	Eye suture during surgery	
	67340	Revise eye muscle add-on	
	67343	Release eye tissue	
	67399	Eye muscle surgery procedure	
0244 Corneal Transplant			T
	65710	Corneal transplant	
	65730	Corneal transplant	
	65750	Corneal transplant	
	65755	Corneal transplant	
	65770	Revise cornea with implant	
	65780	Ocular reconst, transplant	
	65781	Ocular reconst, transplant	
	65782	Ocular reconst, transplant	
0245 Level I Cataract Procedures without IOL Insert			T
	66840	Removal of lens material	
	66940	Extraction of lens	
0246 Cataract Procedures with IOL Insert			T
	66982	Cataract surgery, complex	
	66983	Cataract surg w/IOL, 1 stage	
	66984	Cataract surg wIOL, 1 stage	
	66985	Insert lens prosthesis	
	66986	Exchange lens prosthesis	
0247 Laser Eye Procedures Except Retinal			T
	65855	Laser surgery of eye	
	65860	Incise inner eye adhesions	
	66761	Revision of iris	
	66762	Revision of iris	
	66770	Removal of inner eye lesion	
	66821	After cataract laser surgery	
	67031	Laser surgery, eye strands	
0248 Laser Retinal Procedures			T
	67105	Repair detached retina	
	67145	Treatment of retina	
	67210	Treatment of retinal lesion	
	67228	Treatment of retinal lesion	
0249 Level II Cataract Procedures without IOL Insert			T
	66850	Removal of lens material	
	66852	Removal of lens material	
	66920	Extraction of lens	
	66930	Extraction of lens	
0250 Nasal Cauterization/ Packing			T
	30901	Control of nosebleed	
	30903	Control of nosebleed	
	30905	Control of nosebleed	
	30906	Repeat control of nosebleed	
	42960	Control throat bleeding	
	42970	Control nose/throat bleeding	
0251 Level I ENT Procedures			T
	20500	Injection of sinus tract	
	21089	Prepare face/oral prosthesis	
	21299	Cranio/maxillofacial surgery	
	21310	Treatment of nose fracture	
	21315	Treatment of nose fracture	
	21450	Treat lower jaw fracture	
	21480	Reset dislocated jaw	
	21499	Head surgery procedure	
	21899	Neck/chest surgery procedure	
	30000	Drainage of nose lesion	
	30020	Drainage of nose lesion	
	30560	Release of nasal adhesions	
	30999	Nasal surgery procedure	
	31000	Irrigation, maxillary sinus	
	31299	Sinus surgery procedure	
	31599	Larynx surgery procedure	
	40490	Biopsy of lip	
	40799	Lip surgery procedure	
	40800	Drainage of mouth lesion	
	40806	Incision of lip fold	
	40808	Biopsy of mouth lesion	
	40818	Excise oral mucosa for graft	
	40830	Repair mouth laceration	
	40899	Mouth surgery procedure	
	41005	Drainage of mouth lesion	
	41009	Drainage of mouth lesion	
	41015	Drainage of mouth lesion	
	41250	Repair tongue laceration	
	41251	Repair tongue laceration	
	41599	Tongue and mouth surgery	
	41800	Drainage of gum lesion	
	41899	Dental surgery procedure	
	42000	Drainage mouth roof lesion	
	42180	Repair palate	
	42280	Preparation, palate mold	
	42299	Palate/uvula surgery	
	42310	Drainage of salivary gland	
	42320	Drainage of salivary gland	
	42325	Create salivary cyst drain	
	42660	Dilation of salivary duct	
	42699	Salivary surgery procedure	
	42700	Drainage of tonsil abscess	
	42999	Throat surgery procedure	
	69399	Outer ear surgery procedure	
	69400	Inflate middle ear canal	
	69401	Inflate middle ear canal	

APC/APC Title	CPT/ HCPCS Code	CPT/ HCPCS Description	APC Status Indicator
0251 Level I ENT Procedures Cont'd.			T
	69410	Inset middle ear (baffle)	
	69799	Middle ear surgery procedure	
	69949	Inner ear surgery procedure	
	69979	Temporal bone surgery	
	92502	Ear and throat examination	
0252 Level II ENT Procedures			T
	21110	Interdental fixation	
	21295	Revision of jaw muscle/bone	
	21320	Treatment of nose fracture	
	21400	Treat eye socket fracture	
	21451	Treat lower jaw fracture	
	21493	Treat hyoid bone fracture	
	21494	Treat hyoid bone fracture	
	21685	Hyoid myotomy & suspension	
	30100	Intranasal biopsy	
	30124	Removal of nose lesion	
	30200	Injection treatment of nose	
	30210	Nasal sinus therapy	
	30220	Insert nasal septal button	
	30801	Cauterization, inner nose	
	30802	Cauterization, inner nose	
	31002	Irrigation, sphenoid sinus	
	31603	Incision of windpipe	
	31605	Incision of windpipe	
	40650	Repair lip	
	40652	Repair lip	
	40654	Repair lip	
	40801	Drainage of mouth lesion	
	40805	Removal, foreign body, mouth	
	40819	Excise lip or cheek fold	
	40831	Repair mouth laceration	
	41010	Incision of tongue fold	
	41016	Drainage of mouth lesion	
	41017	Drainage of mouth lesion	
	41018	Drainage of mouth lesion	
	41100	Biopsy of tongue	
	41108	Biopsy of floor of mouth	
	41115	Excision of tongue fold	
	41252	Repair tongue laceration	
	41520	Reconstruction, tongue fold	
	41820	Excision, gum, each quadrant	
	41821	Excision of gum flap	
	42100	Biopsy roof of mouth	
	42140	Excision of uvula	
	42326	Create salivary cyst drain	
	42650	Dilation of salivary duct	
	42900	Repair throat wound	
	43020	Incision of esophagus	
	60000	Drain thyroid/tongue cyst	
	69150	Extensive ear canal surgery	
	69405	Catheterize middle ear canal	
	69420	Incision of eardrum	
	69424	Remove ventilating tube	
	69433	Create eardrum opening	
0253 Level III ENT Procedures			T
	0088T	Rf tongue base vol reduxn	
	21015	Resection of facial tumor	
	21085	Prepare face/oral prosthesis	
	21282	Revision of eyelid	
	21300	Treatment of skull fracture	
	21337	Treat nasal septal fracture	
	21401	Treat eye socket fracture	
	21452	Treat lower jaw fracture	
	21485	Reset dislocated jaw	
	21497	Interdental wiring	
	30110	Removal of nose polyp(s)	
	30115	Removal of nose polyp(s)	
	30117	Removal of intranasal lesion	
	30120	Revision of nose	
	30130	Removal of turbinate bones	
	30310	Remove nasal foreign body	
	30320	Remove nasal foreign body	
	30930	Therapy, fracture of nose	
	31585	Treat larynx fracture	
	31820	Closure of windpipe lesion	
	40500	Partial excision of lip	
	40520	Partial excision of lip	
	40810	Excision of mouth lesion	
	40812	Excise/repair mouth lesion	
	40814	Excise/repair mouth lesion	
	40820	Treatment of mouth lesion	
	41000	Drainage of mouth lesion	
	41007	Drainage of mouth lesion	
	41008	Drainage of mouth lesion	
	41105	Biopsy of tongue	
	41110	Excision of tongue lesion	
	41112	Excision of tongue lesion	
	41113	Excision of tongue lesion	
	41116	Excision of mouth lesion	
	41510	Tongue to lip surgery	
	41806	Removal foreign body, jawbone	
	41822	Excision of gum lesion	
	41825	Excision of gum lesion	
	41826	Excision of gum lesion	
	41828	Excision of gum lesion	
	41830	Removal of gum tissue	
	41850	Treatment of gum lesion	
	41872	Repair gum	
	42104	Excision lesion, mouth roof	
	42106	Excision lesion, mouth roof	
	42160	Treatment mouth roof lesion	
	42235	Repair palate	
	42281	Insertion, palate prosthesis	
	42300	Drainage of salivary gland	
	42305	Drainage of salivary gland	
	42330	Removal of salivary stone	
	42335	Removal of salivary stone	
	42340	Removal of salivary stone	
	42405	Biopsy of salivary gland	
	42408	Excision of salivary cyst	
	42409	Drainage of salivary cyst	
	42600	Closure of salivary fistula	
	42720	Drainage of throat abscess	
	42800	Biopsy of throat	
	42802	Biopsy of throat	
	42804	Biopsy of upper nose/throat	
	42808	Excise pharynx lesion	
	42972	Control nose/throat bleeding	
	43030	Throat muscle surgery	
	69105	Biopsy of external ear canal	
	69222	Clean out mastoid cavity	
	69421	Incision of eardrum	
	69436	Create eardrum opening	
	69540	Remove ear lesion	
0254 Level IV ENT Procedures			T
	21010	Incision of jaw joint	
	21030	Excise max/zygoma b9 tumor	
	21031	Remove exostosis, mandible	
	21032	Remove exostosis, maxilla	
	21040	Excise mandible lesion	
	21076	Prepare face/oral prosthesis	
	21120	Reconstruction of chin	
	21121	Reconstruction of chin	
	21122	Reconstruction of chin	
	21123	Reconstruction of chin	
	21125	Augmentation, lower jaw bone	
	21137	Reduction of forehead	
	21181	Contour cranial bone lesion	

APC/APC Title	CPT/ HCPCS Code	CPT/ HCPCS Description	APC Status Indicator
0254 Level IV ENT Procedures Cont'd.			T
	21235	Ear cartilage graft	
	21296	Revision of jaw muscle/bone	
	21325	Treatment of nose fracture	
	21330	Treatment of nose fracture	
	21335	Treatment of nose fracture	
	21338	Treat nasoethmoid fracture	
	21339	Treat nasoethmoid fracture	
	21345	Treat nose/jaw fracture	
	21356	Treat cheek bone fracture	
	21421	Treat mouth roof fracture	
	21440	Treat dental ridge fracture	
	21445	Treat dental ridge fracture	
	21454	Treat lower jaw fracture	
	30118	Removal of intranasal lesion	
	30140	Removal of turbinate bones	
	30430	Revision of nose	
	30520	Repair of nasal septum	
	30630	Repair nasal septum defect	
	31020	Exploration, maxillary sinus	
	31040	Exploration behind upper jaw	
	31070	Exploration of frontal sinus	
	31300	Removal of larynx lesion	
	31600	Incision of windpipe	
	31601	Incision of windpipe	
	31610	Incision of windpipe	
	31611	Surgery/speech prosthesis	
	31612	Puncture/clear windpipe	
	31613	Repair windpipe opening	
	31785	Remove windpipe lesion	
	31825	Repair of windpipe defect	
	31830	Revise windpipe scar	
	40510	Partial excision of lip	
	40525	Reconstruct lip with flap	
	40527	Reconstruct lip with flap	
	40530	Partial removal of lip	
	40816	Excision of mouth lesion	
	40840	Reconstruction of mouth	
	40842	Reconstruction of mouth	
	40843	Reconstruction of mouth	
	41006	Drainage of mouth lesion	
	41114	Excision of tongue lesion	
	41120	Partial removal of tongue	
	41500	Fixation of tongue	
	41805	Removal foreign body, gum	
	41823	Excision of gum lesion	
	41827	Excision of gum lesion	
	41870	Gum graft	
	41874	Repair tooth socket	
	42107	Excision lesion, mouth roof	
	42145	Repair palate, pharynx/uvula	
	42260	Repair nose to lip fistula	
	42450	Excise sublingual gland	
	42500	Repair salivary duct	
	42665	Ligation of salivary duct	
	42806	Biopsy of upper nose/throat	
	42810	Excision of neck cyst	
	42842	Extensive surgery of throat	
	42950	Reconstruction of throat	
	42955	Surgical opening of throat	
	43130	Removal of esophagus pouch	
	69120	Removal of external ear	
	69140	Remove ear canal lesion(s)	
	69300	Revise external ear	
	69440	Exploration of middle ear	
	69502	Mastoidectomy	
	69610	Repair of eardrum	
	69620	Repair of eardrum	
	69650	Release middle ear bone	
0256 Level V ENT Procedures			T
	21025	Excision of bone, lower jaw	
	21026	Excision of facial bone(s)	
	21029	Contour of face bone lesion	
	21034	Excise max/zygoma mlg tumor	
	21044	Removal of jaw bone lesion	
	21046	Remove mandible cyst complex	
	21047	Excise lwr jaw cyst w/repair	
	21048	Remove maxilla cyst complex	
	21049	Excis uppr jaw cyst w/repair	
	21050	Removal of jaw joint	
	21060	Remove jaw joint cartilage	
	21070	Remove coronoid process	
	21077	Prepare face/oral prosthesis	
	21079	Prepare face/oral prosthesis	
	21080	Prepare face/oral prosthesis	
	21081	Prepare face/oral prosthesis	
	21082	Prepare face/oral prosthesis	
	21083	Prepare face/oral prosthesis	
	21084	Prepare face/oral prosthesis	
	21086	Prepare face/oral prosthesis	
	21087	Prepare face/oral prosthesis	
	21088	Prepare face/oral prosthesis	
	21100	Maxillofacial fixation	
	21127	Augmentation, lower jaw bone	
	21138	Reduction of forehead	
	21139	Reduction of forehead	
	21198	Reconstr lwr jaw segment	
	21199	Reconstr lwr jaw w/advance	
	21206	Reconstruct upper jaw bone	
	21208	Augmentation of facial bones	
	21209	Reduction of facial bones	
	21210	Face bone graft	
	21215	Lower jaw bone graft	
	21230	Rib cartilage graft	
	21240	Reconstruction of jaw joint	
	21242	Reconstruction of jaw joint	
	21243	Reconstruction of jaw joint	
	21244	Reconstruction of lower jaw	
	21245	Reconstruction of jaw	
	21246	Reconstruction of jaw	
	21248	Reconstruction of jaw	
	21249	Reconstruction of jaw	
	21260	Revise eye sockets	
	21261	Revise eye sockets	
	21263	Revise eye sockets	
	21267	Revise eye sockets	
	21270	Augmentation, cheek bone	
	21275	Revision, orbitofacial bones	
	21280	Revision of eyelid	
	21340	Treatment of nose fracture	
	21355	Treat cheek bone fracture	
	21390	Treat eye socket fracture	
	21406	Treat eye socket fracture	
	21407	Treat eye socket fracture	
	21453	Treat lower jaw fracture	
	21461	Treat lower jaw fracture	
	21462	Treat lower jaw fracture	
	21465	Treat lower jaw fracture	
	21470	Treat lower jaw fracture	
	21490	Repair dislocated jaw	
	30125	Removal of nose lesion	
	30150	Partial removal of nose	
	30160	Removal of nose	
	30400	Reconstruction of nose	
	30410	Reconstruction of nose	
	30420	Reconstruction of nose	
	30435	Revision of nose	
	30450	Revision of nose	
	30460	Revision of nose	
	30462	Revision of nose	

APC/APC Title	CPT/ HCPCS Code	CPT/ HCPCS Description	APC Status Indicator
0256 Level V ENT Procedures Cont'd.			T
	30465	Repair nasal stenosis	
	30540	Repair nasal defect	
	30545	Repair nasal defect	
	30580	Repair upper jaw fistula	
	30600	Repair mouth/nose fistula	
	30620	Intranasal reconstruction	
	31030	Exploration, maxillary sinus	
	31032	Explore sinus, remove polyps	
	31050	Exploration, sphenoid sinus	
	31051	Sphenoid sinus surgery	
	31075	Exploration of frontal sinus	
	31080	Removal of frontal sinus	
	31081	Removal of frontal sinus	
	31084	Removal of frontal sinus	
	31085	Removal of frontal sinus	
	31086	Removal of frontal sinus	
	31087	Removal of frontal sinus	
	31090	Exploration of sinuses	
	31200	Removal of ethmoid sinus	
	31201	Removal of ethmoid sinus	
	31205	Removal of ethmoid sinus	
	31320	Diagnostic incision, larynx	
	31400	Revision of larynx	
	31420	Removal of epiglottis	
	31580	Revision of larynx	
	31582	Revision of larynx	
	31586	Treat larynx fracture	
	31588	Revision of larynx	
	31590	Reinnervate larynx	
	31595	Larynx nerve surgery	
	31614	Repair windpipe opening	
	31750	Repair of windpipe	
	31755	Repair of windpipe	
	40700	Repair cleft lip/nasal	
	40701	Repair cleft lip/nasal	
	40702	Repair cleft lip/nasal	
	40720	Repair cleft lip/nasal	
	40761	Repair cleft lip/nasal	
	40844	Reconstruction of mouth	
	40845	Reconstruction of mouth	
	42120	Remove palate/lesion	
	42182	Repair palate	
	42200	Reconstruct cleft palate	
	42205	Reconstruct cleft palate	
	42210	Reconstruct cleft palate	
	42215	Reconstruct cleft palate	
	42220	Reconstruct cleft palate	
	42225	Reconstruct cleft palate	
	42226	Lengthening of palate	
	42227	Lengthening of palate	
	42410	Excise parotid gland/lesion	
	42415	Excise parotid gland/lesion	
	42420	Excise parotid gland/lesion	
	42425	Excise parotid gland/lesion	
	42440	Excise submaxillary gland	
	42505	Repair salivary duct	
	42507	Parotid duct diversion	
	42508	Parotid duct diversion	
	42509	Parotid duct diversion	
	42510	Parotid duct diversion	
	42725	Drainage of throat abscess	
	42815	Excision of neck cyst	
	42844	Extensive surgery of throat	
	42890	Partial removal of pharynx	
	42892	Revision of pharyngeal walls	
	42962	Control throat bleeding	
	60252	Removal of thyroid	
	60260	Repeat thyroid surgery	
	60500	Explore parathyroid glands	
	61330	Decompress eye socket	
	69310	Rebuild outer ear canal	
	69320	Rebuild outer ear canal	
	69450	Eardrum revision	
	69501	Mastoidectomy	
	69505	Remove mastoid structures	
	69511	Extensive mastoid surgery	
	69530	Extensive mastoid surgery	
	69550	Remove ear lesion	
	69552	Remove ear lesion	
	69601	Mastoid surgery revision	
	69602	Mastoid surgery revision	
	69603	Mastoid surgery revision	
	69604	Mastoid surgery revision	
	69605	Mastoid surgery revision	
	69631	Repair eardrum structures	
	69632	Rebuild eardrum structures	
	69633	Rebuild eardrum structures	
	69635	Repair eardrum structures	
	69636	Rebuild eardrum structures	
	69637	Rebuild eardrum structures	
	69641	Revise middle ear & mastoid	
	69642	Revise middle ear & mastoid	
	69643	Revise middle ear & mastoid	
	69644	Revise middle ear & mastoid	
	69645	Revise middle ear & mastoid	
	69646	Revise middle ear & mastoid	
	69660	Revise middle ear bone	
	69661	Revise middle ear bone	
	69662	Revise middle ear bone	
	69666	Repair middle ear structures	
	69667	Repair middle ear structures	
	69670	Remove mastoid air cells	
	69676	Remove middle ear nerve	
	69700	Close mastoid fistula	
	69711	Remove/repair hearing aid	
	69714	Implant temple bone w/stimul	
	69715	Temple bne implnt w/stimulat	
	69717	Temple bone implant revision	
	69718	Revise temple bone implant	
	69720	Release facial nerve	
	69725	Release facial nerve	
	69740	Repair facial nerve	
	69745	Repair facial nerve	
	69801	Incise inner ear	
	69802	Incise inner ear	
	69805	Explore inner ear	
	69806	Explore inner ear	
	69820	Establish inner ear window	
	69840	Revise inner ear window	
	69905	Remove inner ear	
	69910	Remove inner ear & mastoid	
	69915	Incise inner ear nerve	
	69955	Release facial nerve	
	69960	Release inner ear canal	
0258 Tonsil and Adenoid Procedures			T
	42820	Remove tonsils and adenoids	
	42821	Remove tonsils and adenoids	
	42825	Removal of tonsils	
	42826	Removal of tonsils	
	42830	Removal of adenoids	
	42831	Removal of adenoids	
	42835	Removal of adenoids	
	42836	Removal of adenoids	
	42860	Excision of tonsil tags	
	42870	Excision of lingual tonsil	
0259 Level VI ENT Procedures			T
	69930	Implant cochlear device	

APC/APC Title	CPT/ HCPCS Code	CPT/ HCPCS Description	APC Status Indicator
0260 Level I Plain Film Except Teeth			X
	70030	X-ray eye for foreign body	
	70100	X-ray exam of jaw	
	70110	X-ray exam of jaw	
	70120	X-ray exam of mastoids	
	70130	X-ray exam of mastoids	
	70140	X-ray exam of facial bones	
	70150	X-ray exam of facial bones	
	70160	X-ray exam of nasal bones	
	70190	X-ray exam of eye sockets	
	70200	X-ray exam of eye sockets	
	70210	X-ray exam of sinuses	
	70220	X-ray exam of sinuses	
	70240	X-ray exam, pituitary saddle	
	70250	X-ray exam of skull	
	70328	X-ray exam of jaw joint	
	70330	X-ray exam of jaw joints	
	70350	X-ray head for orthodontia	
	70355	Panoramic x-ray of jaws	
	70360	X-ray exam of neck	
	70380	X-ray exam of salivary gland	
	71010	Chest x-ray	
	71015	Chest x-ray	
	71020	Chest x-ray	
	71021	Chest x-ray	
	71022	Chest x-ray	
	71030	Chest x-ray	
	71035	Chest x-ray	
	71100	X-ray exam of ribs	
	71101	X-ray exam of ribs/chest	
	71110	X-ray exam of ribs	
	71120	X-ray exam of breastbone	
	71130	X-ray exam of breastbone	
	72020	X-ray exam of spine	
	72040	X-ray exam of neck spine	
	72069	X-ray exam of trunk spine	
	72070	X-ray exam of thoracic spine	
	72072	X-ray exam of thoracic spine	
	72074	X-ray exam of thoracic spine	
	72080	X-ray exam of trunk spine	
	72100	X-ray exam of lower spine	
	72120	X-ray exam of lower spine	
	72170	X-ray exam of pelvis	
	72190	X-ray exam of pelvis	
	72200	X-ray exam sacroiliac joints	
	72202	X-ray exam sacroiliac joints	
	72220	X-ray exam of tailbone	
	73000	X-ray exam of collar bone	
	73010	X-ray exam of shoulder blade	
	73020	X-ray exam of shoulder	
	73030	X-ray exam of shoulder	
	73050	X-ray exam of shoulders	
	73060	X-ray exam of humerus	
	73070	X-ray exam of elbow	
	73080	X-ray exam of elbow	
	73090	X-ray exam of forearm	
	73092	X-ray exam of arm, infant	
	73100	X-ray exam of wrist	
	73110	X-ray exam of wrist	
	73120	X-ray exam of hand	
	73130	X-ray exam of hand	
	73140	X-ray exam of finger(s)	
	73500	X-ray exam of hip	
	73510	X-ray exam of hip	
	73520	X-ray exam of hips	
	73540	X-ray exam of pelvis & hips	
	73550	X-ray exam of thigh	
	73560	X-ray exam of knee, 1 or 2	
	73562	X-ray exam of knee, 3	
	73564	X-ray exam, knee, 4 or more	
	73565	X-ray exam of knees	
	73590	X-ray exam of lower leg	
	73592	X-ray exam of leg, infant	
	73600	X-ray exam of ankle	
	73610	X-ray exam of ankle	
	73620	X-ray exam of foot	
	73630	X-ray exam of foot	
	73650	X-ray exam of heel	
	73660	X-ray exam of toe(s)	
	74000	X-ray exam of abdomen	
	74010	X-ray exam of abdomen	
	74020	X-ray exam of abdomen	
	74710	X-ray measurement of pelvis	
	76006	X-ray stress view	
	76010	X-ray, nose to rectum	
	76020	X-rays for bone age	
	76040	X-rays, bone evaluation	
	76066	Joint survey, single view	
	76077	Dxa bone density/v-fracture	
	76098	X-ray exam, breast specimen	
	76125	Cine/ video x-rays add-on	
	76150	X-ray exam, dry process	
	76499	Radiographic procedure	
	77417	Radiology port film(s)	
	G0130	Single energy x-ray study	
0261 Level II Plain Film Except Teeth Including Bone Density Measurement			X
	70134	X-ray exam of middle ear	
	70260	X-ray exam of skull	
	71111	X-ray exam of ribs/ chest	
	72010	X-ray exam of spine	
	72050	X-ray exam of neck spine	
	72052	X-ray exam of neck spine	
	72090	X-ray exam of trunk spine	
	72110	X-ray exam of lower spine	
	72114	X-ray exam of lower spine	
	73530	X-ray exam of hip	
	74022	X-ray exam series, abdomen	
	76061	X-rays, bone survey	
	76062	X-rays, bone survey	
	76065	X-rays, bone evaluation	
	76078	Radiographic absorptiometry	
	76100	X-ray exam of body section	
	78350	Bone mineral, single photon	
0262 Plain Film of Teeth			X
	70300	X-ray exam of teeth	
	70310	X-ray exam of teeth	
	70320	Full mouth x-ray of teeth	
0263 Level I Miscellaneous Radiology Procedures			X
	70373	Contrast x-ray of larynx	
	70390	X-ray exam of salivary duct	
	71040	Contrast x-ray of bronchi	
	71060	Contrast x-ray of bronchi	
	74300	X-ray bile ducts/pancreas	
	74301	X-rays at surgery add-on	
	74305	X-ray bile ducts/pancreas	
	74350	X-ray guide, stomach tube	
	74355	X-ray guide, intestinal tube	
	74470	X-ray exam of kidney lesion	
	75809	Nonvascular shunt, x-ray	
	75898	Follow-up angiography	
	75901	Remove CVA device obstruct	
	75902	Remove CVA lumen obstruct	
	75984	X-ray control catheter change	
	76080	X-ray exam of fistula	
	76086	X-ray of mammary duct	
	76088	X-ray of mammary ducts	
	76101	Complex body section x-ray	

APC/APC Title	CPT/ HCPCS Code	CPT/ HCPCS Description	APC Status Indicator
0264 Level II Miscellaneous Radiology Procedures			X
	70170	X-ray exam of tear duct	
	74190	X-ray exam of peritoneum	
	74320	Contrast x-ray of bile ducts	
	74740	X-ray, female genital tract	
	74742	X-ray, fallopian tube	
	75801	Lymph vessel x-ray, arm/leg	
	75803	Lymph vessel x-ray,arms/legs	
	75805	Lymph vessel x-ray, trunk	
	75807	Lymph vessel x-ray, trunk	
	76102	Complex body section x-rays	
0265 Level I Diagnostic Ultrasound			S
	76645	Us exam, breast(s)	
	76802	O US<14 wks, addl fetus	
	76815	Us exam, pg uterus limit	
	76816	Us exam pg uterus repeat	
	76857	Us exam, pelvic, limited	
	76970	Ultrasound exam follow-up	
	76999	Echo examination procedure	
0266 Level II Diagnostic Ultrasound			S
	76506	Echo exam of head	
	76510	Ophth US, b & quant a	
	76511	Ophth US, quant a only	
	76512	Ophth US, b w/non-quant a	
	76513	Echo exam of eye, water bath	
	76516	Echo exam of eye	
	76519	Echo exam of eye	
	76529	Echo exam of eye	
	76536	Us exam of head and neck	
	76604	Us exam, chest, B-scan	
	76700	Us exam, abdom, complete	
	76705	Echo exam of abdomen	
	76770	US exam abdo back wall, comp	
	76775	US exam abdo back wall, lim	
	76778	US exam kidney transplant	
	76800	US exam, spinal canal	
	76801	Ob US < 14 wks, single fetus	
	76805	Ob US >/= 14 wks, sngl fetus	
	76810	Ob US >/= 14 wks, addl fetus	
	76812	Ob US, detailed, addl fetus	
	76817	Transvaginal US, obstetric	
	76818	Fetal biophy profile w/nst	
	76819	Fetal biophys profil w/o nst	
	76830	Transvaginal US, non-ob	
	76831	Echo exam, uterus	
	76856	US exam, pelvic, complete	
	76870	US exam, scrotum	
	76872	US, transrectal	
	76873	Echograp trans r, pros study	
	76880	US exam, extremity	
	76885	US exam infant hips, dynamic	
	76886	US exam infant hips, static	
	76975	GI endoscopic ultrasound	
	76986	Ultrasound guide intraoper	
	93888	Intracranial study	
	93890	TCD, vasoreactivity study	
	93892	TCD, emboli detect w/o inj	
	93893	TCD, emboli detect w/inj	
	93931	Upper extremity study	
0267 Level III Diagnostic Ultrasound			S
	36002	Pseudoaneurysm injection trt	
	75945	Intravascular US	
	75946	Intravascular US add-on	
	76811	Ob US, detailed, sngl fetus	

APC/APC Title	CPT/ HCPCS Code	CPT/ HCPCS Description	APC Status Indicator
	93880	Extracranial study	
	93882	Extracranial study	
	93886	Intracranial study	
	93925	Lower extremity study	
	93926	Lower extremity study	
	93930	Upper extremity study	
	93970	Extremity study	
	93971	Extremity study	
	93975	Vascular study	
	93976	Vascular study	
	93978	Vascular study	
	93979	Vascular study	
	93980	Penile vascular study	
	93981	Penile vascular study	
	93990	Doppler flow testing	
	G0365	Vessel mapping hemo access	
0268 Ultrasound Guidance Procedures			S
	76930	Echo guide, cardiocentesis	
	76932	Echo guide for heart biopsy	
	76936	Echo guide for artery repair	
	76940	Us guide, tissue ablation	
	76941	Echo guide for transfusion	
	76942	Echo guide for biopsy	
	76945	Echo guide, villus sampling	
	76946	Echo guide for amniocentesis	
	76948	Echo guide, ova aspiration	
	76950	Echo guidance radiotherapy	
	76965	Echo guidance radiotherapy	
0269 Level III Echocardiogram Except Transesophageal			S
	93303	Echo transthoracic	
	93307	Echo exam of heart	
	93350	Echo transthoracic	
0270 Transesophageal Echocardiogram			S
	93312	Echo transesophageal	
	93313	Echo transesophageal	
	93315	Echo transesophageal	
	93316	Echo transesophageal	
	93318	Echo transesophageal intraop	
0272 Level I Fluoroscopy			X
	43752	Nasal/orogastric w/stent	
	70370	Throat x-ray & fluoroscopy	
	70371	Speech evaluation, complex	
	71023	Chest x-ray and fluoroscopy	
	71034	Chest x-ray and fluoroscopy	
	71090	X-ray & pacemaker insertion	
	74340	X-ray guide for GI tube	
	76000	Fluoroscope examination	
	76120	Cine/video x-rays	
	76496	Fluoroscopic procedure	
0274 Myelography			S
	70010	Contrast x-ray of brain	
	70015	Contrast x-ray of brain	
	72240	Contrast x-ray of neck spine	
	72255	Contrast x-ray, thorax spine	
	72265	Contrast x-ray, lower spine	
	72270	Contrast x-ray of spine	
	72275	Epidurography	
	76012	Percut vertebroplasty fluor	
	76013	Percut vertebroplasty, ct	
0275 Arthrography			S
	70332	X-ray exam of jaw joint	
	73040	Contrast x-ray of shoulder	
	73085	Contrast x-ray of elbow	
	73115	Contrast x-ray of wrist	
	73525	Contrast x-ray of hip	
	73542	X-ray exam, sacroiliac joint	
	73580	Contrast x-ray of knee joint	
	73615	Contrast x-ray of ankle	

APC/APC Title	CPT/ HCPCS Code	CPT/ HCPCS Description	APC Status Indicator
0276 Level I Digestive Radiology			S
	74210	Contrst x-ray exam of throat	
	74220	Contrast x-ray, esophagus	
	74230	Cine/video x-ray, throat/eso	
	74240	X-ray exam, upper GI tract	
	74241	X-ray exam, upper GI tract	
	74246	Contrst x-ray uppr GI tract	
	74247	Contrst x-ray uppr GI tract	
	74250	X-ray exam of small bowel	
	74270	Contrast x-ray exam of colon	
	74283	Contrast x-ray exam of colon	
	74290	Contrast x-ray, gallbladder	
	74291	Contrast x-rays, gallbladder	
0277 Level II Digestive Radiology			S
	74245	X-ray exam, upper GI tract	
	74249	Contrst x-ray uppr GI tract	
	74251	X-ray exam of small bowel	
	74260	X-ray exam of small bowel	
	74280	Contrast x-ray exam of colon	
0278 Diagnostic Urography			S
	74400	Contrst x-ray, urinary tract	
	74410	Contrst x-ray, urinary tract	
	74415	Contrst x-ray, urinary tract	
	74420	Contrst x-ray, urinary tract	
	74425	Contrst x-ray, urinary tract	
	74430	Contrast x-ray, bladder	
	74440	X-ray, male genital tract	
	74445	X-ray exam of penis	
	74450	X-ray, urethra/bladder	
	74455	X-ray, urethra/bladder	
	74775	X-ray exam of perineum	
0279 Level II Angiography and Venography Except Extremity			S
	75658	Artery x-rays, arm	
	75741	Artery x-rays, lung	
	75746	Artery x-rays, lung	
	75756	Artery x-rays, chest	
	75774	Artery x-ray, each vessel	
	75810	Vein x-ray, spleen/liver	
	75825	Vein x-ray, trunk	
	75827	Vein x-ray, chest	
	75833	Vein x-ray, kidneys	
	75887	Vein x-ray, liver	
	75891	Vein x-ray, liver	
	75992	Atherectomy, x-ray exam	
	75993	Atherectomy, x-ray exam	
	75994	Atherectomy, x-ray exam	
	75995	Atherectomy, x-ray exam	
	75996	Atherectomy, x-ray exam	
0280 Level III Angiography and Venography Except Extremity			S
	75605	Contrast x-ray exam of aorta	
	75625	Contrast x-ray exam of aorta	
	75630	X-ray aorta, leg arteries	
	75650	Artery x-rays, head & neck	
	75662	Artery x-rays, head & neck	
	75665	Artery x-rays, head & neck	
	75671	Artery x-rays, head & neck	
	75676	Artery x-rays, neck	
	75680	Artery x-rays, neck	
	75685	Artery x-rays, spine	

APC/APC Title	CPT/ HCPCS Code	CPT/ HCPCS Description	APC Status Indicator
	75710	Artery x-rays, arm/leg	
	75716	Artery x-rays, arms/legs	
	75722	Artery x-rays, kidney	
	75724	Artery x-rays, kidneys	
	75726	Artery x-rays, abdomen	
	75731	Artery x-rays, adrenal gland	
	75736	Artery x-rays, pelvis	
	75743	Artery x-rays, lungs	
	75885	Vein x-ray, liver	
	75889	Vein x-ray, liver	
0281 Venography of Extremity			S
	75790	Visualize A-V shunt	
	75820	Vein x-ray, arm/leg	
	75822	Vein x-ray, arms/legs	
0282 Miscellaneous Computerized Axial Tomography			S
	76071	CT bone density, peripheral	
	76370	CT scan for therapy guide	
	76375	3d/holograph reconstr add-on	
	76380	CT scan follow-up study	
	76497	CT procedure	
0283 Computerized Axial Tomography with Contrast Material			S
	70460	CT head/brain w/dye	
	70481	CT orbit/ear/fossa w/dye	
	70487	CT maxillofacial w/dye	
	70491	CT soft tissue neck w/dye	
	71260	CT thorax w/dye	
	72126	CT neck spine w/dye	
	72129	CT chest spine w/dye	
	72132	CT lumbar spine w/dye	
	72193	CT pelvis w/dye	
	73201	CT upper extremity w/dye	
	73701	CT lower extremity w/dye	
	74160	CT abdomen w/dye	
	76355	CT scan for localization	
	76360	CT scan for needle biopsy	
0284 Magnetic Resonance Imaging and Magnetic Resonance Angiography with Contract Material			S
	70542	MRI orbit/face/neck w/dye	
	70545	MRI angiography head w/dye	
	70548	MRI angiography neck w/dye	
	70552	MRI brain w/dye	
	70558	MRI brain w/dye	
	71551	MRI chest w/dye	
	72142	MRI neck spine w/dye	
	72147	MRI chest spine w/dye	
	72149	MRI lumbar spine w/dye	
	72196	MRI pelvis w/dye	
	73219	MRI upper extremity w/dye	
	73222	MRI joint upr extrem w/ dye	
	73719	MRI lower extremity w/dye	
	73722	MRI joint of lwr extr w/dye	
	74182	MRI abdomen w/dye	
	75553	Heart MRI for morph w/dye	
	C8900	MRA w/cont, abd	
	C8903	MRI w/cont, breast, uni	
	C8906	MRI w/cont, breast, bi	
	C8909	MRA w/cont, chest	
	C8912	MRA w/cont, lwr ext	
	C8918	MRA w/cont, lwr ext	

APC/APC Title	CPT/ HCPCS Code	CPT/ HCPCS Description	APC Status Indicator
0285 Myocardial Positron Emission Tomography (PET)			S
	G0030	PET imaging prev PET single	
	G0031	PET imaging prev PET multple	
	G0032	PET follow SPECT 78464 singl	
	G0033	PET follow SPECT 78464 mult	
	G0034	PET follow SPECT 76865 singl	
	G0035	PET follow SPECT 78465 mult	
	G0036	PET follow cornry angio sing	
	G0037	PET follow cornry angio mult	
	G0038	PET follow myocard perf sing	
	G0039	PET follow myocard perf mult	
	G0040	PET follow stress echo singl	
	G0041	PET follow stress echo mult	
	G0042	PET follow ventriculogm sing	
	G0043	PET follow ventriculogm mult	
	G0044	PET following rest ECG singl	
	G0045	PET following rest ECG mult	
	G0046	PET follow stress ECG singl	
	G0047	PET follow stress ECG mult	
0287 Complex Venography			S
	75831	Vein x-ray, kidney	
	75840	Vein x-ray, adrenal gland	
	75842	Vein x-ray, adrenal glands	
	75860	Vein x-ray, neck	
	75870	Vein x-ray, skull	
	75872	Vein x-ray, skull	
	75880	Vein x-ray, eye socket	
0288 Bone Density: Axial Skeleton			S
	76070	CT scan, bone density study	
	76075	Dual energy x-ray study	
0289 Needle Localization for Breast Biopsy			X
	76096	X-ray of needle wire, breast	
0296 Level I Therapeutic Radiologic Procedures			S
	74235	Remove esophagus obstruction	
	74327	X-ray bile stone removal	
	74360	X-ray guide, GI dilation	
	74480	X-ray control, cath insert	
	74485	X-ray guide, GU dilation	
0297 Level II Therapeutic Radiologic Procedures			S
	74363	X-ray, bile duct dilation	
	74475	X-ray control, cath insert	
	75894	X-rays, transcath therapy	
	75896	X-rays, transcath therapy	
	75980	Contrast x-ray exam bile duct	
	75982	Contrast x-ray exam bile duct	
0299 Miscellaneous Radiation Treatment			S
	77470	Special radiation treatment	
0300 Level I Radiation Therapy			S
	77401	Radiation treatment delivery	
	77402	Radiation treatment delivery	
	77403	Radiation treatment delivery	
	77404	Radiation treatment delivery	
	77406	Radiation treatment delivery	
	77407	Radiation treatment delivery	
	77408	Radiation treatment delivery	
	77409	Radiation treatment delivery	
	77411	Radiation treatment delivery	
	77750	Infuse radioactive materials	
	77789	Apply surface radiation	

APC/APC Title	CPT/ HCPCS Code	CPT/ HCPCS Description	APC Status Indicator
0301 Level II Radiation Therapy			S
	77412	Radiation treatment delivery	
	77413	Radiation treatment delivery	
	77414	Radiation treatment delivery	
	77416	Radiation treatment delivery	
0302 Level III Radiation Therapy			S
	61795	Brain surgery using computer	
0303 Treatment Device Construction			X
	77332	Radiation treatment aid(s)	
	77333	Radiation treatment aid(s)	
	77334	Radiation treatment aid(s)	
0304 Level I Therapeutic Radiation Treatment Preparation			X
	77280	Set radiation therapy field	
	77300	Radiation therapy dose plan	
	77305	Teletx isodose plan simple	
	77310	Teletx isodose plan intermed	
	77326	Brachytx isodose calc simp	
	77331	Special radiation dosimetry	
	77336	Radiation physics consult	
	77370	Radiation physics consult	
	77399	External radiation dosimetry	
0305 Level II Therapeutic Radiation Treatment Preparation			X
	77285	Set radiation therapy field	
	77290	Set radiation therapy field	
	77315	Teletx isodose plan complex	
	77321	Special teletx port plan	
	77327	Brachytx isodose calc interm	
	77328	Brachytx isodose plan compl	
0310 Level III Therapeutic Radiation Treatment Preparation			X
	77295	Set radiation therapy field	
	77301	Radiotherapy dose plan, IMRT	
0312 Radioelement Applications			S
	77761	Apply intrcav radiat simple	
	77762	Apply intrcav radiat interm	
	77763	Apply intrcav radiat compl	
	77776	Apply interstit radiat simpl	
	77777	Apply interstit radiat inter	
0313 Brachytherapy			S
	77781	High intensity brachytherapy	
	77782	High intensity brachytherapy	
	77783	High intensity brachytherapy	
	77784	High intensity brachytherapy	
	77799	Radium/radioisotope therapy	
0314 Hyperthermic Therapies			S
	77600	Hyperthermia treatment	
	77605	Hyperthermia treatment	
	77610	Hyperthermia treatment	
	77615	Hyperthermia treatment	
	77620	Hyperthermia treatment	
0315 Level II Implantation of Neurostimulator			T
	61886	Implant neurostim arrays	
0320 Electroconvulsive Therapy			S
	90870	Electroconvulsive therapy	
0321 Biofeedback and Other Training			S
	90911	Biofeedback peri/uro/rectal	

APC/APC Title	CPT/ HCPCS Code	CPT/ HCPCS Description	APC Status Indicator
0322 Brief Individual Psychotherapy			S
	90804	Psytx, office, 20-30 min	
	90805	Psytx, off, 20-30 min w/E&M	
	90810	Intac psytx, off, 20-30 min	
	90811	Intac psytx, 20-30, w/E&M	
	90816	Psytx, hosp, 20-30 min	
	90817	Psytx, hosp, 20-30 min w/E&M	
	90823	Intac psytx, hosp, 20-30 min	
	90824	Intac psytx, hsp 20-30 w/E&M	
	90899	Psychiatric service/therapy	
	96150	Assess hlth/behave, init	
	96151	Assess hlth/behave, subseq	
	96152	Intervene hlth/behave, indiv	
	96153	Intervene hlth/behave, group	
	96154	Interv hlth/behave, fam w/pt	
0323 Extended Individual Psychotherapy			S
	90801	Psy dx interview	
	90802	Intac psy dx interview	
	90806	Psytx, off, 45-50 min	
	90807	Psytx, off, 45-50 min w/E&M	
	90808	Psytx, office, 75-80 min	
	90809	Psytx, off, 75-80, w/E&M	
	90812	Intac psytx, off, 45-50 min	
	90813	Intac psytx, 45-50 min w/E&M	
	90814	Intac psytx, off, 75-80 min	
	90815	Intac psytx, 75-80 w/E&M	
	90818	Psytx, hosp, 45-50 min	
	90819	Psytx, hosp, 45-50 min w/E&M	
	90821	Psytx, hosp, 75-80 min	
	90822	Psytx, hosp, 75-80 min w/E&M	
	90826	Intac psytx, hosp, 45-50 min	
	90827	Intac psytx, hsp 45-50 w/E&M	
	90828	Intac psytx, hosp, 75-80 min	
	90829	Intac psytx, hsp 75-80 w/E&M	
	90845	Psychoanalysis	
	90865	Narcosynthesis	
	90880	Hypnotherapy	
0324 Family Psychotherapy			S
	90846	Family psytx w/o patient	
	90847	Family psytx w/patient	
0325 Group Psychotherapy			S
	90849	Multiple family group psytx	
	90853	Group psychotherapy	
	90857	Intac group psytx	
0330 Dental Procedures			S
	D0150	Comprehensve oral evaluation	
	D0240	Intraoral occlusal film	
	D0250	Extraoral first film	
	D0260	Extraoral ea additional film	
	D0272	Dental bitewings two films	
	D0274	Dental bitewings four films	
	D0277	Vert bitewings-sev to eight	
	D0460	Pulp vitality test	
	D0472	Gross exam, prep & report	
	D0473	Micro exam, prep & report	
	D0474	Micro w exam of surg margins	
	D0480	Cytopath smear prep & report	
	D0502	Other oral pathology procedu	
	D0999	Unspecified diagnostic proce	
	D1510	Space maintainer fxd unilat	
	D1515	Fixed bilat space maintainer	
	D1520	Remove unilat space maintain	
	D1525	Remove bilat space maintain	
	D1550	Recement space maintainer	
	D2970	Temporary- fractured tooth	
	D2999	Dental unspec restorative pr	
	D3460	Endodontic endosseous implan	
	D3999	Endodontic procedure	
	D4260	Osseous surgery per quadrant	
	D4263	Bone replce graft first site	
	D4264	Bone replce graft each add	
	D4268	Surgical revision procedure	
	D4270	Pedicle soft tissue graft pr	
	D4271	Free soft tissue graft proc	
	D4273	Subepithelial tissue graft	
	D4355	Full mouth debridement	
	D4381	Localized antimicro delivery	
	D5911	Facial moulage sectional	
	D5912	Facial moulage complete	
	D5983	Radiation applicator	
	D5984	Radiation shield	
	D5985	Radiation cone locator	
	D5987	Commissure splint	
	D6920	Dental connector bar	
	D7111	Extraction coronal remnants	
	D7140	Extraction erupted tooth/exr	
	D7210	Rem imp tooth w mucoper flp	
	D7220	Impact tooth remov soft tiss	
	D7230	Impact tooth remov part bony	
	D7240	Impact tooth remov comp bony	
	D7241	Impact tooth rem bony w/comp	
	D7250	Tooth root removal	
	D7260	Oral antral fistula closure	
	D7261	Primary closure sinus perf	
	D7291	Transseptal fiberotomy	
	D7940	Reshaping bone orthognathic	
	D9630	Other drugs/medicaments	
	D9930	Treatment of complications	
	D9940	Dental occlusal guard	
	D9950	Occlusion analysis	
	D9951	Limited occlusal adjustment	
	D9952	Complete occlusal adjustment	
0332 Computerized Axial Tomography and Computerized Angiography Without Contrast Material			S
	0067T	CT colonography; dx	
	70450	CT head/brain w/o dye	
	70480	CT orbit/ear/fossa w/o dye	
	70486	CT maxillofacial w/o dye	
	70490	CT soft tissue neck w/o dye	
	71250	CT thorax w/o dye	
	72125	CT neck spine w/o dye	
	72128	CT chest spine w/o dye	
	72131	CT lumbar spine w/o dye	
	72192	CT pelvis w/o dye	
	73200	CT upper extremity w/o dye	
	73700	CT lower extremity w/o dye	
	74150	CT abdomen w/o dye	
	76362	CT scan for tissue ablation	
0333 Computerized Axial Tomography and Computerized Angiography Without Contrast Material			S
	70470	CT head/brain w/o&w dye	
	70482	CT orbit/ear/fossa w/o&w dye	
	70488	CT maxillofacial w/o&w dye	
	70492	CT sft tsue nck w/o & w/dye	
	71270	CT thorax w/o&w dye	
	72127	CT neck spine w/o&w dye	
	72130	CT chest spine w/o&w dye	
	72133	CT lumbar spine w/o&w dye	
	72194	CT pelvis w/o&w dye	
	73202	CT uppr extremity w/o&w dye	
	73702	CT lwr extremity w/o&w dye	
	74170	CT abdomen w/o&w dye	

APC/APC Title	CPT/ HCPCS Code	CPT/ HCPCS Description	APC Status Indicator
0335 Magnetic Resonance Imaging, Miscellaneous			S
	70336	Magnetic image, jaw joint	
	75554	Cardiac MRI/function	
	75555	Cardiac MRI/limited study	
	76393	MRI guidance for needle place	
	76394	MRI for tissue ablation	
	76400	Magnetic image, bone marrow	
	76498	MRI procedure	
0336 Magnetic Resonance Imaging and Magnetic Resonance Angiography Without Contrast Material			S
	70540	MRI orbit/face/neck w/o dye	
	70544	MRI angiography head w/o dye	
	70547	MRI angiography neck w/o dye	
	70551	MRI brain w/o dye	
	70557	MRI brain w/o dye	
	71550	MRI chest w/o dye	
	72141	MRI neck spine w/o dye	
	72146	MRI chest spine w/o dye	
	72148	MRI lumbar spine w/o dye	
	72195	MRI pelvis w/o dye	
	73218	MRI upper extremity w/o dye	
	73221	MRI joint upr extrem w/o dye	
	73718	MRI lower extremity w/o dye	
	73721	MRI joint of lwr extre w/o d	
	74181	MRI abdomen w/o dye	
	75552	Heart MRI for morph w/o dye	
	C8901	MRA w/o cont, abd	
	C8904	MRI w/o cont, breast, uni	
	C8907	MRI w/o cont, breast, bi	
	C8910	MRA w/o cont, chest	
	C8913	MRA w/o cont, lwr ext	
	C8919	MRA w/o cont, pelvis	
0337 MRI and Magnetic Resonance Angiography without Contrast Material followed by Contrast Material			S
	70543	MRI orbt/fac/nck w/o&w dye	
	70546	MRI angiograph head w/o&w dye	
	70549	MRI angiograph neck w/o&w dye	
	70553	MRI brain w/o&w dye	
	70559	MRI brain w/o&w/ dye	
	71552	MRI chest w/o&w dye	
	72156	MRI neck spine w/o&w dye	
	72157	MRI chest spine w/o&w dye	
	72158	MRI lumbar spine w/o&w dye	
	72197	MRI pelvis w/o&w dye	
	73220	MRI uppr extremity w/o&w dye	
	73223	MRI joint upr extr w/o&w dye	
	73720	MRI lwr extremity w/o&w dye	
	73723	MRI joint lwr extr w/o&w dye	
	74183	MRI abdomen w/o&w dye	
	C8902	MRA w/o fol w/cont, abd	
	C8905	MRI w/o fol w/cont, brst, un	
	C8908	MRI w/o fol w/cont, breast	
	C8911	MRA w/o fol w/cont, chest	
	C8914	MRA w/o fol w/cont, lwr ext	
	C8920	MRA w/o fol w/cont, pelvis	
0339 Observation			S
	G0244	Observ care by facility to pt	
0340 Minor Ancillary Procedures			X
	0085T	Breath test heart reject	
	11980	Implant hormone pellet(s)	
	11981	Insert drug implant device	
	11982	Remove drug implant device	
	11983	Remove/insert drug implant	
	15852	Dressing change, not for burn	
	20665	Removal of fixation device	
	20975	Electrical bone stimulation	
	30300	Remove nasal foreign body	
	40804	Removal, foreign body, mouth	
	42809	Remove pharynx foreign body	
	46600	Diagnostic anoscopy	
	51798	US urine capacity measure	
	69200	Clear outer ear canal	
	69210	Remove impacted ear wax	
	76514	Echo exam of eye, thickness	
	76977	Us bone density measure	
	78730	Urinary bladder retention	
	G0268	Removal of impacted wax MD	
0341 Skin Tests			X
	86485	Skin test, candida	
	86490	Coccidioidomycosis skin test	
	86510	Histoplasmosis skin test	
	86580	TB intradermal test	
	86585	TB tine test	
	86586	Skin test, unlisted	
0342 Level I Pathology			X
	80500	Lab pathology consultation	
	80502	Lab pathology consultation	
	85060	Blood smear interpretation	
	88125	Forensic cytopathology	
	88160	Cytopath smear, other source	
	88162	Cytopath smear, other source	
	88184	Flowcytometry/tc, 1 marker	
	88185	Flowcytometry/tc, add-on	
	88187	Flowcytometry/read, 2-8	
	88188	Flowcytometry/read, 9-15	
	88299	Cytogenetic study	
	88300	Surgical path, gross	
	88302	Tissue exam by pathologist	
	88311	Decalcify tissue	
	88312	Special stains	
	88313	Special stains	
	88314	Histochemical stain	
	88318	Chemical histochemistry	
	88319	Enzyme histochemistry	
	88321	Microslide consultation	
	88329	Path consult introp	
	88332	Path consult intraop, addl	
	G0364	Bone marrow aspirate & biopsy	
0343 Level II Pathology			X
	85097	Bone marrow interpretation	
	86077	Physician blood bank service	
	86078	Physician blood bank service	
	86079	Physician blood bank service	
	88104	Cytopathology, fluids	
	88106	Cytopathology, fluids	
	88107	Cytopathology, fluids	
	88108	Cytopath, concentrate tech	
	88112	Cytopath, cell enhance tech	
	88161	Cytopath smear, other source	
	88172	Cytopathology eval of fna	
	88173	Cytopath eval, fna, report	
	88304	Tissue exam by pathologist	
	88305	Tissue exam by pathologist	
	88331	Path consult intraop, 1 bloc	
	89220	Sputum specimen collection	
	89230	Collect sweat for test	
0344 Level III Pathology			X
	88182	Cell marker study	
	88189	Flowcytometry/read, 16 & >	
	88307	Tissue exam by pathologist	
	88309	Tissue exam by pathologist	
	88323	Microslide consultation	
	88325	Comprehensive review of data	
	88342	Immunocytochemistry	
	88346	Immunofluorescent study	

APC/APC Title	CPT/ HCPCS Code	CPT/ HCPCS Description	APC Status Indicator
0344 Level III Pathology Cont'd.			X
	88347	Immunofluorescent study	
	88355	Analysis, skeletal muscle	
	88356	Analysis, nerve	
	88358	Analysis, tumor	
	88360	Tumor immunohistochem/manual	
	88361	Tumor immunohistochem/comput	
	88362	Nerve teasing preparations	
	88365	Tissue hybridization	
	88367	Insitu hybridization, auto	
	88368	Insitu hybridization, manual	
0345 Level I Transfusion Laboratory Procedures			X
	86850	RBC antibody screen	
	86891	Autologous blood, op salvage	
	86903	Blood typing, antigen screen	
	86904	Blood typing, patient serum	
	86905	Blood typing, RBC antigens	
	86906	Blood typing, Rh phenotype	
	86921	Compatibility test	
	86970	RBC pretreatment	
	86971	RBC pretreatment	
	86972	RBC pretreatment	
	86975	RBC pretreatment, serum	
	86976	RBC pretreatment, serum	
	86977	RBC pretreatment, serum	
	86978	RBC pretreatment, serum	
	86999	Transfusion procedure	
0346 Level II Transfusion Laboratory Procedures			X
	86860	RBC antibody elution	
	86870	RBC antibody identification	
	86920	Compatibility test	
	86922	Compatibility test	
	86927	Plasma, fresh frozen	
	86945	Blood product/irradiation	
	86965	Pooling blood platelets	
0347 Level III Transfusion Laboratory Procedures			X
	86890	Autologous blood process	
	86930	Frozen blood prep	
	86931	Frozen blood thaw	
	86932	Frozen blood freeze/thaw	
	86950	Leukocyte transfusion	
	86985	Split blood or products	
0348 Fertility Laboratory Procedures			X
	0058T	Cryopreservation, ovary tiss	
	0059T	Cryopreservation, oocyte	
	0087T	Sperm eval hyaluronan	
	89250	Cultr oocyte/embryo <4 days	
	89251	Cultr oocyte/embryo <4 days	
	89253	Embryo hatching	
	89254	Oocyte identification	
	89255	Prepare embryo for transfer	
	89257	Sperm identification	
	89258	Cryopreservation, embryo(s)	
	89259	Cryopreservation, sperm	
	89260	Sperm isolation, simple	
	89261	Sperm isolation, complex	
	89264	Identify sperm tissue	
	89268	Insemination of oocytes	
	89272	Extended culture of oocytes	
	89280	Assist oocyte fertilization	
	89281	Assist oocyte fertilization	
	89290	Biopsy, oocyte polar body	
	89291	Biopsy, oocyte polar body	
	89335	Cryopreserve testicular tiss	
	89342	Storage/year; embryo(s)	
	89343	Storage/year; sperm/semen	
	89344	Storage/year; reprod tissue	
	89346	Storage/year; oocyte	
	89352	Thawing cryopresrved; embryo	
	89353	Thawing cryopresrved; sperm	
	89354	Thaw cryoprsvrd; reprod tiss	
	89356	Thawing cryopresrved; oocyte	
0352 Level I Injections			X
	90799	Ther/prophylactic/dx inject	
	95115	Immunotherapy, one injection	
0353 Level II Allergy Injections			X
	90782	Injection, SC/IM	
	95117	Immunotherapy injections	
0355 Level I Immunizations			K
	90710	Mmrv vaccine, SC	
	90740	Hep B vacc, ill pat 3 dose IM	
	90743	Hep B vacc, adol, 2 dose IM	
	90744	Hep B vacc, ped/adol 3 dose IM	
	90746	Hep B vaccine, adult, IM	
	G0010	Admin Hepatitis B vaccine	
0356 Level IV Immunizations			K
	90376	Rabies Ig, heat treated	
	90393	Vaccine Ig, IM	
	90396	Varicella-zoster Ig, IM	
	90476	Adenovirus vaccine, type 4	
	90586	BCG vaccine, intravesical	
	90636	Hep A/Hep B vacc, adult IM	
	90665	Lyme disease vaccine, IM	
	90675	Rabies vaccine, IM	
	90676	Rabies vaccine, ID	
	90725	Cholera vaccine, injectable	
	90735	Encephalitis vaccine, SC	
	90747	Hep B vacc, ill pat 4 dose IM	
0359 Level II Injections			X
	15860	Test for blood flow in graft	
	90783	Injection, IA	
	90784	Injection, IV	
	90788	Injection of antibiotic	
0360 Level I Alimentary Tests			X
	89100	Sample intestinal contents	
	89105	Sample intestinal contents	
	89130	Sample stomach contents	
	89132	Sample stomach contents	
	89135	Sample stomach contents	
	89136	Sample stomach contents	
	89140	Sample stomach contents	
	89141	Sample stomach contents	
	91040	Esoph balloon distension tst	
	91055	Gastric intubation for smear	
	91060	Gastric saline load test	
	91065	Breath hydrogen test	
	91100	Pass intestine bleeding tube	
	91105	Gastric intubation treatment	
	91132	Electrogastrography	
	91133	Electrogastrography w/test	
	91299	Gastroenterology procedure	
0361 Level II Alimentary Tests			X
	91000	Esophageal intubation	
	91010	Esophagus motility study	
	91011	Esophagus motility study	
	91012	Esophagus motility study	
	91020	Gastric motility	
	91030	Acid perfusion of esophagus	
	91034	Gastroesophageal reflux test	
	91037	Esoph imped function test	
	91038	Esoph imped funct test > 1h	
	91052	Gastric analysis test	
	95075	Ingestion challenge test	

APC/APC Title	CPT/ HCPCS Code	CPT/ HCPCS Description	APC Status Indicator
0362 Contact Lens and Spectacle Services			X
	92311	Contact lens fitting	
	92312	Contact lens fitting	
	92313	Contact lens fitting	
	92315	Prescription of contact lens	
	92316	Prescription of contact lens	
	92317	Prescription of contact lens	
	92325	Modification of contact lens	
	92326	Replacement of contact lens	
	92352	Special spectacles fitting	
	92353	Special spectacles fitting	
	92354	Special spectacles fitting	
	92355	Special spectacles fitting	
	92358	Eye prosthesis service	
	92371	Repair & adjust spectacles	
0363 Level I Otorhinolaryngologic Function Tests			X
	92512	Nasal function studies	
	92541	Spontaneous nystagmus test	
	92542	Positional nystagmus test	
	92544	Optokinetic nystagmus test	
	92545	Oscillating tracking test	
	92547	Supplemental electrical test	
	92587	Evoked auditory test	
	92588	Evoked auditory test	
0364 Level I Audiometry			X
	92552	Pure tone audiometry, air	
	92553	Audiometry, air & bone	
	92555	Speech threshold audiometry	
	92556	Speech audiometry, complete	
	92562	Loudness balance test	
	92563	Tone decay hearing test	
	92564	Sisi hearing test	
	92565	Stenger test, pure tone	
	92567	Tympanometry	
	92568	Acoustic reflex testing	
	92569	Acoustic reflex decay test	
	92571	Filtered speech hearing test	
	92572	Staggered spondaic word test	
	92573	Lombard test	
	92575	Sensorineural acuity test	
	92576	Synthetic sentence test	
	92583	Select picture audiometry	
	92596	Ear protector evaluation	
	92620	Auditory function, 60 min	
	92625	Tinnitus assessment	
	92700	ENT procedure/service	
0365 Level II Audiometry			X
	92557	Comprehensive hearing test	
	92561	Bekesy audiometry, diagnosis	
	92577	Stenger test, speech	
	92579	Visual audiometry (vra)	
	92582	Conditioning play audiometry	
0366 Leve III Audiometry			X
	92601	Cochlear implt f/up exam < 7	
	92602	Reprogram cochlear implt < 7	
	92603	Cochlear implt f/up exam 7 >	
	92604	Reprogram cochlear implt 7 >	
0367 Level I Pulmonary Test			X
	94015	Patient recorded spirometry	
	94150	Vital capacity test	
	94200	Lung function test (MBC/MVV)	
	94250	Expired gas collection	
	94360	Measure airflow resistance	
	94370	Breath airway closing volume	
	94400	CO2 breathing response curve	
	94680	Exhaled air analysis, O2	
	94770	Exhaled carbon dioxide test	
	94799	Pulmonary service/procedure	
0368 Level II Pulmonary Tests			X
	93721	Plethysmography tracing	
	93740	Temperature gradient studies	
	94010	Breathing capacity test	
	94014	Patient recorded spirometry	
	94060	Evaluation of wheezing	
	94240	Residual lung capacity	
	94260	Thoracic gas volume	
	94350	Lung nitrogen washout curve	
	94375	Respiratory flow volume loop	
	94450	Hypoxia response curve	
	94452	Hast w/report	
	94453	Hast w/oxygen titrate	
	94620	Pulmonary stress test/simple	
	94681	Exhaled air analysis, O2/CO2	
	94690	Exhaled air analysis	
	94720	Monoxide diffusing capacity	
	94725	Membrane diffusion capacity	
	94750	Pulmonary compliance study	
0369 Level III Pulmonary Tests			X
	94070	Evaluation of wheezing	
	94621	Pulm stress test/complex	
	94772	Breath recording, infant	
	95070	Bronchial allergy tests	
	95071	Bronchial allergy tests	
0370 Allergy Tests			X
	95004	Percut allergy skin tests	
	95010	Percut allergy titrate test	
	95015	Id allergy titrate-drug/bug	
	95024	Id allergy test, drug/bug	
	95027	Skin end point titration	
	95028	Id allergy test-delayed type	
	95044	Allergy patch tests	
	95052	Photo patch test	
	95056	Photosensitivity tests	
	95060	Eye allergy tests	
	95065	Nose allergy test	
	95078	Provocative testing	
	95180	Rapid desensitization	
	95199	Allergy immunology services	
0371 Level I Allergy Injections			X
	95144	Antigen therapy services	
	95145	Antigen therapy services	
	95146	Antigen therapy services	
	95147	Antigen therapy services	
	95148	Antigen therapy services	
	95149	Antigen therapy services	
	95165	Antigen therapy services	
	95170	Antigen therapy services	
0372 Therapeutic Phlebotomy			X
	99195	Phlebotomy	
0373 Neuropsychological Testing			X
	96100	Psychological testing	
	96110	Developmental test, lim	
	96111	Developmental test, extend	
	96115	Neurobehavior status exam	
	96117	Neuropsych test battery	
0374 Monitoring Psychiatric Drugs			X
	90862	Medication management	
	M0064	Visit for drug monitoring	

APC/APC Title	CPT/ HCPCS Code	CPT/ HCPCS Description	APC Status Indicator
0376 Level II Cardiac Imaging			S
	78473	Gated heart, multiple	
	78483	Heart first pass, multiple	
0377 Level III Cardiac Imaging			S
	78461	Heart muscle blood, multiple	
	78465	Heart image (3D), multiple	
0378 Level II Pulmonary Imaging			S
	78584	Lung V/Q image single breath	
	78585	Lung V/Q imaging	
	78588	Perfusion lung image	
	78596	Lung differential function	
0379 Injection Adenosine 6 mg			K
	J0150	Injection Adenosine 6 Mg	
0380 Dipyridamole Injection			K
	J1245	Dipyridamole injection	
0384 GI Procedures with Stents			T
	43219	Esophagus endoscopy	
	43256	Uppr GI endoscopy w stent	
	43268	Endo cholangiopancreatograph	
	43269	Endo cholangiopancreatograph	
	44370	Small bowel endoscopy/stent	
	44379	S bowel endoscope w/stent	
	44383	Ileoscopy w/stent	
	44397	Colonoscopy w/stent	
	45327	Proctosigmoidoscopy w/stent	
	45345	Sigmoidoscopy w/stent	
	45387	Colonoscopy w/stent	
0385 Level I Prosthetic Urological Procedures			S
	53440	Correct bladder function	
	53444	Insert tandem cuff	
	54400	Insert semi-rigid prosthesis	
0386 Level II Prosthetic Urological Procedures			S
	53445	Insert uro/ves nck sphincter	
	53447	Remove/replace ur sphincter	
	54401	Insert self-contd prosthesis	
	54405	Insert multi-comp penis pros	
	54410	Remove/replace penis prosth	
	54416	Remv/repl penis contain pros	
0387 Level II Hysteroscopy			T
	58560	Hysteroscopy, resect septum	
	58561	Hysteroscopy, remove myoma	
	58563	Hysteroscopy, ablation	
0388 Discography			S
	72285	X-ray c/t spine disk	
	72295	X-ray of lower spine disk	
0389 Non-imaging Nuclear Medicine			S
	78000	Thyroid, single uptake	
	78001	Thyroid, multiple uptakes	
	78003	Thyroid suppress/stimul	
	78190	Platelet survival, kinetics	
	78191	Platelet survival	
	78270	Vit B-12 absorption exam	
	78271	Vit B-12 absrp exam, int fac	
	78272	Vit B-12 absorp, combined	
	78725	Kidney function study	
	78999	Nuclear diagnostic exam	
0390 Level I Endocrine Imaging			S
	78006	Thyroid imaging with uptake	
	78010	Thyroid imaging	
	78011	Thyroid imaging with flow	
	78099	Endocrine nuclear procedure	
0391 Level II Endocrine Imaging			S
	78007	Thyroid image, mult uptakes	
	78070	Parathyroid nuclear imaging	
	78075	Adrenal nuclear imaging	
0393 Red Cell/ Plasma Studies			S
	78110	Plasma volume, single	
	78111	Plasma volume, multiple	
	78120	Red cell mass, single	
	78121	Red cell mass, multiple	
	78122	Blood volume	
	78130	Red cell survival study	
	78135	Red cell survival kinetics	
	78140	Red cell sequestration	
	78160	Plasma iron turnover	
	78162	Radioiron absorption exam	
	78170	Red cell iron utilization	
	78172	Total body iron estimation	
0394 Hepatobiliary Imaging			S
	78201	Liver imaging	
	78202	Liver imaging with flow	
	78205	Liver imaging (3D)	
	78206	Liver image (3D) with flow	
	78215	Liver and spleen imaging	
	78216	Liver & spleen image/flow	
	78220	Liver function study	
	78223	Hepatobiliary imaging	
0395 GI Tract Imaging			S
	78230	Salivary gland imaging	
	78231	Serial salivary imaging	
	78232	Salivary gland function exam	
	78258	Esophageal motility study	
	78261	Gastric mucosa imaging	
	78262	Gastroesophageal reflux exam	
	78264	Gastric emptying study	
	78278	Acute GI blood loss imaging	
	78282	GI protein loss exam	
	78290	Meckel's divert exam	
	78291	Leveen/shunt patency exam	
	78299	GI nuclear procedure	
0396 Bone Imaging			S
	78300	Bone imaging, limited area	
	78305	Bone imaging, multiple areas	
	78306	Bone imaging, whole body	
	78315	Bone imaging, 3 phase	
	78320	Bone imaging (3D)	
	78399	Musculoskeletal nuclear exam	
0397 Vascular Imaging			S
	78445	Vascular flow imaging	
	78455	Venous thrombosis study	
	78456	Acute venous thrombus image	
	78457	Venous thrombosis imaging	
	78458	Ven thrombosis images, bilat	
0398 Level I Cardiac Imaging			S
	78414	Non-imaging heart function	
	78428	Cardiac shunt imaging	
	78460	Heart muscle blood, single	
	78464	Heart image (3D), single	
	78466	Heart infarct image	
	78468	Heart infarct image (EF)	
	78469	Heart infarct image (3D)	
	78472	Gated heart, planar, single	
	78481	Heart first pass, single	
	78494	Heart image, spect	
	78499	Cardiovascular nuclear exam	

APC/APC Title	CPT/ HCPCS Code	CPT/ HCPCS Description	APC Status Indicator
0399 Nuclear Medicine Add-on Imaging			S
	78020	Thyroid met uptake	
	78478	Heart wall motion add-on	
	78480	Heart function add-on	
	78496	Heart first pass add-on	
0400 Hematopoietic Imaging			S
	78102	Bone marrow imaging, ltd	
	78103	Bone marrow imaging, mult	
	78104	Bone marrow imaging, body	
	78185	Spleen imaging	
	78195	Lymph system imaging	
	78199	Blood/lymph nuclear exam	
0401 Level I Pulmonary Imaging			S
	78580	Lung perfusion imaging	
	78586	Aerosol lung image, single	
	78587	Aerosol lung image, multiple	
	78591	Vent image, 1 breath, 1 proj	
	78593	Vent image, 1 proj, gas	
	78594	Vent image, mult proj, gas	
	78599	Respiratory nuclear exam	
0402 Brain Imaging			S
	78600	Brain imaging, ltd static	
	78601	Brain imaging, ltd w/flow	
	78605	Brain imaging, complete	
	78606	Brain imaging, compl w/flow	
	78607	Brain imaging (3D)	
	78610	Brain flow imaging only	
	78615	Cerebral vascular flow image	
	78699	Nervous system nuclear exam	
0403 CSF Imaging			S
	78630	Cerebrospinal fluid scan	
	78635	CSF ventriculography	
	78645	CSF shunt evaluation	
	78647	Cerebrospinal fluid scan	
	78650	CSF leakage imaging	
	78660	Nuclear exam of tear flow	
0404 Renal and Genitourinary Studies Level I			S
	78700	Kidney imaging, static	
	78701	Kidney imaging with flow	
	78704	Imaging renogram	
	78707	Kidney flow/function image	
	78710	Kidney imaging (3D)	
	78715	Renal vascular flow exam	
	78740	Ureteral reflux study	
	78760	Testicular imaging	
	78761	Testicular imaging/flow	
	78799	Genitourinary nuclear exam	
0405 Renal and Genitourinary Studies Level II			S
	78708	Kidney flow/function image	
	78709	Kidney flow/function image	
0406 Tumor/ Infection Imaging			S
	78015	Thyroid met imaging	
	78016	Thyroid met imaging/studies	
	78018	Thyroid met imaging, body	
	78800	Tumor imaging, limited area	
	78801	Tumor imaging, mult areas	
	78802	Tumor imaging, whole body	
	78803	Tumor imaging (3D)	
	78805	Abscess imaging, ltd area	
	78806	Abscess imaging, whole body	
	78807	Nuclear localization/abscess	

APC/APC Title	CPT/ HCPCS Code	CPT/ HCPCS Description	APC Status Indicator
0407 Radionuclide Therapy			S
	79005	Nuclear rx, oral admin	
	79101	Nuclear rx, IV admin	
	79200	Intracavitary nuclear trmt	
	79300	Interstitial nuclear therapy	
	79440	Nuclear joint therapy	
	79445	Nuclear rx, intra-arterial	
	79999	Nuclear medicine therapy	
0409 Red Blood Cell Tests			X
	86880	Coombs test, direct	
	86885	Coombs test, indirect, qual	
	86886	Coombs test, indirect, titer	
	86900	Blood typing, ABO	
	87901	Blood typing, Rh (D)	
0411 Respiratory Procedures			S
	G0237	Therapeutic procd strg endur	
	G0238	Oth resp proc, indiv	
	G0239	Oth resp proc, group	
0412 IMRT Treatment Delivery			S
	0073T	Delivery, comp IMRT	
	77418	Radiation tx delivery IMRT	
0415 Level II Endoscopy Lower Airway			T
	31630	Bronchoscopy dilate/fx repr	
	31631	Bronchoscopy, dilate w/stent	
	31636	Bronchoscopy, bronch stents	
	31638	Bronchoscopy, revise stent	
	31640	Bronchoscopy w/tumor excise	
	31641	Bronchoscopy, treat blockage	
0416 Level I Intravascular and Intracardiac Ultrasound and Flow Reserve			S
	37250	IV US first vessel add-on	
	37251	IV US each add vessel add-on	
	92979	Intravasc US, heart add-on	
	93572	Heart flow reserve measure	
0417 Computerized Reconstruction			S
	G0288	Recon, CTA for surg plan	
0418 Insertion of Left Ventricular Pacing Electrode			T
	33224	Insert pacing lead & connect	
0421 Prolonged Physiologic Monitoring			X
	95250	Glucose monitoring, cont	
0422 Level II Upper GI Procedures			T
	0008T	Upper GI endoscopy, w/ suture	
	43228	Esoph endoscopy, ablation	
	43257	Uppr GI scope w/thrml txmnt	
	43830	Place gastrostomy tube	
0423 Level II Percutaneous Abdominal and Biliary Procedures			T
	47382	Percut ablate liver rf	
0425 Level II Arthroplasty with Prosthesis			T
	23470	Reconstruct shoulder joint	
	24361	Reconstruct elbow joint	
	24363	Replace elbow joint	
	24366	Reconstruct head of radius	
	25441	Reconstruct wrist joint	
	25442	Reconstruct wrist joint	
	25446	Wrist replacement	

APC/APC Title	CPT/ HCPCS Code	CPT/ HCPCS Description	APC Status Indicator
0426 Level II Strapping and Cast Application			S
	29000	Application of body cast	
	29010	Application of body cast	
	29015	Application of body cast	
	29025	Application of body cast	
	29035	Application of body cast	
	29044	Application of body cast	
	29046	Application of body cast	
	29055	Application of shoulder cast	
	29065	Application of long arm cast	
	29075	Application of forearm cast	
	29085	Apply hand/wrist cast	
	29086	Apply finger cast	
	29305	Application of hip cast	
	29325	Application of hip casts	
	29345	Application of long leg cast	
	29355	Application of long leg cast	
	29358	Apply long leg cast brace	
	29365	Application of long leg cast	
	29405	Apply short leg cast	
	29425	Apply short leg cast	
	29435	Apply short leg cast	
	29440	Addition of walker to cast	
	29445	Apply rigid leg cast	
	29710	Removal/revision of cast	
0600 Low Level Clinic Visits			V
	92012	Eye exam established pat	
	99201	Office/outpatient visit, new	
	99202	Office/outpatient visit, new	
	99211	Office/outpatient visit, est	
	99212	Office/outpatient visit, est	
	99241	Office consultation	
	99242	Office consultation	
	99271	Confirmatory consultation	
	99272	Confirmatory consultation	
	99431	Initial care, normal newborn	
	G0101	CA screen; pelvic/breast exam	
	G0245	Initial foot exam pt lops	
	G0246	Follow-up eval of foot pt lops	
	G0264	Assmt otr CHF, CP, asthma	
0601 Mid Level Clinic Visits			V
	92002	Eye exam, new patient	
	99203	Office/outpatient visit, new	
	99213	Office/outpatient visit, est	
	99243	Office consultation	
	99273	Confirmatory consultation	
	G0344	Initial preventive exam	
0602 High Level Clinic Visits			V
	92004	Eye exam, new patient	
	92014	Eye exam & treatment	
	99204	Office/outpatient visit, new	
	99205	Office/outpatient visit, new	
	99214	Office/outpatient visit, est	
	99215	Office/outpatient visit, est	
	99244	Office consultation	
	99245	Office consultation	
	99274	Confirmatory consultation	
	99275	Confirmatory consultation	
	G0175	OPPS service, sched team conf	
0610 Low Level Emergency Visits			V
	99281	Emergency dept visit	
	99282	Emergency dept visit	
0611 Mid Level Emergency Visits			V
	99283	Emergency dept visit	
0612 High Level Emergency Visits			V
	99284	Emergency dept visit	
	99285	Emergency dept visit	
0620 Critical Care			S
	99291	Critical care, first hour	
0648 Breast Reconstruction with Prosthesis			T
	19325	Enlarge breast with implant	
	19342	Delayed breast prosthesis	
	19357	Breast reconstruction	
0651 Complex Interstitial Radiation Source Application			S
	77778	Apply interstit radiat compl	
0652 Insertion of Intraperitoneal Catheters			T
	49420	Insert abdom drain, temp	
	49421	Insert abdom drain, perm	
0653 Vascular Reconstruction/Fistula Repair with Device			T
	35011	Repair defect of artery	
	35261	Repair blood vessel lesion	
	35266	Repair blood vessel lesion	
	35286	Repair blood vessel lesion	
	36870	Percut thrombect AV fistula	
0654 Insertion/ Replacement of a Permanent Dual Chamber Pacemaker			T
	33213	Insertion of pulse generator	
0655 Insertion/ Replacement/Conversion of a Permanent Dual Chamber Pacemaker			T
	33208	Insertion of heart pacemaker	
	33214	Upgrade of pacemaker system	
0656 Transcatheter Placement of Intracoronary Drug-Eluting Stents			T
	G0290	Drug-eluting stents, single	
	G0291	Drug-eluting stents, each add	
0657 Placement of Tissue Clips			S
	19295	Place breast clip, percut	
0658 Percutaneous Breast Biopsies			T
	19103	Bx breast percut w/device	
0659 Hyperbaric Oxygen			S
	C1300	Hyperbaric	
0660 Level II Otorhinolaryngologic Function Tests			X
	92516	Facial nerve function test	
	92520	Laryngeal function studies	
	92543	Caloric vestibular test	
	92546	Sinusoidal rotational test	
	92548	Posturography	
	92584	Electrocochleography	
0661 Level IV Pathology			X
	88348	Electron microscopy	
	88349	Scanning electron microscopy	
0662 CT Angiography			S
	70496	CT angiography, head	
	70498	CT angiography, neck	
	71275	CT angiography, chest	
	72191	CT angiograph pelv w/o&w dye	
	73206	CT angio upr extrm w/o&w dye	
	73706	CT angio lwr extr w/o&w dye	
	74175	CT angio abdom w/o&w dye	
	75635	CT angio abdominal arteries	

APC/APC Title	CPT/ HCPCS Code	CPT/ HCPCS Description	APC Status Indicator
0664 Level I Proton Beam Radiation Therapy			S
	77520	Proton trmt, simple w/o comp	
	77522	Proton trmt, simple w/comp	
0665 Bone Density: Appendicular Skeleton			S
	76076	DEXA peripheral study	
0668 Level I Angiography and Venography Except Extremity			S
	75660	Artery x-rays, head & neck	
	75705	Artery x-rays, spine	
	75733	Artery x-rays, adrenals	
	75960	Transcatheter iv stent rs&i	
	75961	Retrieval, broken catheter	
	75962	Repair arterial blockage	
	75964	Repair artery blockage, each	
	75966	Repair arterial blockage	
	75968	Repair artery blockage, each	
	75970	Vascular biopsy	
	75978	Repair venous blockage	
0670 Intravenous and Intracardiac Ultrasound and Flow Reserve			S
	31620	Endobronchial US add-on	
	92978	Intravasc us, heart add-on	
	93571	Heart flow reserve measure	
	93662	Intracardiac ECG (ice)	
0671 Level II Echocardiogram Except Transesophageal			S
	76825	Echo exam of fetal heart	
	76827	Echo exam of fetal heart	
	93320	Doppler echo exam, heart	
0672 Level IV Posterior Segment Procedures			T
	67040	Laser treatment of retina	
	67107	Repair detached retina	
	67108	Repair detached retina	
	67112	Rerepair detached retina	
0673 Level IV Anterior Segment Eye Procedures			T
	66172	Incision of eye	
	66180	Implant eye shunt	
	66185	Revise eye shunt	
	66225	Repair/graft eye lesion	
0674 Prostate Cryoablation			T
	55873	Cryoablate prostate	
0675 Prostatic Thermotherapy			T
	53850	Prostatic microwave thermotx	
	53852	Prostatic rf thermotx	
0676 Level II Transcatheter Thrombolysis			T
	37201	Transcatheter therapy infuse	
	92973	Percut coronary thrombectomy	
0677 Level I Transcatheter Thrombolysis			T
	36550	Declot vascular device	
	36860	External cannula declotting	
	37202	Transcatheter therapy infuse	
	92977	Dissolve clot, heart vessel	
0678 External Counterpulsation			T
	G0166	Extrnl counterpulse, per tx	
0679 Level II Resuscitation and Cardioversion			S
	92960	Cardioversion electric, ext	
	92961	Cardioversion, electric, int	

APC/APC Title	CPT/ HCPCS Code	CPT/ HCPCS Description	APC Status Indicator
0680 Insertion of Patient Activated Event Recorders			S
	33282	Implant pat-active ht record	
0681 Knee Arthroplasty			T
	27446	Revision of knee joint	
0682 Level V Debridement & Destruction			T
	11044	Debride tissue/muscle/bone	
0683 Level II Photochemotherapy			S
	96913	Photochemotherapy, UV-A or B	
0685 Level III Needle Biopsy/Aspiration Except Bone Marrow			T
	32400	Needle biopsy chest lining	
	32405	Biopsy, lung or mediastinum	
	37200	Transcatheter biopsy	
	47000	Needle biopsy of liver	
	48102	Needle biopsy, pancreas	
	49180	Biopsy, abdominal mass	
	50200	Biopsy of kidney	
	50390	Drainage of kidney lesion	
	62269	Needle biopsy, spinal cord	
0686 Level III Skin Repair			T
	15350	Skin homograft	
0687 Revision/Removal of Neurostimulator Electrodes			T
	61880	Revise/remove neuroelectrode	
	63660	Revise/remove neuroelectrode	
	64585	Revise/remove neuroelectrode	
0688 Revision/Removal of Neurostimulator Pulse Generator Receiver			T
	61888	Revise/remove neuroreceiver	
	63688	Revise/remove neuroreceiver	
	64595	Revise/remove neuroreceiver	
0689 Electronic Analysis of Cardioverter-defibrillators			S
	93741	Analyze ht pace device sngl	
	93742	Analyze ht pace device sngl	
	93743	Analyze ht pace device dual	
	93744	Analyze ht pace device dual	
	93745	Set-up cardiovert-defibrill	
0690 Electronic Analysis of Pacemakers and Other Cardiac Devices			S
	93724	Analyze pacemaker system	
	93727	Analyze ilr system	
	93731	Analyze pacemaker system	
	93732	Analyze pacemaker system	
	93733	Telephone analy, pacemaker	
	93734	Analyze pacemaker system	
	93735	Analyze pacemaker system	
	93736	Telephone analy, pacemaker	
0691 Electronic Analysis of Programmable Shunts/Pumps			S
	62252	CSF shunt reprogram	
	62367	Analyze spine infusion pump	
	62368	Analyze spine infusion pump	
0692 Electronic Analysis of Neurostimulator Pulse Generators			S
	95971	Analyze neurostim, simple	
	95972	Analyze neurostim, complex	
	95973	Analyze neurostim, complex	
	95974	Cranial neurostim, complex	
	95975	Cranial neurostim, complex	
	95978	Analyze neurostim brain/1h	
	95979	Analyze neurostim brain add-on	

APC/APC Title	CPT/ HCPCS Code	CPT/ HCPCS Description	APC Status Indicator
0693 Level II Breast Reconstruction			T
	19162	Remove breast tissue, nodes	
	19318	Reduction of large breast	
	19324	Enlarge breast	
0694 Mohs Surgery			T
	17304	Chemosurgery of skin lesion	
	17305	2 stage Mohs, up to 5 spec	
	17306	3 stage Mohs, up to 5 spec	
	17307	Mohs addl stage up to 5 spec	
	17310	Extensive skin chemosurgery	
0695 Level VII Debridement & Destruction			T
	46917	Laser surgery, anal lesions	
	46922	Excision of anal lesion(s)	
	46924	Destruction, anal lesion(s)	
	54065	Destruction, penis lesion(s)	
	56515	Destroy vulva lesion/s compl	
0697 Level I Echocardiogram Except Transesophageal			S
	76826	Echo exam of fetal heart	
	76828	Echo exam of fetal heart	
	93304	Echo transthoracic	
	93308	Echo exam of heart	
	93321	Doppler echo exam, heart	
	93325	Doppler color flow add-on	
0698 Level II Eye Tests & Treatments			S
	65205	Remove foreign body from eye	
	65210	Remove foreign body from eye	
	65220	Remove foreign body from eye	
	65222	Remove foreign body from eye	
	67820	Revise eyelashes	
	67938	Remove eyelid foreign body	
	68040	Treatment of eyelid lesions	
	68760	Close tear duct opening	
	68801	Dilate tear duct opening	
	92140	Glaucoma provocative tests	
	92284	Dark adaptation eye exam	
	92286	Internal eye photography	
	92287	Internal eye photography	
0699 Level IV Eye Tests & Treatment			T
	67350	Biopsy eye muscle	
	68110	Remove eyelid lining lesion	
	68810	Probe nasolacrimal duct	
	92019	Eye exam & treatment	
	92018	New eye exam & treatment	
	92230	Eye exam with photos	
0700 Antepartum Manipulation			T
	59412	Antepartum manipulation	
0701 SR 89 Chloride, per mCi			K
	A9600	Strontium-89 chloride	
0702 SM 153 Lexidronam, 50 mCi			K
	A9605	Samarium sm153 Lexidronamm	
0703 Butorphanol Tartrate			K
	J0595	Butorphanol tartrate 1 mg	
0704 IN 111 Satumomab Pendetide Per Dose			K
	A4642	Satumomab Pendetide per dose	
0705 Technetium TC99M Tetrofosmin			K
	A9502	Technetium TC99M tetrofosmin	
0726 Dexrazoxane HCl Injection			K
	J1190	Dexrazoxane HCl injection	
0728 Filgrastim Injection			K
	J1440	Filgrastim 300 mcg injection	
0729 Injection, Meropenem			K
	J2185	Meropenem	
0730 Pamidronate Disodium			K
	J2430	Pamidronate disodium/30 mg	
0731 Sargramostim Injection			K
	J2820	Sargramostim injection	
0732 Mesna Injection			K
	J9209	Mesna injection	
0733 Non ESRD Epoetin alpha Injection			K
	Q0136	Non ESRD epoetin alpha inj	
0734 Injection, Darbepoetin alfa (for non-ESRD), per 1 mcg			K
	Q0137	Darbepoetin alfa, non-ESRD	
0735 Ampho B Cholesteryl Sulfate			K
	J0288	Ampho B cholesteryl sulfate	
0736 Amphotericin B Liposome Injection			K
	J0289	Amphotericin B liposome inj	
0737 Ammonia N-13, Per Dose			K
	A9526	Ammonia N-13, per dose	
0738 Rasburicase			G
	J2783	Rasburicase	
0750 Dolasetron Mesylate			K
	J1260	Dolasetron mesylate	
0763 Dolasetron Mesylate Oral			K
	Q0180	Dolasetron mesylate oral	
0764 Granisetron HCl Injection			K
	J1626	Granisetron HCl injection	
0765 Granisetron HCl 1 mg Oral			K
	Q0166	Granisetron HCl 1 mg oral	
0768 Ondansetron HCl Injection			K
	J2405	Ondansetron HCl injection	
0769 Ondansetron HCl Oral			K
	Q0179	Ondansetron HCl 8 mg oral	
0800 Leuprolide Acetate			K
	J1950	Leuprolide acetate/3.75 mg	
0802 Etoposide Oral			K
	J8560	Etoposide oral 50 mg	
0807 Aldesleukin/ Single Use Vial			K
	J9015	Aldesleukin/single use vial	
0809 BCG Live Intravesical Vaccine			K
	J9031	BCG live intravesical vac	
0810 Goserelin Acetate Implant			K
	J9202	Goserelin acetate implant	
0811 Carboplatin Injection			K
	J9045	Carboplatin injection	
0812 Carmus Bischl Nitro Injection			K
	J9050	Carmus bischl nitro inj	
0813 Cisplatin Injection			K
	J9060	Cisplatin 10 mg injection	

APC/APC Title	CPT/ HCPCS Code	CPT/ HCPCS Description	APC Status Indicator
0814 Asparaginase Injection			K
	J9020	Asparaginase injection	
0815 Cyclophosphamide Injection			K
	J9070	Cyclophosphamide 100 mg inj	
0816 Cyclophosphamide Lyophilized			K
	J9093	Cyclophosphamide lyophilized	
0817 Cytarabine HCl Injection			K
	J9100	Cytarabine HCl 100 mg injection	
0819 Decarbazine Injection			K
	J9130	Decarbazine 100 mg injection	
0820 Daunorubicin			K
	J9150	Daunorubicin	
0821 Daunorubicin Citrate Liposom			K
	J9151	Daunorubicin citrate liposom	
0822 Diethylstilbestrol Injection			K
	J9165	Diethylstilbestrol injection	
0823 Docetaxel			K
	J9170	Docetaxel	
0824 Etoposide Injection			K
	J9181	Etoposide 10 mg injection	
0827 Floxuridine Injection			K
	J9200	Floxuridine injection	
0828 Gemcitabine HCl			K
	J9201	Gemcitabine HCl	
0830 Irinotecan Injection			K
	J9206	Irinotecan injection	
0831 Ifosfomide Injection			K
	J9208	Ifosfomide injection	
0832 Idarubicin HCl Injection			K
	J9211	Idarubicin HCl injection	
0834 Interferon Alfa-2a Injection			K
	J9213	Interferon Alfa-2a inj	
0836 Interferon Alfa-2b Injection Recombinant			K
	J9214	Interferon Alfa-2b inj	
0838 Interferon Gamma 1-b Injection			K
	J9216	Interferon Gamma 1-b inj	
0840 Melphalan HCl			K
	J9245	Inj melphalan HCl 50 mg	
0842 Fludarabine Phosphate Injection			K
	J9185	Fludarabine phosphate inj	
0843 Pegaspargase			K
	J9266	Pegaspargase/singl dose vial	
0844 Pentostatin Injection			K
	J9268	Pentostatin injection	
0845 Phentolaine Mesylate Injection			K
	J2760	Phentolaine mesylate inj	
0846 Cilastatin Sodium Injection			K
	J0743	Cilastatin sodium injection	
0847 Doxorubic HCl Chemotherapy			K
	J9000	Doxorubic HCl 10 mg vl	
0848 Testosterone Enanthate Injection			K
	J0900	Testosterone enanthate inj	
0849 Rituximab			K
	J9310	Rituximab cancer treatment	
0851 Thiotepa Injection			K
	J9340	Thiotepa injection	
0852 Topotecan			K
	J9350	Topotecan	
0855 Vinorelbine Tartrate			K
	J9390	Vinorelbine tartrate/10 mg	
0856 Porfimer Sodium			K
	J9600	Porfimer sodium	
0857 Bleomycin Sulfate Injection			K
	J9040	Bleomycin sulfate injection	
0858 Cladribine			K
	J9065	Inj Cladribine per 1 mg	
0860 Plicamycin (Mithramycin) Injection			K
	J9270	Plicamycin (Mithramycin) inj	
0861 Leuprolide Acetate Injection			K
	J9218	Leuprolide acetate injection	
0862 Mitomycin			K
	J9280	Mitomycin 5 mg inj	
0863 Paclitaxel Injection			K
	J9265	Paclitaxel injection	
0864 Mitoxantrone HCl			K
	J9293	Mitoxantrone HCl 5 mg	
0865 Interferon Alfa-n3 Injection, Human Leukocyte Derived, 2			K
	J9215	Interferon Alfa-n3 inj	
0866 Foscarnet Sodium Injection			K
	J1455	Foscarnet sodium injection	
0867 Methacholine Chloride, Nebulizer			K
	J7674	Methacholine chloride, neb	
0887 Azathioprine Parenteral			K
	J7501	Azathioprine parenteral	
0888 Cyclosporine Oral			K
	J7502	Cyclosporine oral 100 mg	
0890 Lymphocyte Immune Globulin			K
	J7504	Lymphocyte immune globulin	
0891 Tacrolimus Oral			K
	J7507	Tacrolimus oral per 1 mg	
0900 Alglucerase Injection			K
	J0205	Alglucerase injection	
0901 Alpha 1 Proteinase Inhibitor			K
	J0256	Alpha 1 proteinase inhibitor	
0902 Botulinum Toxin A, Per Unit			K
	J0585	Botulinum toxin a per unit	
0903 Cytomegalovirus Imm IV/Vial			K
	J0850	Cytomegalovirus Imm IV/vial	
0905 Immune Globulin			K
	J1563	IV immune globulin	
0906 RSV-IV Ig			K
	J1565	RSV-IV Ig	
0910 Interferon Beta-1b			K
	J1830	Interferon beta-1b/0.25 mg	
0911 Streptokinase			K
	J2995	Inj Streptokinase/250,000 IU	
0916 Injection Imiglucerase /Unit			K
	J1785	Injection imiglucerase/unit	
0917 Adenosine			K
	J0152	Adenosine injection	
0925 Factor VIII			K
	J7190	Factor VIII	
0926 Factor VIII (Porcine)			K
	J7191	Factor VIII (porcine)	

APC/APC Title	CPT/ HCPCS Code	CPT/ HCPCS Description	APC Status Indicator
0927 Factor VIII Recombinant			K
	J7192	Factor VIII recombinant	
0928 Factor IX Complex			K
	J7194	Factor IX complex	
0929 Anti-inhibitor Per IU			K
	J7198	Anti-inhibitor	
0931 Factor IX Non-recombinant			K
	J7193	Factor IX non-recombinant	
0932 Factor IX Recombinant			K
	J7195	Factor IX recombinant	
0949 Plasma, Pooled Multiple Donor, Solvent/Detergent T			K
	P9023	Frozen plasma, pooled, sd	
0950 Blood (Whole) For Transfusion			K
	P9010	Whole blood for transfusion	
0952 Cryoprecipitate			K
	P9012	Cryoprecipitate each unit	
0954 RBC Leukocytes Reduced			K
	P9016	RBC leukocytes reduced	
0955 Plasma, Fresh Frozen			K
	P9059	Plasma, frz between 8-24 hour	
0956 Plasma Protein Fraction			K
	P9043	Plasma protein fract, 5%, 50 ml	
0957 Platelet Concentrate			K
	P9019	Platelets, each unit	
0958 Platelet Rich Plasma			K
	P9020	Platelet rich plasma unit	
0959 Red Blood Cells			K
	P9021	Red blood cells unit	
0960 Washed Red Blood Cells			K
	P9022	Washed red blood cells unit	
0961 Infusion, Albumin (Human) 5%			K
	P9041	Albumin (human), 5%, 50 ml	
0963 Albumin (human), 5%			K
	P9045	Albumin (human), 5%, 250 ml	
0964 Albumin (human), 25%			K
	P9046	Albumin (human), 25%, 20 ml	
0965 Albumin (human), 25%			K
	P9047	Albumin (human), 25%, 50 ml	
0966 Plasmaprotein Fract, 5%			K
	P9048	Plasmaprotein fract, 5%, 250 ml	
0967 Split Unit of Blood			K
	P9011	Blood split unit	
0968 Platelets Lleukocyte Reduced Irradiated			K
	P9033	Platelets leuko reduced irrad	
0969 Red Blood Cell Leukocyte Reduced Irradiated			K
	P9040	RBC leuko reduced irradiated	
1009 Cryoprecipitate Reduced Plasma			K
	P9044	Cryoprecipitate reduced plasma	
1010 Blood, L/R, CMV-Neg			K
	P9051	Blood, L/R, CMV-neg	
1011 Platelets, HLA-m, L/R, Unit			K
	P9052	Platelets, HLA-m, L/R, unit	
1013 Platelet Concentrate, L/R, Unit			K
	P9031	Platelets leukocytes reduced	
1016 Blood, L/R, Froz/Deglycerol/Washed			K
	P9054	Blood, L/R, froz/degly wash	
1017 Platelets, Aph/pher, L/R, CMV-Neg, Unit			K
	P9055	Plt, aph/pherL/R,CMV-neg	
1018 Blood, L/R, Irradiated			K
	P9056	Blood, L/R, irradiated	
1019 Platelets, Aph/pher, L/R, Irradiated, Unit			K
	P9037	Plate phere leukoredu irrad	
1020 Plt, Pher, L/R,CMV, Irrad			K
	P9053	Plt, pher, L/R, CMV neg, irrad	
1021 RBC, Frz/Deg/Wsh, L/R, Irrad			K
	P9057	RBC, frz/deg/wsh, L/R, irrad	
1022 RBC, L/R, CMV Neg, Irrad			K
	P9058	RBC, L/R, CMV neg, irrad	
1045 Lobenguane Sulfate I-131			K
	A9508	Lobenguane sulfate I-131	
1046 Inj, Moxifloxacin			K
	J2280	Inj, Moxifloxacin 100 mg	
1049 Thiamine HCl			K
	J3411	Thiamine HCl 100 mg	
1050 Pyridoxine HCl			K
	J3415	Pyridoxine HCl 100 mg	
1052 Injection, Voriconazole			K
	J3465	Injection, Voriconazole	
1062 Acyclovir			K
	Q4075	Acyclovir, 5 mg	
1064 I-131 Sodium Iodide Capsule			K
	A9517	Th I131 so iodide cap millic	
	A9528	Dx I131 so iodide cap millic	
1065 I-131 Sodium Iodide Solution			K
	A9529	Dx I131 so iodide sol millic	
	A9530	Th I131 so iodide sol millic	
1070 Dopamine HCl			K
	Q4076	Dopamine HCl, 40 mg	
1079 CO 57/58			K
	C1079	CO 57/58 per 0.5 uCi	
1080 I-131 Tositumomab, Dx			K
	C1080	I-131 Tositumomab, dx	
1081 I-131 Tositumomab, Tx			K
	C1081	I-131 Tositumomab, tx	
1082 Treprostinil			K
	Q4077	Treprostinil, 1 mg	
1083 Injection, Adalimumab			K
	J0135	Adalimumab injection	
1084 Denileukin Diftitox			K
	J9160	Denileukin diftitox, 300 mcg	
1085 Injection, Gallium Nitrate			K
	J1457	Gallium nitrate injection	

APC/APC Title	CPT/ HCPCS Code	CPT/ HCPCS Description	APC Status Indicator
1086 Temozolomide, Oral			K
	J8700	Temozolmide	
1089 Cyanocobalamin Cobalt co57			K
	Q3012	Cyanocobalamin Cobalt co57	
1091 IN 111 Oxyquinoline			K
	C1091	IN 111 Oxyquinoline,per 0.5 mCi	
1092 IN 111 Pentetate			K
	C1092	IN 111 Pentetate per 0.5 mCi	
1093 TC 99M Fanolesomab			K
	C1093	TC 99M Fanolesomab	
1095 Technetium TC 99M Depreotide			K
	A9511	Technetium TC 99m depreotide	
1096 TC 99M Exametazime, Per Dose			K
	A9521	Technetium TC 99m	
1122 TC 99M Arcitumomab, Per Vial			K
	C1122	TC 99M Arcitumomab per vial	
1167 Epirubicin HCl			K
	J9178	Inj, Epirubicin HCl, 2 mg	
1178 Busulfan IV			K
	C1178	Busulfan IV, 6 mg	
1201 TC 99M Succimer, Per Vial			K
	C1201	TC 99M succimer, per vial	
1203 Verteporfin for Injection			K
	J3395	Verteporfin injection	
1207 Octreotide Injection, Depot			K
	J2353	Octreotide injection, depot	
1305 Apligraf			K
	C1305	Apligraf	
1409 Factor VIIIa Recombinant			K
	Q0187	Factor VIIa recombinant	
1501 New Technology – Level I ($0-$50)			S
	0003T	Cervicography	
1502 New Technology – Level II ($50-$100)			S
	C9722	KV imaging w/LR tracking	
	G0294	Non-cov proc, clinical trial	
1503 New Technology – Level III ($100-$200)			S
	G0248	Demonstrate use home INR mon	
	G0249	Provide test material,equipm	
1504 New Technology – Level IV ($200-$300)			S
	G0304	Pre-op service LVRS 1-9 dos	
	G0305	Post op service LVRS min 6	
1505 New Technology – Level V ($300-$400)			S
	G0293	Noncov surg proc, clin trial	
1506 New Technology – Level VI ($400-$500)			S
	91035	G-esoph reflx tst w/electrod	
1507 New Technology – Level VII ($500-$600)			S
	79403	Hematopoetic nuclear therapy	
	G0303	Pre-op service LVRS 10-15 dos	
1508 New Technology – Level VIII ($600-$700)			S
	78804	Tumor imaging, whole body	
1509 New Technology – Level IX ($700-$800)			S
	G0302	Pre-op service LVRS complete	
1510 New Technology – Level X ($800-$900)			S
	77523	Proton trmt, intermediate	
	77525	Proton treatment, complex	
1511 New Technology – Level XI ($900-$1000)			S
	95967	MEG, evoked, each add'l	
1513 New Technology - Level XIII ($1100 - $1200)			S
	G0125	PET image pulmonary nodule	
	G0210	PET img wholebody dxlung	
	G0211	PET img wholbody init lung	
	G0212	PET img wholebod restag lung	
	G0213	PET img wholbody dx	
	G0214	PET img wholebod init	
	G0215	PETimg wholebod restag	
	G0216	PET img wholebod dx melanoma	
	G0217	PET img wholebod init melan	
	G0218	PET img wholebod restag mela	
	G0220	PET img wholebod dx lymphoma	
	G0221	PET imag wholbod init lympho	
	G0222	PET imag wholbod resta lymph	
	G0223	PET imag wholbod reg dx head	
	G0224	PET imag wholbod reg ini hea	
	G0225	PET whol restag headneckonly	
	G0226	PET img wholbody dx esophagl	
	G0227	PET img wholbod ini esophage	
	G0228	PET img wholbod restg esopha	
	G0229	PET img metaboloc brain pres	
	G0230	PET myocard viability post	
	G0231	PET WhBD colorec; gamma cam	
	G0232	PET whbd lymphoma; gamma cam	
	G0233	PET whbd melanoma; gamma cam	
	G0234	PET WhBD pulm nod; gamma cam	
	G0251	Linear acc based stero radio	
	G0296	PET imge restag thyrod cance	
	G0338	Linear accelerator stero pln	
1516 New Technology - Level XVI ($1400 - $1500)			S
	95966	MEG, evoked, single	
	G0242	Multisource photon ster plan	
	G0253	PET image brst dection recur	
	G0254	PET image brst eval to tx	
	G0330	PET image initial dx cervcal	
	G0331	PET image restage ovarian ca	
	G0336	PET imaging brain Alzheimers	
1519 New Technology - Level IXX ($1700-$1800)			S
	C9716	RF energy to anus	
1522 New Technology – Level XXII ($2000-$2500)			S
	G3001	Admin + supply, Tositumomab	
1523 New Technology - Level XXIII ($2500-$3000)			S
	19297	Place breast cath for rad	
1524 New Technology - Level XIV ($3000-$3500)			S
	19296	Place po breast cath for rad	
	19298	Place breast rad tube/caths	
1525 New Technology – Level XXV – ($3500-$4000)			S
	33225	L ventric pacing lead add-on	
	C9713	Non-contact laser vap prosta	
	G0340	Robt lin-radsurg fractx 2-5	
1528 New Technology – Level XXVIII ($5000-$5500)			S
	95965	MEG, spontaneous	
	G0173	Stereo radoisurgery,complete	
	G0243	Multisour photon stero treat	
	G0339	Robot lin-radsurg com, first	

APC/APC Title	CPT/ HCPCS Code	CPT/ HCPCS Description	APC Status Indicator
1547 New Technology – Level X ($800-$900)			T
	0027T	Endoscopic epidural lysis	
	C9720	HE ESW tx, tennis elbow	
	C9721	HE ESW tx, plantar fasciitis	
1555 New Technology – Level XVIII ($1600-$1700)			T
	61623	Endovasc tempory vessel occl	
1556 New Technology – Level XIX ($1700-$1800)			T
	C9704	Inj inert subs upper GI	
1557 New Technology – Level XX ($1800-$1900)			T
	20982	Ablate, bone tumor(s) perq	
1559 New Technology – Level XXII ($2000-$2500)			T
	92974	Cath place, cardio brachytx	
	93580	Transcath closure of ASD	
	93581	Transcath closure of VSD	
1564 New Technology – Level XXVII ($4500-$5000)			T
	36566	Insert tunneled CV cath	
1600 Technetium TC 99m Sestamibi			K
	A9500	Technetium TC 99m	
1602 Technetium TC 99m Apcitide			K
	A9504	Technetium TC 99m apcitide	
1603 Thallous Chloride TL 201			K
	A9505	Thallous chloride TL 201/mci	
1604 IN 111 Capromab Pendetide, Per Dose			K
	A9507	Indium/111 capromab pendetid	
1605 Abciximab Injection			K
	J0130	Abciximab injection	
1606 Anistreplase			K
	J0350	Injection Anistreplase 30 U	
1607 Eptifibatide Injection			K
	J1327	Eptifibatide injection	
1608 Etanercept Injection			K
	J1438	Etanercept injection	
1609 Rho(D) Immune Globulin H, SD			K
	J2792	Rho(D) immune globulin H, SD	
1611 Hylan G-F 20 Injection			K
	J7320	Hylan G-F 20 injection	
1612 Daclizumab, Parenteral			K
	J7513	Daclizumab, parenteral	
1613 Trastuzumab			K
	J9355	Trastuzumab	
1615 Basiliximab			K
	Q2019	Basiliximab	
1618 Vonwillebrand Factor Complex, Per IU			K
	Q2022	VonWillebrand factr cmplx per IU	
1619 Gallium GA 67			K
	Q3002	Gallium GA 67	
1620 Technetium TC 99m Bicisate			K
	Q3003	Technetium TC 99m bicisate	
1622 Technetium TC 99m Mertiatide			K
	Q3005	Technetium TC 99m mertiatide	
1624 Sodium Phosphate p32			K
	Q3007	Sodium phosphate p32	
1625 Indium 111-in Pentetreotide			K
	Q3008	Indium 111-in pentetreotide	
1628 Chromic Phosphate p32			K
	Q3011	Chromic phosphate p32	
1716 Brachytx Source, Gold 198			H
	C1716	Brachytx source, Gold 198	
1717 Brachytx Source, HDR Ir-192			H
	C1717	Brachytx source, HDR Ir-192	
1718 Brachytx Source, Iodine 125			H
	C1718	Brachytx source, Iodine 125	
1719 Brachytx Source, Non-HDR Ir-192			H
	C1719	Brachytx source,Non-HDR Ir-192	
1720 Brachytx Source, Palladium 103			H
	C1720	Brachytx source, Palladium 103	
1775 FDG, per dose (4-40 mCi/ml)			K
	C1775	FDG, per dose (4-40 mCi/ml)	
1814 Retinal Tamp, Silicone Oil			H
	C1814	Retinal tamp, silicone oil	
1818 Integrated Keratoprosthesis			H
	C1818	Integrated keratoprosthesis	
1819 Tissue Localization – Excision Device			H
	C1819	Tissue localization - excision	
2616 Brachytx Source, Yttrium-90			H
	C2616	Brachytx source, Yttrium-90	
2632 Brachytx Sol, I-12 Per mCi			H
	C2632	Brachytx sol, I-125, per mCi	
2633 Brachytx Source, Cesium-131			H
	C2633	Brachytx source, Cesium-131	
2634 Brachytx Source, HA, I-125			H
	C2634	Brachytx source, HA, I-125	
2635 Brachytx Source, HA, P-103			H
	C2635	Brachytx source, HA, P-103	
2636 Brachytx Linear Source, P-103			H
	C2636	Brachytx linear source, P-103	
7000 Amifostine			K
	J0207	Amifostine	
7003 Epoprostenol Injection			K
	J1325	Epoprostenol injection	
7005 Gonadorelin Hydrochloride			K
	J1620	Gonadorelin hydroch/100 mcg	
7007 Inject Milrinone Lactate			K
	J2260	Inj Milrinone lactate, per 5 mg	
7011 Oprelvekin Injection			K
	J2355	Oprelvekin injection	
7015 Busulfan, Oral			K
	J8510	Oral Busulfan	
7019 Aprotinin			K
	Q2003	Aprotinin, 10,000 kIU	

APC/APC Title	CPT/ HCPCS Code	CPT/ HCPCS Description	APC Status Indicator
7022 Elliotts B Solution Per Ml			K
	Q2002	Elliotts B solution per ml	
7024 Corticorelin Ovine Triflutat			K
	Q2005	Corticorelin ovine triflutat	
7025 Digoxin immune FAB (Ovine)			K
	Q2006	Digoxin immune fab (ovine)	
7026 Ethanolamine Oleate			K
	Q2007	Ethanolamine oleate 100 mg	
7027 Fomepizole			K
	Q2008	Fomepizole, 15 mg	
7028 Fosphenytoin			K
	Q2009	Fosphenytoin, 50 mg	
7030 Hemin			K
	Q2011	Hemin, per 1 mg	
7031 Octreotide Acetate Injection			K
	J2352	Octreotide acetate injection	
7034 Somatropin Injection			K
	J2941	Somatropin injection	
7035 Teniposide			K
	Q2017	Teniposide, 50 mg	
7036 Urokinase Injection			K
	J3365	Urokinase 250,000 IU inj	
7037 Urofollitropin			K
	Q2018	Urofollitropin, 75 IU	
7038 Monoclonal Antibodies			K
	J7505	Monoclonal antibodies	
7040 Pentastarch 10% Solution			K
	Q2013	Pentastarch 10% solution	
7041 Tirofiban HCl			K
	J3245	Tirofiban HCl	
7042 Capecitabine, Oral			K
	J8520	Capecitabine, oral, 150 mg	
7043 Infliximab Injection			K
	J1745	Infliximab injection	
7045 Trimetrexate Glucoronate			K
	J3305	Inj Trimetrexate glucoronate	
7046 Doxorubicin HCl Liposome Injection			K
	J9001	Doxorubicin HCl liposome inj	
7048 Alteplase Recombinant			K
	J2997	Alteplase recombinant	
7049 Filgrastim Injection			K
	J1441	Filgrastim 480 mcg injection	
7051 Leuprolide Acetate Implant			K
	J9219	Leuprolide acetate implant	
7308 Aminolevulinic Acid HCl Top			K
	J7308	Aminolevulinic acid HCl top	
7316 Sodium Hyaluronate Injection			K
	J7317	Sodium hyaluronate injection	
9001 Linezolid Injection			K
	J2020	Linezolid injection	
9002 Tenecteplase			K
	J3100	Tenecteplase injection	
9003 Palivizumab			K
	C9003	Palivizumab, per 50 mg	
9004 Gemtuzumab Ozogamicin			K
	J9300	Gemtuzumab Ozogamicin	
9005 Reteplase Injection			K
	J2993	Reteplase injection	
9008 Baclofen Refill Kit			K
	C9008	Baclofen refill kit-500 mcg	
9009 Baclofen Refill Kit Per 2000 mcg			K
	C9009	Baclofen refill Kit-2000 mcg	
9012 Arsenic Trioxide			K
	J9017	Arsenic trioxide	
9013 CO 57 Cobaltous Chloride			K
	C9013	CO 57 cobaltous chloride	
9015 Mycophenolate Mofetil Oral			K
	J7517	Mycophenolate Mofetil oral	
9018 Botulinum Toxin B			K
	J0587	Botulinum toxin type B	
9019 Caspofungin Acetate			K
	J0637	Caspofungin acetate	
9020 Sirolimus Tablet			K
	J7520	Sirolimus, oral	
9021 Immune Globulin			K
	J1564	Immune globulin 10 mg	
9022 IM Injection Interferon beta 1-a			K
	Q3025	IM inj Interferon beta 1-a	
9023 Rho d Immune Globulin			K
	J2788	Rho d immune globulin 50 mcg	
9024 Amphotericin B Lipid Complex			K
	J0287	Amphotericin B lipid complex	
	J0288	Amph B cholesteryl sulfate	
	J0289	Amphotericin B liposome inj	
9025 Rubidium-Rb-82			K
	Q3000	Rubidium-Rb-82	
9026 High Dose Contrast MRI			K
	A4643	High dose contrast MRI	
9027 Supp-paramagnetic Contrast Material			K
	A4647	Supp-paramagnetic contr mat	
9028 Tetracycline Injection			K
	J0120	Tetracycline injection	
9029 Amiodarone HCl			K
	J0282	Amiodarone HCl	
9030 Amphotericin B			K
	J0285	Amphotericin B	
9031 Arbutamine HCl Injection			K
	J0395	Arbutamine HCl injection	
9032 Baclofen 10 Mg Injection			K
	J0475	Baclofen 10 mg injection	
9033 Cidofovir Injection			K
	J0740	Cidofovir injection	
9034 Brompheniramine Maleate Injection			K
	J0945	Drompheniramine maleate injection	
9035 Medroxyprogesterone Injection			K
	J1051	Medroxyprogesterone injection	
9036 Dimethyl Sulfoxide 50%			K
	J1212	Dimethyl sulfoxide 50% 50 ml	
9037 Methadone Injection			K
	J1230	Methadone injection	
9038 Injection, Estrogen Conjugate			K
	J1410	Inj estrogen conjugate 25 mg	

APC/APC Title	CPT/ HCPCS Code	CPT/ HCPCS Description	APC Status Indicator
9040 Intraocular Fomivirsen Na	J1452	Intraocular Fomivirsen Na	K
9041 Gamma Globulin Injection	J1460	Gamma globulin 1 cc injection	K
9042 Glucagon Hydrochloride	J1610	Glucagon hydrochloride/1 mg	K
9044 Ibutilide Fumarate Injection	J1742	Ibutilide fumarate injection	K
9045 Iron Dextran	J1750	Iron dextran	K
9046 Iron Sucrose Injection	J1756	Iron sucrose injection	K
9047 Itraconazole Injection	J1835	Itraconazole injection	K
9048 Inject Desmopressin Acetate	J2597	Inj desmopressin acetate	K
9049 Inject Protirelin	J2725	Inj Protirelin per 250 mcg	K
9050 Na Ferric Gluconate Complex	J2916	Na ferric gluconate complex	K
9051 Urea Injection	J3350	Urea injection	K
9053 Nasal Vaccine Inhalation	J3530	Nasal vaccine inhalation	K
9054 Metabolically Active Tissue	J7342	Metabolically active tissue	K
9055 Injectable Human Tissue	J7350	Injectable human tissue	K
9057 Lepirudin	Q2021	Lepirudin	K
9104 Anti-thymocycte Gobulin Rabbit	J7511	Antithymocyte globuln rabbit	K
9105 Hep B Immune Globulin	C9105	Hep B imm glob, per 1 ml	K
9108 Thyrotropin Allfa	J3240	Thyrotropin Injection	K
9109 Tirofliban HCl	C9109	Tirofiban hcl, 6.25 mg	K
9110 Alemtuzumab	J9010	Alemtuzumab injection	K
9111 Injection, Bivalirudin	J0583	Bivalirudin	K
9112 Perflutren Lipid Micro	C9112	Perflutren lipid micro, 2 ml	K
9114 Nesiritide	J2324	Nesiritide	K
9115 Injection, Zoledronic Acid	J3487	Zoledronic acid	K
9117 Yttrium 90 Ibritumomab Tiuxetan	C1083	Yttrium 90 Ibritumomab Tiuxetan	K
9118 In-III Ibritumomab Tiuxetan	C1082	In-111 Ibritumomab Tiuxetan	K
9119 Pegfilgrastim	J2505	Injection, Pegfilgrastim 6 mg	K
9120 Injection, Fulvestrant	J9395	Injection, Fulvestrant	K
9121 Injection, Argatroban	C9121	Injection, Argatroban	K
9122 Injection, Triptorelin Pamoate	J3315	Triptorelin pamoate	K
9123 Transcyte	C9123	Transcyte, per 247 sq cm	G
9124 Injection, Daptomycin	J0878	Daptomycin injection	G
9125 Risperidone, Long Acting	J2794	Risperidone, long acting	G
9200 Orcel	C9200	Orcel, per 36 cm^2	G
9201 Dermagraft	C9201	Dermagraft, per 37.5 sq cm	G
9202 Octafluoropropane	C9202	Octafluoropropane	K
9203 Perflexane Lipid Micro	C9203	Perflexane lipid micro	G
9204 Ziprasidone Mesylate	J3486	Ziprasidone mesylate	G
9205 Oxaliplatin	C9205	Oxaliplatin	G
9206 Integra	C9206	Integra, per cm^2	K
9207 Bortezomib Injection	J9041	Bortezomib injection	G
9208 Agalsidase beta Injection	J0180	Agalsidase beta injection	G
9209 Laronidase Injection	J1931	Laronidase injection	G
9210 Palonosetron HCl Injection	J2469	Palonosetron HCl injection	G
9211 Injection, Alefacept IV	C9211	Alefacept IV inj	G
9212 Injection, Alefacept IM	C9212	Alefacept IM inj	G
9213 Injection, Pemetrexed	J9305	Pemetrexed injection	G
9214 Injection, Bevacizumab	J9035	Bevacizumab injection	G
9215 Injection, Cetuximab	J9055	Cetuximab injection	G
9216 Abarelix, Inject Suspension	J0128	Abarelix Injection	G
9217 Leuprolide Acetate Suspension	J9217	Leuprolide acetate suspension	K
9218 Injection, Azacitidine	C9218	Injection, Azacitidine	G
9219 Mycophenolic Acid	J7518	Mycophenolic acid	G
9220 Sodium Hyaluronate	C9220	Sodium hyaluronate	G
9221 Graftjacket Reg Matrix	C9221	Graftjacket Reg Matrix	G

APC/APC Title	CPT/ HCPCS Code	CPT/ HCPCS Description	APC Status Indicator
9222 Graftjacket Soft Tissue			G
	C9222	Graftjacket SftTis	
9300 Injection, Omalizumab			G
	J2357	Omalizumab injection	
9400 Thallous chloride, brand			K
	C9400	Thallous chloride, brand	
9401 Strontium-89 chloride, brand			K
	C9401	Strontium-89 chloride, brand	
9402 Th I-131 So Iodide cap, brand			K
	C9402	Th I131 so iodide cap, brand	
9403 Dx I131 So Iodide cap, brand			K
	C9403	Dx I131 so iodide cap, brand	
9404 Dx I-131 So Iodide sol, brand			K
	C9404	Dx I131 so iodide sol, brand	
9405 Th I131 So iodide sol, brand			K
	C9405	Th I131 so iodide sol, brand	
9410 Dexrazoxane HCl Inj, brand			K
	C9410	Dexrazoxane HCl inj, brand	
9411 Pamidronate disodium, brand			K
	C9411	Pamidronate disodium, brand	
9413 Sodium hyaluronate Inj, brand			K
	C9413	Sodium hyaluronate inj, bran	
9414 Etoposide oral, brand			K
	C9414	Etoposide oral, brand	
9415 Doxorubic HCl chemo, brand			K
	C9415	Doxorubic HCl chemo, brand	
9417 Bleomycin sulfate inj, brand			K
	C9417	Bleomycin sulfate inj, brand	
9418 Cisplatin inj, brand			K
	C9418	Cisplatin inj, brand	
9419 Inj cladribine, brand			K
	C9419	Inj cladribine, brand	
9420 Cyclophosphamide Inj, brand			K
	C9420	Cyclophosphamide inj, brand	
9421 Cyclophosphamide lyo, brand			K
	C9421	Cyclophosphamide lyo, brand	
9422 Cytarabine HCl Inj, brand			K
	C9422	Cytarabine HCl inj, brand	
9423 Dacarbazine Inj, brand			K
	C9423	Dacarbazine inj, brand	
9424 Daunorubicin, brand			K
	C9424	Daunorubicin, brand	
9425 Etoposide Inj, brand			K
	C9425	Etoposide inj, brand	
9426 Floxuridine Inj, brand			K
	C9426	Floxuridine inj, brand	
9427 Ifosfomide Inj, brand			K
	C9427	Ifosfomide inj, brand	
9428 Mesna Injection, brand			K
	C9428	Mesna injection, brand	
9429 Idarubicin HCl Inj, brand			K
	C9429	Idarubicin hcl inj, brand	
9430 Leuprolide Acetate Inj, brand			K
	C9430	Leuprolide acetate inj, brand	
9431 Paclitaxel Inj, brand			K
	C9431	Paclitaxel inj, brand	
9432 Mitomycin Inj, Brand			K
	C9432	Mitomycin inj, brand	
9433 Thiotepa Inj, brand			K
	C9433	Thiotepa inj, brand	
9435 Gonadorelin Hydroch, brand			K
	C9435	Gonadorelin hydroch, brand	
9436 Azathioprine Parenteral, Brand			K
	C9436	Azathioprine parenteral, brnd	
9437 Carmus Bischl Nitro Injection			K
	C9437	Carmus bischl nitro inj	
9438 Cyclosporine Oral, Brand			K
	C9438	Cyclosporine oral, brand	
9439 Diethylstilbesterol Injection			K
	C9439	Diethylstilbesterol injection	
9500 Platelets, Irradiated			K
	P9032	Platelets, irradiated	
9501 Platelets, Pheresis Leukocytes Reduced			K
	P9035	Platelet pheres leukoreduced	
9502 Platelet Pheresis Irradiated			K
	P9036	Platelet pheresis irradiated	
9503 Fresh Frozen Plasma, Each Unit			K
	C9503	Fresh frozen plasma, ea unit	
	P9060	Fr frz plasma donor retested	
9504 RBC Deglycerolized			K
	P9039	RBC deglycerolized	
9505 RBC Irradiated			K
	P9038	RBC irradiated	
9506 Granulocytes, Pheresis			K
	P9050	Granulocytes, pheresis unit	
9507 Platelets, Pheresis			K
	P9034	Platelets, pheresis	
9508 Plasma, Frozen w/in 8 Hours			K
	P9017	Plasma 1 donor frz w/in 8 hr	

Notes

Index

Instructions for the Use of the CPT Index

Main Terms

The index is organized by main terms. Each main term can stand alone, or be followed by up to three modifying terms. There are four primary classes of main entries:

1. Procedure or service.
   For example: Endoscopy; Anastomosis; Splint
2. Organ or other anatomic site.
   For example: Tibia; Colon; Salivary Gland
3. Condition.
   For example: Abscess; Entropion; Tetralogy of Fallot
4. Synonyms, Eponyms and Abbreviations.
   For example: EEG; Bricker Operation; Clagett Procedure

Modifying Terms

A main term may be followed by a series of up to three indented terms that modify the main term. When modifying terms appear, one should review the list, as these subterms do have an effect on the selection of the appropriate code for the procedure.

Code Ranges

Whenever more than one code applies to a given index entry, a code range is listed. If several non-sequential codes apply, they will be separated by a comma. For example:

Esophagus
  Reconstruction 43300, 43310, 43313

If two or more sequential codes apply, they will be separated by a hyphen. For example:

Debridement
  Burns 01951-01953, 16010-16030

Conventions

As a space saving convention, certain words infer some meaning. This convention is primarily used when a procedure or service is listed as a subterm. For example:

Knee
  Incision (of)

In this example, the word in parentheses (of) does not appear in the index, but it is inferred. As another example:

Pancreas
  Anesthesia (for procedures on)

In this example, as there is no such entity as pancreas anesthesia, the words in parentheses are inferred. That is, anesthesia for procedures on the pancreas.

The alphabetic index is NOT a substitute for the main text of *CPT*. Even if only one code appears, the user must refer to the main text to ensure that the code selection is accurate.

A

B

C

D

Exploration, Larynx by Incision

Exploratory Laparotomy

Expression

Exteriorization, Small Intestine

External Auditory Canal

External Cephalic Version 59412

External Ear

External Extoses

External Fixation

Extirpation, Lacrimal Sac

Extracorporeal Circulation 33960-33961

Extracorporeal Dialyses

Extracorporeal Membrane Oxygenation

Extracorporeal Photochemotherapies

Extracorporeal Shock Wave Therapy

Extracranial

Extraction

Extraction, Cataract

Extradural Anesthesia

Extradural Injection

Extraocular Muscle

Extrauterine Pregnancy

Extravasation Blood

Extremity

Eye

G

I

Incision and Drainage

Inkblot Test

Inner Ear

Innominate

Innominate Arteries

Inorganic Sulfates

Insemination

Insertion

Inspiratory Positive Pressure Breathing

Instillation

J

K

L

N

O

Q

R

Rectal Bleeding

Rectal Prolapse

Rectal Sphincter

S

Skin Graft and Flap

Skull

Skull Base Surgery

Tunica Vaginalis

Turbinate

U

W

X

Y

Z